Diagnostic Imaging: Abdomen and Pelvis

Diagnostic Imaging: Abdomen and Pelvis

Edited by Nicolas Berry

AMERICAN
MEDICAL PUBLISHERS
www.americanmedicalpublishers.com

American Medical Publishers,
41 Flatbush Avenue,
1st Floor, New York,
NY 11217, USA

Visit us on the World Wide Web at:
www.americanmedicalpublishers.com

ISBN: 978-1-63927-069-9

Cataloging-in-Publication Data

Diagnostic imaging : abdomen and pelvis / edited by Nicolas Berry.
p. cm.
Includes bibliographical references and index.
ISBN 978-1-63927-069-9
1. Diagnostic imaging. 2. Abdomen--Imaging. 3. Pelvis--Imaging.
4. Imaging systems in medicine. I. Berry, Nicolas.
RC78.7.D53 D53 2022
616.075 4--dc23

Table of Contents

Preface

Diagnostic imaging, also called medical imaging, is the technique and process of imaging the interior of a body for clinical intervention. It is also used to visually represent the function of organs and tissues. Diagnostic imaging reveals the internal structures hidden by the skin and the bones using technologies like electromagnetic radiation, ultrasonic waves, radiopharmaceuticals, etc. Other technologies which are used in diagnostic imaging include endoscopy, elastography and thermography. Imaging procedures like computed tomography (CT) of the abdomen and pelvis is used to detect diseases of the small bowel, colon and other internal organs and is often used to determine the cause of unexplained pain. This book outlines the processes and applications of diagnostic imaging of the abdomen and the pelvis in detail. It traces the progress in this field and highlights some of its key concepts and applications. This book includes contributions of experts and scientists which will provide innovative insights into this field.

The information contained in this book is the result of intensive hard work done by researchers in this field. All due efforts have been made to make this book serve as a complete guiding source for students and researchers. The topics in this book have been comprehensively explained to help readers understand the growing trends in the field.

I would like to thank the entire group of writers who made sincere efforts in this book and my family who supported me in my efforts of working on this book. I take this opportunity to thank all those who have been a guiding force throughout my life.

Editor

1

Urinary Obstruction, Stone Disease, and Infection

Refky Nicola and Christine O. Menias

Learning Objectives

- To review the pathogenesis of urinary infection, obstruction, and stones
- To discuss the imaging features of acute urologic infections such as renal abscess, acute pyelonephritis, and emphysematous pyelonephritis or chronic infections such as renal tuberculosis
- To illustrate the imaging of struvite or infection stones as well as highlight their complications

Urinary Infection

Introduction

Urinary tract infection is the most common urologic ailment, reported to affect 150 million patients annually worldwide. The diagnosis is usually based on clinical symptoms and urinalysis. In general, imaging is not necessary for the diagnosis of uncomplicated urinary tract infections in adult patients. However, diagnostic imaging can play an important role in the evaluation of patient's infections who do not respond to antibiotic treatment in the first 72 h. It also helps to look for structural abnormalities of the urinary tract, which guide appropriate medical or surgical therapy. Various imaging modalities, including ultrasound (US), computed tomography (CT), and magnetic resonance imaging (MRI), are useful in the diagnosis and depiction of urinary tract infections. This section highlights the imaging features of acute pyelonephritis, renal and perinephric abscess, pyonephrosis, emphysematous pyelonephritis, xanthogranulomatous pyelonephritis, and renal tuberculosis, using multimodality approach.

Ultrasound

Ultrasound (US) is a readily available imaging modality to serve as the initial modality in the evaluation of patients who have the clinical diagnosis of pyelonephritis. US serves as a good screening modality to evaluate for structural anatomic anomalies or complications of urinary tract infection, such as hydronephrosis and obstructive uropathy. Gray-scale imaging features of pyelonephritis include renal enlargement, hydronephrosis, loss of renal sinus fat due to edema, loss of corticomedullary differentiation, areas of hypoperfusion on color Doppler, and abscess formation [1]. There may be changes in the renal echogenic pattern and the involved kidney which can be either hyperechoic or hypoechoic. The urinary bladder may also be evaluated in this setting and can show amount of residual urine volume, presence of bladder wall thickening, or potentially a stone. However, ultrasound is limited in its ability to differentiate calcification from gas within the collecting system or parenchyma, visualization of small abscesses, and perinephric extension of infection which are all common in early infections. In one study, ultrasound findings were noted in only 24% of patients, while other studies report

R. Nicola, M.Sc. D.O.
Division of Abdominal Imaging, SUNY-Upstate Medical Center, Syracuse, NY, USA

C. O. Menias, M.D. (✉)
Department of Radiology, Mayo Clinic in Arizona, Scottsdale, AZ, USA
e-mail: Menias.Christine@mayo.edu

only 20% of patients [2, 3]. However, new techniques such as tissue harmonics have showed sensitivity and specificity of 97% and 80% [3].

CT Technique

CT is the preferred imaging modality for the evaluation of complicated pyelonephritis because it provides both physiologic and anatomic detail and identifies both extrarenal and intrarenal pathology [4]. An unenhanced CT is excellent for identifying gas in the urinary tract, stones, hemorrhage, and dilatation of the urinary tract [5]. Regions of higher attenuation on non-contrast CT are associated with hemorrhage, while areas of lower attenuation represent edema. Following intravenous contrast administration, pyelonephritis manifests as "wedge shaped" or linear regions of decreased enhancement that spans from the renal sinus to the renal cortex. The excretory phase, obtained between 3 and 5 min after the administration of contrast, should be performed in suspected urinary obstruction [2]. CT also can evaluate for additional features of renal inflammation and its complications, including inflammation of the perinephric fat, thickening of Gerota's fascia, and abscess formation.

Acute Renal Infection

Acute Pyelonephritis

CT is indicated when complications of renal infection are suspected. Predisposing conditions, including urinary calculi, neurogenic bladder, immune system compromise, diabetes, IV drug abuse, or chronic debilitating disease, increase the risk of complications that require intervention. Most urinary tract infections are caused by gram-negative bacilli, but the incidence of fungal and tuberculous infections is rising. Acute pyelonephritis is a multifocal infection of one or both kidneys, which can result from either hematogenous spread or from ascending infection from the bladder and usually resolves after appropriate antibiotic therapy. Adults who fail to improve should be imaged to detect complications.

CT signs of acute bacterial infection of the kidneys include wedge-shaped areas of decreased parenchymal enhancement due to decreased blood flow caused by edema. A striated pattern of linear alternating increased and decreased attenuation ("striated nephrogram") on enhanced scans is classic [6]. This differential enhancement is contributed by various factors, namely, tubular obstruction by inflammatory debris, interstitial edema, and vasospasm which tend to decrease the flow of contrast through tubules [7, 8].

Acute Renal/Perirenal Abscess

Untreated or inadequately treated pyelonephritis can lead to suppuration, liquefaction, and parenchymal necrosis that eventually leads to abscess. Patients at risk of abscess formation include those with diabetes, chronic diseases, immunocompromised state, urinary tract obstruction, and intravenous drug abusers. Renal abscesses tend to be solitary and may decompress into the perinephric space or collecting system. On US, they usually are hypoechoic with through transmission, mobile debris, and occasional air pockets and on color Doppler lack internal flow. US is less sensitive in determining the presence and extent of perinephric extension relative to CT; however, it is an appropriate modality for follow-up imaging to look for response to treatment and as a guide for percutaneous drainage. CT demonstrates a fluid collection with an enhancing rim which may contain gas. Large abscesses usu-ally require catheter or surgical drainage (Fig.). Extension of infection into the perirenal space is common, and perirenal abscesses may develop. Extra- parenchymal collections can extend to the psoas muscle, pelvis, or groin [4, 6].

Emphysematous Pyelonephritis

Emphysematous pyelonephritis is a severe life-threatening necrotizing type of pyelonephritis that develops in mostly diabetics (90%), but also in immunocompromised patients,

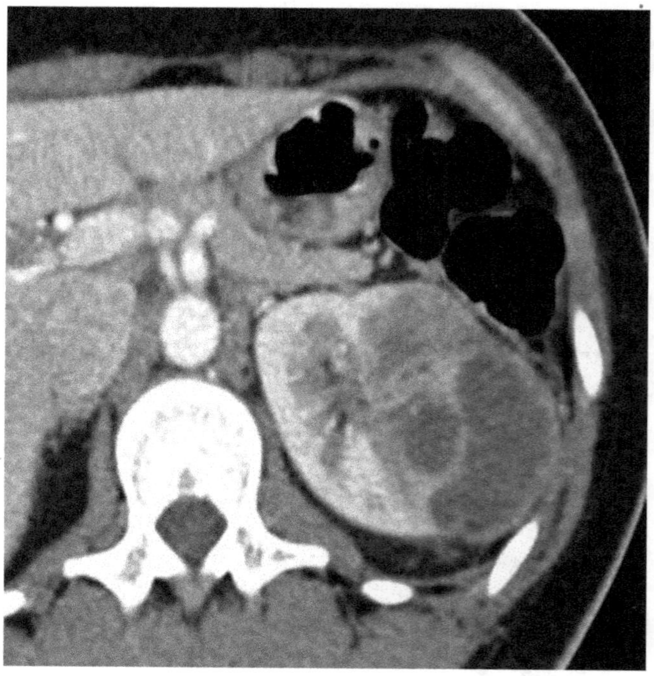

Fig. Renal Abscess in a 37-year-old female with HIV and fever. Axial contrast-enhanced CT image of the left kidney shows a complex peripherally enhancing fluid collection and associated perinephric stranding. Subsequent drained fluid grew *Staphylococcus aureu*

and patients with urinary obstruction. Gas is produced from metabolism of glucose by gram-negative bacteria. CT shows gas in the renal parenchyma in addition to signs of renal inflammation. The most common gas-forming organisms are *E. coli*, *Klebsiella pneumoniae*, and *Proteus mirabilis* which are also the same organisms associated with struvite stones. US shows an enlarged kidney with nondependent echoes (gas) in the parenchyma or collecting system, with "dirty shadowing" that helps differentiate from stones. US is limited in evaluating the extent of the disease. CT is the imaging modality of choice for emphysematous pyelonephritis with findings of parenchymal enlargement and destruction without or with abscess formation, small streaks of gas, or fluid collections [4, 9, 10].

Emphysematous pyelonephritis is classified into two types based on imaging features and prognosis.

Type 1 emphysematous pyelonephritis is renal parenchymal destruction with streaky or mottled areas of gas without an extrarenal fluid collection. Type 2 is renal or perirenal fluid collections that are directly associated with a loculated gas or gas within the collecting system. The mortality for type 1 and type 2 is 69% and 18%, respectively.

Pyonephrosis

Pyonephrosis is an acute infection with pus within an obstructed collecting system. Renal destruction is rapid, and urgent drainage of the collecting system is required. The obstruction can be due to tumor, stricture, sloughed papilla, tumor, or stones. If patients are left untreated, patients may develop loss of renal function and septic shock [11, 12]. US features include dilatation of the pelvicalyceal system, internal collecting system fluid-fluid levels, echogenic debris, and occasionally dirty echoes of gas. CT features may show a dilated but thick-walled collecting system, distended with high attenuation pus-filled fluid, and thinning of the renal cortex, and typically source of obstruction.

Renal Tuberculosis

Tuberculosis (TB) remains the leading global cause of death from infectious disease [4]. The urinary tract is the most common extra-pulmonary site of infection and results from hematogenous dissemination in 15–20% of cases [4]. The rise of tuberculosis within developed countries is caused by the spread of HIV (human immunodeficiency viral) infection and antibiotic-resistant strains of mycobacterium. The urinary tract may be involved even though chest radiographs do not show evidence of TB. Multiple caseous granulomas form in the cortex because of its favorable blood supply. These may remain dormant or reactivate, spreading organisms to the tubules, resulting in papillary necrosis. Progressive infection will eventually destroy the kidney. The common imaging findings of renal tuberculosis are due to papillary necrosis which is followed by parenchymal destruction. Parenchymal lesions lead to corticomedullary scarring and renal contour scarring. Pelvoinfundibular stricture, cortical low-attenuation lesions, scarring, and papillary necrosis and calcifications are findings which are all associated with renal tuberculosis [13, 14]. Calcification is very commonly seen and varies from granular, amorphous, and curvilinear which can replace segments or the entire renal parenchyma resulting in the end stage "putty kidney" [14].

Urinary Stones and Obstruction

Introduction

The most common cause of urinary obstruction in the emergent setting is urolithiasis, but chronic urinary obstruction has multiple etiologies such as lymphadenopathy or retroperitoneal fibrosis. Also, the patients with a history of urothelial, cervical, prostate, or colon carcinoma are also susceptible to chronic urinary obstruction due to neoplastic obstruction [15]. Therefore, the role of the radiologist is pivotal in differentiating between acute and chronic urinary obstruction because an accurate diagnosis is essential in avoiding serious complications such as sepsis or chronic renal insufficiency.

Epidemiology

Urolithiasis has become a problem which transcends geography, culture, and gender. Approximately, 1.2 million Americans are affected each year. About 12% of men and 5% of women will develop urolithiasis during their lifetime. However, the prevalence is estimated to be higher in more developed countries [16–20]. Stone disease is also one of America's costliest health issues, accounting for approximately $2 billion annual health-care dollars [21].

Stone Composition

There are several dietary, hereditary, and environmental factors which play an integral role in stone disease, such as hypercalciuria, renal tubular acidosis, and chronic diarrhea and gout [20]. The composition of most upper urinary tract stones is either calcium (i.e., calcium oxalate dehydrate, calcium oxalate monohydrate, calcium phosphate), struvite, or uric acid with calcium being the most common. Less common compositions include protein matrix, cystine, brushite, or stones due to drug-related therapies such as indinavir. Even though most stones are visible on CT, the struvite stones and uric acid stones are radiolucent on radiography [22]. Due to the difference in composition of renal stones, there is a wide variation in the attenuation on multidetector CT. For example, calcium monohydrate and brushite measure 1700–2800 HU, calcium phosphate 1200–1600 HU, cystine 600–1100 HU, struvite 600–900 HU, and uric acid 200–450 HU [23–25].

The importance of identifying the stone composition is directly related to management. Uric acid stones are managed with medical therapy. Cystine- and calcium-based stones cannot be easily fragmented with shock wave lithotripsy (SWL) [22].

Clinical Perspective

The most common complaint in patients with urolithiasis is acute flank pain which is eventually relieved with the passage of the stone. If the stone is lodged at the ureteropelvic junction (UPJ), the pain will radiate to the groin. However, if the stone is located distally at the ureterovesical junction (UVJ), it will cause suprapubic discomfort and voiding urgency. Pain typically radiates to the testis or labium [26]. In addition, patients will complain of vomiting, nausea, and microscopic hematuria. However, staghorn calculus which is caused by urease-producing bacteria such *Proteus mirabilis*, *Pseudomonas aeruginosa*, *Klebsiella pneumoniae*, and *E. coli* can manifest as a recurrent urinary tract infection instead of an obstruction [20]. If there is an infection and an obstructed collecting system, patients can present with sepsis [27]. Microscopic or macroscopic hematuria can occur regardless of urinary obstruction. Usually, a urinalysis and complete blood count is done to evaluate for infection.

CT Technique

Since 1995 unenhanced MDCT is the primary modality of choice in the evaluation of patients with renal colic and accounts for 20% of all CT examinations which are performed for acute abdominal pain. Thin (1–3 mm) reconstruction sections are helpful for detection of small stones. However, 5 mm MDCT with 3 mm coronal reformatted images has been found to improve stone detection while maintaining radiation dose benefits [28]. A tube potential of 100–120 kvp and automatic tube current modulation is performed with a tube current of 80 to 500 mAs. Typically, intravenous contrast administration is not required for the evaluation of renal calculi at CT.

Unlike MDCT which uses a single energy source, dual-energy CT (DECT) allows for acquisition of CT images at two different energies. With MDCT, stone composition is difficult to assess since there is significant overlap in attenuation for each of the stone subtypes. By comparing the attenuation of a stone at two different energy levels, the mystery of the stone's composition is somewhat mitigated. For example, this becomes particularly useful in differentiating uric acid from calcium-based stones, since both have similar attenuation coefficient on single-energy CT [26].

Struvite Stone and their Complications

Struvite stones, which are also known as *infection stones*, are composed of magnesium ammonium phosphate and comprise 15–20% of all renal calculi. Struvite stones develop more frequently in a patient with urinary stasis or recurrent urinary tract infections. Struvite stones with superimposed pyelonephritis are caused by bacteria entering the renal tubules and inciting an inflammatory response which involves the tubules and renal interstitium [7]. CT is useful in assessing intra- and extrarenal inflammation such as gas, calculus, and hemorrhage [4]. CT shows the inciting staghorn calculus with superimposed pyelonephritis with wedge-shaped areas of decreased enhancement corresponding to the striated nephrogram and perinephric stranding [7, 8]. Another complication is pyonephrosis, which is a dilated, obstructed, and infected collecting system. Struvite calculi can obstruct the pelvicalyceal system with superimposed infection and can lead to significant morbidity if not adequately treated.

Xanthogranulomatous Pyelonephritis

Xanthogranulomatous pyelonephritis is a rare form of chronic pyelonephritis which develops from chronic obstruction due to struvite/infected renal stones resulting in a chronic granulomatous inflammatory response and eventual destruction and replacement of the renal parenchyma, by lipid-laden macrophages. The most common inciting organisms are *E. coli* and *Proteus mirabilis* which are organisms associated with struvite/infection stones. XGPN classically presents in mid-aged female patients with recurrent urinary tract infection, diabetes, or obstructing urinary stones [2, 5]. XGPN may involve the entire kidney (diffuse) or related to an obstructed upper or lower pole (focal), which at times is difficult to differentiate from tumor or abscess.

Imaging of XGPN

US features of XGPN are nonspecific and include focal or diffuse enlargement of the kidney with renal cortical thinning, and echogenicity within the calyces, and typically a large UPJ stone with posterior acoustic shadowing due to

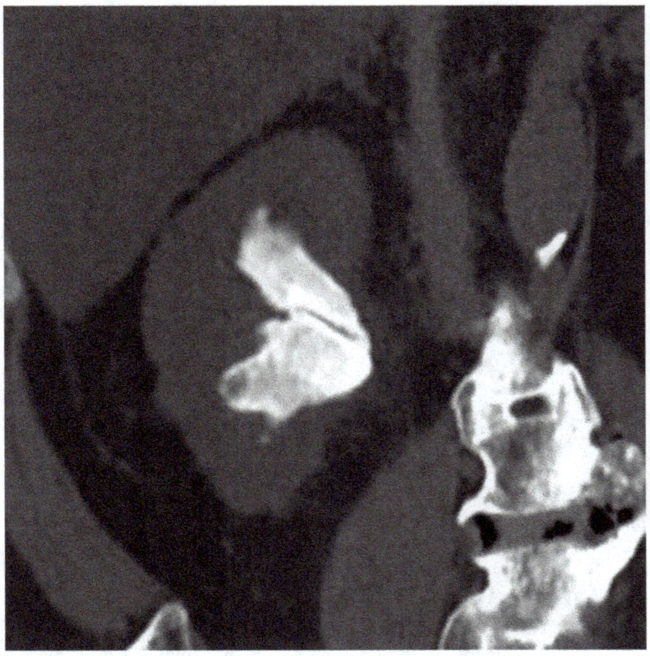

Fig. XGPN in a 56-year-old female with flank pain and urinary tract infection. Axial contrast-enhanced CT image shows an enlarged non-functioning left kidney with blown-out calyces and "bear paw" appearance, with a large central staghorn struvite/infection stone. Subsequent nephrectomy specimen confirmed XGPN

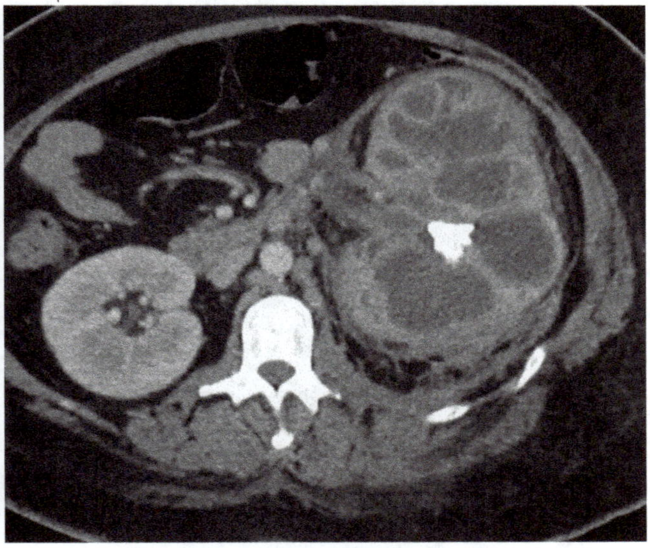

Fig. Staghorn calculus in a 68-year-old female with flank pain. Coronal non-contrast CT image in bone windows shows a large stone filling in the right renal pelvocalyceal system with a staghorn appearance consistent with an infection stone. Stone analysis subsequently showed struvite/magnesium ammonium phosphate. Note the subtle perinephric inflammatory stranding

the stone, obscuring detail of the kidney. Contrast-enhanced CT is the modality of choice in the evaluation of XGPN; however, MR serves as a useful alternative when IV contrast cannot be administered. CT may show an enlarged kidney replaced with low-attenuation dilated/blown-out calyces resulting in renal cortical thinning, resulting in the classic "bear paw sign" [4]. These blown-out calyces are thought to represent dilated calyces filled with hemorrhage, debris, or pus (Fig.). XGPN results in a non-functioning enlarged kidney, with typically a large central staghorn/infected stru-vite stone that fails to excrete on the excretory phase [4] (Fig.). Extrarenal extension of XGPN is often present with inflammatory changes and abscess that track from the kidney and dissect through the posterior flank, psoas mus-cle, and adjacent viscera like the liver and spleen.

Renal Replacement Lipomatosis

Another end-spectrum complication of long-standing stone disease is complete destruction and atrophy of the renal sinus, perinephric space, and hilum with subsequent fatty replacement, known as renal sinus or replacement lipomatosis (RRL) [29]. In the most extensive form of RRL, there is total atrophy of the renal parenchyma and complete fibro-fatty replacement. RRL is typically unilateral and linked to renal stones in 76–79% and results from severe renal atrophy or destruction due to chronic stone disease, chronic pyelonephritis, and renal tuberculosis [29]. US findings may demonstrate a large hyperechoic fatty mass which may suggest the diagnosis; however, parenchymal and renal sinus fat deposition may not be well visualized on ultrasound, and the echogenicity of fat may obscure detection of its associated stone. CT is the modality of choice, to confirm the end stage renal atrophy and fatty proliferation in the renal sinus and perinephric space, and helps differentiate RRL from fat-containing neoplasms.

Concluding Remarks

Ultrasound and CT play an important role in the evaluation of patients who present with acute urinary tract infection, obstruction, and stone disease. Familiarity with the pathogenesis, imaging features, and treatment of these entities can aid radiologic diagnoses and guide appropriate patient management.

Take-Home Message

- Ultrasound and CT play an important role in the evaluation of patients who present with acute urinary tract infection, obstruction, and stone disease. Familiarity with the pathogenesis, imaging features, and treatment of these entities can aid radiologic diagnoses and guide appropriate patient management.

References

1. Rigsby CM, Rosenfield AT, Glickman MG, Hodson J. Hemorrhagic focal bacterial nephritis: findings on gray-scale sonography and CT. AJR Am J Roentgenol. 1986;146(6):1173–7. https://doi.org/10.2214/ajr.146.6.1173.
2. Stunell H, Buckley O, Feeney J, Geoghegan T, Browne RF, Torreggiani WC. Imaging of acute pyelonephritis in the adult. Eur Radiol. 2007;17(7):1820–8. https://doi.org/10.1007/s00330-006-0366-3.
3. Kim B, Lim HK, Choi MH, Woo JY, Ryu J, Kim S, Peck KR. Detection of parenchymal abnormalities in acute pyelonephritis by pulse inversion harmonic imaging with or without microbubble ultrasonographic contrast agent: correlation with computed tomography. J Ultrasound Med. 2001;20(1):5–14.
4. Craig WD, Wagner BJ, Travis MD. Pyelonephritis: radiologic-pathologic review. Radiographics. 2008;28(1):255–77; quiz 327-258. https://doi.org/10.1148/rg.281075171.
5. Goldman SM, Fishman EK. Upper urinary tract infection: the current role of CT, ultrasound, and MRI. Semin Ultrasound CT MR. 1991;12(4):335–60.
6. Kawashima A, Sandler CM, Goldman SM, Raval BK, Fishman EK. CT of renal inflammatory disease. Radiographics. 1997;17(4):851–66; discussion 867–858. https://doi.org/10.1148/radiographics.17.4.9225387.
7. Talner LB, Davidson AJ, Lebowitz RL, Dalla Palma L, Goldman SM. Acute pyelonephritis: can we agree on terminology? Radiology. 1994;192(2):297–305. https://doi.org/10.1148/radiology.192.2.8029384.
8. Dalla-Palma L, Pozzi-Mucelli F, Pozzi-Mucelli RS. Delayed CT findings in acute renal infection. Clin Radiol. 1995;50(6):364–70.
9. Silver TM, Kass EJ, Thornbury JR, Konnak JW, Wolfman MG. The radiological spectrum of acute pyelonephritis in adults and adolescents. Radiology. 1976;118(1):65–71. https://doi.org/10.1148/118.1.65.
10. Wan YL, Lee TY, Bullard MJ, Tsai CC. Acute gas-producing bacterial renal infection: correlation between imaging findings and clinical outcome. Radiology. 1996;198(2):433–8. https://doi.org/10.1148/radiology.198.2.8596845.
11. Yoder IC, Pfister RC, Lindfors KK, Newhouse JH. Pyonephrosis: imaging and intervention. AJR Am J Roentgenol. 1983;141(4):735–40. https://doi.org/10.2214/ajr.141.4.735.
12. Subramanyam BR, Raghavendra BN, Bosniak MA, Lefleur RS, Rosen RJ, Horii SC. Sonography of pyonephrosis: a prospective study. AJR Am J Roentgenol. 1983;140(5):991–3. https://doi.org/10.2214/ajr.140.5.991.
13. Kenney PJ. Imaging of chronic renal infections. AJR Am J Roentgenol. 1990;155(3):485–94. https://doi.org/10.2214/ajr.155.3.2117344.
14. Muttarak M, ChiangMai WN, Lojanapiwat B. Tuberculosis of the genitourinary tract: imaging features with pathological correlation. Singap Med J. 2005;46(10):568–74; quiz 575.
15. Farrell TA, Hicks ME. A review of radiologically guided percutaneous nephrostomies in 303 patients. J Vasc Interv Radiol. 1997;8(5):769–74.
16. Curhan GC. Epidemiology of stone disease. Urol Clin North Am. 2007;34(3):287–93. https://doi.org/10.1016/j.ucl.2007.04.003.
17. Stamatelou KK, Francis ME, Jones CA, Nyberg LM, Curhan GC. Time trends in reported prevalence of kidney stones in the United States: 1976–1994. Kidney Int. 2003;63(5):1817–23. https://doi.org/10.1046/j.1523-1755.2003.00917.x.
18. Johnson CM, Wilson DM, O'Fallon WM, Malek RS, Kurland LT. Renal stone epidemiology: a 25-year study in Rochester, Minnesota. Kidney Int. 1979;16(5):624–31.
19. Soucie JM, Thun MJ, Coates RJ, McClellan W, Austin H. Demographic and geographic variability of kidney stones in the United States. Kidney Int. 1994;46(3):893–9.
20. Cheng PM, Moin P, Dunn MD, Boswell WD, Duddalwar VA. What the radiologist needs to know about urolithiasis: part 1—pathogenesis, types, assessment, and variant anatomy. AJR Am J Roentgenol. 2012;198(6):W540–7. https://doi.org/10.2214/AJR.10.7285.
21. Pearle MS, Calhoun EA, Curhan GC, Urologic Diseases of America P. Urologic diseases in America project: urolithiasis. J Urol. 2005;173(3):848–57. https://doi.org/10.1097/01.ju.0000152082.14384.d7.
22. Kambadakone AR, Eisner BH, Catalano OA, Sahani DV. New and evolving concepts in the imaging and management of urolithiasis: urologists' perspective. Radiographics. 2010;30(3):603–23. https://doi.org/10.1148/rg.303095146.
23. Saw KC, McAteer JA, Monga AG, Chua GT, Lingeman JE, Williams JC Jr. Helical CT of urinary calculi: effect of stone composition, stone size, and scan collimation. AJR Am J Roentgenol. 2000;175(2):329–32. https://doi.org/10.2214/ajr.175.2.1750329.
24. Bellin MF, Renard-Penna R, Conort P, Bissery A, Meric JB, Daudon M, Mallet A, Richard F, Grenier P. Helical CT evaluation of the chemical composition of urinary tract calculi with a discriminant analysis of CT-attenuation values and density. Eur Radiol. 2004;14(11):2134–40. https://doi.org/10.1007/s00330-004-2365-6.
25. Mostafavi MR, Ernst RD, Saltzman B. Accurate determination of chemical composition of urinary calculi by spiral computerized tomography. J Urol. 1998;159(3):673–5.
26. Masch WR, Cronin KC, Sahani DV, Kambadakone A. Imaging in Urolithiasis. Radiol Clin N Am. 2017;55(2):209–24. https://doi.org/10.1016/j.rcl.2016.10.002.
27. Conrad S, Busch R, Huland H. Complicated urinary tract infections. Eur Urol. 1991;19(Suppl 1):16–22.
28. Lin WC, Uppot RN, Li CS, Hahn PF, Sahani DV. Value of automated coronal reformations from 64-section multidetector row computerized tomography in the diagnosis of urinary stone disease. J Urol. 2007;178(3 Pt 1):907–11. https://doi.org/10.1016/j.juro.2007.05.042; discussion 911.
29. Chang SD, Coakley FV, Goldstein RB. Case report: renal replacement lipomatosis associated with renal transplantation. Br J Radiol. 2005;78(925):60–1. https://doi.org/10.1259/bjr/31723131.

2

Disease of the Gallbladder and Biliary Tree

Jeong Min Lee and Daniel T. Boll

Learning Objectives

- To discuss typical imaging features of common cholangiopathies.
- To discuss the imaging diagnosis of premalignant tumors of the gallbladder and bile duct.
- To explain the classical and emerging classification systems of cholangiocarcinoma.
- To discuss the strengths and weaknesses of imaging modalities and the role of multimodality and multiparametric approaches in the diagnostic work-up of biliary malignancies.

Biliary Tract

Jeong Min Lee, M.D.

Congenital Biliary Anomalies

Choledochal Cyst

Choledochal cyst involves congenital cystic dilatation of any portion of the extrahepatic bile ducts, and most choledochal cysts are diagnosed in childhood; however, up to 20% of cysts manifest in adults. It is classified based on the spectrum of morphologic changes in the bile ducts. The most common classification scheme is the Todani modification of the Alonso-Lej classification.

Todani type I—single cystic dilatation of the extrahepatic bile duct (EBD).
Todani Type II—true diverticula of the EBD.
Todani Type III—choledochocele or ectasia of an intramural EBD segment.
Todani Type IV—multiple and can have both intrahepatic and extrahepatic components.
Todani Type V (Caroli disease)—cystic dilatation of the intrahepatic bile ducts (IBDs).

Complications of choledochal cysts in adults include rupture with bile peritonitis, stone formation, cholangitis, liver abscess, and cholangiocarcinoma (CC). CC arising in a choledochal cysts appears as an intracystic soft tissue density mass or irregular thickening of the cyst wall [1].

Choledocholithiasis

Regardless of whether bile duct dilatation is present, the visible ducts should be scrutinized to identify and characterize filling defects, the vast majority of which represent stones [2]. Detectability of a bile duct stone on CT depends on the calcium content and requires precontrast CT. Depending on the composition, stones may show soft tissue attenuation, near-water attenuation, or fat attenuation with peripheral calcification. Stones are manifested as a signal void on T2-weighted imaging or MRCP (Fig.). On T1-weighted imaging, cholesterol stones are generally iso- or hypointense, while pigment stones are hyperintense due to the presence of metal ions. ERCP is highly accurate for the detection of small choledocholithiasis and also provides access for therapeutic intervention.

J. M. Lee, M.D.
Department of Radiology, Seoul National University Hospital, Seoul, Republic of Korea
e-mail: jmsh@snu.ac.kr

D. T. Boll, M.D. (✉)
Department of Radiology and Nuclear Medicine, University Hospital of Basel, Basel, BS, Switzerland
e-mail: Daniel.Boll@usb.ch

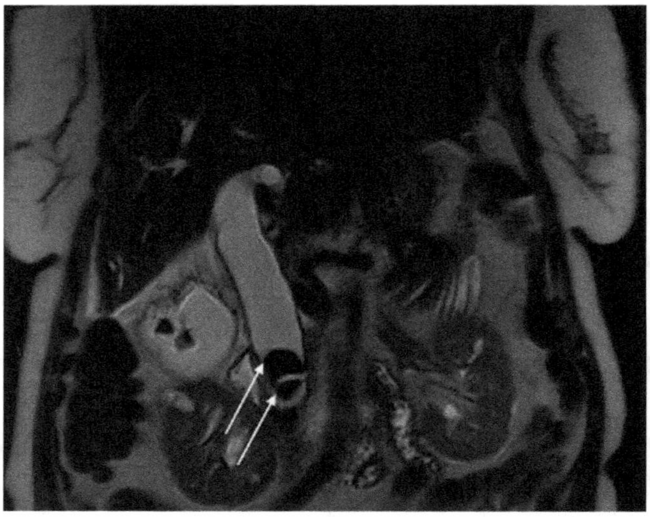

Fig. . 70-year-old male patient with choledocholithiasis (arrows) in the retropancreatic portion of the hepatocholedochal duct as seen on coronal T2-weighted breathheld MR sequences. Note the distention of the DHC and further concrements in the chronically inflamed gallbladder

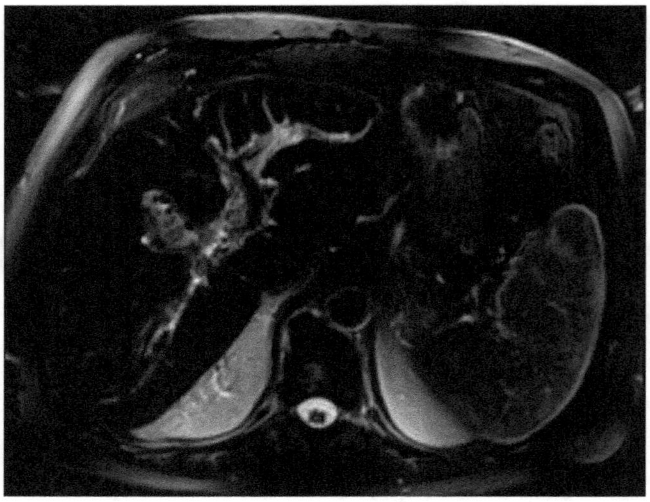

25-year-old male patient post liver transplant with chronic cholangitis showing multiple concrements and sludge in the intrahepatic biliary system with widening of the biliary ducts and surrounding inflammatory changes as seen on axial T2-weighted fat-saturated MR images

Inflammatory Disorders (Cholangitis)

Suppurative Cholangitis

Acute bacterial cholangitis is a potentially life-threatening infection, usually arising in the setting of bile duct obstruction, with ensuing bacterial contamination, stagnant bile, and increased biliary pressures. Choledocholithiasis accounts for up to 80% of cases of acute cholangitis (Fig.). CT or MRI shows diffuse, concentric wall thickening of the bile duct with associated periductal edema and mural enhancement, with or without pneumobilia [3]. Marked inhomogeneous parenchymal enhancement in the arterial is frequently present in patients with acute suppurative cholangitis [4].

Recurrent Pyogenic Cholangitis

Recurrent pyogenic cholangitis is characterized by stenosis or strictures of the peripheral ducts, with decreased branching and abrupt tapering ("arrowhead appearance") associated with disproportionate dilatation of the central and extrahepatic bile ducts [5]. Sonography, CT, and MRCP not only allow the correct diagnosis to be made but also serve as a vital road map for subsequent intervention by illustrating the location and extent of disease [6]. MRCP findings of RPC include IBD or EBD stones, multiple strictures of IBD, short-segment focal EBD stricture, localized dilatation of lobar or segmental bile ducts with a predilection for the lateral segment of the left lobe and the posterior segment of the right lobe, bile duct wall thickening, abrupt tapering, and decreased arborization of the IBDs [7]. CC associated with RPC most frequently occurs in segments with a high stone burden or at atrophied segments, and suggestive imaging features of CC development include progressive atrophy of affected hepatic segments or lobes and narrowing or obliteration of the portal vein [8, 9].

Primary Sclerosing Cholangitis

PSC is a progressive cholestatic disease characterized by inflammation and fibrosis of the bile duct which is commonly associated with inflammatory bowel disease [10]. Diagnosis of primary sclerosing cholangitis can be made by typical cholangiographic findings and the exclusion of secondary causes. The typical cholangiographic features include diffuse, multifocal short-segmental strictures and mild dilatation in the intrahepatic and extrahepatic bile ducts alternating with normal ducts, which sometimes produce "beaded" appearance [5] (Fig.). Patients with PSC have a 10–15% lifetime risk of developing CC [11], and CC in PSC usually presents as a periductal infiltrating type CC associated with dominant stenosis [11]. Suggestive imaging findings of CC in PSC include irregular dominant stricture with a shouldered margin, prominent mural thickening, and rapidly progressed dilatation of the bile duct proximal to the stricture.

IgG4-Related Cholangitis

IgG4-related sclerosing cholangitis is the biliary manifestation of IgG4 sclerosing disease, a recently recognized disease entity that manifests histologically as infiltration by abundant IgG4-positive plasma cells [7]. Differentiation of IgG4-SC from other types of sclerosing cholangitis, espe-

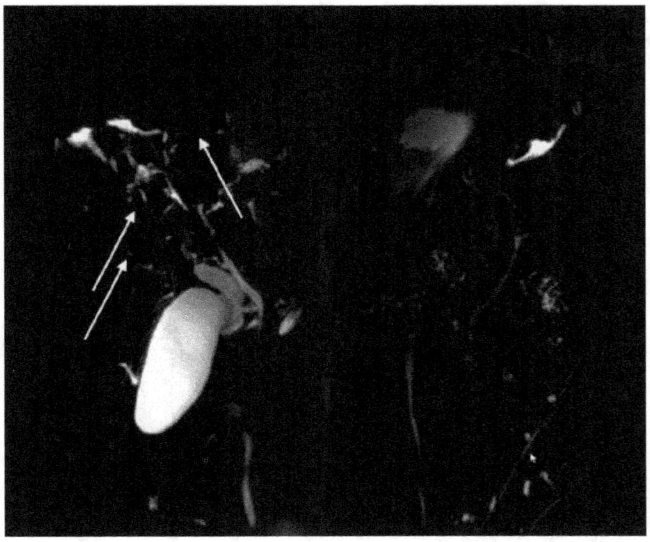

Fig. 52-year-old female patient with primary sclerosing cholangitis and typical beading of the intrahepatic biliary system (arrows) as seen on coronal MRCP images. Note the normally configured extrahepatic biliary duct

cially from PSC or bile duct cancers, is clinically important as IgG4-SC shows a dramatic response to steroid therapy [12]. Unlike in PSC, multifocal strictures in IgG4-related sclerosing cholangitis are long and continuous and are associated with prestenotic dilatation. An elevated serum IgG4 level and the presence of extrabiliary IgG4 sclerosing disease (e.g., involvement of the pancreas, kidneys, thyroid gland, and salivary glands) are strongly suggestive of IgG4-related sclerosing cholangitis [7]. In cases of IgG4-SC, CT or MR imaging demonstrates long-segmental, symmetrical, circumferential wall thickening and delayed contrast enhancement of the involved bile ducts [5].

Neoplasms

Benign Tumors of the Bile Ducts

Common benign tumors of the bile ducts include bile duct hamartoma, adenoma, biliary papillomatosis, and biliary cystadenoma.

Biliary Hamartoma

Biliary hamartoma, also known as von Meyenburg complex, manifests as multiple or innumerable cysts, typically less than 1.5 cm, distributed in both lobes of the liver [13, 14].

Biliary Cystadenoma (Biliary Mucinous Cystic Neoplasms)

Biliary cystadenomas and cystadenocarcinomas are rare, multilocular cystic tumors of biliary origin, and more than 85% of these tumors occur in middle-aged women [15]. Biliary cystadenomas typically appear as cystic masses with a well-marginated capsule, internal septa, and mural nodules, with rare capsular calcification [14]. Although imaging features of cystadenomas and cystadenocarcinomas overlap, malignant cystadenocarcinomas tend to have a thicker wall and thicker internal septa and more often contain intratumoral papillary and polypoid projections [13].

Intraductal Papillary Neoplasm of the Bile Duct (IPNB)

Two major premalignant bile duct tumors include biliary intraepithelial neoplasia (BilIN) and intraductal papillary neoplasms of the bile duct (IPNB), both of which can progress to CC. IPNB shows a diverse spectrum of premalignant lesions toward invasive CC according to the location of the origin and presence of mucin hypersecretion. Typical imaging features of IPNB are the presence of intraductal tumors and bile duct dilatation [16]. IPNB with mucin secretion often causes dilatation of the downstream duct and patulous ampulla of Vater due to mucin hypersecretion [17]. On imaging, this can be seen as aneurysmal dilatation of the bile duct with or without visible intraductal mucin-secreting tumors, and the upstream duct can also be dilated [18, 19].

Malignant Tumors of the Bile Ducts

Cholangiocarcinoma is an adenocarcinoma arising from the bile ducts (Fig.). On the basis of macroscopic growth patterns, CC can be categorized into mass-forming (MF), periductal-infiltrating (PI), and intraductal-growing (IDG) types according to the classification proposed by the Liver Cancer Study Group of Japan (LCSGJ) [20]. Not only diagnosis of cholangiocarcinoma but also appropriate categorization of bile duct tumors based on their morphologic features and location on cross-sectional imaging studies, including computed tomography and magnetic resonance imaging, is

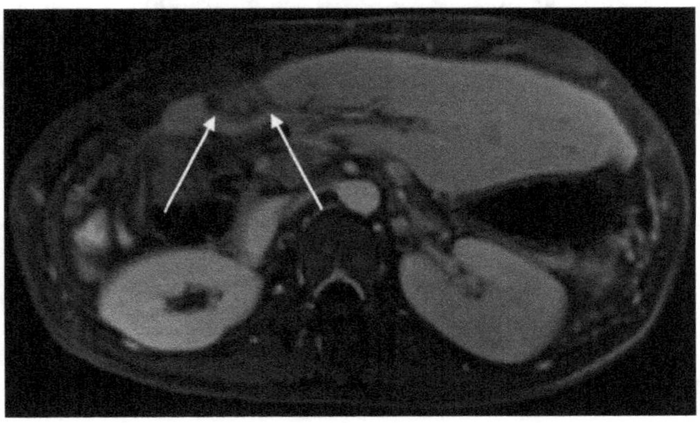

Fig. 73-year-old female patient with recurrence of cholangiocarcinoma (arrows) following right-sided hemihepatectomy with hepaticojejunal anastomosis, on equilibrium phase contrast-enhanced MR imaging

important to predict their biologic behaviors and choose relevant treatment strategies [16]. MF-type ICC typically manifests as a large non-encapsulated mass of lobulated or irregular contour, which typically shows early peripheral rim enhancement with progressive centripetal enhancement on a CT and MR imaging, and is frequently accompanied by hepatic capsular retraction and dilated peripheral bile ducts [16]. IDG-type CC appears as a polypoid or papillary tumor within the dilated bile duct lumen and has a growth pattern of superficial mucosal spreading [16].

Perihilar CC usually presents as a narrowed perihilar duct with irregular wall thickening which typically shows progressively delayed enhancement and upstream bile duct dilatation on CT or MRI [21]. Long-segmental involvement (>12 mm), a thickened (>1.5 mm) wall, luminal irregularity or asymmetry, and incremental enhancement may favor a malignant stricture, while benign strictures often involve short segments and a smooth transition [7, 22]. For perihilar cholangiocarcinomas, the local extent of the tumor is most commonly described using the Bismuth-Corlette (BC) system. Tumors are classified into type I (tumor involving only the common hepatic duct below the first confluence), type II (tumor involving the first confluence without involvement of second confluences), type III (tumor involving either right (IIIA) or left (IIIB) second confluence), and type IV (tumor involving both right and left second confluence). In general, BC type IV, BC type III with contralateral liver atrophy or contralateral vascular invasion, invasion of the main portal vein or common hepatic artery, and the presence of distant metastases are regarded to be unresectable [23]. As surgical complete resection is the only potentially curative treatment, it is critical to determine the type and extent of surgery for selection of the most appropriate surgical candidates with imaging. However, accurate staging of many CCs still remains challenging due to the small size of the tumors involved and the complex anatomy of the bile duct and adjacent structures as well as the high frequency of anatomical variations [24]. A multimodality approach using CT, MRI with MRCP, direct cholangiography, endoscopic ultrasound, and positron emission tomography has most frequently been applied to surgical candidates [24].

Gallbladder

Daniel T. Boll, M.D.

Normal Anatomy

Located along the undersurface of the liver in the plane of the interlobar fissure between the right and left hepatic lobes, the gallbladder is a round tubular structure with a cross-sectional diameter of up to 5 cm and a normal wall thickness of 1–3.5 mm [25, 26].

The bile-filled lumen of the gallbladder measures water isodensity (0–20 Hounsfield units) on CT and water-isointense signal characteristics on T2-weighted MR imaging; formation and retention of sludge may create gradients of signal intensity/density, resulting in a parfait-like appearance. The vicarious excretion of CT contrast material from prior contrast-enhanced CT imaging as well as utilization of hepatocyte-specific contrast materials in hepatic MR imaging may alter the imaging appearance of bile on CT as well as MR imaging [27, 28].

Congenital Variants and Anomalies

Agenesis of the Gallbladder

Being a rare malformation (0.01–0.2% in autopsy series), agenesis of the gallbladder results from a developmental failure of the caudal division of the primitive hepatic diverticulum or failure of vacuolization. It may result in biliary tract symptoms and formation of extrahepatic and intrahepatic gallstones in up to 50% of patients [25, 29].

Duplication of the Gallbladder

The duplication of the gallbladder is an equally rare malformation (0.02% in autopsy series), resulting in a longitudinal septum, divides the gallbladder cavity, and each cavity drains through its own cystic duct. Embryologically, duplication of the gallbladder is the result of an incomplete revacuolization of the primitive gallbladder. Differentiation from gallbladder folds, a bilobed gallbladder, a choledochal cyst, or a gallbladder diverticulum may be challenging on imaging studies [30].

Phrygian Cap of the Gallbladder

This most common anomaly of the gallbladder through a septation between the body and the distal fundus may be seen in up to 6% of all patients. Two types have been described: the retroserosal more concealed type and the serosal type with the peritoneum outlining the fundus reflecting on itself and overlying the body of the gallbladder [25, 31].

Multiseptate Gallbladder

Septations throughout the gallbladder, creating communicating chambers, may lead to stasis of bile and formation of gallstones [32].

Diverticula of the Gallbladder

True gallbladder diverticula are congenital in nature and contain all three muscle layers. Pseudodiverticula are developmental in nature and are usually associated with adenomyomatosis and contain little or no smooth muscle layers in their walls. (Pseudo)Diverticula can occur at any location throughout the gallbladder wall [25, 33].

Ectopic Gallbladder

Various locations of the gallbladder have been described; of particular interest is the intrahepatic location of the gallbladder, which is entirely surrounded by hepatic parenchyma. Intrahepatic subcapsular locations may particularly complicate the diagnosis of an acute cholecystitis as secondary signs of inflammation may be subtle or masked entirely. Shrinkage of the liver in patients with cirrhosis, as well as patients with chronic obstructive pulmonary disease, may show gallbladders interposed between the liver surface and diaphragm [25, 34].

Pathologic Conditions

Gallstones

The appearance of gallstones in cross-sectional imaging is primarily composition based; most gallstones contain various admixtures of bile pigment, cholesterol, and calcium. Larger proportions of calcium may render gallstones hyperdense on CT imaging, while pure cholesterol stones may be lower in CT density than surrounding bile; central inclusions of gas mostly consist of nitrogen and may lead to flotation of gallstones.

The high signal intensity of bile on T2-weighted images allows better delineation of hypointense gallstones compared to T1-weighted sequences. While cholesterol stones are usually hypointense in appearance on T1-weighted images, pigment stones tend to have higher signal intensities. Central areas of T2 hyperintensity usually corresponds to fluid-filled clefts [25, 35, 36].

Acute Cholecystitis

An obstruction of either the gallbladder neck or the cystic duct may lead to increased intraluminal pressures and eventually result in an inflammation of the gallbladder wall. Gallstones lodged in the neck of the gallbladder or the cystic duct leading to biliodynamic obstruction as well as pressure-induced mucosal ischemia and injury are the preeminent reason for acute cholecystitis. Ultrasound, CT, and MRI may show distinct features of acute cholecystitis, such as cholecystolithiasis, gallbladder wall thickening, pericholecystic fluid and inflammation, thickened bile, an indistinct interface between the gallbladder wall and liver capsule, and potentially gallbladder perforation (Fig.). Gallbladder perforations can be subdivided into acute, subacute, and chronic stages; a subacute perforation with a surrounding abscess is the most frequently encountered type of gallbladder perforation. The use of hepatobiliary contrast agents in MR imaging may provide additional functional information about cystic duct patency [25, 37, 38].

In emphysematous cholecystitis, an additional vascular compromise of the cystic artery is hypothesized to accelerate the development of gas-forming organisms in the resultant anaerobic environment with eventual penetration of gas into the gallbladder wall. A more frequent occurrence in diabetic patients, as well as the male population with an acalculous gallbladder, potentially hints at a separate pathogenesis in contrast to calculous cholecystitis [39].

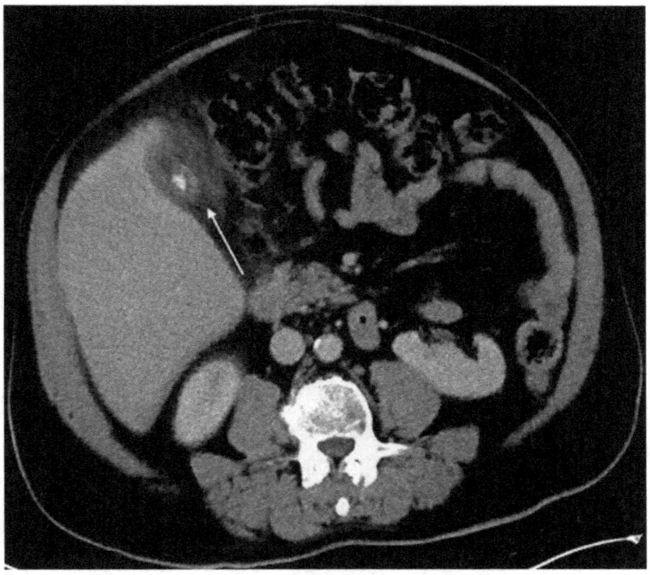

Fig. 49-year-old male patient with acute calculous cholecystitis as seen on portal venous contrast-enhanced CT imaging. Note the gallbladder wall thickening and surrounding fluid (arrow) as well as the intraluminal gallstone

Inflammation causing ulceration of the mucosal lining and subsequent necrosis may lead to hemorrhagic cholecystitis. The intraluminal hematoma that may be seen on CT and MRI may, however, be difficult to differentiate from high-intensity/high-density bile. An accompanying perforation of the gallbladder wall may lead to hemoperitoneum [40].

Coexisting cardiovascular disease predisposes patients with acute cholecystitis to develop gangrenous wall segments. Intraluminal membranes and irregularity of the gallbladder wall intermittently perforated and potentially surrounded by a pericholecystic abscess are key imaging features.

Acalculous Cholecystitis

In approximately 5% of all patients with acute cholecystitis, no intraluminal stones can be found. Long stays in intensive care units and abdominal trauma may lead to increased viscosity and subsequent stasis of bile leading to obstruction and mucosal ischemia [25, 41].

Chronic Cholecystitis

Repetitive mucosal trauma through preexisting gallstones as well as recurrent attacks of multiple acute cholecystitic episodes may contribute to the poorly understood pathogenesis of this fairly common disease. A florid inflammatory response to irritations may also indicate a genetic predisposition. While cross-sectional imaging of chronic cholecystitis may not substantially differ from acute cholecystitis, the greatest difference appears to be a contracted state of the gallbladder in chronic cholecystitis compared to the acute scenario. A decreased gallbladder ejection fraction is oftentimes associated with chronic cholecystitis [25].

Microperforations through mucosal ulcers as well as ruptured Rokitansky-Aschoff sinuses may lead to penetration of bile into the gallbladder wall, resulting in the formation of xanthogranulomas representing the hallmark of xanthogranulomatous cholecystitis. Gallstones are almost always present, and an irregular configuration of the gallbladder wall is frequently observed. Xanthogranulomatous lesions in the wall can also lead to interim mural abscess formations. These may appear hypodense on contrast-enhanced CT imaging as well as hyperintense nodules on T2-weighted MR imaging sequences. Differentiation from gallbladder cancer may be challenging; however, a patent mucosal lining/luminal surface is more indicative of xanthogranulomatous cholecystitis [25].

Impaction of gallstones inside the cystic duct with subsequent compression of the common hepatic duct and resultant inflammation are mechanisms leading to the Mirizzi syndrome. A fairly low insertion of the cystic duct into the common hepatic duct may predispose this patient subpopulation. Differentiating the inflammatory origin of the stricture of the common hepatic duct from a neoplastic process may be challenging; the lack of lymphadenopathy, as well as a distinct focal mass, may be helpful secondary signs. Erosion of gallstones through the gallbladder wall directly into the adjacent bowel via a cholecystoenteric fistula is the most common mechanism to form a gallstone ileus, in particular within the distal ileum [25, 42].

Chronic inflammatory changes of the gallbladder wall may lead to dystrophic calcifications associated with thick fibrous tissue layers of the gallbladder wall, indicating a porcelain gallbladder. The porcelain gallbladder is frequently associated with gallbladder carcinoma [17] (Fig.).

Hyperplastic Cholecystosis

A benign proliferation of normal gallbladder wall tissue characterizes this noninflammatory condition.

A deposition of cholesterol-laden macrophages into the lamina propria of the gallbladder wall may lead to formation of cholesterol polyps and other hallmark cholesterolosis. Due to their small size, these polyps are best seen on ultrasound imaging [25, 43].

A hypertrophy of the muscular wall with corresponding mucosal overgrowth and formation of intramural diverticula and sinus tracts, then called Rokitansky-Aschoff sinuses, is the hallmark of adenomyomatosis. This disease can be seen diffusely infiltrating the gallbladder wall, may have an annular appearance, or may be very focal. Detection of a thickened gallbladder wall in addition to small cystic spaces on CT and MR imaging helps to differentiate adenomyomatosis from gallbladder cancer [43].

Gallbladder Neoplasms

Benign neoplasms of the gallbladder are rare and usually represent adenomas, which are, incidentally, (0.3–0.5%) found during cholecystectomies [25].

During the sixth or seventh decades of life with a female predilection of 2:1–3:1, gallbladder carcinomas, occur histopathologically usually as adenocarcinomas; however, adenosquamous, squamous, or neuroendocrine carcinomas can also be found, may arise from the gallbladder wall. Predisposing factors associated with gallbladder carcinoma are gallstones (75% of patients with gallbladder carcinomas have gallstones), porcelain gallbladder, genetic factors, as well as pancreaticobiliary ductal unions (reflux of pancreatic juice into the common bile duct leading to chronic inflammation) (Fig.). On cross-sectional imaging, either a mass is seen replacing the gallbladder fossa or the mass is noted filling most of the enlarged and deformed gallbladder. In invasion of surrounding structures, in particular the liver, the hepatoduodenal ligament, the right hepatic flexure, or the duodenum is frequently observed. Lymphatic spread to the regional and distant lymph nodes is very common, and gallbladder carcinoma hematogenous metastasis to the liver, intraductal tumor spread, as well as

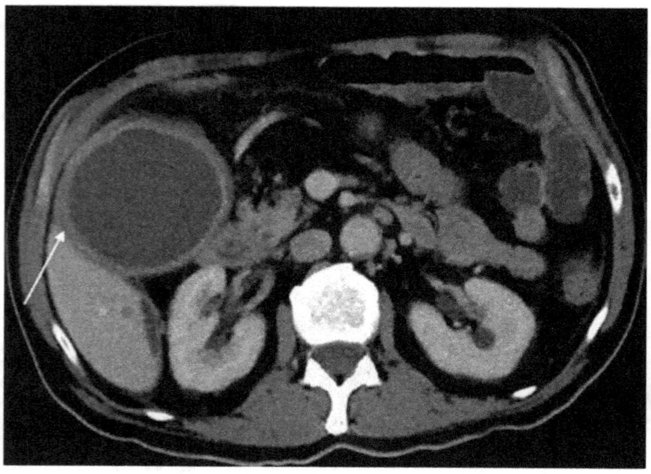

Fig. 69-year-old female patient with chronic cholecystitis with thickening of the gallbladder wall (arrow) without substantial pericholecystic fluid surrounding this acalculous gallbladder as seen on portal venous phase contrast-enhanced CT imaging

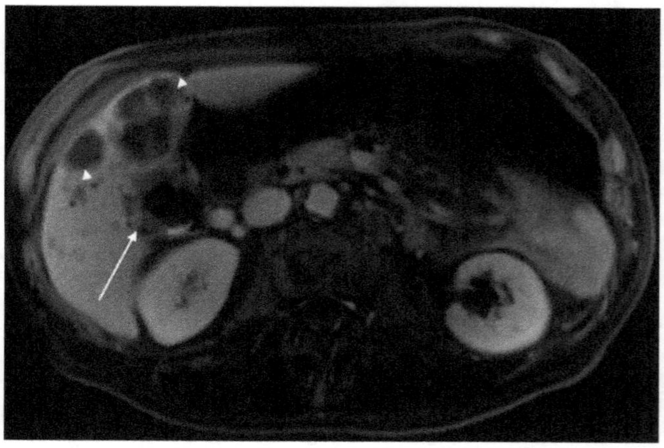

Fig. 65-year-old female patient with gallbladder carcinoma, infiltrating the liver (arrow), and multiple intrahepatic metastases (arrowheads) with gallstones on T1-weighted contrast-enhanced MR imaging using a hepatocyte-specific contrast agent in a 5-min delayed phase

peritoneal seeding is also fairly common. Biliary obstruction may be observed in up to 50% of patients [25, 44, 45].

Secondary lymphoma to the gallbladder is rare and may be seen in disseminated lymphomatous stages; primary lymphoma involving the gallbladder is extremely rare [46].

Metastases to the gallbladder is also a rare disease and can originate from any source; however, malignant melanoma is the most common cause of metastatic tumors, accounting for more than 50% of all cases of gallbladder metastases [47].

Concluding Remarks

Familiarity with the typical clinical and radiologic appearances of various etiologies of gallbladder disease, cholangiopathies, and biliary malignancies is important for accurate image interpretation, and thus enabling optimal clinical and surgical management.

Take-Home Messages

- An appreciation of the pathologic basis of gallbladder and biliary disease, combined with careful inspection of the imaging appearances, is vital for the correct interpretation of biliary studies.
- Differential diagnosis of various cholangiopathies is important because specific management exists and prognosis can be different according to the type of disease.
- Awareness of the underlying risk factors and morphologic characteristics of gallbladder disease and cholangiocarcinoma is important for accurate diagnosis and for differentiation from other hepatic tumorous and non-tumorous lesions.
- Imaging studies play important roles in the diagnosis and treatment planning of patients with biliary malignancies, and multimodality and multiparametric imaging approaches can provide complementary information in evaluating the tumor extent and resectability.

Key Points

- Imaging of gallbladder and biliary disease often requires a multimodality imaging approach.
- Sclerosing cholangitis is a spectrum of chronic progressive cholestatic liver disease characterized by inflammation, fibrosis, and stricture of the bile ducts, which can be classified as primary and secondary sclerosing cholangitis. A systematic approach combined with the appropriate clinical settings and imaging findings can be helpful for differentiating the various causes of sclerosing cholangitis.
- Although tissue biopsy or surgery is needed for the definitive diagnosis of many of biliary strictures, certain imaging characteristics of the narrowed segment (e.g., thickened wall, long-segment involvement, asymmetry, indistinct outer margin, luminal irregularity, and hyperenhancement relative to the liver parenchyma) may favor a malignant cause.
- Biliary malignancies typically demonstrate arterial phase enhancement with persistent enhancement into the portal venous phase, related to the fibrotic nature of these neoplasms.
- In the resectability assessment of perihilar CC, longitudinal tumor extent, vascular invasion, anatomical variation of the bile duct and vessels, future remnant volume, and presence or absence of distant metastasis should be considered.
- Intraductal papillary mucinous neoplasms of the bile duct (IPMN-B) bear a striking similarity to IPMN of the pancreas with regard to its histopathologic features and frequently show intraductal tumors, mucobilia, and diffuse dilatation of upstream and downstream bile ducts.
- Knowledge of congenital variants and anomalies of the gallbladder anatomy is essential to understand and characterize gallbladder disease.
- Pathogenesis of gallstone formation and resultant acute and chronic cholecystitis and their complications influences treatment decisions.
- Differentiating inflammatory gallbladder disease from gallbladder neoplasms can be challenging in early stages; recognizing imaging features which raise the suspicion for potential underlying neoplasms is essential in guiding potential treatment options.

References

1. Mortele KJ, Rocha TC, Streeter JL, Taylor AJ. Multimodality imaging of pancreatic and biliary congenital anomalies. Radiographics. 2006;26:715–31.
2. Yeh BM, Liu PS, Soto JA, Corvera CA, Hussain HK. MR imaging and CT of the biliary tract. Radiographics. 2009;29:1669–88.
3. Lee NK, Kim S, Lee JW, et al. Discrimination of suppurative cholangitis from nonsuppurative cholangitis with computed tomography (CT). Eur J Radiol. 2009;69:528–35.
4. Bader TR, Braga L, Beavers KL, Semelka RC. MR imaging findings of infectious cholangitis. Magn Reson Imaging. 2001;19:781–8.
5. Seo N, Kim SY, Lee SS, et al. Sclerosing cholangitis: Clinicopathologic features, imaging Spectrum, and systemic approach to differential diagnosis. Korean J Radiol. 2016;17:25–38.
6. Heffernan EJ, Geoghegan T, Munk PL, Ho SG, Harris AC. Recurrent pyogenic cholangitis: from imaging to intervention. AJR Am J Roentgenol. 2009;192:W28–35.
7. Katabathina VS, Dasyam AK, Dasyam N, Hosseinzadeh K. Adult bile duct strictures: role of MR imaging and MR cholangiopancreatography in characterization. Radiographics. 2014;34:565–86.

8. Kim JH, Kim TK, Eun HW, et al. CT findings of cholangiocarcinoma associated with recurrent pyogenic cholangitis. AJR Am J Roentgenol. 2006;187:1571–7.
9. Al-Sukhni W, Gallinger S, Pratzer A, et al. Recurrent pyogenic cholangitis with hepatolithiasis--the role of surgical therapy in North America. J Gastrointest Surg. 2008;12:496–503.
10. Eaton JE, Talwalkar JA, Lazaridis KN, Gores GJ, Lindor KD. Pathogenesis of primary sclerosing cholangitis and advances in diagnosis and management. Gastroenterology. 2013;145:521–36.
11. Khaderi SA, Sussman NL. Screening for malignancy in primary sclerosing cholangitis (PSC). Curr Gastroenterol Rep. 2015;17:17.
12. Ponsioen CY. Diagnosis, differential diagnosis, and epidemiology of primary Sclerosing cholangitis. Dig Dis. 2015;33(Suppl 2):134–9.
13. Buetow PC, Midkiff RB. MR imaging of the liver. Primary malignant neoplasms in the adult. Magn Reson Imaging Clin N Am. 1997;5:289–318.
14. Yam BL, Siegelman ES. MR imaging of the biliary system. Radiol Clin N Am. 2014;52:725–55.
15. Devaney K, Goodman ZD, Ishak KG. Hepatobiliary cystadenoma and cystadenocarcinoma. A light microscopic and immunohistochemical study of 70 patients. Am J Surg Pathol. 1994;18:1078–91.
16. Joo I, Lee JM. Imaging bile duct tumors: pathologic concepts, classification, and early tumor detection. Abdom Imaging. 2013;38:1334–50.
17. Kane RA, Jacobs R, Katz J, Costello P. Porcelain gallbladder: ultrasound and CT appearance. Radiology. 1984;152:137–41.
18. Lim JH, Yoon KH, Kim SH, et al. Intraductal papillary mucinous tumor of the bile ducts. Radiographics. 2004;24:53–66.
19. Takanami K, Yamada T, Tsuda M, et al. Intraductal papillary mucininous neoplasm of the bile ducts: multimodality assessment with pathologic correlation. Abdom Imaging. 2011;36:447–56.
20. Yamasaki S. Intrahepatic cholangiocarcinoma: macroscopic type and stage classification. J Hepato-Biliary-Pancreat Surg. 2003;10:288–91.
21. Valls C, Ruiz S, Martinez L, Leiva D. Radiological diagnosis and staging of hilar cholangiocarcinoma. World J Gastrointest Oncol. 2013;5:115–26.
22. Kim JY, Lee JM, Han JK, et al. Contrast-enhanced MRI combined with MR cholangiopancreatography for the evaluation of patients with biliary strictures: differentiation of malignant from benign bile duct strictures. J Magn Reson Imaging. 2007;26:304–12.
23. Jarnagin WR, Fong Y, DeMatteo RP, et al. Staging, resectability, and outcome in 225 patients with hilar cholangiocarcinoma. Ann Surg. 2001;234:507–17.
24. Corona-Villalobos CP, Pawlik TM, Kamel IR. Imaging of the patient with a biliary tract or primary liver tumor. Surg Oncol Clin N Am. 2014;23:189–206.
25. Lim JH, Kim KW, Choi D-i. Biliary tract and gallbladder. In: Haaga JR, Boll DT, editors. CT and MRI of the whole body. 6th ed. Philadelphia: Elsevier; 2017. p. 1192–267.
26. Smathers RL, Lee JK, Heiken JP. Differentiation of complicated cholecystitis from gallbladder carcinoma by computed tomography. AJR Am J Roentgenol. 1984;143:255–9.
27. Havrilla TR, Reich NE, Haaga JR, Seidelmann FE, Cooperman AM, Alfidi RJ. Computed tomography of the gallbladder. AJR Am J Roentgenol. 1978;130:1059–67.
28. Strax R, Toombs BD, Kam J, Rauschkolb EN, Patel S, Sandler CM. Gallbladder enhancement following angiography: a normal CT finding. J Comput Assist Tomogr. 1982;6:766–8.
29. Al-Fallouji MA. Perforated posterior peptic ulcer associated with gallbladder agenesis and midgut malrotation. Br J Clin Pract. 1983;37:353–6. 358
30. Udelsman R, Sugarbaker PH. Congenital duplication of the gallbladder associated with an anomalous right hepatic artery. Am J Surg. 1985;149:812–5.
31. Foster DR. Triple gall bladder. Br J Radiol. 1981;54:817–8.
32. Toombs BD, Foucar E, Rowlands BJ, Strax R. Multiseptate gallbladder. South Med J. 1982;75:610–2.
33. Kochhar R, Nagi B, Mehta SK, Gupta NM. ERCP diagnosis of a gallbladder diverticulum. Gastrointest Endosc. 1988;34:150–1.
34. Gore RM, Ghahremani GG, Joseph AE, Nemcek AA Jr, Marn CS, Vogelzang RL. Acquired malposition of the colon and gallbladder in patients with cirrhosis: CT findings and clinical implications. Radiology. 1989;171:739–42.
35. Brink JA, Ferrucci JT. Use of CT for predicting gallstone composition: a dissenting view. Radiology. 1991;178:633–4.
36. Tsai HM, Lin XZ, Chen CY, Lin PW, Lin JC. MRI of gallstones with different compositions. AJR Am J Roentgenol. 2004;182:1513–9.
37. Bennett GL, Balthazar EJ. Ultrasound and CT evaluation of emergent gallbladder pathology. Radiol Clin N Am. 2003;41:1203–16.
38. Paulson EK. Acute cholecystitis: CT findings. Semin Ultrasound CT MR. 2000;21:56–63.
39. Jacob H, Appelman R, Stein HD. Emphysematous cholecystitis. Am J Gastroenterol. 1979;71:325–30.
40. Jenkins M, Golding RH, Cooperberg PL. Sonography and computed tomography of hemorrhagic cholecystitis. AJR Am J Roentgenol. 1983;140:1197–8.
41. Mirvis SE, Vainright JR, Nelson AW, et al. The diagnosis of acute acalculous cholecystitis: a comparison of sonography, scintigraphy, and CT. AJR Am J Roentgenol. 1986;147:1171–5.
42. Koehler RE, Melson GL, Lee JK, Long J. Common hepatic duct obstruction by cystic duct stone: Mirizzi syndrome. AJR Am J Roentgenol. 1979;132:1007–9.
43. JUTRAS JA. Hyperplastic cholecystoses; hickey lecture, 1960. Am J Roentgenol Radium Therapy, Nucl Med. 1960;83:795–827.
44. Hamrick RE Jr, Liner FJ, Hastings PR, Cohn I Jr. Primary carcinoma of the gallbladder. Ann Surg. 1982;195:270–3.
45. Yoshimitsu K, Honda H, Shinozaki K, et al. Helical CT of the local spread of carcinoma of the gallbladder: evaluation according to the TNM system in patients who underwent surgical resection. AJR Am J Roentgenol. 2002;179:423–8.
46. Mitropoulos FA, Angelopoulou MK, Siakantaris MP, et al. Primary non-Hodgkin's lymphoma of the gall bladder. Leuk Lymphoma. 2000;40:123–31.
47. Guida M, Cramarossa A, Gentile A, et al. Metastatic malignant melanoma of the gallbladder: a case report and review of the literature. Melanoma Res. 2002;12:619–25.

3

Diseases of the Colon and Rectum: CT Colonography

C. Dan Johnson and Perry J. Pickhardt

Learning Objectives

- To implement proper technique for obtaining a high-quality CT colonography examination
- To educate others regarding the safety and performance of CT colonography
- To participate in a quality improvement program related to CT colonography
- To recognize difficult-to-detect lesions at CT colonography

The public health need for colorectal cancer screening is compelling. Colorectal cancer is common, accounting for approximately 50,000 deaths yearly in the USA [1]. The benign precursor adenoma can be detected by several different imaging techniques, and, if removed, can prevent malignant transformation. The approximately 10-year polyp dwell time allows ample opportunity for patients to be screened and polyps detected and removed. Potentially, under ideal screening circumstances, an entire class of cancers could be prevented. Unfortunately, barriers exist to ideal screening, including suboptimal performance of many existing colorectal screening tests, reluctant compliance by patients to follow recommended screening guidelines, and variable insurance coverage of examination charges. In many ways, CT colonography (CTC) approaches an ideal screening test by addressing issues and problems inherent with other techniques. This syllabus will highlight many key issues for CT colonography today.

C. Dan Johnson, M.D. (✉)
Mayo Clinic, Scottsdale, AZ, USA
e-mail: johnson.daniel2@mayo.edu

P. J. Pickhardt, M.D.
University of Wisconsin, Madison, WI, USA

Technique

Proper technique at CT colonography is imperative for high performance. The three main steps include preparation, CT scanning, and interpretation.

Preparation

1. *Dietary restriction*. Preparation begins with a recommendation for patients to consume clear liquids or a low-residue diet for at least 1 day prior to beginning the cathartic bowel preparation. Although this step is optimal, it can be skipped if patients are following the subsequent instructions carefully.
2. *Stool tagging*. 10–20 mL of barium or iodinated contrast material is administered orally for three meals prior to beginning the cathartic preparation. This contrast agent mixes with stool and ideally is evacuated with the cathartic preparation. Residual stool will contain high-attenuation contrast and can be easily discriminated from soft tissue attenuation polyps. Some prefer to perform stool tagging after the cathartic agent, but before fluid tagging.
3. *Cathartic*. The cathartic preparation can be performed with a number of different formulations including polyethylene glycol electrolyte solution and magnesium citrate or bisacodyl tablets. Phospho-soda agents are not recommended because of prior issues with renal insufficiency and sodium retention. Bisacodyl tablets require the patient to be well hydrated for the purgation process to be successful. Bisacodyl tablets are easy to consume and well tolerated by patients. Polyethylene glycol electrolyte solution provides the cleanest colon, but some patients find it more difficult to consume in its entirety.
4. *Fluid tagging*. Following the cathartic preparation, the small bowel will continue to secrete soft tissue attenuation fluid into the colon. This fluid can obscure immersed pol-

yps. Tagging of this fluid is accomplished by drinking 60 ml of iodinated contrast material (either hyperosmolar or iso-osmolar) at bedtime, on the day before the exam. The high attenuation tagging allows inspection of the immersed portions of the colon wall and visualization of any colon lesions within this fluid.

5. *Insufflation*. The colon must be fully distended with air or carbon dioxide for optimal visualization at CT. Commercially available insufflation devices are available instilling CO_2 at a predefined rate and pressure. Excess intraluminal colonic pressure during a colonic contraction will result in venting of gas into the room—thereby reducing patient discomfort and the risk of perforation. As the pressure is reduced, the machine automatically refills the colon. Turning the patient on the CT table is helpful in creating a well-distended colon.
6. *Spasmolytics* [2]. The use of spasmolytics is controversial. Although it has not been shown to improve image quality, there are some that believe the exam is more comfortable for patients [3].

CT Scanning

Acquisition of CT data using thin collimation and isotropic reconstruction intervals will result in high-quality images in any desired plane. The colon and rectum data should be acquired in a single breath-hold, using a low-dose technique. Generally, we use a 1 mm collimation, reconstructing every 0.8 mm, 50 mAs. Optimally, new reconstruction software should be employed to enable ultralow-dose acquisition. Ideally, average patients should receive an effective dose equivalent of less than 5 mSv [4].

Interpretation

There are two main ways to interpret a CTC examination: either a primary 2D with 3D problem-solving or primary 3D with 2D problem-solving approaches. Both methods have been shown to have equal effectiveness. Most authorities advocate that each exam should have both a 2D and 3D review. Small polyps are more easily detected with a 3D (endoluminal) review, whereas obstructing cancers and flat lesions are better detected with a 2D review. There is no proven difference between software manufacturers in lesion detection [5] (Fig.).

Performance

The performance of CT colonography has undergone exhaustive testing. The Department of Defense (DoD) trial by Pickhardt et al. demonstrated sensitivity similar to colonoscopy [6], but concerns were raised that community practices might not be able to achieve these results. The National CT Colonography Trial findings were similar to the Pickhardt's trial and have reassured many groups [7] that the test can be performed with high accuracy in both academic and private practice settings.

Training and preferably testing of radiologists are requirements for optimal reader performance [8]. Participation in a dedicated training program is recommended. These training sessions should provide enough time for the radiologist to become facile with a specific colonography software package and experience interpreting at least 50 proven cases. Polyp detection testing will allow individuals an opportunity to assess if additional training is needed before clinical implementation. In order to continue to improve reader performance, it is recommended that patients who are undergoing both CTC and subsequent colonoscopy be reviewed retrospectively to assess for CTC false-positive and false-negative detections. This quality improvement review offers a rich experience for learning and gaining expertise, confidence, and competence. Strict adherence to state-of-the art CTC protocol requirements is also recommended including stool and fluid tagging regimens, mechanical insufflation of the colon, thin-section data acquisition, and low-dose CT techniques [9]. It is clear that meticulous attention to all aspects of the examination and interpretation is required to achieve the best results.

Acceptance

Today, nearly 40 million US adults age 50 or older have not undergone a sigmoidoscopy or colonoscopy within the previous 10 years or had used a fecal occult blood test (FOBT) home test kit within the preceding year [10]. The major disincentive for patients undergoing a full structural colorectal examination is the laxative purgation [11]. Work is being done to reduce the burden of laxation either with the use of a partial colon preparation [12] or without cathartic preparation [13]. Although not considered standard of care, evidence from feasibility trials is promising and may translate to better patient acceptance in the future.

Despite a full cathartic bowel preparation, the advantages of CTC include the lack of required sedation and intravenous line placement, a quick return to work following the examination, and the convenience of no driving restrictions following the test.

The disadvantage of CTC includes the fact that if a significant polyp is identified, patients must undergo colonoscopy and polypectomy. If same-day colonoscopy is not offered, then the patient must undergo a second bowel preparation, spend another day away from work, and experience added worry and inconvenience. In a screening population (including false-positive interpretations), the prevalence of patients being referred from CTC to colonoscopy for polypectomy is 12% when a 6 mm threshold is applied [6, 7]. This translates into an 88% chance that an individual patient will

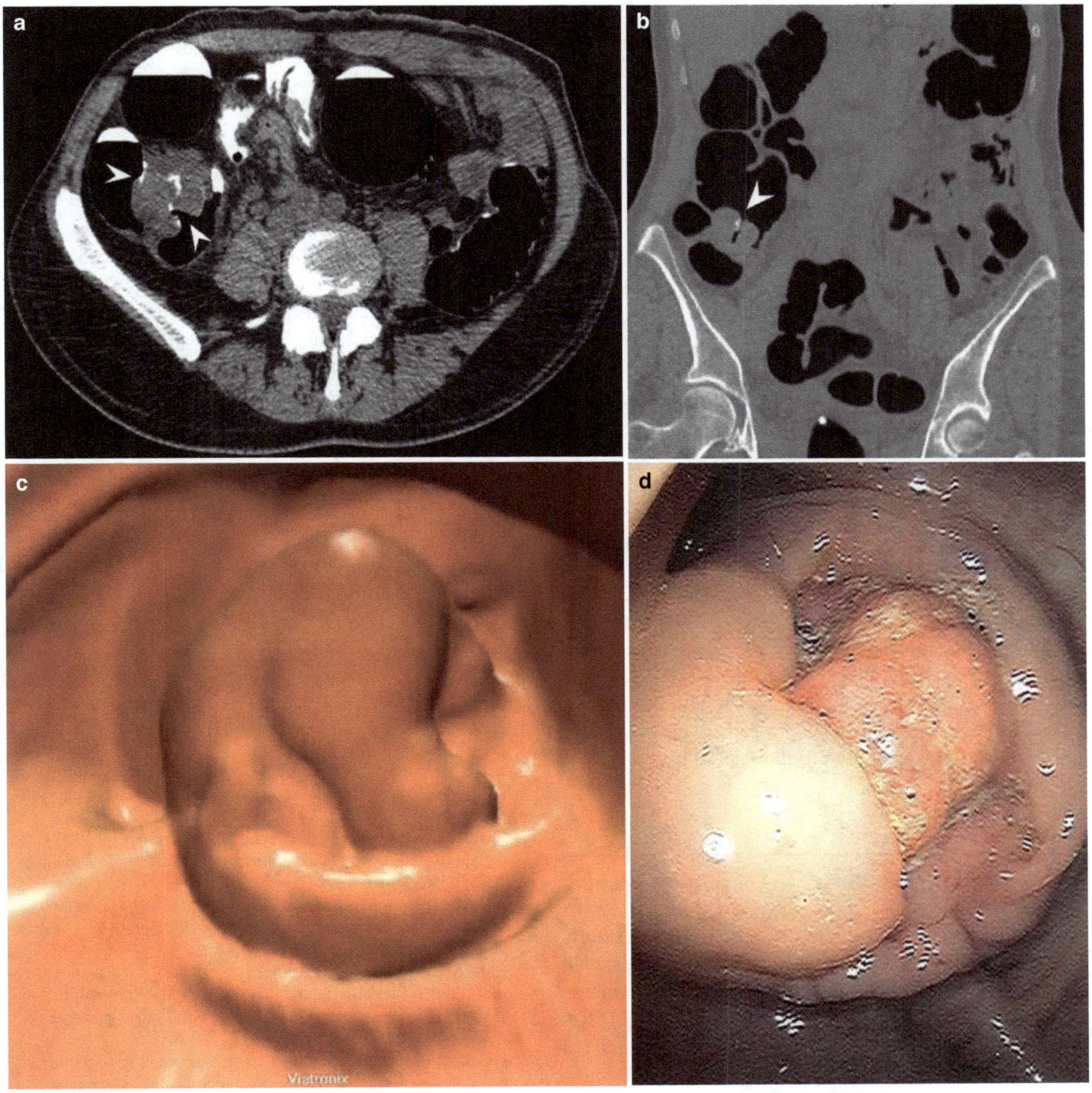

Fig. Unsuspected colon cancer in 56-year-old asymptomatic woman undergoing CTC screening. Transverse (**a**) and coronal (**b**) 2D images from CTC show a bulky soft tissue mass in the right colon (arrowheads). 3D endoluminal CTC image (**c**) correlates with the image from subsequent same-day colonoscopy (**d**)

not require a second procedure—thereby mitigating concerns for redundancy. Those with a high likelihood of polyps may best be triaged to colonoscopy screening.

Safety

The main risk for patients at CTC is the risk of colorectal perforation. The symptomatic perforation rate has been estimated to be 1:20,000 examinations and likely safer among screening patients [14]. In contrast, colonoscopy perforation rates have been recorded to be in the range of 1:1000 [15], often but not always related to biopsy procedures. Bleeding can also follow colonoscopy intervention and is more common than perforation.

Radiation risk from a CTC examination has been of public concern. It is unfortunate that the risk associated with the low radiation dose required for CTC has been misunderstood. The standard dose at CTC represents about 25–50% of the dose used for a standard body CT examination. This results in an average dose of approximately 2.5–5 mSv, similar to annual environmental exposures in many locales that is without known adverse health effects. The doses at CTC can be reduced significantly even further using new noise reduction software (iterative reconstruction). The real risk of this small dose is unknown, but the Health Physics Society has stated that doses in this range are associated with risks for the development of radiation-induced cancer that are either too small to measure or are nonexistent [16]. Even if a very small risk is assumed from radiation exposure at CT, it must be balanced against the risk of developing colon cancer (1:13) and the risks of other alternative procedures including colonoscopy [17].

ExtracolonicFindings

Extracolonic abnormalities are common in patients of screening age [18, 19]. Although lifesaving findings can be identified, most incidental findings are of little clinical significance but can potentially increase the cost of care if additional testing and treatment are recommended. A pragmatic approach to these findings is needed. Radiologists should only recommend follow-up studies for those findings most likely to be of clinical significance. Clinicians will be grateful if additional testing is minimized and for those that might benefit from additional studies to include recommendations for optimal follow-up within the radiologic report.

Individual Responsibility

Maintaining high-quality interpretations is a responsibility that each individual, each practice, and our specialty should assume. The ACR has established a national CTC database within the National Radiology Data Registry (NRDR) [20]. Selected process and outcome metrics can be quickly entered online and compared to national benchmarks. These measures include process metrics related to the CT technique and the adequacy of patient preparation, outcome metrics related to colon perforation, true positive and false-positive rates for large (≥1 cm) polyps, and the prevalence of significant extracolonic findings. Practices seriously interested in providing the best care should be encouraged to participate in this data registry and manage their practice so benchmark metrics are achieved.

A spirit of cooperation between radiologists and gastroenterologists is needed for optimal patient care. Guidelines will need to be jointly developed for the proper use of colonography and colonoscopy and for processes to efficiently transfer patients with polyps to colonoscopy. Those practices that are able to do this effectively will offer patients a service of high value and will likely find themselves very busy.

Key Point

- CT colonography is a well-validated examination and should be available clinically. Radiologists committed to performing the examination to the highest quality must obtain the education and equipment needed. We have an obligation to educate and to collaborate with referring physicians on the correct use of the technique. We must be vigilant that extracolonic findings are properly reported so that only highly suspicious lesions have recommended additional follow-up testing. Lastly, a commitment to incorporate ongoing quality measures within your daily practice will ensure that patients continue to receive the highest standards of care. Radiology has an exciting opportunity to serve the public and potentially reduces the incidence of a common cancer killer.

References

1. Siegel R, Naishadham D, Jemal A. Cancer statistics, 2012. CA Cancer J Clin. 2012;62:10–29.
2. Yee J, Hung RK, Akerkar GA, Wall SD. The usefulness of glucagon hydrochloride for colonic distention in CT colonography. AJR. 1999;173:169–72.
3. Laghi A. Computed tomography Colonography in 2014: an update on technique and indications. World J Gastroenterol. 2014;20:16858–67.
4. Flicek KT, Hara AK, Silva AC, et al. Reducing the radiation dose for CT colonography using adaptive statistical iterative reconstruction: a pilot study. AJR. 2010;195:126–31.
5. Hara AK, Blevins M, Chen MH, et al. ACRIN CT Colonography trial: does reader's preference for primary two-dimensional versus primary three-dimensional interpretation affect performance? Radiology. 2011;259:435–41.
6. Pickhardt PJ, Choi JR, Hwang I, et al. Computed tomographic virtual colonoscopy to screen for colorectal neoplasia in asymptomatic adults. N Engl J Med. 2003;349:2191–200.
7. Johnson CD, Chen MH, Toledano A, et al. Accuracy of CT colonography for detection of large adenomas and cancer. N Engl J Med. 2008;359:1207–17.
8. Fletcher JG, Chen MH, Herman BA, et al. Can radiologist training and testing ensure high performance in CT colonography? Lessons from the National CT Colonography Trial. Am J Roentgenol. 2010 Jul;195(1):117–25.
9. Robbins JB, Kim DH. Computed tomographic Colonography: evidence and techniques for screening. Semin Roentgenol. 2013 Jul;48:264–72.
10. Centers for Disease Control and Prevention. Vital signs: colorectal cancer screening among adults aged 50-75 years—United States, 2008. MMWR Morb Mortal Wkly Rep. 2010:808–12.
11. Beebe TJ, Johnson CD, Stoner SM, Anderson KJ, Limburg PJ. Assessing attitudes toward laxative preparation in colorectal

cancer screening and effects on future testing: potential receptivity to computed tomographic colonography. Mayo Clin Proc. 2007;82:666–71.
12. Johnson CD, Kriegshauser JS, Lund JT, et al. Partial preparation computed tomographic colonography: a feasibility study. Abdom Imaging. 2011;36:707–12.
13. Johnson CD, Manduca A, Fletcher JG, et al. Noncathartic CT colonography with stool tagging: performance with and without electronic subtraction. Am J Roentgenol. 2006;190:361–6.
14. Pickhardt PJ. Incidence of colonic perforation at CT colonography: review of existing data and implication for screening of asymptomatic adults. Radiology. 2006;239:313–6.
15. Waye JD, Kahn O, Auerbach ME. Complications of colonoscopy and flexible sigmoidoscopy. Gastrointest Endosc Clin N Am. 1996;6:342–77.
16. Radiation risk in perspective. *Position Statement of the Health Physics Society* July 2010. http://hps.org/documents/risk_ps010-2.pdf
17. Hendee WR, O'Connor MK. Radiation risks of medical imaging: separating fact from fantasy. Radiology. 2012;264:312–21.
18. Gluecker TM, Johnson CD, Wilson LA, et al. Extracolonic findings at CT colonography: evaluation of prevalence and cost in a screening population. Gastroenterology. 2003;124:911–6.
19. Pickhardt PJ, Kim DH, Meiners RJ, et al. Colorectal and extracolonic cancers detected at screening CT colonography in 10,286 asymptomatic adults. Radiology. 2010;255:83–8.
20. American College of Radiology. National Radiology Data Registry for CT Colonography. https://nrdr.acr.org/Portal/CTC/Main/page.aspx

4

Urogenital Pathologies in Children Revisited

Jeanne S. Chow and Annemieke S. Littooij

Learning Objectives

- To describe the normal findings of the pediatric urogenital tract
- To list the potential causes of urinary tract dilatation
- To discuss the subtypes of congenital female tract anomalies

Part I

Urinary Tract by Ultrasound: The BUK Approach

A systematic approach to the urinary tract by ultrasound: the BUK approach.

Introduction

In the past, most imaging evaluations of the infant or child with signs or symptoms of a urinary tract abnormality began with a plain X-ray of the abdomen, a so-called KUB, with the letters standing for, from "top to bottom," kidneys, ureters, and bladder. Today, however, imaging usually begins with an ultrasound of the fetus, and the standard approach is to survey the urinary tract of the infant and child from the "bottom to top" that is, to begin with the bladder and then to look at the ureters and finally the kidneys, in other words, a BUK instead of a KUB approach.

J. S. Chow (✉)
Department of Radiology, Boston Children's Hospital, Boston, MA, USA
e-mail: jeanne.chow@childrens.harvard.edu

A. S. Littooij
Department of Radiology, University Medical Center Utrecht, Utrecht, The Netherlands

Bladder

The bladder is a urine-filled structure in the fetal pelvis seen as early as 8 weeks gestation by transvaginal ultrasound. Usually two (occasionally one) umbilical arteries encircle the normal bladder and provide a landmark for finding the bladder. The bladder fills and empties periodically as the fetus voids, so an "absent" bladder may actually be an empty bladder which becomes "present" as it refills.

After birth, the normal urinary bladder appears as an anechoic urine-filled structure surrounded by a thin wall. The layers of the wall include the echogenic outer serosa, the central hypoechoic muscularis, and the inner echogenic mucosa. Wall thickness depends on the degree of distension. During and at the end of voiding, a normal bladder wall can appear thick and irregular. The bladder is pliable and thus the shape depends on adjacent structures. Whereas a full bladder is spherical, a partially full bladder can assume many shapes and tends to be trapezoidal in the transverse plane. It is centered posterior to the rectus abdominis muscles and its midline linea alba. The rectum is posterior to the bladder in boys and girls with the vagina/uterus interposed between the rectum and bladder in girls. The bladder is often imaged first in infants because that is the most likely time to see a full bladder, before excitement or irritation leads to urination (Fig.).

Radiologists often assume that the bladder is normal or that the fluid-filled structure in the pelvis is automatically the bladder. This leads to mistakes. For example, bladder exstrophy, a rare condition in which the bladder forms as a plate on the anterior pelvic wall, is diagnosed by noticing the absence of a normal bladder on fetal ultrasound. However, 50% of children born with bladder exstrophy are diagnosed postnatally because people fail to check if a normal bladder is present.

Other fluid-filled structures in the pelvis can be mistaken for the bladder. These include large ureteroceles, ovarian cysts or masses, and the dilated (obstructed) vagina.

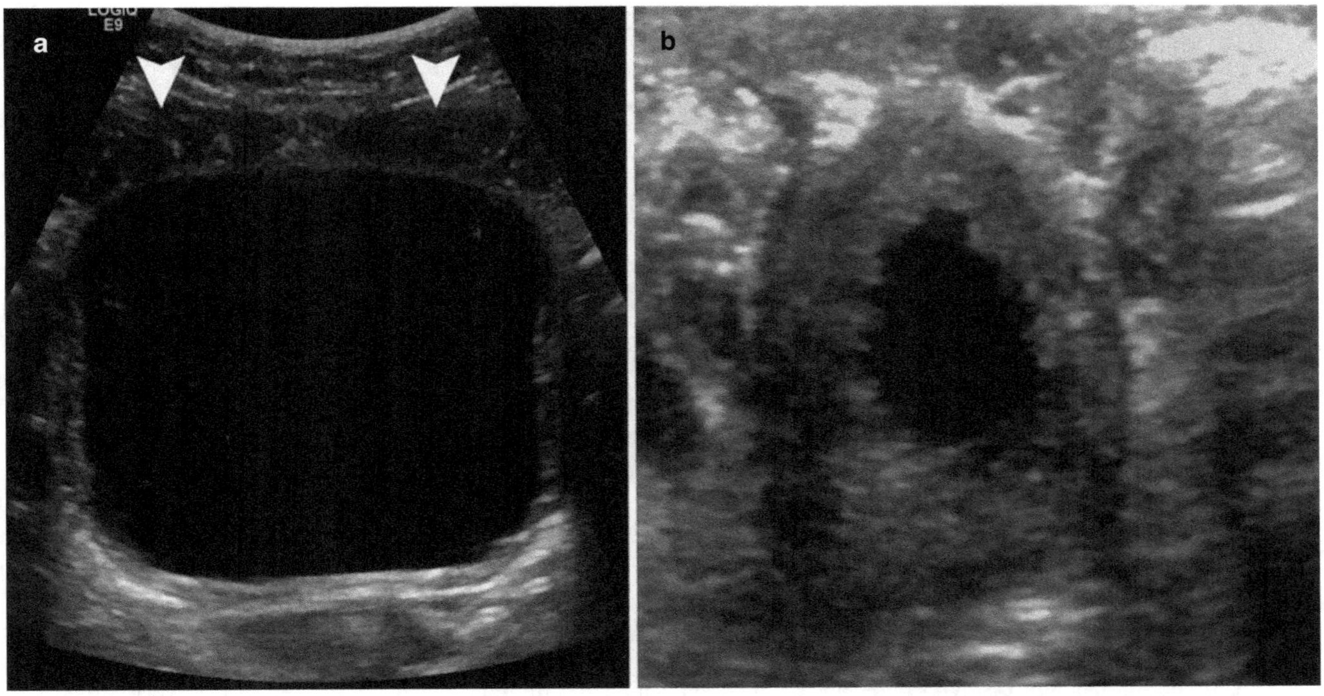

Fig. (**a**, **b**) Two transverse images of the bladder demonstrate (**a**) a full urinary bladder. Note the square or trapezoidal configuration. The rectus abdominis muscles (arrowheads) are anterior to the bladder wall. During or just after micturition (**b**), the wall can appear thick and irregular

Ureters

The ureters start at the renal pelvis, course down on the psoas muscles, cross the internal iliac vessels, and then enter the bladder posterolaterally. The fetal ureters are typically invisible unless they are dilated. The more dilated the ureter, the more tortuous it becomes because dilation increases width and also length. Extremely dilated ureters can be mistaken for dilated loops of bowel (Fig.).

In children, dilated ureters are often first noticed as tubular anechoic structures located posterolaterally while imaging the bladder. Peristalsing boluses of urine or "ureteral jets" are seen entering the bladder by color Doppler. There are no established values for normal or abnormal ureteral widths by ultrasound. However, a normal ureter in a child is 3–4 mm in diameter. Normal fluid-filled ureters can be seen peristalsing. Visualizing the ureter does not mean that it is abnormal.

Ureteral dilation is due to vesicoureteral reflux (VUR), obstruction, or both reflux and obstruction. Vesicoureteral reflux is the reverse flow of urine from the bladder to the kidney. Reflux of infected urine leads to pyelonephritis. Dilated ureters continue to peristalse and the changing diameter is commonly seen by ultrasound. The most common test to distinguish obstruction from reflux is a voiding cystourethrogram (VCUG), also called a micturating cystourethrogram (MCUG). If the VCUG shows reflux, the dilatation of the ureters and kidneys is due to reflux. If the refluxed material does not drain well at the end of the test, then either reflux coexists with obstruction. Drainage films are important to make this distinction [1]. If there is no reflux, then the dilation is due to obstruction.

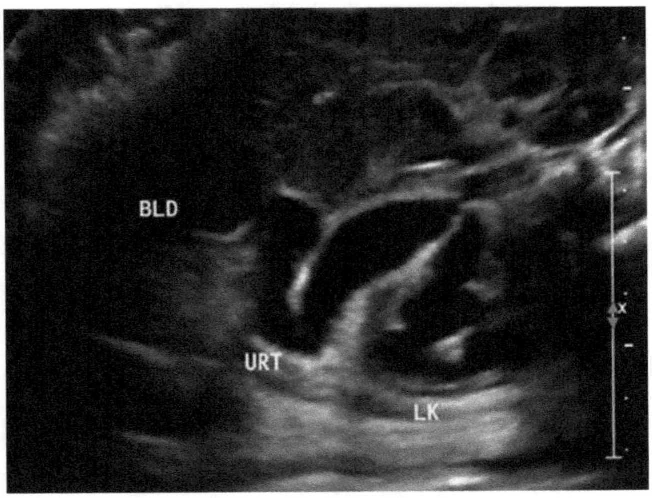

Fig. A dilated fetal ureter can be confused with dilated bowel. However, the ureter (URT) connects the bladder (BLD) to the kidney (LK). Normally, a fetal ureter is not visualized. In infants and children, a normal peristalsing ureter can be visualized and not necessarily abnormal

The most common congenital cause of ureteral obstruction is primary megaureter. This is due to a functional obstruction at the orthotopic ureterovesical junction. Seventy percent of patients with primary megaureter improve with time. The width of the diameter of the ureter can help to predict resolution [2]. Obstructed ureters may also be ectopic, as what occurs with the upper pole of a duplex kidney or, more rarely, a single ectopic ureter.

When the reflux is severe, the megacystis-megaureter association may lead to enlargement of the bladder (megacystis) and dilation of the ureter or ureters (megaureter) [3]. The bladder enlarges because there is recycling of urine so that the bladder never fully empties and is constantly refilling with refluxed urine from the ureters, and it eventually dilates. Severe megacystis-megaureter can lead to urinary retention.

Kidneys

Kidneys normally migrate from the fetal pelvis to the normal renal fossae at 4–6 weeks gestation. The renal fossae are paraspinous, centered at the lumbar vertebral level of L1–L2. Kidneys are first seen in utero at 10 weeks gestation. Nearby landmarks include the echogenic spine, and the suprarenal hypoechoic boomerang-shaped adrenal glands, and the liver and spleen. The adrenal cortex is hypoechoic and the medulla echogenic. The normal suprarenal or adrenal gland can be up to one-third the size of the kidney in the second trimester.

When the kidney does not migrate to the normal location, it is ectopic. Since kidneys normally ascend from the fetal pelvis to the renal fossae, ectopic kidneys are typically somewhere in-between. Occasionally, when the liver or diaphragm has not formed normally, ectopic kidneys may be present in the chest. Kidneys may also fuse while ascending, forming cross-fused ectopic kidneys, horseshoe kidneys, or lump kidneys.

When a kidney is absent from the renal fossa in utero, 50% are ectopic and 50% are absent [4]. When there is a solitary kidney, 23% are associated with other congenital anomalies, including those in the VACTERL association. Thirty percent of these patients have vesicoureteral reflux (personal unpublished data).

The normal echogenicity of a kidney in an infant or child is more variable than in an adult. In adults, normal kidneys are hypoechoic compared to the liver. In infants and children, normal kidneys may be relatively isoechoic or hypoechoic. In newborns and premature infants, relatively echogenic kidneys may still be normal. In addition, kidneys are separated into lobes, with a central hypoechoic medulla and a peripheral relatively hypoechoic cortex. The adjacent lobes create an undulating cortex which is described as normal fetal lobation. The normal indentations between renal lobes are distinguished from scarring as the indentation is between the pyramids, versus centered at the tip of the pyramids in scarring. The hypoechoic pyramids become isoechoic to adjacent renal parenchyma over time and are occasionally confused for masses or cysts (Fig.).

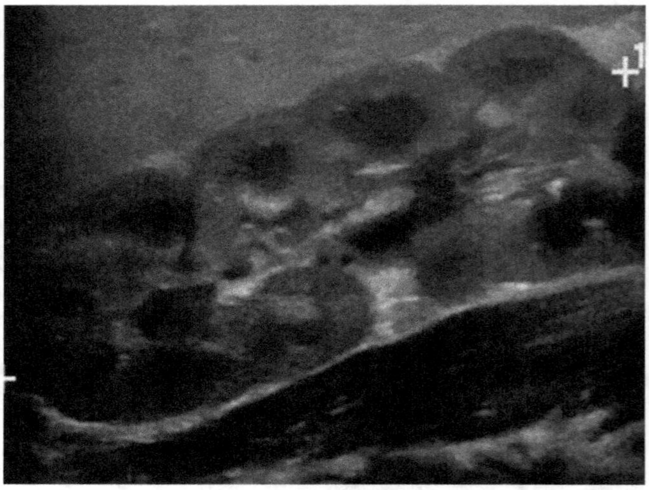

Fig. The typical characteristics of a kidney in an infant are hypoechoic medullary pyramids and fetal lobulation which gives a lobular contour to the kidneys

Compared to adults, renal masses are relatively uncommon in children. Renal tumors tend to be very large. The most common solid tumor in an infant is a mesoblastic nephroma. Despite their large size, they tend to be benign. The most common childhood renal tumor is Wilms' tumor. In the past three decades, the survival rate of children with these tumors approaches 90% [5]. Simple cysts are relatively uncommon compared to adults. If more than one simple cyst is identified, cystic renal disease should be considered, including autosomal dominant polycystic disease. Cystic tumors, including cystic nephroma or focal cystic dysplasia, are uncommon. When the whole kidney develops as abnormal, cysts with no normal renal parenchyma, a multicystic dysplastic kidney is formed.

The collecting tubules in the medullary pyramids drain into the minor calyces which drain into the major calyces and into the renal pelvis. When there is urinary tract dilation, there is progressive dilation of the pelvis and calyces. This is described by many terms, including pyelectasis in utero and hydronephrosis in fetuses and children.

There are many ways of describing the dilated urinary tract. The only system which unifies prenatal and postnatal imaging into one system is the Urinary Tract Dilation System (UTD) which was created by radiologists, urologists, and nephrologists. The six common descriptions are (1) anterior posterior renal pelvic diameter, (2) calyceal dilation, (3) ureteral dilation, (4) renal parenchymal thickness, (5) renal parenchymal echogenicity, and (6) bladder appearance. In fetuses, oligohydramnios which may be due to urinary tract abnormalities is also described [6–8].

Prenatal urinary tract dilation or hydronephrosis is common, present in 1–4% of pregnancies. Most prenatal hydronephrosis is mild and resolves [9, 10]. The most common pathology to cause pelvic and calyceal dilation without ureteral dilation is ureteropelvic junction obstruction. This is due to an intrinsic obstruction at the ureteropelvic junction or occasionally is due to a crossing anomalous renal vessel. The vessel causes obstruction when there is increased urine production and the vessel kinks the ureteropelvic junction. These obstructions, unlike intrinsic ureteropelvic junction obstructions, are intermittent and cause pain only during obstruction.

The greater the degree of prenatal or postnatal hydronephrosis, the greater the likelihood of ureteropelvic junction obstruction. The likelihood of vesicoureteral reflux is the same regardless of the degree of dilation [11]. MAG-3 and MRU examinations are both useful for quantifying the degree of obstruction and relative renal function [12].

There are certain entities that tend to affect the entire urinary tract: the bladder, ureters, and kidneys. The three most common entities are duplex kidneys with complete ureteral duplication, posterior urethral valves, and prune belly syndrome.

When there is complete ureteral duplication, the upper pole ureteral orifice is ectopic (the Weigert-Meyer rule). The ectopic upper pole ureter terminates anywhere from the trigone of the bladder, inferiorly and medially to the base of the bladder (the so-called ectopic pathway). In boys, ectopic ureters terminate above the urethral sphincter in the proximal urethra and Wolffian duct remnants including the ejaculatory ducts, vasa, and seminal vesicles. In females, ectopic ureters can extend below the urethral sphincter or into the vagina and can cause daytime and nighttime wetting. When the ectopic ureter is obstructed or ends in a ureterocele, it dilates. A ureterocele is cystic dilation of the intramural portion of the ureter, which appears as a thin-walled cyst in the bladder and is continuous with the ureter. The more ectopic the ureter, the more dysplastic the associated upper pole parenchyma. The lower pole is the analog of the single system ureter. There may be coexisting lower pole reflux or ureteropelvic junction obstruction.

Posterior urethral valves are thin leaflets which cause obstruction in the posterior urethra, at the base of the verumontanum, in boys. The valves cause a variable degree of bladder outlet obstruction, bladder wall thickening, and variable hydroureteronephrosis. Often the degree of left and right urinary tract dilation is asymmetric. The hydroureteronephrosis may be due to reflux, obstruction, or both. VCUG/MCUG diagnoses both the posterior urethral valves and reflux. Although this diagnosis can be suspected in utero, milder cases present in childhood with infection or milder hydroureteronephrosis. In severe cases, the kidneys may be dysplastic and high pressures may lead to forniceal rupture, urinomas, and urine ascites (Fig.).

Prune belly syndrome can mimic posterior urethral valves. The triad of cryptorchism, dysplastic kidneys, and severe reflux can appear radiographically similar to posterior urethral valves. The bladder is dilated but thinner than in boys with valves, the ureters are severely dilated, and the kidneys are dysplastic. However, children with prune belly syndrome have lax anterior abdominal wall musculature and no posterior urethral valves despite a dilated posterior urethra. The anterior urethra may also be dilated, the so-called megalourethra.

Summary

If one systematically looks at the bladder, ureters, and kidneys (BUK), the urinary tract will be evaluated completely. The most common mistake is that people assume that the bladder is normal. Ureteral dilation should be evaluated carefully, as dilation distinguishes hydronephrosis (typically due to ureteropelvic junction obstruction) from hydroureteronephrosis (typically caused by primary megaureter or reflux). An MCUG/VCUG distinguishes reflux from obstruction. When evaluating the kidney, carefully assess its

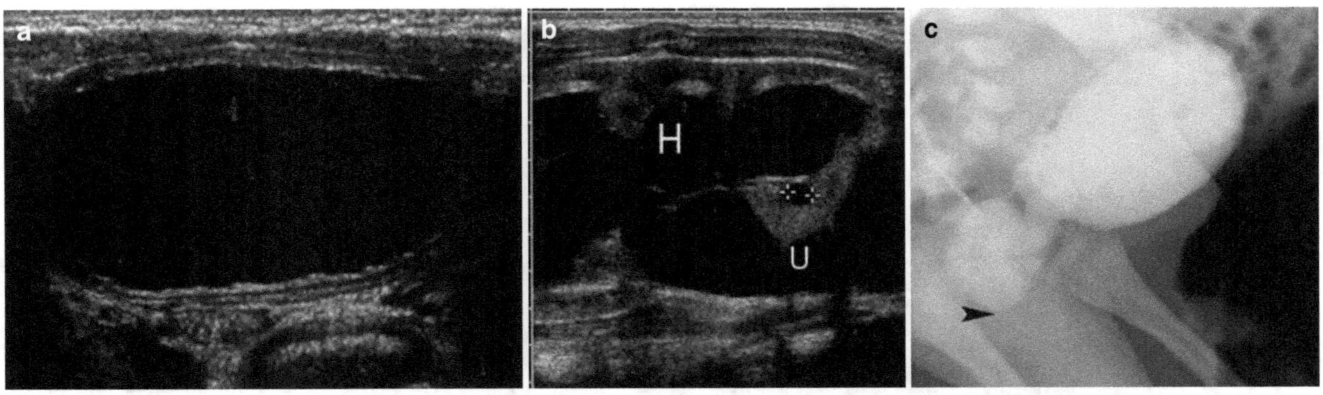

Fig. (**a–c**) Posterior urethral valves, depending on severity, can affect the appearance of the bladder, ureters, and kidney. In this example of severe posterior urethral valves, (**a**) the bladder wall is thick and irregular; (**b**) there is severe hydronephrosis (H) characterized by pelvic and peripheral calyceal dilation, thinning and cystic dysplasia of the renal parenchyma, and ureteral dilation (U); and (**c**) A VCUG demonstrates posterior urethral valves (arrowhead) with severe dilation of the posterior urethra presence, echogenicity, and for the presence and degree of urinary tract dilation. The common entities which affect the bladder, kidney, and ureters are duplex kidneys with complete ureteral duplication, posterior urethral valves, and prune belly syndrome.

Part II

FemaleGenital Tract

Ultrasound is the most important imaging technique in childhood pelvic imaging. MRI is only used in complex cases.

NormalDevelopment

The paramesonephric (Müllerian) ducts are paired structures that undergo fusion and resorption that form the uterus, proximal fallopian tubes, and upper vagina. The distal segments of the Müllerian ducts fuse in the midline forming the uterovaginal canal. The development of the uterus is complete by 12 weeks' gestation. Interruption of normal fusion and resorption of the Müllerian ducts give rise to a broad spectrum of Müllerian duct anomalies. Lower part of the vagina and ovaries arises from the urogenital sinus and the primitive yolk sac, respectively [13].

Uterus

In the newborn girl, the female internal genitalia are prominent due to the maternal and placental hormone exposure in utero. The endometrium is normally clearly seen as an echogenic stripe at the center of the uterus. After 2–3 months until puberty, the uterus is relatively small and tubular in configuration (2–4 cm) with the cervix being as large and as thick as the fundus (<1 cm). The endometrium lining is relatively inconspicuous. During puberty the fundus of the uterus enlarges and becomes bulbous in contour. The postpubertal uterus is around 5–8 cm in length and has a pear-shaped appearance. The endometrial lining undergoes cyclic changes associated with the menstrual cycle [14] (Fig.).

CongenitalAbnormalities

Female genital tract anomalies may result from agenesis, hypoplasia, or abnormalities related to disorders in lateral fusion, vertical fusion, or resorption. Congenital Müllerian anomalies occur in around 1.5% of females and are strongly associated with renal anomalies (in 30–50%) [15]; however congenital Müllerian anomalies are not associated with ovarian anomalies.

Ultrasound examination of the uterus should be performed in all female neonates with MCDK, unilateral renal dysplasia, single kidney, or adrenal hyperplasia due to the high risk of associated female tract anomalies.

Additional MRI can be valuable as MRI provides great anatomical detail of both the endometrium and outer contour of the uterus [14].

Imperforate hymen is the most common obstructive anomaly of the female pelvis [16]. Usually there are no other associated abnormalities. Ultrasound shows fluid distention of the vagina with a lesser degree of cervical/uterine distention. Echogenic debris within the fluid is due to mucous secretions in neonates and blood in postmenarcheal girls. This fluid-debris level helps to distinguish a dilated vagina from the bladder or other cystic pelvic masses.

Partial or complete failure of resorption of the septum between the two Müllerian ducts results in a septate uterus. The external surface has a normal configuration and there are two endometrial cavities. The septum is complete if it extends to the cervical os. There is a single cervix.

Bicornuate uterus results from partial non-fusion of the Müllerian ducts. The external surface is deeply indented. A common challenge is to differentiate between a bicornuate uterus and a septate uterus. This distinction is clinically important because the septate uterus carries a high risk of miscarriage. The absence of the indentation of the external contour (<1 cm cleft) with the presence of duplicated endometrial cavity is the key feature to diagnose a septate uterus rather than a bicornuate uterus [17].

Complete non-fusion leads to a didelphys uterus. Two cervices are inevitably present. Unicornuate uterus occurs when there is a complete or near-complete arrested

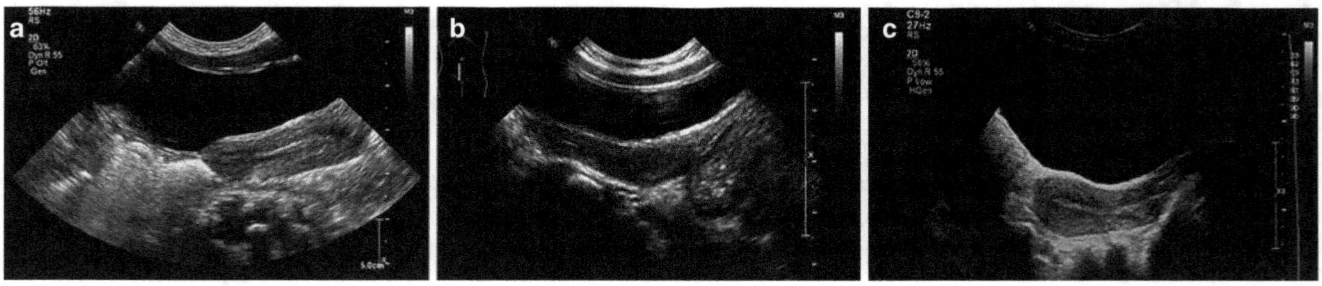

Fig. (**a**–**c**) Sagittal image of a neonate (**a**), 4-year-old (**b**) and 18-year-old (**c**) girl, illustrates the relative large uterus in the newborn, the more tubular appearance in a child and the pear-shape appearance in the adolescent girl

development of one of the Müllerian ducts resulting in a single-horned uterus with a single round ligament and fallopian tube [16]. Presence of endometrium in a rudimentary horn is a clinically important finding because there is an increased prevalence of endometriosis, pelvic pain and higher risk of problems during pregnancy (miscarriage, ectopic pregnancy, preterm labor, and uterine rupture).

Complete arrested development of both Müllerian ducts is also known as the Mayer-Rokitansky-Kuster-Hauser syndrome. In this syndrome there is a congenital absence of the proximal vagina, cervix, and uterus with normal external genitalia [17]. Primary amenorrhea is the most common clinical presentation.

Ovaries

Ovaries can be distinguished from other pelvic structures by identifying small follicle cysts within the ovaries that can be seen from birth. The size of the follicles decreases during a hormonally quiescent period. The conspicuity and number of follicle cysts increases after adrenarche (around 10–11 years of age) and puberty [18].

Ovarian Cysts and Other Lesions

In the fetus and in the neonatal period, large ovarian cysts are occasionally detected due to maternal and placental hormone exposure. Most neonatal cysts are asymptomatic and resolve within the first year of life. Complications from larger ovarian cysts include torsion, bleeding, and strangulation in an inguinal hernia [14].

Ovarian Torsion

Torsion is caused by partial or complete rotation of the ovary and/or fallopian tube around the infundibulopelvic ligament. In the neonate ovarian torsion occurs due to a cyst. During childhood torsion is most often caused by an ovarian mass (cystic teratoma). The sonographic features of ovarian torsion include enlarged ovary with peripherally located follicles. Often the ovary is located in the midline of the lower abdomen with the uterus deviated toward the affected side. Sometimes the whirlpool sign of twisted vascular pedicle can be seen. Doppler findings can be widely variable related to the dual blood supply of the ovaries (uterine and ovary artery) [14].

OvarianNeoplasm

Ovarian neoplasms are extremely rare in the neonate and infant. The most common benign ovarian tumor in childhood is a cystic teratoma, accounting more than 90% of all benign ovarian tumors. Most cystic teratomas have a complex appearance on sonographic imaging that depends on the relative amount of fat, calcium, serous fluid, and hair within the lesion [19].

Part III

MaleGenital Tract

NormalDevelopment

The descent of the testis occurs at two stages. The intra-abdominal descent takes place at 10–15 weeks' and the inguinoscrotal descent occurs at 26–40 weeks' gestation [13]. At ultrasound, the testis is a homogenous bean-shaped structure, which has an echogenic mediastinum as one of its landmarks. Blood flow is normally homogeneous.

CongenitalAbnormalities

Ultrasound is often used to identify the location of the undescended testis (also called cryptorchidism) with variable success. Some people advocate the use of MRI. However, the appearance of a smaller, ectopic testis is often similar to lymph node with either ultrasound or MRI. The echogenic mediastinum and the homogeneous blood flow can be useful ultrasound characteristics to distinguish the testis from an inguinal node.

Testicular Torsion

Testicular torsion can occur in newborns and infants. They will present with an enlarged, discolored scrotum. The testis is often unsalvageable because the torsion is discovered too late. Extravaginal torsions are more common in infancy, compared to intravaginal torsions, which occurs during puberty.

Ultrasound findings of testicular torsion are complete absence of blood flow in the testis in comparison to the other side. With prolonged torsion the affected testis becomes hypoechoic. Most often the testis lies more cranially within the scrotal sac and the twisted spermatic cord can be seen. The most important part of the examination is to compare the findings with the normal side (Fig.) [20].

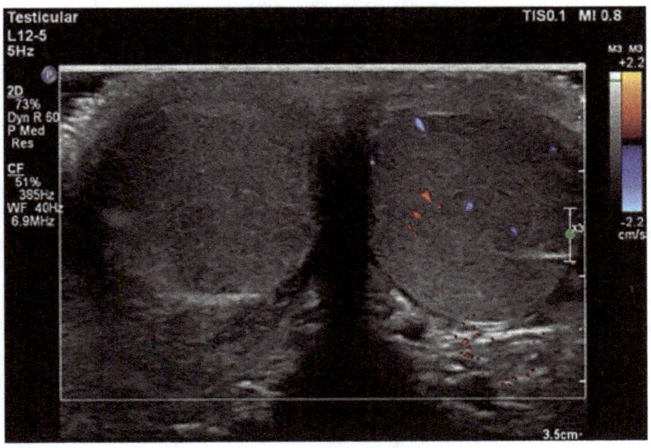

Fig. Sagittal ultrasound image shows an inguinal hernia in a female infant that contains uterus and both ovaries

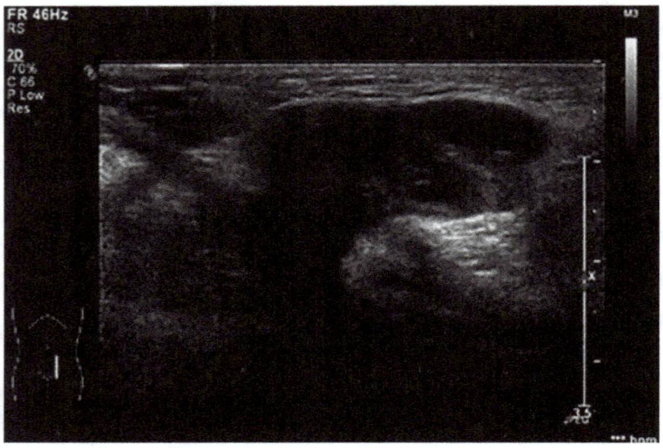

Fig. Transverse image of both testes in a 14-year-old boy shows absent vascularity of the right testis consistent with torsion. Comparison with the normal side is an important part of the ultrasound study

Inguinal Hernia

Indirect, sliding hernia inguinalis is an uncommon finding in male and female neonates, especially in premature infants (up to 30%) due to a patent processus vaginalis (Fig.). The bowel, ovaries, and fallopian tubes are the organs that are most commonly incarcerated. Ultrasound is an accurate method to determine the content of inguinal hernia. Peristalsis with the herniated bowel loops suggests viability.

Key Points

- Ultrasound is an essential tool in the evaluation of the urogenital tract in infants and children.
- Look systematically at the bladder, ureters, and kidneys to evaluate congenital urinary tract anomalies.
- The finding of dilated ureter distinguishes UPJ obstruction from reflux/primary megaureter.
- In the newborn girl, the female internal genitalia are prominent due to the maternal and placental hormone exposure in utero.
- Female genital tract anomalies are strongly associated with renal anomalies.
- Indirect, sliding hernia inguinalis is a common finding in male and female neonates, especially in premature infants (up to 30%) due to a patent processus vaginalis.

References

1. Lebowitz RL. The coexistence of obstruction and reflux in children. Australas Radiol. 1984;28:124–5.
2. McLellan DL, Retik AB, Bauer SB, et al. Rate and predictors of spontaneous resolution of prenatally diagnosed primary nonrefluxing megaureter. J Urol. 2002;168:2177–80; discussion 2180
3. Mandell J, Lebowitz RL, Peters CA, et al. Prenatal diagnosis of the megacystis-megaureter association. J Urol. 1992;148:1487–9.
4. Chow JS, Benson CB, Lebowitz RL. The clinical significance of an empty renal fossa on prenatal sonography. J Ultrasound Med. 2005;24:1049–54; quiz 1055-1047
5. Smets AM, de Kraker J. Malignant tumours of the kidney: imaging strategy. Pediatr Radiol. 2010;40:1010–8.
6. Nguyen HT, Benson CB, Bromley B, et al. Multidisciplinary consensus on the classification of prenatal and postnatal urinary tract dilation (UTD classification system). J Pediatr Urol. 2014;10:982–98.
7. Chow JS, Darge K. Multidisciplinary consensus on the classification of antenatal and postnatal urinary tract dilation (UTD classification system). Pediatr Radiol. 2015;45:787–9.
8. Chow JS, Koning JL, Back SJ, et al. Classification of pediatric urinary tract dilation: the new language. Pediatr Radiol. 2017;47:1109–15.
9. Tombesi MM, Alconcher LF. Short-term outcome of mild isolated antenatal hydronephrosis conservatively managed. J Pediatr Urol. 2012;8:129–33.
10. Alconcher LF, Tombesi MM. Natural history of bilateral mild isolated antenatal hydronephrosis conservatively managed. Pediatr Nephrol. 2012;27:1119–23.
11. Lee RS, Cendron M, Kinnamon DD, et al. Antenatal hydronephrosis as a predictor of postnatal outcome: a meta-analysis. Pediatrics. 2006;118:586–93.
12. Dickerson EC, Dillman JR, Smith EA, et al. Pediatric MR urography: indications, techniques, and approach to review. Radiographics. 2015;35:1208–30.
13. Servaes S, Epelman M. The current state of imaging pediatric genitourinary anomalies and abnormalities. Curr Probl Diagn Radiol. 2013;42:1–12.
14. Muller LS. Ultrasound of the paediatric urogenital tract. Eur J Radiol. 2014;83:1538–48.
15. Chan YY, Jayaprakasan K, Zamora J, et al. The prevalence of congenital uterine anomalies in unselected and high-risk populations: a systematic review. Hum Reprod Update. 2011;17:761–71.
16. Paltiel HJ, Phelps A. US of the pediatric female pelvis. Radiology. 2014;270:644–57.
17. Behr SC, Courtier JL, Qayyum A. Imaging of mullerian duct anomalies. Radiographics. 2012;32:E233–50.
18. Herter LD, Golendziner E, Flores JA, et al. Ovarian and uterine sonography in healthy girls between 1 and 13 years old: correlation of findings with age and pubertal status. AJR Am J Roentgenol. 2002;178:1531–6.
19. Epelman M, Chikwava KR, Chauvin N, et al. Imaging of pediatric ovarian neoplasms. Pediatr Radiol. 2011;41:1085–99.
20. Munden MM, Trautwein LM. Scrotal pathology in pediatrics with sonographic imaging. Curr Probl Diagn Radiol. 2000;29:185–205.

5

Diagnostic Imaging of Urinary Obstruction, Stone Disease and Infection

S. O. Schönberg, J. Budjan, and D. Hausmann

Learning Objectives

- To understand indications for imaging and choice of cross-sectional imaging method depending on pathology
- To identify "high-risk" patients to develop severe and/or chronic urogenital inflammations
- To learn about sequence composition of a "standard" MRI protocol and additional potentially useful functional sequences
- To see the MRI appearance of various acute and chronic inflammatory urogenital pathologies
- To think of the differential diagnosis (e.g., lymphoma or posttransplant lymphoproliferative disorder)

Background

Uncomplicated Versus ComplicatedUrinary Tract Infection

Acute infection is mostly diagnosed based on clinical presentation and laboratory tests without imaging examinations [1]. Urinary tract infections are regarded as uncomplicated in otherwise healthy patients without structural or functional urinary abnormalities. Complicated urinary tract infections are accompanied by factors that potentially decrease therapy effectiveness, such as immunocompromission, unusually virulent pathogen, and patient-related factors (Table). Imaging of uncomplicated cystitis or pyelonephritis is regarded as unnecessary by most authors. In contrary, patients who suffer from complicated urinary tract infections may benefit from imaging [1, 2].

S. O. Schönberg, M.D., Ph.D. (✉) · J. Budjan, M.D.
Medical Faculty Mannheim, Heidelberg University, Mannheim, Germany
e-mail: stefan.schoenberg@umm.de

D. Hausmann, M.D.
Institute of Radiology, Kantonsspital Baden AG, Switzerland

Imaging

MRI plays an increasingly important role in the diagnostic work-up of urological patients as an alternative or complementary imaging of CT. However, on the one hand, the availability of MRI scanners is lower than that of CT scanners, and on the other hand, the cost of an MRI is significantly higher than that of a CT scan. In emergency situations, such as trauma, acute bleeding, or renal colic with suspected underlying urolithiasis, CT is the imaging modality of choice.

MRI examinations usually require more patient cooperation than CT examinations. Non-compliance can significantly affect the image quality and thus the diagnostic confidence.

Moreover, in the first trimester of pregnancy, MRI should only be performed when absolutely necessary and at low-field strengths only (1.5 T or less). Certain questions can only be answered to a limited extent, as contrast agents are contraindicated during pregnancy.

The narrowing of the MRI tube may lead to additional problems in emergency situations, on the one hand, caused by claustrophobia (if necessary, a premedication with an anxiolytic drug may be considered) and, on the other hand, by obesity.

Despite these limitations, owing to the superior soft tissue contrast, MRI can provide useful information as a supplementary modality in the assessment of inflammatory urinary tract diseases.

Table Complicated urinary tract infection (Patient-related factors)

Complicated urinary tract infection (Patient-related factors)
• Delayed therapy
• Male
• Childhood urinary tract infections
• Immunocompromised (e.g., HIV)
• Leukemia
• Pregnant
• Elderly patients
• Diabetes
• Failed antibiotic treatment
• Prolonged symptoms

MRI

Standard Protocol

In clinical routine, there is currently no "universal protocol" as the sequences or the image contrasts can differ between MRI scanners (especially depending on field strength and manufacturers). The examination of the kidneys is performed as a standard procedure in supine position using body coils, which are placed directly on the abdomen.

A typical protocol for the evaluation of structural and inflammatory kidney disease consists of morphological sequences such as T2-weighted sequences with or without fat saturation in different plane orientations and non-contrast-enhanced T1-weighted sequences with or without fat saturation. In this context, most readers prefer the axial and coronal plane directions for the evaluation of the urinary tract. In addition, normally in-phase and opposed-phase sequences ("chemical-shift imaging") are obtained to detect intracellular fat proportions. Increasingly, this "standard imaging" is flanked by functional techniques, which generate information beyond pure morphology (e.g., dynamic contrast-enhanced imaging (DCE) or diffusion-weighted imaging (DWI)).

For most MRI examinations, intravenous contrast medium is injected. After contrast, dynamic axial fat-saturated T1-weighted sequences are acquired in arterial, venous, and later contrast agent phases. In addition to the axial plane direction, a coronal T1-weighted fat-saturated sequence is recommended. If, moreover, inflammatory disease in the course of the ureters is suspected, additional late phases are advisable. These urographic phases are acquired between 10 and 20 min after contrast medium injection. In order to optimize the urographic images, an additional administration of a diuretic or an i.v. water bolus and a parasympatheticolytic may be useful.

Additional Protocols

Stone Disease

Concrements have no intrinsic MRT signal and consequently appear hypointense on T1- and T2-weighted images. In addition to T2-weighted sequences, late urographic phases can be used for the detection of concrements in the urinary tract. In the latter, stones may be detected indirectly as a filling defect in the course of the ureter.

Diffusion-Weighted Imaging (DWI)

In principle, DWI is a technique which enables the visualization of diffusion properties (= uniform distribution of particles) of water molecules in vivo. The average spatial mobility of a water molecule per time unit is measured in a defined volume. Water diffusion is based on the Brownian molecular motion (= temperature-induced movement of particles in liquids) and can be quantified by measuring the "apparent diffusion coefficient (ADC)." A decrease in the space between individual cells in tissue, e.g., due to cell swelling, leads to reduced mobility of the free water. DWI allows indirect estimations of the cell density; this can be used to differentiate pathologies with increased cell density (e.g., tumors or abscesses). "Zoomed" single-shot echo-planar imaging (EPI)-DWI performed with a small FOV in the phase-encoding direction by employment of two independent radiofrequency transmit channels ("parallel transmit") to generate spatially tailored 2D parallel radiofrequency (RF). RF excitation pulses have been proven useful to increase image quality at 3 T. In clinical practice, DWI should now become an integral part of the standard MRI protocol renal zoomed EPI-DWI with spatially selective radiofrequency excitation pulses in two dimensions [3].

Advanced T1-Weighted Contrast-Enhanced Sequences

Isotropic, highly accelerated (e.g., by "compressed-sensing"), dynamic ("4D") post-contrast T1-weighted sequences with a temporal resolution below 10 s may be employed to generate perfusion maps in a "one-stop-shop" approach for the quantitative analysis of various perfusion parameters (e.g., to assess renal function or scarring) aside from high-resolution morphologic images. In this context, radial T1-weighted sequences are particularly useful in patients with impaired breath-hold capabilities as they help to reduce motion-induced artifacts. Sequences that combine speed and radial acquisition will soon be commercially available. To date, the clinical value of these sequences to assess renal inflammatory disease has not been assessed, and limitations include time-consuming image reconstructions that need to be carried out on an external server [4].

Blood Oxygenation Level-Dependent (BOLD) Imaging

BOLD imaging is a noninvasive procedure that allows a relative assessment of the oxygen partial pressure in tissue. The signal of BOLD imaging is based on the different magnetic properties of oxyhemoglobin and deoxyhemoglobin and thus allows an indirect estimation of the relative local oxygen concentration. This technique is currently subject of research and has not yet established itself in clinical routine [5, 6].

Sodium

In the future, completely new technical approaches could also play an increasing role. In studies, the extent to which sodium imaging is suitable for detecting and differentiating kidney pathologies is investigated. Sodium MRI uses the protons of sodium-23 for imaging instead of the hydrogen proton (H-1) used in the conventional MRI. Sodium nuclei occur much less frequently than H-1 nuclei in the human body. At the same time, they exhibit less favorable physical properties for MR imaging, which makes this process technically very demanding (e.g., the use of own coils and optimized sequences). The technique may also enable to assess kidney function (e.g., posttherapeutic after radiation therapy of retroperitoneal sarcomas). This method has not yet entered clinical routine [7, 8].

Acute and Chronic Inflammatory Renal Diseases

Spectrum of Kidney Infections

Renal inflammations range from acute to chronic and mild to severe.

Acute pyelonephritis can be diffuse or focal and may resolve or exacerbate to abscess-forming pyelonephritis. Immunocompromission might predispose patients to more severe or even life-threatening clinical courses like emphysematous pyelonephritis. Renal infections can develop into a permanently damaging chronic pyelonephritis or xanthogranulomatous pyelonephritis [1]. Prolonged untreated tuberculosis may lead to scarring, fibrosis, and stricture of the urinary collective system. Immunocompromised patients are particularly prone to fungal infections (mostly *Candida* and *Aspergillus*). Some rare infections include malakoplakia and eosinophilic cystitis (Table).

Table Spectrum of kidney infections

Acute	Chronic	Others
Acute pyelonephritis Focal nephritis Abscess Emphysematous pyelonephritis Papillary necrosis Pyonephrosis	Chronic pyelonephritis Xanthogranulomatous pyelonephritis Malakoplakia Eosinophilic cystitis	Tuberculosis Fungal

Pyelonephritis

Acute pyelonephritis is the most frequent inflammatory change in the kidneys and is usually caused by gram-negative bacteria. The incidence of acute pyelonephritis parallels that of lower urinary tract infections. It occurs around five times more often in females with a steep increase after puberty. The parenchyma often enhances inhomogeneously, especially in the nephrographic contrast medium phase, with wedge-shaped zones of lower contrast as an indication of an inflammatory process. Unfortunately, a "striated nephrogram" is unspecific and can also be present in other conditions like contusion as well as obstruction or renal vein thrombosis. Diffuse acute pyelonephritis can lead to renal enlargement and poor enhancement of the parenchyma, absence or reduced excretion of contrast, and fat imbibition in fat-saturated T2-weighted sequences as a sign of inflammation.

MRI is superior to CT in the detection of nephritic components since the inflammatory changes in the (high) b values can present as signal elevations by means of DWI or as corresponding reductions of the ADC [9]. Furthermore, pus can be detected in the kidney globule system (the signal behavior is also signal elevation in b-value images and ADC reduction corresponding to dark areas on the ADC map), although differentiation from tumor or blood coagulation is often impossible (Fig.).

In the protracted course of pyelonephritis, the renal parenchyma may become scarred and lose function. Chronic pyelonephritis can also be triggered by urine infections in childhood, reflux, or frequent infections. MRI shows polar scars with underlying calyceal distortion and atrophy as well as hypertrophy of healthy parenchyma. Fetal lobulations can be discriminated by depressions located in between calyces rather than overlying calyces. Lobar infarctions are distinguished by absence of calyceal involvement [1].

Abscess

Abscesses of the kidneys usually develop in the context of pyelonephritis, when several small abscesses fuse. All ages can be affected, and there is no recognized gender predilec-

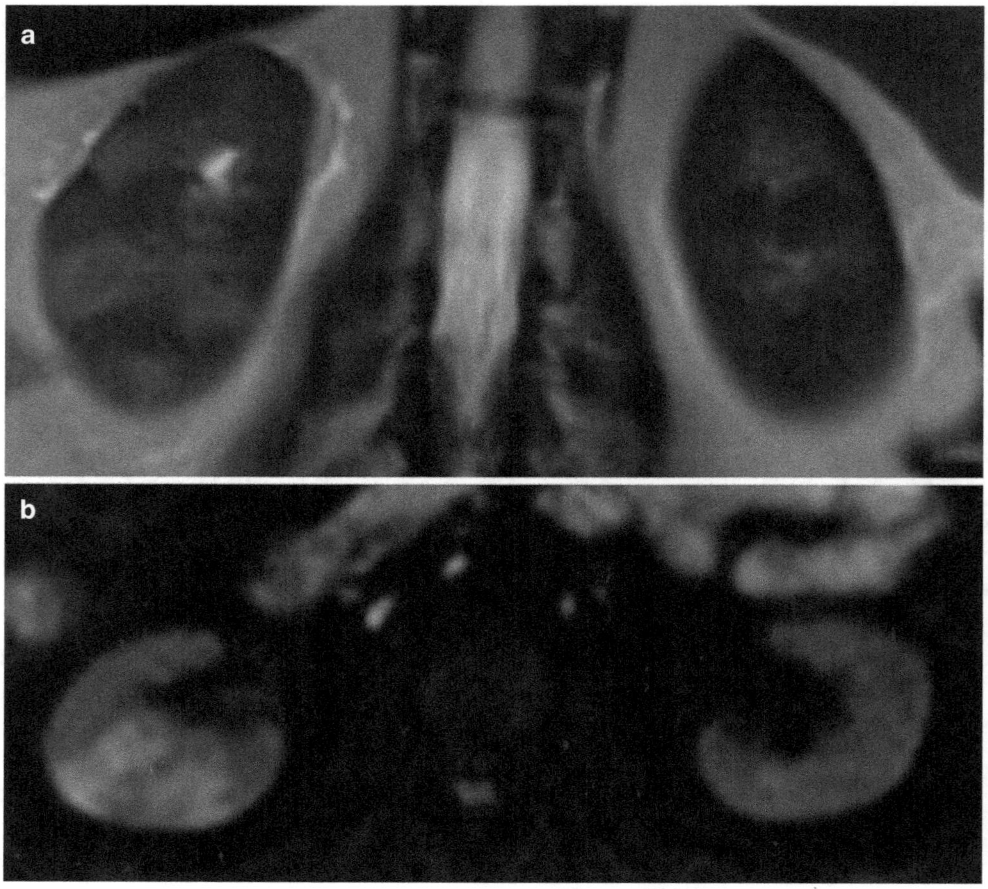

Fig. A 54-year-old female patient presenting with fever and abdominal pain. Coronal T2 haste (**a**) depicting wedge-shaped areas of increased signal intensity in the renal parenchyma and organ enlargement. Fluid imbibition of the surrounding fat tissue is also seen. High b-value DWI (**b**) shows corresponding signal elevations in the affected areas

tion. Predisposing factors are diabetes and vesicoureteral reflux. Peripheral rim enhancement is frequently seen in contrast-enhanced T1-weighted MRT sequences. Abscesses may also contain air inclusions, for the detection of which CT is significantly more sensitive than MRI; in the latter air can only be detected indirectly as areas of signal loss. However, MRI allows a reliable detection of kidney abscesses, especially through the implementation of DWI into clinical routine, and is the imaging method of choice in case of unclear findings. Differentiation from renal cell carcinoma or lymphoma can, however, be difficult in some cases. In particular, the patient's history as well as short-term follow-ups may help.

Pyonephrosis

Pyonephrosis is an infection of the kidney which leads to pus deposition in the upper collecting system which can progress to obstruction. The most likely cause is concrements, but tumors or fibrotic changes can also trigger pyonephrosis. A contrast medium level in urine above pus is indicative of pyonephrosis. Since pyonephrosis is an emergency, which can be diagnosed well by means of CT, MRI is used less frequently.

Xanthogranulomatous Pyelonephritis

Xanthogranulomatous pyelonephritis (XPN) is a chronic granulomatous disease of the renal parenchyma, in which the parenchyma is progressively replaced by fat-containing macrophages, other inflammatory cells and cell detritus. Recurrent *E. coli* and *Proteus mirabilis* infection affecting middle-aged females and rarely diabetes are associated [10, 11]. In the overwhelming majority of cases, this inflammatory change arises from a chronic urinary obstruction, such as a ureteral constriction. In most patients (90%), a staghorn calculus is found. Atypical characteristics comprise lack of calculi (10%), focal instead of diffuse involvement (10%), and renal atrophy instead of enlargement. Chronic inflammation may develop into fistulae formation to adjacent organs. XPN is usually one-sided. Ureteral or renal pelvic stones can often be detected only unilaterally in affected patients. In addition to ureteral stones, however, subpelvic ureteral stenoses and ureteral masses may also be responsible for the chronic urinary accumulation.

The more frequent generalized form of the XPN shows the image of an extended renal pelvis and rarefied renal parenchyma with the tissue consisting of xanthoma cells (lipid-containing macrophages). This is also described as the "bear claw." In addition, the perirenal fat tissue exhibits an inflammatory co-reaction, which is characterized, in particular, by fluid collections.

MRI is particularly useful in patients with chronic renal dysfunction leading to renal impairment. The fat-containing cells appear iso-hyperintense in T1- and T2-weighted and a signal decrease is seen in fat-saturated sequences.

The diagnosis of the focal form of XPN is often difficult, whose appearance resembles that of renal cell carcinoma. In these cases, histologic confirmation of the diagnosis must be obtained.

Tuberculosis

Renal tuberculosis arises from hematogenous dissemination of the disease. In about 50% of the patients, lung involvement cannot be detected. Caliectasis is seen in early stages in urographic phases with a feathery contour; in the protracted course, a "phantom calyx" or a cavity communicating with a malformed calyx can be present [1]. Later, the granulomas coalesce forming mass-like lesions (tuberculoma) which may rupture into the pelvic collective system. Fibrosis leading to infundibular stenosis can also occur. The end stage is characterized by a shrunken ("putty") and/or calcified kidney or an enlarged sac with caseous material ("case cavernous-type autonephrectomy"). Involvement of the ureters is associated with wall thickening with strictures and shortening of the ureters. Bladder involvement leads multiple diverticula and organ contraction [1].

Fungal Infection

Immunocompromission in patients with HIV, hematooncological diseases, or diabetes is the main risk factor for fungal infection of the urinary tract that is mostly very severe and potentially life-threatening. The most common organisms found are *Candida* and *Aspergillus* which are usually acquired by hematogenous spread or urinary tract infection [1]. Multiple renal abscesses and striated nephrogram can be seen indicating acute pyelonephritis. Irregular defects in the collecting system may correspond to conglomerations of fungal hyphae and fungal balls. Fungal infections with mucor are rare, in which vessel invasion resulting in infarctions with high mortality can be present. Diffuse punctate calcifications, barely visible on MRI, in the kidneys or organs of the reticuloendothelial system can be indicative of a *Pneumocystis carinii* infection in HIV patients.

Stone Disease

MRI is the cross-sectional imaging method if, in case of a negative result of CT regarding the presence of calculi, a secondary imaging of the urinary tract is necessary to assess other soft tissue-related (e.g., urogenital malignancies) causes of urinary obstruction. Due to the low proton content, calculi have no MRI signal and can thus only be detected indirectly as a signal-free lesion. In T2-weighted sequences or contrast-enhanced MR urography, filling defects appear as indirect indicators for a calculus. A "perinephric imbibition," that is, fluid around the kidneys or ureters, can often be observed.

Retroperitoneum

Retroperitoneal Fibrosis

Retroperitoneal fibrosis, often referred to as Ormond's disease, is a probably autoimmune, in some cases, medically mediated chronic inflammation in the retroperitoneum which leads to an increasing fibrosis of the structures located there (Fig.). Correspondingly, in the majority of cases, the

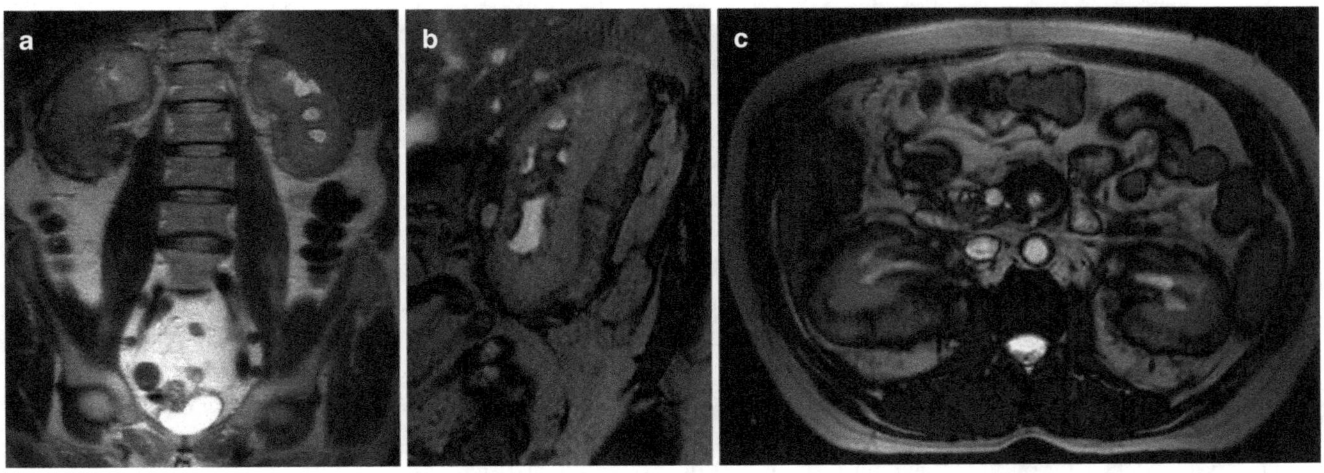

Fig. Coronal (**a**), sagittal (**b**), and axial (**c**) T2-weighted images showing a rare case of entrapment of both kidneys by histopathologically proven retroperitoneal fibrosis leading to hydronephrosis

ureters running here are also affected. The fibrotic tissue, which usually spreads out cranially and caudally starting at the level of the lower lumbar spine, can be directly visualized with sectional imaging. A pannus-like growth around the aorta, iliac vessels, and ureters is typical. The ureters are displaced in a characteristic manner to the medial direction. The middle third of the ureter is most frequently affected, but all ureteral sections may be involved. In the regions surrounding the fibrotic tissue, a stenosis of the ureters with a consecutive dilatation of the upper sections can occur. Contrast-enhanced images indicate the activity of the inflammation since a strong contrast agent uptake of the fibrotic tissue indicates active inflammation.

Inflammations of the Bladder

Bladder Infection

The detection of an inflammatory bladder wall change is a diagnostic challenge, since it is mostly indicated only by an irregular thickening, possibly with an inflammatory reaction of the adjacent fat tissue. However, this is a primarily unspecific finding and initially does not permit a reliable differentiation between malignancies, benign inflammatory changes, or posttherapeutic changes. Therefore, it is absolutely necessary to take into account the clinic presentation, the history of the patient, and the further development of the patient's disease for a differential diagnosis. In MRI, high-resolution sequences for assessing the bladder wall or DWI can help resolve the diagnostic dilemma.

Another factor which affects the wall thickness of the bladder is the filling state. False-positive, pathological conditions can be simulated in a nearly empty bladder. In order to achieve a comparable filling state and to increase the detection of a potential tumor infiltration of the bladder wall, filling of the bladder is possible via a catheter with dilute contrast medium before an MRI examination. However, from a practical point of view, it should be noted that filling of the urinary bladder during a longer examination can lead to a reduced image quality in case of movement artifacts due to the urge to urinate.

Bladder infections often appear as nodular, irregular wall thickenings of the urinary bladder, since these can cause a bullous edema of the urinary bladder wall. Chronic infections, on the other hand, can lead to fibrotic changes with a subsequent contraction of the bladder wall.

Cystitis is defined by a bacterial count above 100,000 per mL urine and is most frequently caused by *E. coli*. In sectional imaging, this often impresses by a wall thickening of the urinary bladder. A rare, life-threatening form of cystitis found in diabetics and immunosuppressed patients is emphysematous cystitis. This shows gas accumulations in the bladder wall, which can expand into the ureter.

Likewise in diabetics the candida infection of the bladder is found. The fermentation of sugars in the urinary bladder can lead to detectable air, sometimes also to fungus balls.

In irradiated patients, radiation cystitis may occur. Here, in the acute phase, there is often a wall edema and hemorrhage. In the long term, ulceration, fibrosis, and shrinkage can develop. In imaging, the changes are often unspecific.

Schistosomiasis

Schistosomiasis, also referred to as bilharzia, is caused by parasitic worms. Over 200 million people are infected, with the majority in Africa. It is a major health concern in rural areas of developing countries predisposing individuals to squamous cell carcinoma and urothelial carcinoma. The infection generally occurs in the bladder but can spread to the ureters and kidneys via reflux. In the acute phase, nodular bladder wall thickening is seen in urography or MRI. Dystrophic, typically curvilinear calcifications, best seen on CT, in the bladder wall or ureter are common findings and are caused by calcified dead ova. Typical additional appearances are strictures of the ureters or reflux.

Fistula

Fistula formation can be attributed to various underlying pathologies. The most common cause of fistula in Europe is a secondary fistula in Crohn's disease. In smaller fistulae, the only clinical indicator can be a chronic cystitis. Frequently, larger fistulae lead to air or feces excretion via the urine. In MRI, fistula detection can be achieved directly (by filling the fistula with contrast medium) or indirectly (only by showing the connection of two structures or by air detection in the fistula). For fistula detection MRI is superior to CT, since the fistulae can be detected relatively specific, on the one hand, via T2-weighted sequences with fat suppression and after contrast agent application in fat-saturated T1-weighted sequences. Furthermore, MRI can be used to detect a concomitant abscess via diffusion-weighted imaging with high specificity. A direct (via a catheter) or an indirect (urographic late phase) filling of the urinary bladder can be performed. Depending on the localization of the presumed fistula, rectal contrast can also be helpful, although from a practical point of view a simultaneous filling does not appear to be useful (possibly at different time points).

Differential Diagnosis

Lymphoma

Retroperitoneal lymphomas are an important differential diagnosis of both, abscess-forming inflammatory disease of the kidneys and Ormond's disease. Renal lymphomas appear T1-hypointense and T2-iso–/hyperintense to normal parenchyma with poor enhancement relative to healthy renal tissue and may mimic acute pyelonephritis. Typically, renal lymphomas are associated with restricted diffusion and extremely low ADC values similar to those of abscesses (Fig.). In renal transplants posttransplant lymphoproliferative disorders (PTLD) are quite common and an important differential diagnosis to abscess-forming pyelonephritis and graft-versus-host disease.

Retroperitoneal lymphomas, in contrast to retroperitoneal fibrosis, show a rather mass-forming growth, and structures (e.g., ureters) are rather laterally displaced. In doubt, CT can be used to guide biopsy, since the diagnosis of retroperitoneal fibrosis is ultimately made by means of histopathology, despite typical image criteria.

Posttherapeutic Change

Patients with gynecologic tumors and rectal or prostatic cancers are often treated surgically and/or with chemoradiation, which can lead to ureteric strictures. The ureter may be injured in the process of pelvic surgery or transected, potentially causing hydronephrosis or urinoma. Strictures or fibrosis leading to ureteric obstruction is common, as well as bowel and urinary tract fistulae. Lymphoceles may lead to an external compression of the ureter and/or bladder.

Take-Home Messages

- Sectional imaging, MRI in particular, may be useful in complicated urogenital infections.
- Clinical history of patients may help to differentiate certain pathologies and to identify "high-risk" patients.
- Acute and chronic inflammatory changes can be assessed with CT and MRI; MRI is possibly with greater significance in some differential diagnosis,

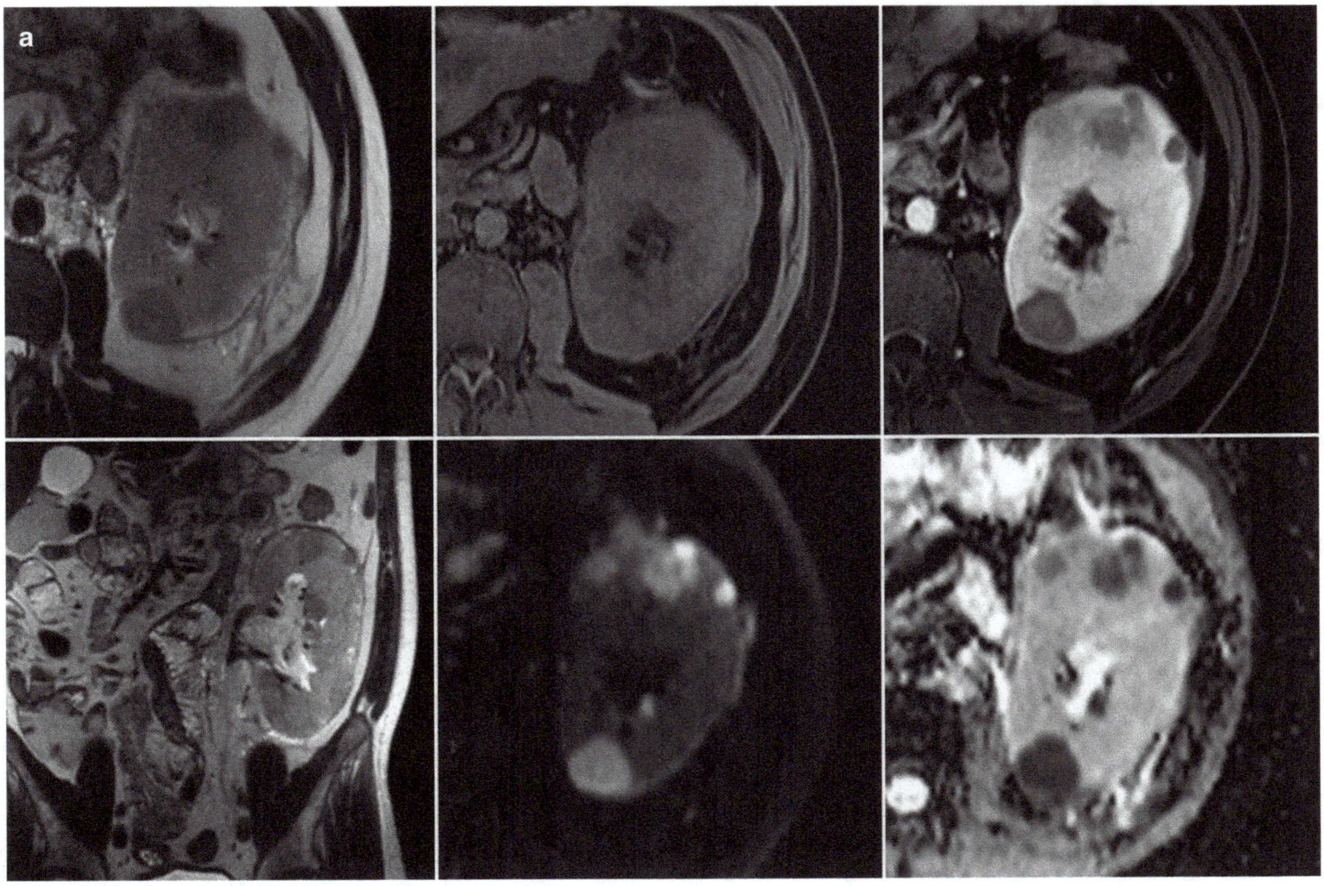

Fig. A 35-year-old male patient with focal T2-hypointense/T1-isointense lesions showing poor enhancement. Lesions display very high signal on high b-value DWI and significantly reduced ADC values (**a**). Lymphoma was diagnosed based on histopathology. Patient responded to chemotherapy, which is indicated by increase of ADC values and decrease of signal on high b-value images (**b**)

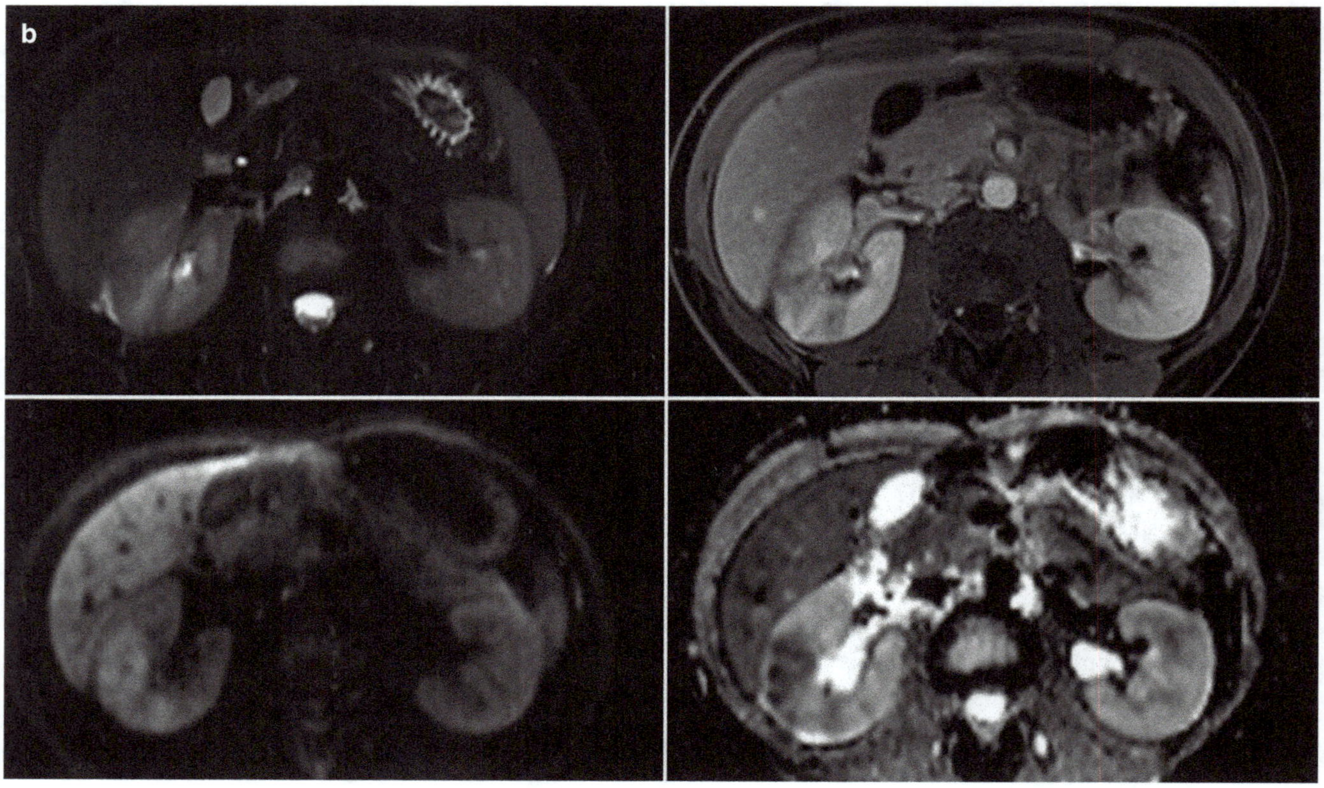

Fig. (continued)

whereas CT offers the possibility of direct intervention, e.g., installation of abscess drainage.

- Standard sequences should be accompanied by functional imaging (e.g., DWI).
- CT is the modality of choice for imaging of urolithiasis; MRI may help in the further work-up of certain patients (e.g., to rule out malignancies if no calculi are detectable).
- In the investigation of retroperitoneal or ureteral pathologies, urographic phases are useful.
- Lymphoma should be considered as a differential diagnosis of lower and upper urogenital tract inflammation.

References

1. Das CJ, Ahmad Z, Sharma S, Gupta AK. Multimodality imaging of renal inflammatory lesions. World J Radiol. 2014;6(11):865–73.
2. Sandler CM, Amis ES Jr, Bigongiari LR, Bluth EI, Bush WH Jr, Choyke PL, et al. Imaging in acute pyelonephritis. American College of Radiology. ACR appropriateness criteria. Radiology. 2000;215(Suppl):677–81.
3. He YL, Hausmann D, Morelli JN, Attenberger UI, Schoenberg SO, Riffel P. Renal zoomed EPI-DWI with spatially-selective radiofrequency excitation pulses in two dimensions. Eur J Radiol. 2016;85(10):1773–7.
4. Riffel P, Zoellner FG, Budjan J, Grimm R, Block TK, Schoenberg SO, et al. "One-stop shop": free-breathing dynamic contrast-enhanced magnetic resonance imaging of the kidney using iterative reconstruction and continuous golden-angle radial sampling. Investig Radiol. 2016;51(11):714–9.
5. Michaely HJ, Metzger L, Haneder S, Hansmann J, Schoenberg SO, Attenberger UI. Renal BOLD-MRI does not reflect renal function in chronic kidney disease. Kidney Int. 2012;81(7):684–9.
6. Nissen JC, Mie MB, Zollner FG, Haneder S, Schoenberg SO, Michaely HJ. Blood oxygenation level dependent (BOLD)—renal imaging: concepts and applications. Z Med Phys. 2010;20(2):88–100.
7. Haneder S, Kettnaker P, Konstandin S, Morelli JN, Schad LR, Schoenberg SO, et al. Quantitative in vivo 23Na MR imaging of the healthy human kidney: determination of physiological ranges at 3.0T with comparison to DWI and BOLD. MAGMA. 2013;26(6):501–9.
8. Haneder S, Konstandin S, Morelli JN, Nagel AM, Zoellner FG, Schad LR, et al. Quantitative and qualitative (23)Na MR imaging of the human kidneys at 3 T: before and after a water load. Radiology. 2011;260(3):857–65.
9. Henninger B, Reichert M, Haneder S, Schoenberg SO, Michaely HJ. Value of diffusion-weighted MR imaging for the detection of nephritis. ScientificWorldJournal. 2013;2013:348105.
10. Craig WD, Wagner BJ, Travis MD. Pyelonephritis: radiologic-pathologic review. Radiographics. 2008;28(1):255–77; quiz 327–8.
11. Quinn FM, Dick AC, Corbally MT, McDermott MB, Guiney EJ. Xanthogranulomatous pyelonephritis in childhood. Arch Dis Child. 1999;81(6):483–6.

6

MRI of the Pelvic Floor and MR Defecography

Francesca Maccioni and Celine D. Alt

Learning Objectives

- To gain a basic knowledge on anatomy and pathophysiology of the pelvic floor unit
- To get familiar with the recently published general recommendations for standardized imaging and reporting of pelvic floor disorder using MRI
- To discuss how to apply these recommendations in case-based evaluations

Introduction

The female pelvic floor is a complex functional and anatomic system. It is composed of an active muscular component and a passive support system. Furthermore, it is topographically divided in three main functional and anatomic compartments: the anterior, supporting the bladder and urethra; the middle, supporting the vagina and uterus; and the posterior or anorectal compartment [1]. When the pelvic floor is damaged in its fascial, muscular, or neural components at the level of any of its three compartments, several pelvic floor dysfunctions or disorders (PFD) may arise [2]. As pelvic floor muscles and fasciae act like a unique functional entity, dysfunction of one compartment is commonly associated with various dysfunctions of the other compartments as well. Hence, a multidisciplinary team, often called a pelvic floor unit, is strongly recommended that includes urogynecologists, urologists, gastroenterologists, proctologists, physicians, radiologists, physiotherapists, and specialized nurses. Additionally, the correct diagnosis of the specific PFD and the identification of all associated disorders are mandatory for an effective conservative or surgical treatment. Dynamic MRI provides excellent morphological and functional display of the pelvic floor and is therefore additionally applied for a comprehensive overview of the pelvic floor and the entire pelvic structures. Evaluation is best done by performing a standardized MRI procedure and using a systemic approach to report the MRI findings [3]. To improve effective communication between the radiologist and the clinician, it is also relevant to understand the specific lesions underlying PFD and to explain the frequent association of disorders in different pelvic compartments.

F. Maccioni (✉)
Department of Radiological Sciences, Oncology and Pathology, Sapienza University of Rome, Rome, Italy
e-mail: francesca.maccioni@uniroma1.it

C. D. Alt
Department of Diagnostic and Interventional Radiology, University Duesseldorf, Medical Faculty, Duesseldorf, Germany
e-mail: celine.alt@med.uni-duesseldorf.de

Functional Anatomy of the Pelvic Floor

Pathogenesis

The pelvic floor is an integrated system composed of an active component, the striated muscles, and a passive support system, the suspensory ligaments and fascial coverings, and is associated with an intricate neural network. It not only provides support for the pelvic viscera (bladder, bowel, uterus) but maintains their functioning, thanks to the combined action of the two major pelvic floor structures: the levator ani muscle (LAM), and the endopelvic fascia [1, 2, 4].

Levator Ani Muscle (LAM)

The LAM has two main components: the iliococcygeus and pubococcygeus muscles. Various muscle subdivisions of the LAM are assigned to the medial portions of the pubococcygeus in order to reflect the attachments of the muscle to the urethra, vagina, anus, and rectum. These subdivisions of the LAM are referred to as the Mm. pubourethralis, pubovaginalis, puboanalis, and puborectalis or, collectively, as the M. pubovisceralis. More posteriorly, the pelvic diaphragm becomes continuous with the ischiococcygeus muscle. The LAM contracts continuously, providing tone to the pelvic floor against stress coming from gravity and intra-abdominal pressure. LAM contraction closes the urogenital hiatus and compresses the urethra, vagina, and anorectal junction (ARJ) in the direction of the pubic bone. Furthermore, the puborectalis component of the LAM, called the puborectal muscle, is an intrinsic and relevant part of the anal sphincter complex. It plays a primary role in the defecation process, acting as a sling that opens and closes access to the anal canal. Relaxation of the puborectal muscle, in fact, opens the anorectal angle (ARA); its contraction closes this angle, thus impeding defecation.

EndopelvicFascia

The endopelvic fascia is a layer of connective tissue that connects and attaches the uterus and vagina to the pelvic bones [1]. Pelvic organs are supported by a series of fascial (ligamental) and elastic condensations of the endopelvic fascia, which support the uterus and vagina, preventing genital organ prolapse.

PubocervicalFascia

The anterior portion of the endopelvic fascia, the pubocervical fascia, extends from the anterior vaginal wall to the pubis and supports the bladder. Damage to this ligament may cause urethral hypermobility and urinary incontinence.

RectovaginalFascia

The posterior portion of the endopelvic fascia forms the rectovaginal fascia, called Denonvilliers aponeurosis, composed of thin, connective tissue in the rectovaginal septum. It further extends, along with the cardinal and uterosacral ligaments (parametrium), from the posterior cervix and vaginal wall toward the sacrum [1]. Damage to or weakness of this fascia represents a major cause of rectocele.

Etiology of Pelvic Floor Failure

Obstetric lesions are considered primary causes of pelvic floor damage. Lesions of the iliococcygeus muscles are more frequent in the first phase of delivery, whereas the pubococcygeus muscles may be damaged in the second phase; midline episiotomy or forceps delivery are associated with anal sphincter rupture [2, 5]. During delivery, damage to the anterior portion of the endopelvic fascia (pubocervical fascia) may determine urethral hypermobility and/or cystocele, whereas a lesion of its posterior portion, the rectovaginal fascia, may result in an anterior rectocele or enterocele [5]. Pudendal nerve impairment during vaginal delivery for ischemic and mechanical factors diminishes the LAM's capability for providing adequate pelvic support. Other causes of pelvic floor weakness include aging, obesity, hysterectomy, and the patient's genetic predisposition.

Indication for Dynamic Pelvic Floor Imaging

A pelvic floor disorder (PFD) is characterized by a variable association of pelvic organ prolapse (POP) and functional disturbances involving the bladder (e.g., urinary incontinence and/or voiding dysfunction), the vagina and/or uterus (e.g., sexual dysfunctions), and the rectum (e.g., obstructed defecation syndrome (ODS)) [4]. The most common PFD are ODS, POP, and urinary incontinence. Nearly 50% of multiparous women >50 years of age are affected by these disorders, with a negative impact on their quality of life and a frequent need of invasive surgical treatments [2, 4].

Key Point

- The pelvic floor should be considered as one unit since the three compartments work as one entity. Therefore, combined defects of the pelvic floor are common and the entire pelvis should be evaluated for PFD diagnosis.

Diagnosis of PFD Using Dynamic MRI

Dynamic pelvic floor (DPF)-MRI has emerged a valuable alternative technique for assessing PFD and grading POP, especially in the posterior compartment [6, 7]. Thanks to its multiplanar capability and high soft tissue contrast, MRI allows comprehensive morphologic and functional evaluation of all three compartments at the same time, without the use of ionizing radiation. It enables real-time assessment of functional diseases with dynamic acquisitions, similar to conventional defecography [6]. The main limit of MRI is the obliged supine position for patient imaging, which is necessary if a closed 1.5-Tesla magnet is used. The supine position of MR defecography has been criticized because defecation evaluation is not under physiological conditions [8, 9].

Comparative studies performed with open and closed magnets have ultimately established a good concordance between results obtained in the sitting and the supine position, thus validating the use of closed MRI for assessing defecation [8]. For over 25 years, since its early clinical introduction, dynamic MRI for the evaluation of pelvic floor dysfunction has been performed with extremely heterogeneous techniques due to the variability of patient preparation, MRI equipments, and image evaluation systems [10, 11]. Recently a standardized technique for DPF-MRI performance evaluation has been proposed by a ESUR-ESGAR working group of experts [3].

Key Point

- There is no difference in the detection of clinically relevant pathologies regarding PFD when performing dynamic MRI in sitting position (open magnet) or in supine position (closed magnet).

GeneralPreparation

According to the recommendations on MR defecography, the patient should void for about 2 h before the examination to have the bladder moderately filled [3]. A rectal cleansing enema the evening before the examination might be helpful but is not obligatory needed. To decrease patients' discomfort and to increase patients' compliance during dynamic and evacuation phases, a protective pad or a diaper pant should be offered to the patient. Prior to the examination, the full history of pelvic floor disorder should be taken, and the patient should be trained on how to correctly perform the dynamic phases of the examination and the evacuation phase. The patient should be informed that the full extent of pelvic organ prolapse (POP) and certain abnormalities are only visible during defecation, which makes evacuation of the gel mandatory [3].

DPF-MRI Procedure

Patients' Positioning and Preparation

The given technical aspects of MRI of the pelvic floor relate to conventional closed configuration magnets for MR imaging allowing patient positioning in lying body position only [3]. The MR defecography should preferably be performed with at least 1.5 T using a phased array coil centered low on the pelvis to ensure complete visualization of prolapsed organs [3]. The patient is placed in the supine position with the knees elevated (e.g., on a pillow with firm consistency) which facilitates straining and evacuation. No oral or intravenous contrast is necessary. Vaginal filling with 20 cm^3 ultrasound gel is helpful for better demarcation, but its application may be limited due to social or religious backgrounds. However, the rectum should be distended with ultrasound gel, especially in order to clearly diagnose an intussusception and to evaluate the efficacy of rectal evacuation [3].

MRI Sequences

The recommended MR-defecography protocol consists of static MR sequences (high-resolution T2-weighted images (T2WI), e.g., TSE, FSE, RARE) in three planes and dynamic MR sequences (steady state, e.g., FISP, GRASS, FFE, PSIF, SSFP, and T2-FFE, or balanced-state-free precession sequence, e.g., TrueFISP, FIESTA, b-FFE) in sagittal plane (squeezing, straining, defecation). Adequate pelvic stress during the dynamic sequences is important in order to assess the full extent of pelvic floor disorder. Therefore, a clear movement of the abdominal wall and the small bowel must be seen during dynamic phases. The dynamic sequences "squeezing" and "straining" require breath holding, wherefore the duration should not exceed 20 seconds each [3]. The "defecation" sequence should be repeated until the rectum is emptied (total time duration around 2–3 min) to show full extent of POP and to exclude rectal intussusception [3].

Key Point

- Adequate pelvic stress during straining (clear movement of the abdominal wall and small bowel is seen) and the evacuation of the rectal gel during defecation are crucial so that the examination can be considered diagnostic.

MRI Interpretation

The static images should be analyzed for detection and classification of structural abnormalities, while the dynamic images should be analyzed with regard to functional abnormalities assessed by metric measurements of the three compartments of the pelvic floor. Due to the different views of the clinical specialists involved in the treatment of pelvic floor disorder, it is suggested to consider adapting the MRI reporting scheme according to the specialty of the referring physician [3].

Measurement and Grading

The pubococcygeal line (PCL) is the recommended **reference line** to measure POP as it practically represents the level of the pelvic floor [3]. It is drawn on sagittal plane from the inferior aspect of the pubic symphysis to the last coccygeal joint [10]. After defining the PCL, the distance from each reference point is measured perpendicularly to the PCL at rest and at maximum strain.

The **organ-specific reference point** in the anterior, middle, and posterior compartment is the most inferior aspect of the bladder base (B), the anterior cervical lip (most distal edge of the cervix) (C), or the vaginal vault in case of previous hysterectomy (V), the pouch of Douglas (P), and the anorectal junction (ARJ) (Fig.) [3]. Measured values above the reference line have a minus sign, values below a plus sign [12].

The **anorectal angle (ARA)** should be drawn along the posterior border of the rectum and a line along the central axis of the anal canal on sagittal plane at rest, squeezing and maximum straining (Fig.) [3].

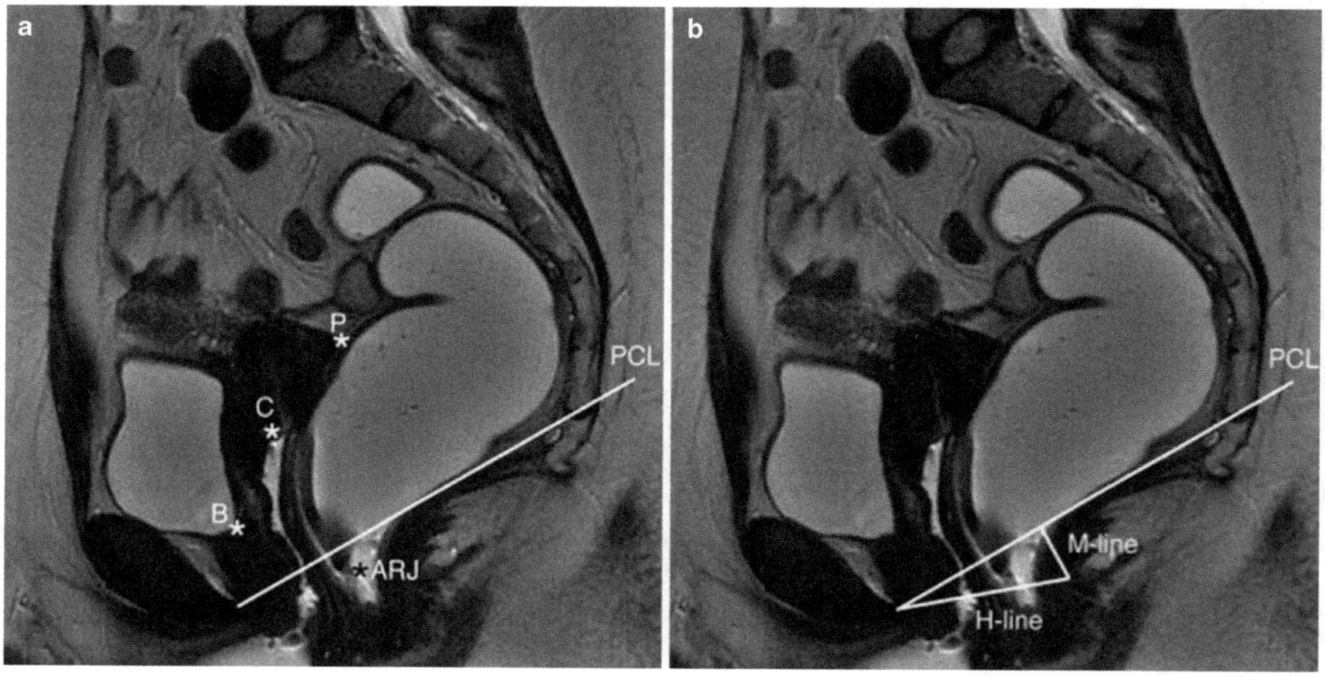

Fig. (**a**, **b**) Presentation of the metric measurements on sagittal plane at rest. (**a**) The reference points are marked according to the PCL. This image at rest presents all reference points in a normal location without protrusion or descent. (**b**) The hiatus at rest presents with a normal width and is located in a normal position according to the pelvic floor level (PCL) without descent (M-line). *PCL* pubococcygeal line, *B* bladder neck, *C* anterior cervical lip, *P* douglas pouch, *ARJ* anorectal junction, *H-line* hiatal width, *M-line* hiatal descent

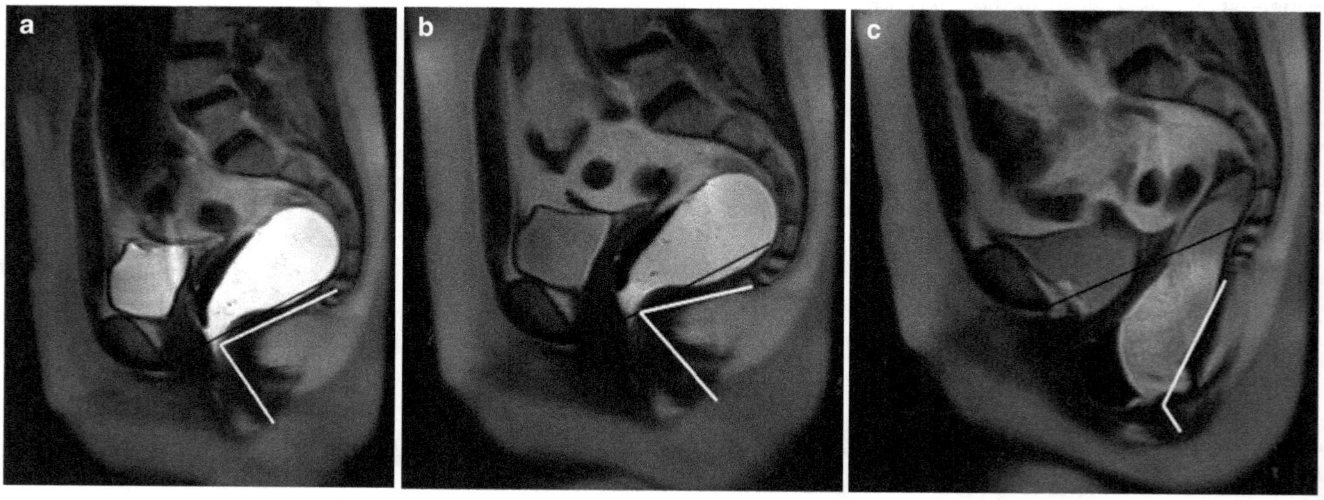

Fig. . (**a–c**) Anorectal angle variations. (**a**) Sagittal T2-weighted image at rest after rectal filling with gel. The anorectal angle (white line) is approximately 85°. The anorectal junction corresponds to the apex of the angle, and it is placed at the level of the PCL. (**b**) Sagittal T2-weighted image during squeezing of the pelvic floor. The anorectal angle (white line) is reduced to 80°. The anorectal junction remains at the level of the PCL. (**c**) Sagittal T2-weighted image during straining. The anorectal angle (white line) opens to 130° due to rectal prolapse (160°) and is associated with severe prolapse of the anorectal junction (6 cm). *PCL* pubococcygeal line (black line)

To **grade pelvic organ prolapse in the anterior and middle compartment**, the recommended grading system starts at +1 cm below the PCL based on the fact that the pelvic floor may normally descend and widen up to 2 cm during abdominal pressure and the pelvic organs consequently follow the movement of the pelvic floor inferiorly [13]. The recommended grading system for cystoceles and uterine descent is as follows: °0 = up to +1 cm below the PCL, °I = +1 to +3 cm below the PCL, °II = +3 to +6 cm below the PCL, and °III = more than +6 cm below the PCL [3].

The **position of the anorectal junction** is stated to be normal up to +3 cm below the PCL. The recommended grading system for rectal descent is therefore as follows [14]: °0 = up to +3 cm below the PCL, °I = between +3 and +5 cm below the PCL, and °II = more than +5 cm below the PCL [3, 14].

The anterior rectal wall bulge in **rectoceles** should be reported as pathological from grade °II, as a grade °I rectocele can be observed in nearly 78–99% of parous women, while rarely in men [7, 15, 16]: °0 = no outpouching, °I = outpouching up to 2 cm, °II = outpouching between 2 and 4 cm, and °III = outpouching at least 4 cm [3].

2.3.3.2 Further Evaluation

If a **cystocele** is present, the differentiation of a distention (central defect) or a displacement (lateral defect) cystocele can be made, which is relevant for therapy planning [17].

If a **herniation of the pelvic peritoneal sac** into the rectogenital pouch (pouch of Douglas) is present, the report should include the content of the peritoneal sac [3]. It may contain fat (called peritoneocele), small-bowel loops (properly defined as enterocele), or sigmoid colon (defined as sigmoidocele).

The **change of the ARA** expresses the functioning of the puborectal muscle. In healthy individuals in the supine position, the ARA at rest is between 85 and 95° [6]. During squeezing pelvic organs elevate in relationship to the PCL, sharpening the ARA by 10–15° (due to contraction of the puborectal muscle), while during straining and defecation, the ARA becomes more obtuse, typically by 15–25°, than when measured at rest (Fig.) [6].

Anismus is characterized by lack or insufficient relaxation of the puborectal muscle and external anal sphincter during defecation [6]. Anismus determines constipation and incomplete defecation due to a paradoxical contraction of the puborectal muscle during straining and defecation, without significant variation in the ARA in the different functional phases.

If no **evacuation of rectal content** at all or a delayed evacuation time is present although the compliance is good (more than 30 seconds to evacuate 2/3 of the rectal content), anismus should be considered [3, 18].

Functional abnormalities like loss of urine through the urethra during maximum straining, urethral hypermobility, urethral funneling, or a contrary movement of the puborectal muscle should be reported if present [3].

Reporting of **pelvic organ mobility** (the movement of the organs compared to their location at rest) can give more valuable information than a grading system alone, taking into consideration that each woman has a unique straining of her pelvic floor and the grade of prolapse alone may not fully depict individual manifestation of POP or PFD [19].

Pelvic floor relaxation often coexists with pelvic organ prolapse. For quantification of the weakness of the levator ani and to reflect pelvic floor laxity, the length of the hiatus (H-line; extending from the inferior aspect of the pubic bone to the posterior wall of the rectum), the descent of the levator plate (M-line), and the levator plate angle can be evaluated on sagittal plane at rest and during maximal straining (Fig.) [3]. Generalized pelvic floor weakness is also defined as **descending perineal syndrome**. One of the main causes is thought to be excessive anismus.

Structural defects and anatomical abnormalities like urethral ligament defect and/or distortion; puborectalis muscle detachment, disruption, atrophy, or avulsion; or diffuse or focal iliococcygeus muscle abnormality are commonly assessed on static T2-weighted images and should be reported if present [3].

Overview on Compartment-Based Symptoms

AnteriorCompartment

Stress urinary incontinence (SUI) is the most common type of urinary incontinence in women, commonly caused by a defect in the urethral support system [20]. Other pathological causes have been attributed to urethral hypermobility, intrinsic sphincter deficiency, or urethral trauma (e.g., resulting from childbearing, surgical trauma, prolonged increased abdominal pressure) [21–23]. Women suffering from SUI often fear urinary leakage and are therefore impaired in their social or physical activities [24].

MiddleCompartment

Women affected by levator ani trauma (e.g., caused by vaginal childbirth) may suffer from non-specific complaints as abnormal emptying of the bladder, frequency and urgency, organ protrusion, pelvic pain, or pressure, as well as from dyspareunia and urinary or fecal incontinence [13, 25]. POP of the middle compartment may arise from damages of the connective tissue or vaginal supporting structures due to age or collagen defects. However, an avulsion of the pubovisceral muscle at its inferior aspect or the detachment from its insertion on the arcus tendineus fasciae pelvis band during vaginal delivery causes laxity and is propagated as the most common cause of pelvic floor dysfunction [26].

PosteriorCompartment

The obstructed defecation syndrome (ODS) is the most frequent symptom related to the posterior compartment and may be sustained either by mechanical causes (e.g., rectal prolapse, rectal descent, rectal invagination, rectocele, enterocele) or by a functional disorder (puborectalis syndrome, dyssynergic defecation) [6, 27].

Common symptoms of rectal prolapse include constipation, sensation of incomplete evacuation, fecal incontinence, and rectal ulceration with bleeding.

An intrarectal intussusception (invagination of the rectal wall) may produce a sensation of incomplete emptying, whereas an intra-anal invagination rather produces a sensation of incomplete or obstructed defecation due to outlet obstruction. High-grade intussusceptions are frequently associated with a rectocele (Figs. and 2.4) [28, 29].

Enteroceles may be symptomatic, causing a sense of fullness and incomplete evacuation and occasionally lower abdominal pain (Fig.). However, an enterocele does not usually impair evacuation [6].

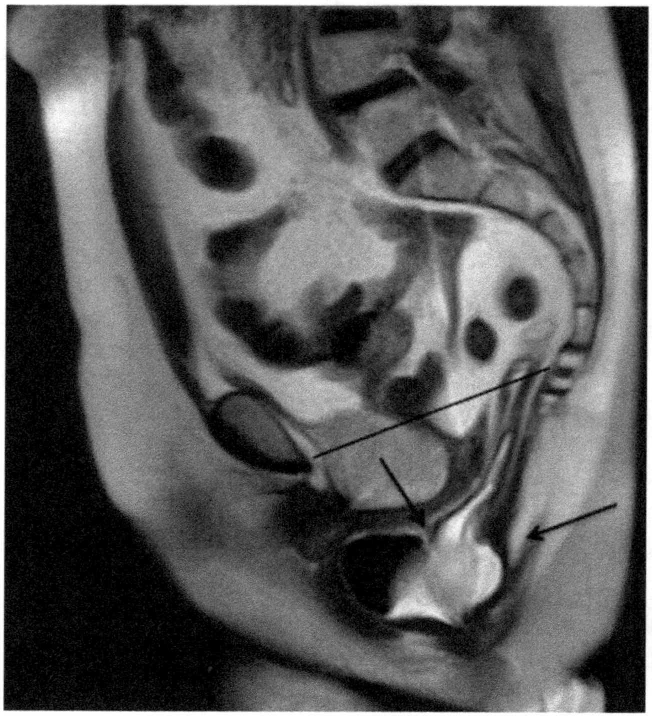

Fig. . Tricompartment prolapse in a patient with obstructed defecation syndrome. In the evacuation phase, a large anterior rectocele develops (>4 cm) associated with rectal invagination, severe descent of the ARJ (>6 cm), cystocele (>4 cm), and vaginal vault prolapse after hysterectomy

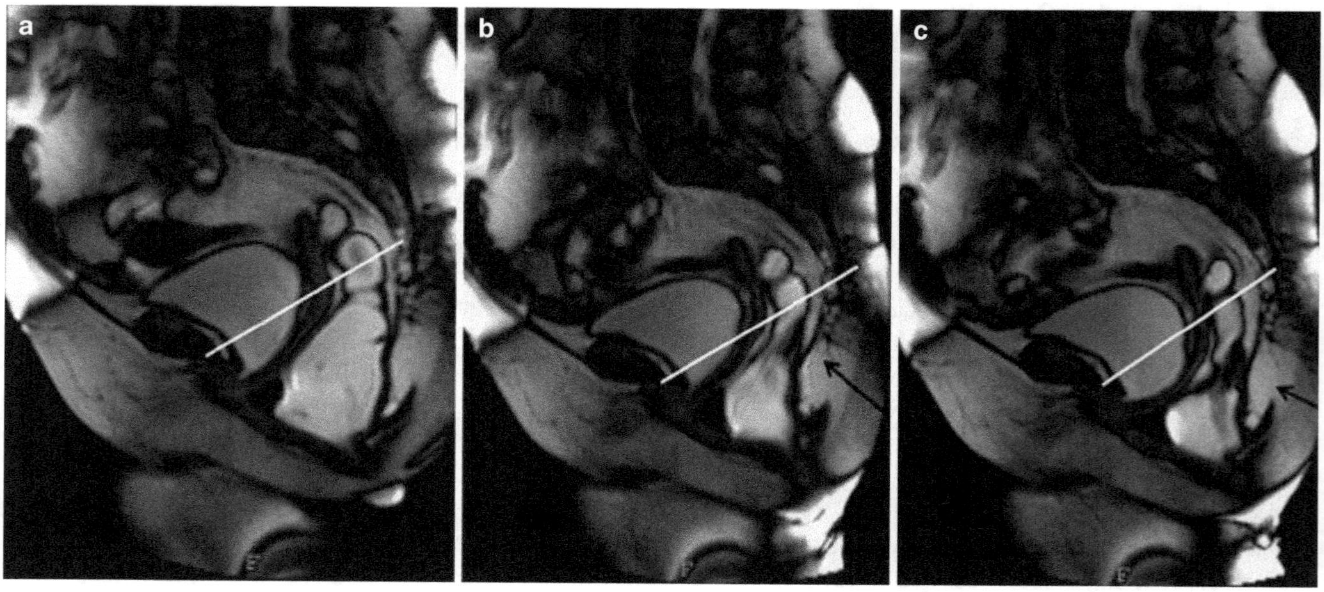

Fig. (**a–c**) Rectocele with rectal invagination during progressive straining. (**a**) Sagittal balanced image after filling with rectal gel shows an anterior rectocele (3 cm) associated with prolapsed anorectal junction (5 cm). (**b**) Progressive straining shows rectal invagination above the rectocele. (**c**) Rectal invagination and rectocele are more evident at maximum straining during evacuation

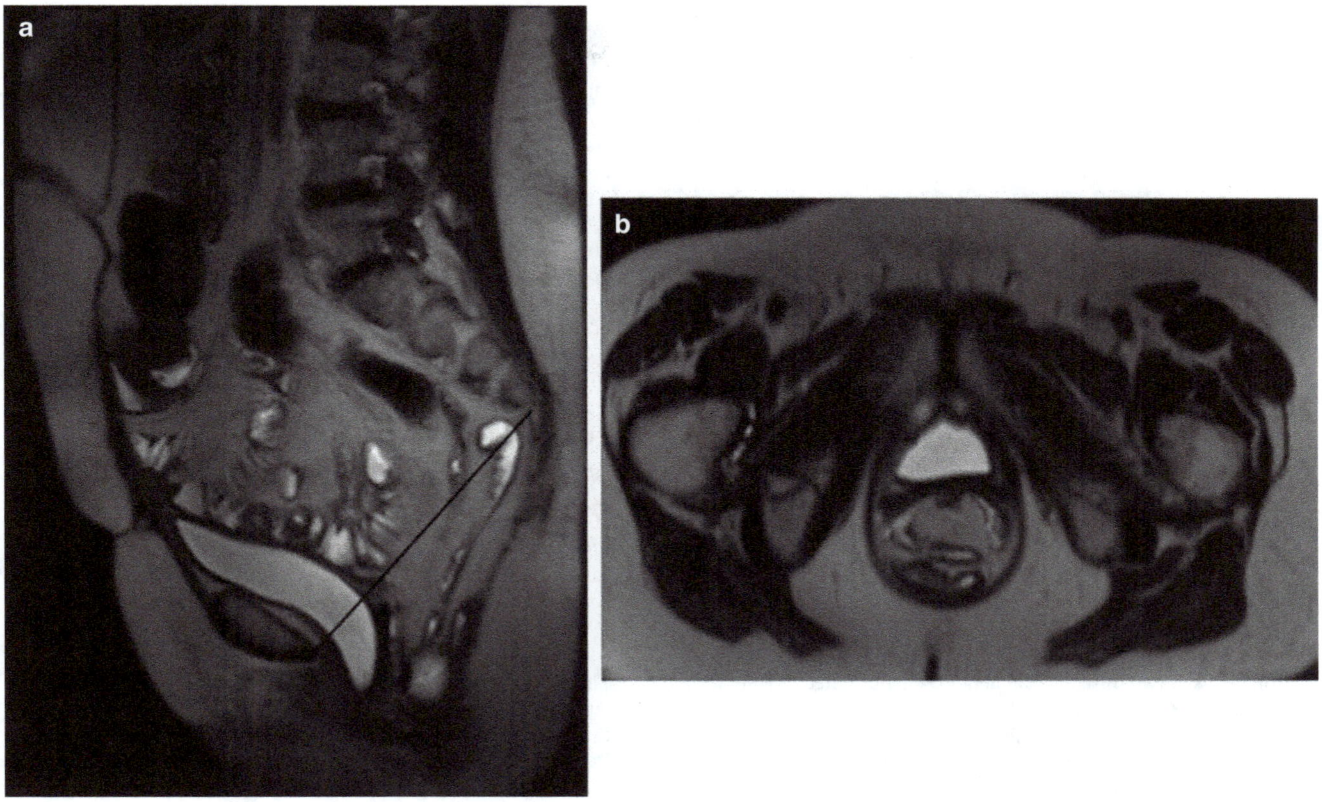

Fig. . (**a, b**) Tricompartment pelvic organ prolapse with cystocele, enterocele, and rectal prolapse. In the rectum, a balloon catheter is visible. (**a**) T2-weighted sagittal image. (**b**) Axial view, with clear opening of the pelvic hiatus and prolapse of the bladder base and small-bowel loops (cystocele and enterocele)

Symptoms related to a rectocele include vaginal bulging, dyspareunia, the sensation of a mass in the vagina, defecatory dysfunction, constipation, or the sensation of incomplete evacuation. The fecal trapping in the rectocele leads many patients to empty their bowels by digitating and pressing on the posterior wall of the vagina or perineum.

Key Point

- An intussusception is commonly only visible at the end of defecation phase, when the gel is evacuated; therefore it is mandatory to extend the defecation sequence in time or repeat the sequence if necessary.

Concluding Remarks

Dynamic pelvic floor MRI provides relevant morphological and functional information on pelvic floor structures for the diagnosis of pelvic floor disorder. However, knowledge about anatomy and pathogenesis of the pelvic floor unit as well as information about patients' history are crucial for the interpretation of dynamic pelvic floor MRI. Additionally, a systemic approach to perform and report dynamic pelvic floor MRI is crucial to enhance effective communication between the radiologist and the clinician for the sake of patients' benefit. The recently published recommendations on MR defecography by experts of the ESUR/ESGAR should be used, and all patients should undergo the same preparation and protocol, regardless of the leading symptoms of PFD to guarantee a complete documentation of the pelvic floor.

References

1. DeLancey JO. The anatomy of the pelvic floor. Curr Opin Obstet Gynecol. 1994;6(4):313–6.
2. Olsen AL, Smith VJ, Bergstrom JO, Colling JC, Clark AL. Epidemiology of surgically managed pelvic organ prolapse and urinary incontinence. Obstet Gynecol. 1997;89(4):501–6.
3. El Sayed RF, Alt CD, Maccioni F, Meissnitzer M, Masselli G, Manganaro L, et al. Magnetic resonance imaging of pelvic floor

dysfunction— joint recommendations of the ESUR and ESGAR Pelvic Floor Working Group. Eur Radiol. 2017;27(5):2067–85.
4. Elneil S. Complex pelvic floor failure and associated problems. Best Pract Res Clin Gastroenterol. 2009;23(4):555–73.
5. Mortele KJ, Fairhurst J. Dynamic MR defecography of the posterior compartment: Indications, techniques and MRI features. Eur J Radiol. 2007;61(3):462–72.
6. Maccioni F. Functional disorders of the ano-rectal compartment of the pelvic floor: clinical and diagnostic value of dynamic MRI. Abdom Imaging. 2013;38(5):930–51.
7. Elshazly WG, El Nekady Ael A, Hassan H. Role of dynamic magnetic resonance imaging in management of obstructed defecation case series. Int J Surg. 2010;8(4):274–82.
8. Bertschinger KM, Hetzer FH, Roos JE, Treiber K, Marincek B, Hilfiker PR. Dynamic MR imaging of the pelvic floor performed with patient sitting in an open-magnet unit versus with patient supine in a closed-magnet unit. Radiology. 2002;223:501–8.
9. Roos JE, Weishaupt D, Wildermuth S, Willmann JK, Marincek B, Hilfiker PR. Experience of 4 years with open MR defecography: pictorial review of anorectal anatomy and disease. Radiographics. 2002;22(4):817–32.
10. Yang A, Mostwin JL, Rosenshein NB, Zerhouni EA. Pelvic floor descent in women: dynamic evaluation with fast MR imaging and cinematic display. Radiology. 1991;179(1):25–33.
11. Maccioni F, Al Ansari N, Buonocore V, et al. Prospective comparison between two different magnetic resonance defecography techniques for evaluating pelvic floor disorders: air-balloon versus gel for rectal filling. Eur Radiol. 2016;26(6):1783–91.
12. Singh K, Jakab M, Reid WM, Berger LA, Hoyte L. Three-dimensional magnetic resonance imaging assessment of levator ani morphologic features in different grades of prolapse. Am J Obstet Gynecol. 2003;188(4):910–5.
13. Boyadzhyan L, Raman SS, Raz S. Role of static and dynamic MR imaging in surgical pelvic floor dysfunction. Radiographics. 2008;28(4):949–67.
14. Halligan S, Bartram C, Hall C, Wingate J. Enterocele revealed by simultaneous evacuation proctography and peritoneography: Does "defecation block" exist? Am J Roentgenol. 1996;167(2):461–6.
15. Morren GL, Balasingam AG, Wells JE, Hunter AM, Coates RH, Perry RE. Triphasic MRI of pelvic organ descent: sources of measurement error. Eur J Radiol. 2005;54(2):276–83.
16. Woodfield CA, Hampton BS, Sung V, Brody JM. Magnetic resonance imaging of pelvic organ prolapse: comparing pubococcygeal and midpubic lines with clinical staging. Int Urogynecol J Pelvic Floor Dysfunct. 2009;20(6):695–701.
17. Elsayed RF. Anterior compartment. In: Shaaban AM, editor. Diagnostic imaging: gynecology. 2nd ed. Amirsys: Elsevier; 2015. p. 8-40–68.
18. Halligan S, Bartram CI, Park HJ, Kamm MA. Proctographic features of anismus. Radiology. 1995;197(3):679–82.
19. Alt CD, Brocker KA, Lenz F, Sohn C, Kauczor HU, Hallscheidt P. MRI findings before and after prolapse surgery. Acta Radiol. 2014;55(4):495–504.
20. Deutchman M, Wulster-Radcliffe M. Stress urinary incontinence in women: diagnosis and medical management. MedGenMed. 2005;7(4):62.
21. Koelbl H, Mowstin J, Boiteux JP. Pathophysiology. In: Abrams P, Cardozo L, Koury S, Wein A, editors. Incontinence. Plymouth: Health Publications Ltd.; 2002. p. 165–201.
22. Kim JK, Kim YJ, Choo MS, Cho KS. The urethra and its supporting structures in women with stress urinary incontinence: MR imaging using an endovaginal coil. AJR Am J Roentgenol. 2003;180(4):1037–44.
23. Mostwin JL, Yang A, Sanders R, Genadry R. Radiography, sonography, and magnetic resonance imaging for stress incontinence. Contributions, uses, and limitations. Urol Clin North Am. 1995;22(3):539–49.
24. Abrams P, Cardozo L, Fall M, Griffiths D, Rosier P, Ulmsten U, et al. The standardisation of terminology of lower urinary tract function: report from the Standardisation Sub-committee of the International Continence Society. NeurourolUrodyn. 2002;21(2):167–78.
25. Petros P. The female pelvic floor: function, dysfunction, and management according to the integral theory. 2nd ed. Heidelberg: Springer; 2007. p. xix. 260 p
26. DeLancey JO, Kearney R, Chou Q, Speights S, Binno S. The appearance of levator ani muscle abnormalities in magnetic resonance images after vaginal delivery. Obstet Gynecol. 2003;101(1):46–53.
27. Zbar AP. Posterior pelvic floor disorders and obstructed defecation syndrome: clinical and therapeutic approach. Abdom Imaging. 2013;38(5):894–902.
28. Felt-Bersma RJ, Cuesta MA. Rectal prolapse, rectal intussusception, rectocele, and solitary rectal ulcer syndrome. Gastroenterol Clin North Am. 2001;30(1):199–222.
29. Kenton K, Shott S, Brubaker L. The anatomic and functional variability of rectoceles in women. Int Urogynecol J Pelvic Floor Dysfunct. 1999;10(2):96–9.

7

Imaging of Diffuse and Inflammatory Liver Disease

Pablo R. Ros

Learning Objectives

- To describe the pathophysiology of common and unusual diffuse diseases of the liver
- To learn to differentiate the overstorage of fat, iron, copper, and amyloid in the liver based on cross-sectional imaging
- To review diffuse hepatic manifestations of extrahepatic neoplasms
- To illustrate typical imaging findings of diffuse and focal liver infections including fungal, viral, parasitic, and bacterial etiology

Introduction

The role of imaging in the detection, characterization, and follow-up of diffuse liver disease has increased due to advances in cross-sectional imaging.

Diffuse liver disease is classified classically along pathogenesis into cirrhosis, vascular diseases, congenital, metabolic and storage, and neoplastic [1–5]. This chapter discusses the last three categories and in addition includes both diffuse and focal inflammatory/infectious diseases. Elsewhere in this syllabus, cirrhosis and vascular diseases are reviewed.

P. R. Ros
Department of Radiology, University Hospitals Health System/
Case Western Reserve University, Cleveland, OH, USA
e-mail: Pablo.Ros@UHhospitals.org

Metabolic and Storage Diseases

Steatosis and Steatohepatitis

Hepatic steatosis results from a variety of abnormal processes including increased production or mobilization of fatty acids (e.g., obesity, steroid use) or decreased hepatic clearance of fatty acids due to hepatocellular injury (e.g., alcoholic liver disease, viral hepatitis). Histopathologically, the hallmark of all forms of fatty liver is the accumulation of fat globules within the hepatocytes. The distribution of steatosis can be variable, ranging from focal, to regional, to diffuse. Diffuse steatosis is common and estimated to occur in approximately 30% of obese patients. Patients with steatosis are usually asymptomatic although some individuals may present with right upper quadrant pain or abnormal liver function parameters. Non-alcohol-related liver steatosis is also known as nonalcoholic fatty liver disease (NAFLD). Histopathologic findings of NAFLD vary from steatosis alone to steatosis with inflammation, necrosis, and fibrosis. At the most severe end of the NAFLD spectrum resides nonalcoholic steatohepatitis (NASH), with or without cirrhosis. Histopathologic findings of NASH include steatosis (predominately macrovesicular), mixed lobular inflammation, and hepatocellular ballooning. Unlike steatosis alone, NASH may progress to cirrhosis.

CT easily identifies diffuse steatosis. The attenuation value of normal liver is usually on average 8 HU greater than that of spleen on non-contrast CT images. In patients with fatty change, however, an abnormally decreased density will be demonstrated, typically 10 and 25 HU less than the spleen on non-contrast CT and contrast-enhanced CT images, respectively. The diagnosis of hepatic steatosis is more reliably made on non-contrast images.

Key Points

- The extent of fatty changes, iron deposition, and fibrotic remodeling can be quantified using MRI although their simultaneous presence can influence each other's results.
- Metastatic liver disease demonstrates mostly a multifocal disease, diffuse, and subtle presentation, requiring awareness and interpretation of indirect features.
- The liver is one of the most affected organs in parasitic diseases. Radiologists should be able to recognize and suspect the most relevant parasitic diseases, including hepatic schistosomiasis and echinococcosis.
- Acute hepatitis results in increased T1 and T2 relaxation times as well as periportal edema. Chronic hepatitis doesn't necessarily show distinct imaging features before developing into cirrhotic changes at long term.
- Imaging in infectious diseases might be crucial as they can be fatal if not promptly treated. With the help of CT and MRI, entities that may manifest with similar clinical and laboratory findings can be excluded.

Undoubtedly the most sensitive technique to detect fatty change of the liver is the use of inphase and out-of-phase gradient echo MR pulse sequences (Fig.). Multi-echo sequences, MR spectroscopy, and other MR techniques have been proposed to quantify the fat burden in the liver with success. Conjoint iron deposition, however, may be a confounding factor in estimating the fat fraction based on dual-echo chemical shift imaging. The fat fraction may be overestimated, and, therefore, the component of iron deposition requires correction as suggested by Kang et al.

Hepatic fatty change is, however, not always uniform but can present as a focal area of steatosis in an otherwise normal liver (focal steatosis) or as subtotal fatty change with sparing of certain areas (focal sparing) (Fig.). On imaging, sev-eral features allow the correct identification of focal fatty change or focal spared areas: (1) the typical periligamentous and periportal location, (2) lack of mass effect, (3) sharply angulated boundaries of the area, (4) nonspherical shape, (5) absence of vascular displacement or distorsion, and (6) lobar or segmental distribution [6, 7].

IronOverload

Iron overload states are categorized in hemochromatosis, where the iron accumulates preferentially within the hepatocytes, and hemosiderosis, where it is deposited in the Kupffer cells.

Primary Hemochromatosis

Hereditary or primary hemochromatosis is an autosomal recessive disorder of iron metabolism characterized by abnormal absorption of iron from the gut with subsequent excessive deposition of iron into the hepatocytes, pancreatic acinar cells, myocardium, joints, endocrine glands, and skin. In addition, the reticuloendothelial system (RES) cells in patients with primary hemochromatosis are abnormal and unable to store processed iron effectively. As a consequence, patients with primary hemochromatosis don't accumulate iron into the RES. Clinical findings of cirrhosis and its complications (portal hypertension, development of HCC) predominate in patients with long-lasting disease.

On CT excessive storage of iron into the hepatocytes will result in an overall *increased* density. However, this CT appearance of a hyperdense liver is nonspecific since similar features can be seen with gold deposition and in Wilson's disease, type IV glycogen storage disease, and following amiodarone administration. Performing non-contrast CT in patients with suspected hemochromatosis is important because excessive iron cannot be detected in the setting of enhancing parenchyma. However, the sensitivity of CT for iron is often insufficient as there is.

(a) A minimum threshold for liver iron detection that is five times higher than the normal liver iron level.
(b) Concomitant liver steatosis (hypodense appearance) may be similar to the CT appearance of early iron overstorage.

MRI is far more specific than any other imaging modalities for the characterization of iron overload due to the paramagnetic properties of iron. The superparamagnetic effect of accumulated iron in the hepatocytes results in significant reduction of T2 or T2* relaxation times which diminish the signal intensity on T2-weighted or on T1-weighted multi-echo spoiled gradient-echo images. Conversely to excessive storage of fat, in iron deposition, there will be an increase of signal intensity in chemical shift imaging from the in phase to the opposed phase. The amount of iron can be quantified using gradient-echo sequences with T2* weighting and progressively longer echo times. In general, comparison of the signal intensity of liver with that of paraspinal muscles provides a useful internal control. Hepatocellular carcinomas, complicating 35% of patients with advanced hemochromatosis, are usually easily detected on both T1- and T2-weighted images due to the background of decreased signal intensity of the liver [8, 9].

Hemosiderosis

In patients with hemosiderosis or siderosis, either due to transfusional iron overload states or dyserythropoiesis (e.g., thalassemia major, sideroblastic anemia, pyruvate kinase deficiency, chronic liver disease), the excessive iron is

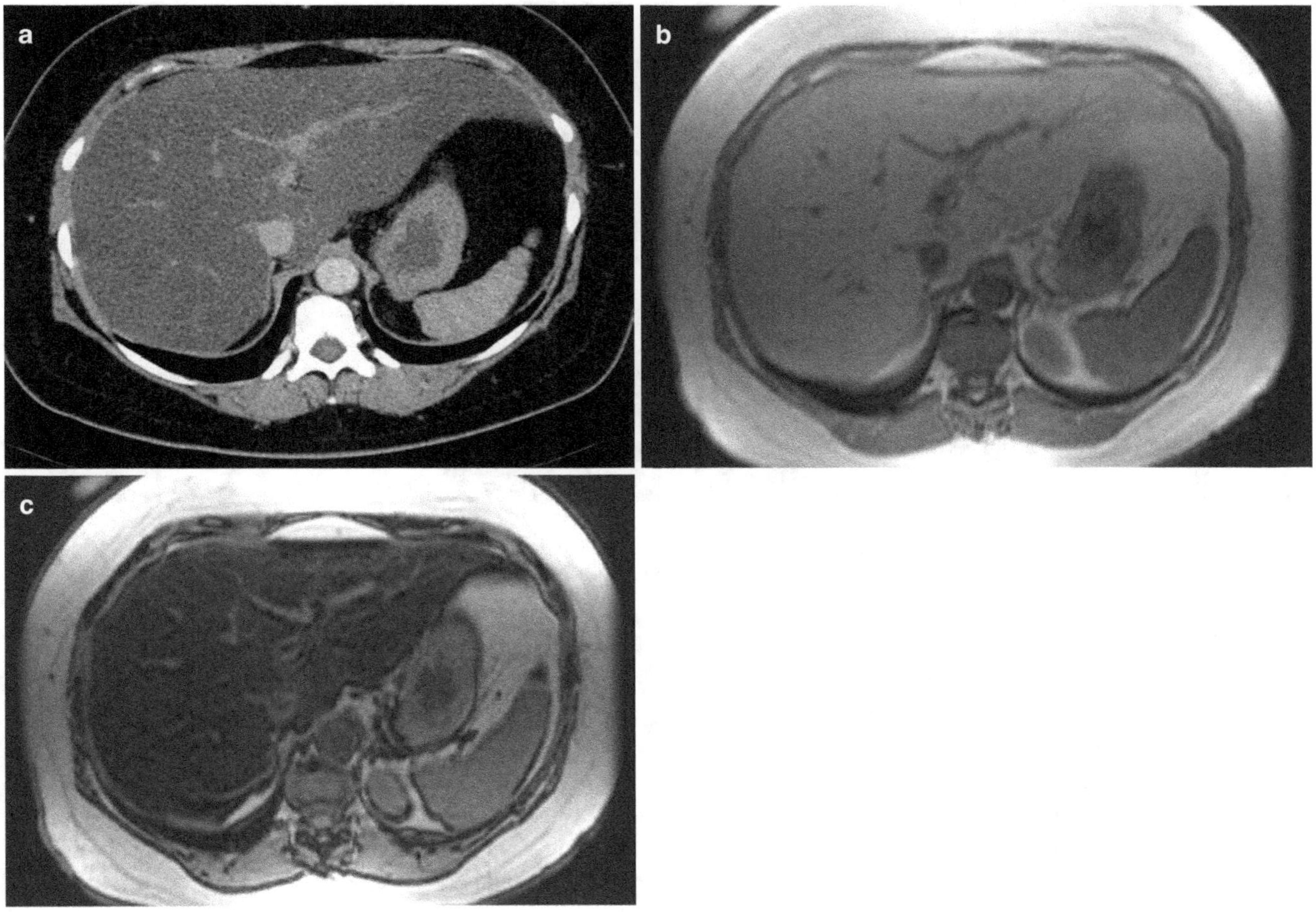

Fig. Diffuse fatty liver. 41-year-old female presenting with epigastric pain. Axial CECT image (**a**) demonstrates diffuse low attenuation of the liver without displacement of the hepatic vessels. In- (**b**) and out-of-phase (**c**) T1-weighted new MRI images show significant signal drop in the liver on the out-of-phase images

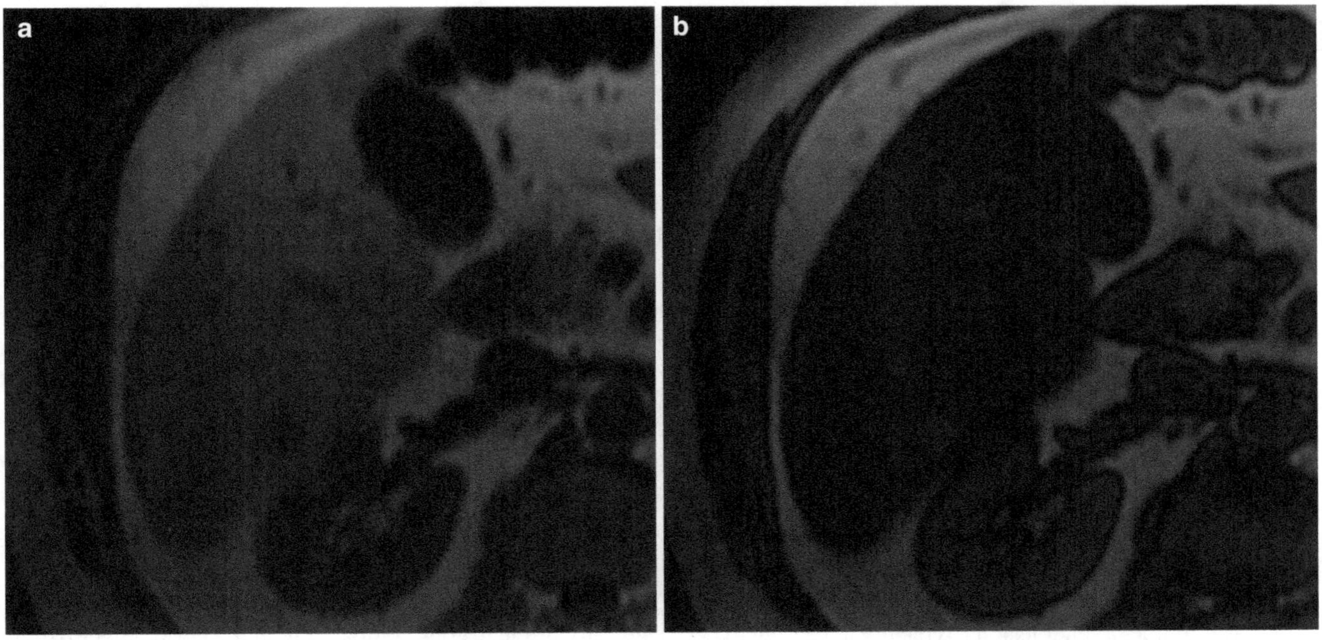

Fig. Hemosiderosis. Focal fatty sparing. 59-year-old male with right upper quadrant pain and elevated liver function tests. Axial chemical shift MRI images show signal drop of the entire steatotic liver from in- (**a**) to out-of-phase (**b**) with focal fatty sparing in liver segment 6

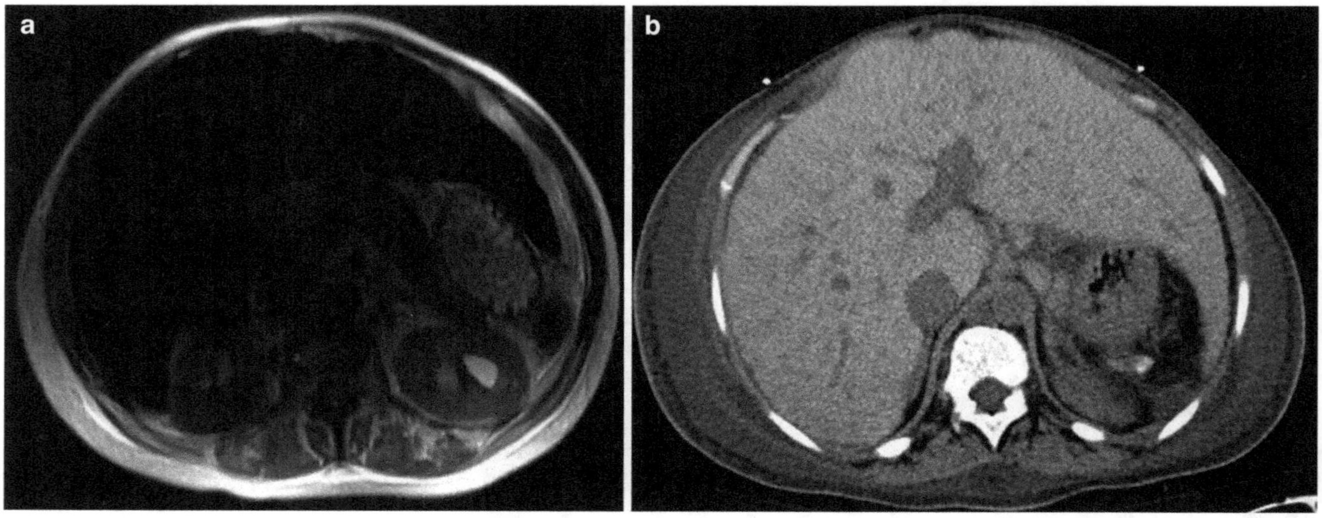

Fig. 29-year-old female with long history of sickle cell anemia requiring multiple transfusions. Axial T2-weighted MRI demonstrates significantly decreased liver-signal intensity and NECT increased attenuation in the liver due to the iron overload

processed and accumulates in organs containing reticuloendothelial cells, including liver, spleen, and bone marrow.

By CT, there is diffuse, increased attenuation of liver and spleen (Fig.). In MRI, the extrahepatic signal intensity changes in the spleen and bone marrow allow MR imaging to distinguish primary hemochromatosis from hemosiderosis. Although in general the clinical significance of transfusional iron overload states is negligible, patients with chronic hemosiderosis can develop symptoms similar to those of the primary form as well as cirrhosis and HCC.

Wilson Disease

Wilson disease, also known as hepatolenticular degeneration, is a rare autosomal recessive abnormality of copper metabolism characterized by accumulation of toxic levels of copper in the brain, cornea (Kayser-Fleischer rings), and liver, the latter due to impaired biliary excretion. Hepatic deposition of copper, predominantly seen in periportal areas and along the hepatic sinusoids, evokes an inflammatory reaction resulting in acute hepatitis with fatty change. Subsequently, chronic hepatitis may result in liver fibrosis and eventually macronodular cirrhosis.

Due to the high atomic number of copper, a hyperdense liver may be seen on unenhanced CT scans. However, this finding is not universally present, and usually only nonspecific signs such as hepatomegaly, fatty change, and, in advanced cases, cirrhosis are observed. During the early stage of the disease due to the paramagnetism of ionic copper, MR imaging can be valuable by demonstrating focal copper depositions as multiple nodular lesions, typically appearing hyperintense and hypointense on T1- and T2-weighted images, respectively, as described by Cheon JE et al [10].

Amyloidosis

Amyloidosis consists of deposition of fibrils of protein-mucopolysaccharide complexes throughout the body and is classified based on the biochemical composition of the amyloid fibrils. Primary amyloidosis is due to the deposition of immunoglobulin light chains and is associated with multiple myeloma and monoclonal gammopathy. Secondary amyloidosis is due to deposition of amyloid A protein and is associated with chronic infection, rheumatoid arthritis, and malignancies. Exceeded only by the spleen and kidney, the liver is the third most common solid organ prone to this deposition.

Hepatic amyloidosis has a nonspecific imaging appearance. The most common finding is diffuse hepatomegaly. CT sporadically demonstrates focal areas of low attenuation within the liver corresponding to sites of amyloid deposition (amyloid pseudotumor). Patients may present with a picture of jaundice which is due to intrahepatic cholestasis [11, 12].

NeoplasticDiseases

Metastatic Disease

Neoplastic infiltration due to diffuse metastatic disease can occur with many primary tumors. Melanoma, malignant neuroendocrine tumors, pancreatic adenocarcinoma, breast carcinoma, and colonic adenocarcinoma are some of the more commonly encountered causes of diffuse hepatic metastatic disease.

CT appearances of hepatic metastases depend on the vascularity of the lesions compared with the normal liver parenchyma. Diffuse metastatic involvement may produce only subtle imaging findings and be only detectable through

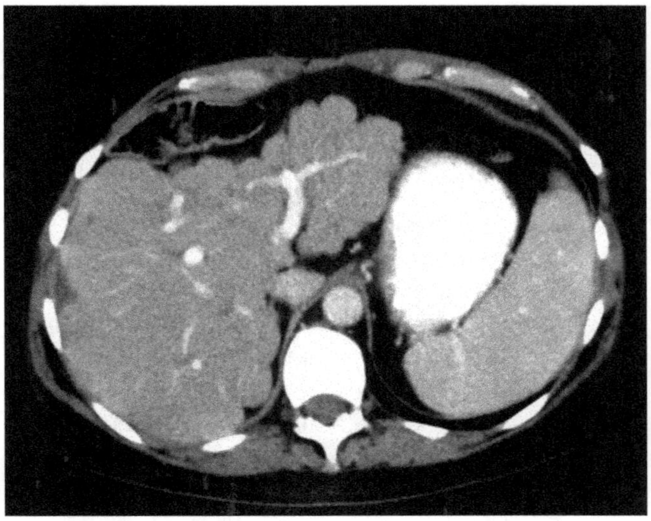

Fig. Diffuse metastatic breast cancer (pseudocirrhosis pattern). 43-year-old female treated for metastatic breast cancer. Axial CECT image demonstrates several small low-density lesions in the liver and a nodular contour of the liver due to hepatic capsular retraction

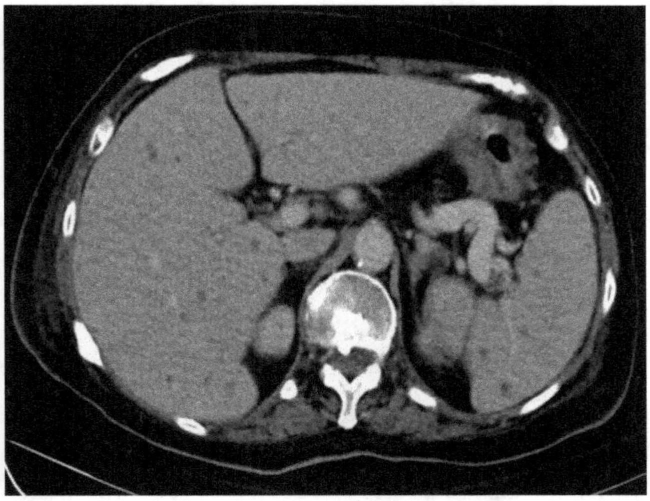

Fig. Hepatic candidiasis. 66-year-old female with leukemia presenting with abnormal liver function tests. Axial CECT image demonstrates multiple small low-attenuation lesions seen throughout the liver and spleen. Splenomegaly and bilateral pleural effusions are also present

indirect features, such as diffuse parenchymal heterogeneity, vascular and architectural distortion, or alterations of the liver contour. The latter, particularly seen in patients with treated breast cancer metastases, has been reported as the "pseudocirrhosis" sign (Fig.). In addition, treated breast cancer metastases may mimic the appearance of liver hemangiomata.

Lymphoma

Lymphoma can infiltrate the liver both primarily and secondarily. Primary lymphoma of the liver is extremely rare. Conversely the liver is often secondarily involved in both Hodgkin's and non-Hodgkin's lymphoma. Typically, the liver parenchyma is diffusely infiltrated with microscopic nests of neoplastic cells without significant architectural distortion, and, therefore, lymphomatous involvement is difficult to detect by imaging alone. Associated abnormalities, such as splenomegaly and lymphadenopathy, may narrow the differential diagnosis.

Diffuse Infectious and Inflammatory Diseases

Fungal Infections

Hepatosplenic fungal infection is a clinical manifestation of disseminated fungal disease in patients with hematologic malignancies or compromise of the immunologic system. The reported prevalence of fungal dissemination ranges from 20% to 40%. Most hepatic fungal microabscesses occur in leukemia patients and are caused by *Candida albicans* [16].

Candidiasis

Candida albicans, in the liver, may evoke little or no inflammatory reaction, cause a superlative response, or occasionally produce granulomas. The typical histologic pattern of hepatic candidiasis is characterized by microabscesses, with the yeast or pseudohyphal forms of the fungus in the center of the lesion and a surrounding area of necrosis and polymorphonuclear infiltrate.

At contrast-enhanced CT, fungal microabscesses usually appear as multiple rounds, discrete areas of low attenuation, generally ranging from 2 to 20 mm (Fig.). These micro-abscesses usually enhance centrally after intravenous admin-istration of contrast medium, although peripheral enhancement may occur.

At MR imaging, the untreated nodules are rounded lesions less than 1 cm in diameter that are minimally hypointense on T1-weighted and gadolinium-enhanced images and markedly hyperintense on T2-weighted images. After treatment, lesions appear mildly to moderately hyperintense on T1- and T2-weighted images and demonstrate enhancement on gadolinium-enhanced images. A dark ring is usually seen around these lesions with all sequences. Completely treated lesions are minimally hypointense on T1-weighted images, isointense to mildly hyperintense on T2-weighted images, moderately hypointense on early gadolinium-enhanced images, and minimally hypointense on delayed gadolinium-enhanced images. MR imaging is superior to CT and US in the detection of these fungal foci [17].

GranulomatousDiseases

Granulomatous hepatitis is associated with a wide variety of conditions, most commonly with sarcoidosis, tuberculosis, and histoplasmosis. Hepatic granulomas usually appear as discrete, sharply defined nodules consisting of aggregates of epithelioid cells by a rim of mononuclear cells, predominantly lymphocytes.

Sarcoidosis

Sarcoidosis is a multisystem disorder of unknown pathogenesis, characterized by noncaseating granulomas. Although it may involve almost any organ in the body, pulmonary sarcoidosis is most common. Sarcoidosis of the liver is also relatively frequently seen, but the granulomas are usually not macroscopically detectable and thus may not produce focal abnormalities on imaging studies. Classically, the granulomas develop in a periportal location resulting in periportal fibrosis, cirrhosis, and eventually portal hypertension.

Hepatic contrast-enhanced CT may typically reveal multiple, diffuse small low-density areas in both the liver and spleen (Fig.). MRI features of hepatic sarcoidosis are also nonspecific and include organomegaly, multiple low- signal- intensity lesions relative to background paren-chyma with all sequences, increased periportal signal, irregularity of the portal and hepatic vein branches, and patchy areas of heterogeneous signal. Recent literature by Ferreira et al. confirms the nonspecific appearance but describes as a characteristic feature with large central regenerative nodules and wedge-shaped areas of peripheral parenchymal atrophy [18, 19].

Tuberculosis

Tuberculosis is one of the most common infectious diseases worldwide. Generally, tuberculosis in the liver presents as either miliary or focal form. Focal hepatic TB is further subdivided into nodular (i.e., tuberculous abscess and tuberculoma) and tubular or hepatobiliary tuberculosis (i.e., tuberculosis involving the intrahepatic ducts). Hepatic miliary tuberculosis is the most common and is reported to occur in 50–80% of all patients with terminal pulmonary tuberculosis. Miliary tuberculosis is usually not detected by imaging. Hepatomegaly may be the only radiological abnormality.

In the healing stage of tuberculosis, CT may show diffuse hepatic calcifications (approximately 50% of cases). Reported CT findings of nodular tuberculosis are nonspecific and include hypoattenuating lesions both before and after intravenous contrast administration.

At MR imaging, the lesions are hypointense on T1-weighted images and hypo- to isointense on T2-weighted images. Tuberculosis lesion differently enhances after gadolinium administration. Because of these rather nonspecific findings with all imaging techniques, percutaneous liver biopsy is necessary [20].

Histoplasmosis

Histoplasmosis is the most common cause of fungal infection in the Ohio River Valley of the United States. Fortunately, 99% of patients exposed to histoplasmosis develop only subclinical infections. Liver involvement is common in disseminated histoplasmosis, which usually originates in the lungs. The most common hepatic findings include portal lymphohistiocytic inflammation and discrete, well-delineated granu-

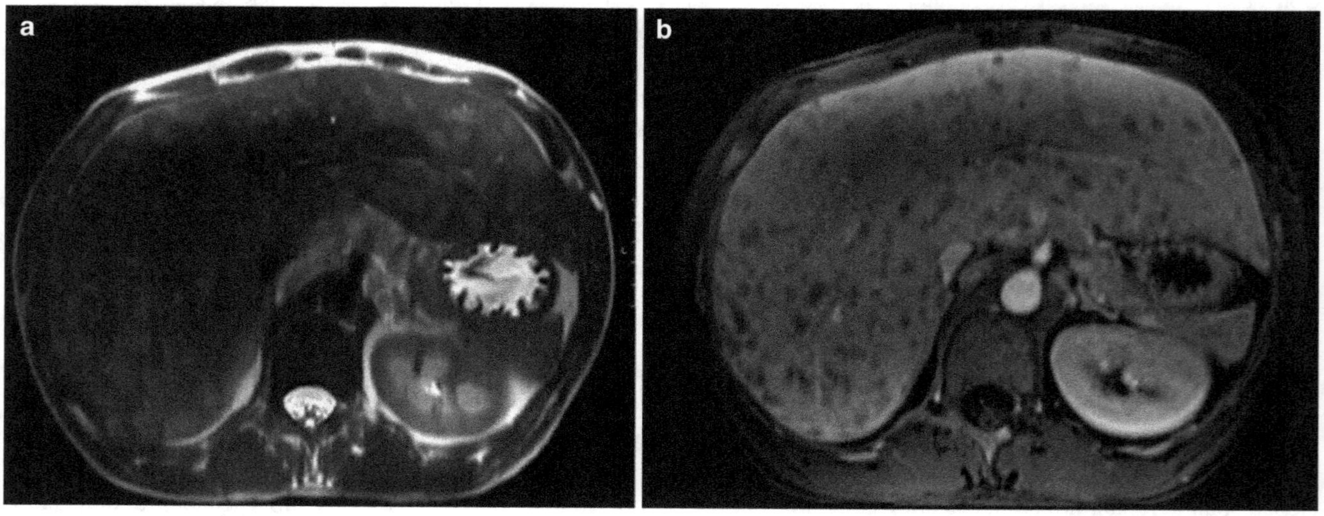

Fig. Hepatic sarcoidosis. 44-year-old male with fever and hilar adenopathy on chest X-ray. Axial T2-weighted (left) and T1-weighted post-contrast (right) MR images show multiple small T2-hyperintense, T1-hypointense, ring-enhancing lesions throughout the liver. Note the small spleen that is consistent with chronic auto infarction from coexisting sickle cell anemia lomas. In patients with healed histoplasmosis, the presence of small, punctate calcifications scattered throughout the liver and spleen is typical but nonspecific finding [21].

ParasiticInfections

Schistosomiasis

Schistosoma japonicum, *S. haematobium*, and *S. mansoni* are the three most important species that infect humans. The schistosomas live in the bowel lumen and lay eggs in the mesenteric veins. The eggs may then embolize to the portal vein. The eggs themselves do not survive and subsequently calcify. Chronic infections with either *S. japonicum* or *S. mansoni* result in the formation of cirrhosis and the risk of development of hepatocellular carcinoma. Histologically, schistosomiasis is characterized by white, pinhead-sized granulomas scattered throughout the liver. At the center of each granuloma is a schistosome egg. Periportal fibrosis is the major pathological consequence of the *Schistosoma mansoni* infection. In severe infections, the surface of the liver shows granulomatous involvement and widespread fibrous portal enlargement ("pipestem" fibrosis).

At CT, the most pathognomonic pattern is the presence of calcified septa, usually aligned perpendicular to the liver capsule ("tortoiseshell" or "turtleback" appearance).

Viral Infections

Viral Hepatitis

Acute viral hepatitis is a systemic infection that affects the liver and is usually caused by one of five viral agents: hepatitis A virus, hepatitis B virus (HBV), hepatitis C virus, the HBV-associated delta agent or hepatitis D virus, and hepatitis E virus. A vast array of other viruses may also produce hepatitis, including herpes viruses, yellow-fever virus, rubella virus, Coxsackievirus, and adenovirus. The diagnosis of acute hepatitis is usually based on serologic, virologic, and clinical findings. Probably the most important role of radiology in patients with acute hepatitis is to help rule out other diseases that produce similar clinical and biochemical abnormalities, such as extrahepatic cholestasis, diffuse metastatic disease, and cirrhosis.

At CT and MR imaging, findings in acute viral hepatitis are nonspecific and include hepatomegaly and periportal edema. At CT, heterogeneous enhancement and well-defined regions of low attenuation may be present. At MR imaging, periportal edema appears as high-signal-intensity areas on T2-weighted images. Involved areas may be normal or demonstrate decreased signal intensity on T1-weighted images and increased signal intensity on T2-weighted images. There is also impaired uptake of liver-specific agents. Extrahepatic findings in patients with severe acute hepatitis include gallbladder wall thickening due to edema and, infrequently, ascites. In chronic hepatitis, the CT and MR imaging features resemble those of early-stage liver cirrhosis. Periportal lymphadenopathy may be the sole detectable abnormality in both acute and chronic hepatitis.

HIV Infection

The liver and biliary tracts are frequent sites of involvement during the course of HIV infection. Coinfection with hepatitis B and C viruses is particularly common due to the shared means of transmission of these viruses with HIV. AIDS-related cholangiopathy is the newest common manifestation. At CT, inflammation of the gallbladder or biliary tree manifests as mural thickening or abnormal contrast enhancement. MRCP is more sensitive and specific than US or CT in depicting the mural irregularity of the extrahepatic ducts that result from the exuberant periductal inflammation, focal mucosal ulcers, and interstitial edema found in AIDS-related cholangitis.

Uncommon Hepatic Infections

Cat-Scratch Disease

Cat-scratch disease is an infection that affects immunocompetent children or adolescents. It is caused by *Bartonella henselae*, a gram-negative bacillus that is usually introduced by the scratch of a cat. Cat-scratch disease takes many forms, from regional lymphadenitis to disseminated infection. The typical clinical manifestation of cat-scratch disease is painful lymphadenopathy proximal to the site of inoculation. Disseminated infection is seen in 5–10% of cases. In the abdomen, multiple granulomas ranging from 3 to 30 mm may form in the liver and spleen, with or without hepatosplenomegaly. Histopathologic findings include vascular proliferative lesions (peliosis hepatis) and necrotizing granulomatous lesions.

At unenhanced CT, the lesions are hypoattenuating relative to normal parenchyma. Three different patterns at contrast-enhanced CT have been described: *(a)* persistent hypoattenuation relative to the liver, *(b)* isoattenuation relative to surrounding tissues, and *(c)* marginal enhancement. Only a few MR imaging studies of cat-scratch disease have been described. The lesions appear as low-signal-intensity nodules on T1-weighted MR images and as high-signal-intensity nodules on T2-weighted images. Peripheral enhancement may be seen on gadolinium-enhanced T1-weighted images [23, 24].

Bacillary Angiomatosis

Bacillary angiomatosis is also a manifestation of infection by *Bartonella henselae in* immunocompromised patients.

This is the same organism that causes cat-scratch disease in noncompromised patients. It is characterized by localized areas of vascular proliferation that may affect the skin, airway, mucous membranes, visceral organs, bone, and brain. Contrast-enhanced CT may demonstrate multiple diffuse low- or high-attenuation lesions less than 1 cm scattered throughout the hepatic parenchyma. Ascites, mild periportal edema, and intrahepatic biliary ductal dilatation may occur. These imaging features are nonspecific and must be distinguished, especially in AIDS patients, from hepatic abscesses related to other bacteria, viruses, or fungi; AIDS-related lymphoma; Kaposi sarcoma; and, less commonly, disseminated *Pneumocystis carinii* infection [25].

Focal Infections

Bacterial (Pyogenic) Abscess

Pyogenic abscess, although uncommon in the antibiotic era, is still challenging clinically since its presentation is quite variable, from profound septicemia to chronic, indolent symptoms.

Enhanced CT can reliably diagnose over 90% of hepatic pyogenic abscesses, revealing two main patterns: multiple microabscesses (disseminated or clustered) and large macroabscesses. By virtue of its good spatial and contrast resolution, computed tomography (CT) is the single best method for detecting hepatic abscess, with a sensitivity as high as 97%. On CT scans, abscesses appear as generally rounded masses that are hypodense on both contrast and non-contrast scans. Central gas, either as air bubbles or an air-fluid level, is a specific sign, but it is present in less than 20% of cases. A thick, enhancing, peripheral rim is also noted.

At MR imaging, air within the abscess appears as a signal void and is therefore more difficult to differentiate from calcifications. However, the shape and location (air-fluid level) should enable the correct diagnosis. After administration of gadolinium-DTPA, abscesses typically show rim enhancement (the "double-target" sign). Small lesions (<1 cm) may enhance homogeneously mimicking hemangiomas. Percutaneous, image-guided aspiration followed by drainage is the method of choice for definitive diagnosis and treatment with success in over 90% of cases.

Amebic Abscess

Hepatic abscess is the most common extraintestinal manifestation of amebiasis, affecting approximately 10% of patients with amebiasis. Although rare in the continental United States, 10% of the world's population is infected with *Entamoeba histolytica*. Clinically, patients with amebic abscess are more acutely ill than patients with pyogenic abscess, with high fever and right upper quadrant pain. Diagnosis is made by positive serologic amebic titers, although they have false-negative rates of almost 20%.

CT demonstrates well the extrahepatic extensions to chest wall, pleura, or adjacent viscera. Percutaneous catheter drainage of an amebic abscess is rarely necessary because of the effectiveness of amebicidal therapy. Occasionally, percutaneous drainage is needed in large, symptomatic abscesses with poor response to medical therapy, suspected bacterial superinfection, and threatening intrapericardial rupture. The CT appearance of amebic abscess is variable and nonspecific. The lesions are usually peripheral, round, or oval areas of low attenuation (10–20 Hounsfield units). A peripheral rim of slightly higher attenuation can be seen on non-contrast scans and shows marked enhancement after administration of contrast material.

On MR imaging, amebic liver abscesses are spherical and usually solitary lesions with a hyperintense center on T2-weighted images and a hypointense center on T1-weighted images. The abscess wall is thick, and on gadolinium-enhanced images, the enhancement pattern is similar to that of pyogenic abscess [26].

Echinococcal Disease

Hydatid disease has two main forms affecting humans *Echinococcus granulosus* and *Echinococcus multilocularis or alveolaris*. These infections have well-defined and different geographic distributions. The pathologic and imaging findings differ dramatically between these parasites.

On CT scans, *E. granulosus* appears as unilocular or multilocular, well-defined cysts with either thick or thin walls. Daughter cysts are usually seen as areas of lower attenuation than the mother cyst and are usually in the periphery of the lesion. Daughter cysts can also float free in the lumen of the mother cyst, so altering the patient's position may change the position of these cysts, confirming the diagnosis of echinococcal disease. Curvilinear ring-like calcification is also a common feature.

On MR studies, the cyst component of echinococcal cysts is similar to that of other cysts, with long T1 and T2 relaxation times. However, MR imaging best demonstrates the pericyst, the matrix and hydatid sand (debris consisting of freed scolices), and the daughter cysts. The pericyst usually has low-signal intensity on T1- and T2-weighted images, because of its fibrous component. This rim and a multiloculated or multicystic appearance are distinctive features. The

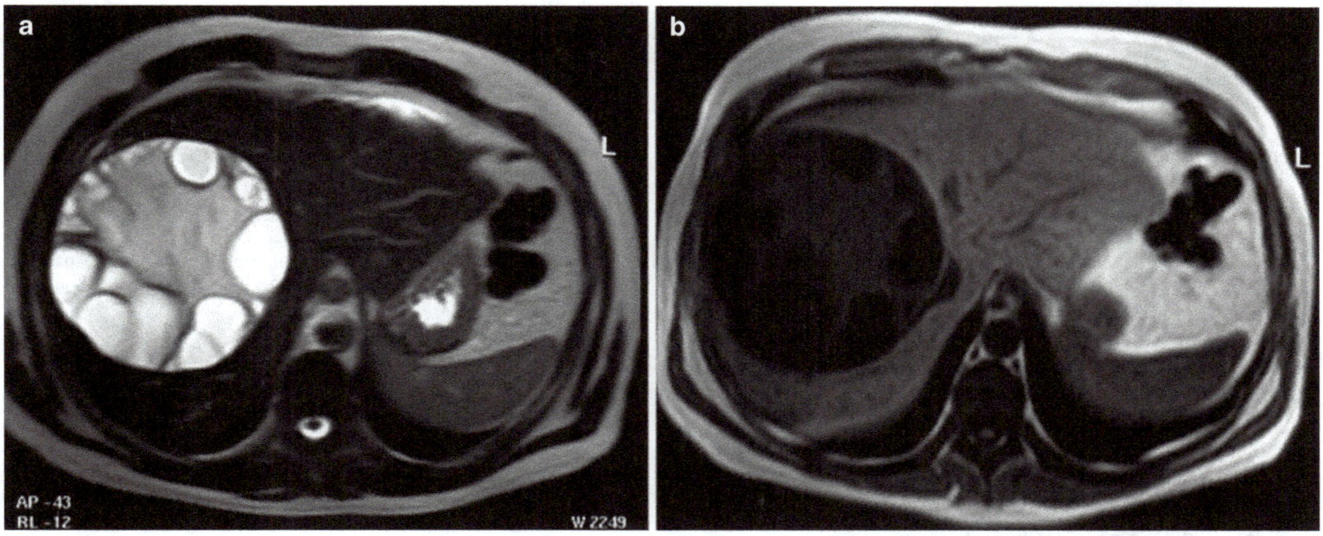

Fig. Echinococcus granulosus cyst. 28-year-old man with right upper quadrant pain. Axial (**a**) T2-weighted image demonstrates a large cystic mass in the right lobe of the liver which is surrounded by a hypointense rim and contains more hyperintense smaller cysts in its periphery. On the axial T1-weighted image (**b**), the hypointense rim is well visualized, and the peripheral cysts are hypointense relative to the center of the lesion

hydatid matrix appears hypointense on T1-weighted images and markedly hyperintense on T2-weighted images. When present, daughter cysts are hypointense relative to the matrix on both T1- and T2-weighted images (Fig.). Floating membranes have low-signal intensities on T1- and T2-weighted images.

E. multilocularis appears as a solid large mass or masses, with minimal to no enhancement after intravenous administration of contrast material and possible small punctate calcification [27–29].

Concluding Remarks

The spectrum of diffuse liver diseases includes a broad range of different entities including metabolic, storage, neoplastic, infectious, and inflammatory disorders. They may have unique or overlapping image findings. Knowing the typical features of the different diffuse and inflammatory liver diseases with CT and MRI techniques allows radiologists to play a key role in the diagnosis and management of diffuse liver diseases. Likewise, focal inflammatory diseases such as abscesses and hydatid disease can be characterized by imaging [14, 22, 30].

Acknowledgments We appreciate the contributions of Verena Obmann, MD, in updating this manuscript from it's prior version (cite: Hodler J, Kubik-Huch R, von Schulthess GK, Zollikofer ChL, editors. Diseases of the abdomen and pelvis 2014–2017. Springer 2014. pp. 87–94).

Take-Home Messages

- Storage diseases generally involve the liver diffusely but can also manifest as focal alterations and can mimic other pathologies including malignancy.
- Diffuse neoplastic involvement may produce subtle imaging findings and be only detectable through indirect features, such as hepatomegaly, diffuse parenchymal heterogeneity, vascular and architectural distortion, or alterations of the liver contour.
- Imaging in infectious diseases might be crucial as they can be fatal if not promptly treated. CT and MRI play a crucial role to differentiate and characterize diffuse and inflammatory liver disease.

References

1. Hamm B, Ros PR, editors. Abdominal imaging, vol. 1–4. Berlin: Springer; 2013.
2. Ros PR, Mortele KJ, Pelsser V, Thomas S. CT/MRI of the abdomen and pelvis: a teaching file. 3rd ed. Philadelphia, PA: Wolters Klumer/Lippincott, Williams and Wilkins; 2013.
3. Ros PR. Hepatic imaging and intervention. In clinics in liver disease. Philadelphia, PA: W.B. Saunders; 2002.
4. Mortele KJ, Ros PR. Imaging of diffuse liver disease. Semin Liver Dis. 2001;21(2):195–212.
5. Chundru S, Kalb B, Arif-Tiwari H, Sharma P, Costello J, Martin DR. MRI of diffuse liver disease: the common and uncommon etiologies. Diagn Interv Radiol. 2013;19(6):479–87.

6. Other GB. Diffuse liver diseases: steatosis, hemochromaosis, etc. In: Hamm B, Ros PR, editors. Abdominal imaging, vol. 70. Berlin: Springer; 2013. p. 1027–44. Volume II Sec. V.
7. Kang BK, Yu ES, Lee SS, Lee Y, Kim N, Sirlin CB, Cho EY, Yeom SK, Byun JH, Park SH, Lee MG. Hepatic fat quantification: a prospective comparison of magnetic resonance spectroscopy and analysis methods for chemical-shift gradient echo magnetic resonance imaging with histologic assessment as the reference standard. Investig Radiol. 2012;47(6):368–75.
8. Queiroz-Andrade M, Blasbalg R, Ortega CD, Rodstein MAM, Baroni RH, Rocha MS, Cerri GG. MR imaging findings of iron overload. Radiographics. 2009;29:1575–89.
9. Wood JC, Ghugre N. Magnetic resonance imaging assessment of excess iron in thalassemia, sickle cell disease and other iron overload diseases. Hemoglobin. 2008;32:85–96.
10. Cheon JE, Kim IO, Seo JK, Ko JS, Lee JM, Shin CI, Kim WS, Yeon KM. Clinical application of liver MR imaging in Wilson's disease. Korean J Radiol. 2010;11(6):665–72.
11. Ros PR, Sobin LH. Amyloidosis: the same cat, with different stripes. Radiology. 1994;190:14–5.
12. Marmoloya G, Karlins NL, Petrelli M, McCullough A. Unusual computed tomography findings in hepatic amyloidosis. Clin Imaging. 1990;14:248.
13. Bachler P, Baladron MJ, Menias C, Beddings I, Loch R, Zalaquett E, et al. Multimodality imaging of liver infections: differential diagnosis and potential pitfalls. Radiographics. 2016;36(4):1001–23.
14. Erturk SM, Yapici O. Liver inflammatory and infectious diseases. In: Hamm B, Ros PR, editors. Abdominal imaging, vol. 68. Berlin: Springer; 2013. p. 1001–12. Volume II Sec. V.
15. Mortele KJ, Segatto E, Ros PR. The infected liver: radiologic-pathologic correlation. Radiographics. 2004;24:937–55.
16. Semelka RC, Kelekis NL, Sallah S, Worawattanakul S, Ascher SM. Hepatosplenic fungal disease: diagnostic accuracy and spectrum of appearances on MR imaging. AJR. 1997;169(5):1311–6.
17. Pastakia B, Shawker TH, Thaler M, O'Leary T, Pizzo PA. Hepatosplenic candidiasis: wheels within wheels. Radiology. 1988;166:417–44.
18. Ferreira A, Ramalho M, de Campos RO, Heredia V, Roque A, Vaidean G, Semelka RC. Hepatic sarcoidosis: MR appearances in patients with chronic liver disease. Magn Reson Imaging. 2013;31(3):432–8.
19. Palmucci S, Torrisi SE, Caltabiano DC, Puglisi S, Lentini V, Grassedonio E, et al. Clinical and radiological features of extra-pulmonary sarcoidosis: a pictorial essay. Insights Imaging. 2016;7(4):571–87.
20. Karaosmanoglu AD, Onur MR, Sahani DV, Tabari A, Karcaaltincaba M. Hepatobiliary tuberculosis: imaging findings. AJR Am J Roentgenol. 2016:1–11.
21. Monzawz S, Ohtomo K, Oba H, et al. Septa in the liver of patients with chronic hepatic Schistosomiasis japonica: MR appearance. AJR. 1994;162:1347–51.
22. Mortele KJ, Ros PR. MR imaging in chronic hepatitis and cirrhosis. Semin Ultrasound CT MR. 2002;23(1):79–100.
23. Danon O, Duval-Arnould M, Osman Z, et al. Hepatic and splenic involvement in cat-scratch disease: imaging features. Abdom Imaging. 2000;25:182–3.
24. Rappaport DC, Cumming WA, Ros PR. Disseminated hepatic and splenic lesions in cat-scratch disease: imaging features. AJR. 1991;156:1227–8.
25. Moore EH, Russell LA, Klein JS, et al. Bacillary angiomatosis in patients with AIDS: multiorgan imaging findings. Radiology. 1995;197:67–72.
26. Van Allen RJ, Katz MD, Johnson MB, Laine LA, Liu Y, Ralls PW. Uncomplicated amebic liver abscess: prospective evaluation of percutaneous therapeutic aspiration. Radiology. 1992;183:827–30.
27. Czermak BV, Akhan O, Hiemetzberger R, Zelger B, Vogel W, Jaschke W, et al. Echinococcosis of the liver. Abdom Imaging. 2008;33(2):133–43.
28. Kantarci M, Bayraktutan U, Karabulut N, Aydinli B, Ogul H, Yuce I, et al. Alveolar echinococcosis: spectrum of findings at cross-sectional imaging. Radiographics. 2012;32(7):2053–70.
29. Alghofaily KA, Saeedan MB, Aljohani IM, Alrasheed M, McWilliams S, Aldosary A, et al. Hepatic hydatid disease complications: review of imaging findings and clinical implications. Abdom Radiol (NY). 2017;42(1):199–210.
30. Boll DT, Merkle EM. Diffuse liver disease: strategies for hepatic CT and MR imaging. Radiographics. 2009;29:1591–614.

8

Diseases of the Upper GI Tract

Richard M. Gore and Marc S. Levine

Learning Objectives

- To review the key double-contrast upper GI examination features of benign infectious and inflammatory esophagitis
- To identify the double-contrast barium features of the various gastritides
- To review the role of MDCT, endoscopic ultrasound, MR, PET/CT, PET-MR, and functional imaging in the staging and follow-up of esophageal cancer
- To understand the role of MDCT, endoscopic ultrasound, MR, PET/CT, PET-MR, and functional imaging in the staging and follow-up of gastric cancer

NonneoplasticConditions

Gastroesophageal Reflux Disease

Early reflux esophagitis typically is characterized on double-contrast studies by granularity of the distal esophagus secondary to mucosal edema and inflammation [1]. Shallow ulcers appear as punctate, linear, or serpiginous barium collections, sometimes associated with radiating folds [1]. This ulceration almost always extends proximally from the gastroesophageal junction as a continuous area of disease, so ulcers that are confined to the upper or midesophagus should suggest another cause for the patient's disease. Scarring from reflux esophagitis can lead to the development of reflux-induced (peptic) strictures, typically seen as smooth, tapered areas of distal esophageal narrowing or as asymmetric ringlike strictures above a hiatal hernia [1].

Barrett'sEsophagus

Barrett's esophagus is a premalignant condition in which the usual squamous epithelium in the distal esophagus is replaced my metaplastic columnar epithelium secondary to chronic reflux esophagitis. This condition develops in 10% of patients with reflux esophagitis and 20–40% with peptic strictures [1]. Barrett's esophagus sometimes can be recognized on barium studies by the development of a tapered or ringlike stricture in the midesophagus [1]. Other patients may develop a distinctive reticular pattern of the mucosa [2]. In the presence of a hiatal hernia and reflux, a high stricture or reticular pattern should be strongly suggestive of Barrett's esophagus. Another recently reported finding of Barrett's esophagus is a high Z line at the level of an elevated squamocolumnar mucosal junction above long-segment columnar metaplasia [3].

InfectiousEsophagitis

Candida esophagitis typically is manifested on double-contrast barium studies by multiple discrete linear or irregular plaquelike defects separated by normal mucosa [4]. Patients with AIDS occasionally may develop a more fulminant form of candidiasis characterized by a grossly irregular or shaggy esophagus secondary to trapping of barium between innumerable plaques and pseudomembranes [5].

R. M. Gore, M.D. (✉)
North Shore University Health System, Evanston, IL, USA

Pritzker School of Medicine at the University of Chicago, Chicago, IL, USA

M. S. Levine, M.D.
Hospital of the University of Pennsylvania, Philadelphia, PA, USA

Perelman School of Medicine at the University of Pennsylvania, Philadelphia, PA, USA

In an immunocompromised patient with dysphagia or odynophagia, these findings should be highly suggestive of *Candida* esophagitis. In contrast, herpes esophagitis usually is characterized by multiple small, discrete ulcers in the upper or midesophagus without associated plaque formation (Fig.) [ ].

Patients with AIDS occasionally may develop CMV esophagitis, manifested by giant ulcers greater than 1 cm in size [7]. Because herpetic ulcers rarely become this large, giant ulcers should suggest CMV in patients with AIDS. Human immunodeficiency virus (HIV) has also been recognized as a cause of giant esophageal ulcers indistinguishable from those in CMV [8]. Unlike CMV ulcers, however, HIV ulcers may undergo rapid healing on treatment with oral steroids, so endoscopy is required to differentiate these infections.

EosinophilicEsophagitis

Eosinophilic esophagitis (EoE) has been recognized as a chronic inflammatory disease causing dysphagia and recurrent food impactions in young men, who often have a history of allergies, asthma, or peripheral eosinophilia. EoE may be manifested on esophagography by segmental strictures, discrete ringlike indentations (the so-called ringed esophagus) [9], or a small-caliber esophagus with smooth, long-segment narrowing of virtually the entire thoracic esophagus (Fig.) [ ]. Recently, lichen planus involving the esophagus has been recognized as another cause of a small-caliber esophagus indistinguishable from that in EoE [11]. Unlike EoE, however, lichen planus typically occurs in elderly women with a skin rash

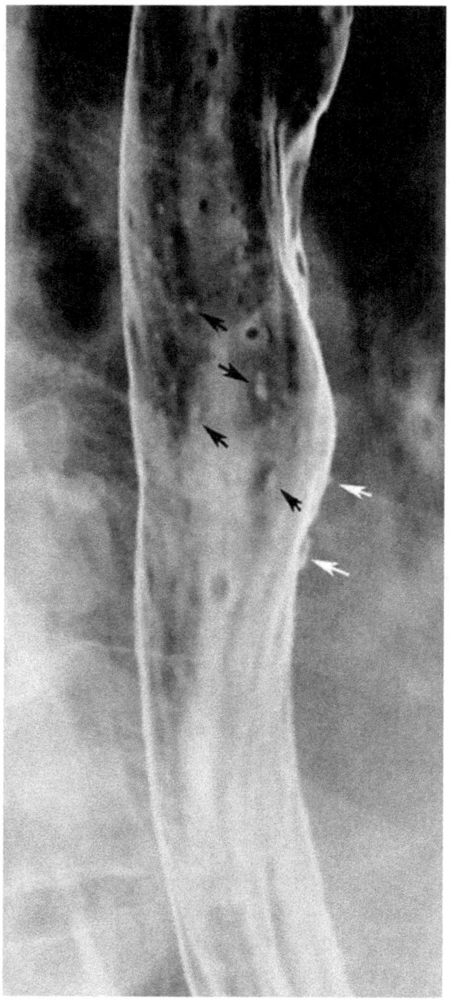

Fig. Herpes esophagitis. Double-contrast esophagram shows multiple small, discrete ulcers both en face (black arrows) and in profile (white arrows) in the midesophagus. In the appropriate clinical setting, these findings are highly suggestive of herpes esophagitis

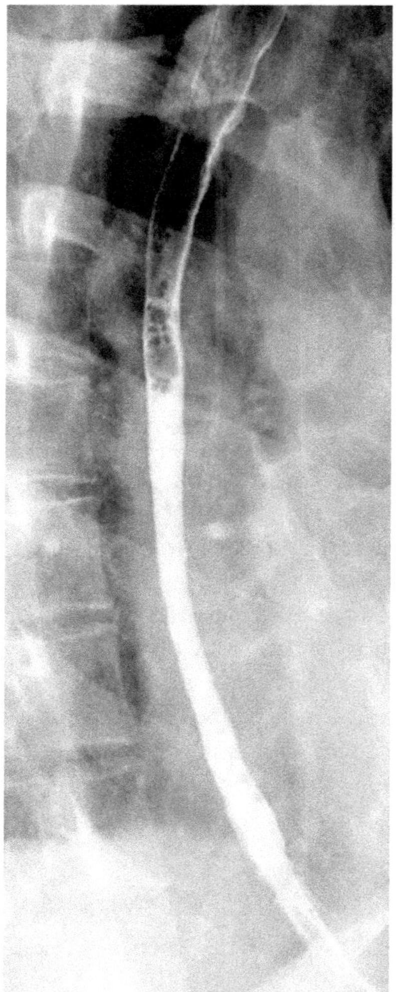

Fig. Eosinophilic esophagitis with a small-caliber esophagus. Barium esophagram shows diffuse narrowing of the entire thoracic esophagus, which has a smooth, uniform contour. This was a young man with long-standing dysphagia and asthma. Lichen planus involving the esophagus may produce identical findings, but these patients tend to be elderly woman, often presenting with dysphagia and a skin rash and is not associated with allergies, asthma, or peripheral eosinophilia [11].

Drug-InducedEsophagitis

Drug-induced esophagitis is caused by various medications, including tetracycline, doxycycline, potassium chloride, quinidine, alendronate, and nonsteroidal anti-inflammatory drugs (NSAIDs) [12]. Affected individuals often ingest the medication with little or no water immediately before going to bed, so the medication lodges in the midesophagus, causing a focal contact esophagitis. Double-contrast studies may reveal a focal cluster of small, discrete ulcers in the mid-esophagus indistinguishable from those in herpes esophagitis [12], but the correct diagnosis usually is suggested by the clinical history.

ErosiveGastritis

Erosive gastritis is characterized on double-contrast studies by multiple punctate or slitlike collections of barium surrounded by radiolucent halos of edematous mucosa [13]. The erosions tend to be located in the gastric antrum and often are aligned on the crests of the folds. NSAIDs are by far the most common cause of erosive gastritis, accounting for more than 50% of cases. Occasionally, however, NSAID-induced erosive gastritis may be manifested by multiple distinctive linear or serpiginous erosions that tend to be clustered in the gastric antrum or body, often near the greater curvature [14]. These erosions are thought to result from localized mucosal injury as the dissolving NSAID capsules collect by gravity in the most dependent portion of the stomach. Whatever the explanation, detection of this finding should lead to careful questioning about recent NSAID use, and if confirmed, the offending medication should be withdrawn.

Helicobacter Pylori Gastritis

Helicobacter pylori gastritis can be diagnosed on barium studies by thickened folds in the antrum, body, or, less commonly, fundus of the stomach [15]. Other patients with *H. pylori* may have a polypoid form of gastritis characterized by grossly thickened, lobulated folds, mimicking the appearance of Ménétrier's disease, lymphoma, or even a submucosally infiltrating carcinoma [15]. In these cases, endoscopy and biopsy are required for a definitive diagnosis.

GastricUlcers

Benign gastric ulcers classically appear en face as round or ovoid barium collections with a smooth, surrounding mound of edema and/or thin, straight folds radiating to the edge of the ulcer crater [16]. When viewed in profile, benign ulcers project beyond the gastric wall and are often associated with an ulcer mound or collar. In contrast, malignant ulcers appear en face as irregular craters in a discrete mass with nodularity or clubbing of adjoining folds [16]. When viewed in profile, malignant ulcers project inside the lumen within a mass that forms acute angles with the wall rather than the obtuse angles expected for a benign mound of edema [16].

Most benign ulcers are located on the lesser curvature or posterior wall of the gastric antrum of the body [16]. Occasionally, however, benign ulcers may occur on the greater curvature of the distal antrum, and nearly all of these ulcers are found to be caused by NSAIDs [16]. As NSAID-induced greater curvature ulcers enlarge, they can penetrate inferiorly via the gastrocolic ligament into the transverse colon, producing a gastrocolic fistula [17]. In today's pill-oriented society, these NSAID-induced ulcers are the most common cause of gastrocolic fistulas.

NeoplasticConditions

EsophagealCancer

On double-contrast barium studies, early squamous cell carcinomas of the esophagus present as small sessile polypoid lesions with smooth or slightly lobulated contours; plaque-like lesions that often have flat, central ulcers that are best visualized in profile; or as superficial spreading lesions with a nodular appearance of the mucosa without a discrete mass. Advanced squamous cell carcinomas may appear infiltrative, ulcerative (Fig.), polypoid, or, less commonly, varicoid. Advanced carcinomas most commonly have an infiltrative appearance because they tend to grow circumferentially in the esophageal wall [18].

Early adenocarcinomas of the esophagus arising from Barrett's mucosa can manifest as small sessile polyps, plaque-like lesions, or superficial spreading lesions that cause focal nodularity of the mucosa without a discrete mass. These early cancers can also cause focal irregularity, flattening, or nodularity in a pre-existing peptic stricture. Accordingly, early endoscopy and biopsy are necessary to exclude adenocarcinoma whenever any of these suspicious features develop in a region of a peptic stricture. Advanced adenocarcinoma of the esophagus can appear infiltrating, polypoid, ulcerative, or, less commonly, varicoid on barium studies [18].

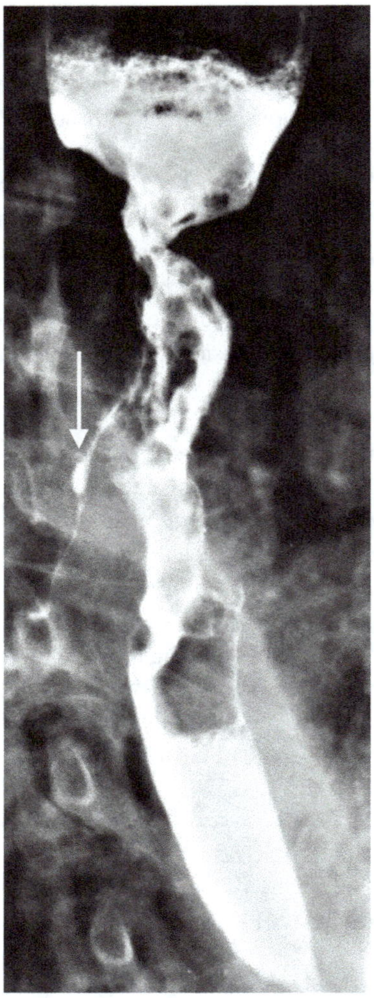

Fig. Squamous cell carcinoma of the midesophagus. Double-contrast esophagram demonstrates a long, ulcerating, malignant appearing esophageal stricture associated with an esophago-bronchial fistula (arrow). Note the dilation of the esophagus proximal to the neoplasm

Squamous cell carcinomas of the esophagus tend to be located in the upper or midthoracic esophagus and only rarely invade the adjacent stomach by contiguous spread. Adenocarcinomas of the esophagus develop primarily in the distal thoracic esophagus and have a marked tendency to invade the gastric cardia and fundus (Fig.). It may not always be possible to differentiate gastric adenocarcinoma of the gastric cardia invading the distal esophagus from a Barrett's-related cancer arising from the distal esophagus [18].

Since a multimodality approach is presently used to treat esophageal cancer, a precise histologic diagnosis and highly accurate tumor staging are prerequisites for selecting the most suitable treatment options. This requires histologic classification of the tumor type, the exclusion of distant organ metastases, localization of the primary tumor in relation to the tracheobronchial tree, and determination of the penetration of the primary tumor through the esophageal wall into the surrounding tissues [19].

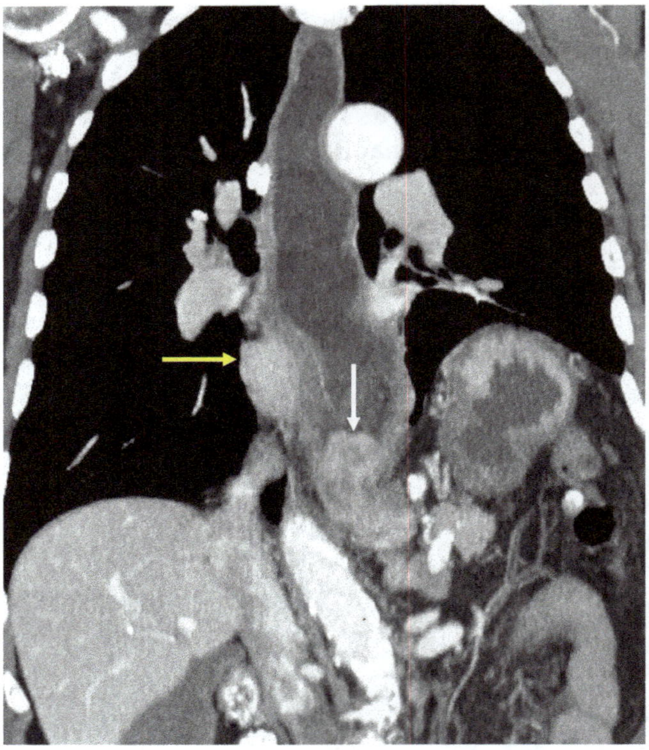

Fig. Adenocarcinoma of the gastroesophageal junction. Coronal reformatted CT image shows a partially obstructing mass at the gastroesophageal junction (white arrow). Notice the paraesophageal adenopathy (yellow arrow)

CT is useful in distinguishing between patients with early cancer (T1 and T2) who need further evaluation with EUS and those with T3 and T4 disease. For local staging of esophageal cancer using CT, 3 mm is considered the upper limit of normal mural thickness. The following comprise radiologic T stage criteria for esophageal cancer:

T1: focal or circumferential wall thickening of >3 and ≤10 mm and/or intense enhancement of the esophageal wall, without stenosis, and the outer borders of the tumor are smooth.

T2: focal, polypoid, or diffuse circumferential thickening of the esophageal wall >10 and ≤15 mm and the outer borders of the tumor are either smooth or show stranding for less than one-third of the tumor extension.

T3: tumor appears symmetric or asymmetric, and markedly diffuse or circumferential wall thickening of ≥15 mm, with mild-to-severe stenosis, and marked stranding for over one-third of the tumor extension, or extensive blurring of the outer border.

T4: tumor shows invasion into one of the adjacent structures: pericardium, the diaphragm, the pleura (T4a), the tracheobronchial tree, or the aorta and spine (T4b) [20].

Lymphatic spread is found in 74–88% of patients with esophageal carcinoma. Accurate lymph node assessment for metastatic spread is challenging, even with PET/MDCT. Diagnostic accuracy is improved if morphology, including size and shape, contrast enhancement pattern, and tracer uptake of lymph nodes are considered. N staging is as follows: **N0,** no regional lymph node metastasis; **N1,** 1–2 positive regional lymph nodes; **N2,** 3–6 positive regional lymph nodes; and **N3,** ≥7 positive regional lymph nodes [21].

Hematogenous metastases from esophageal carcinoma may involve the liver, lungs, adrenal glands, kidneys, bones, and brain. Lymph node involvement outside the periesophageal location is considered M1 disease [21].

GastricCancer

On double-contrast barium studies, Type I early gastric cancers typically appear as small protruded lesions in the stomach. Type II early gastric cancers are relatively flat lesions with elevated, superficial, or protruded components. These lesions may present as plaque-like elevations, mucosal nodularity, shallow ulcers, or some combination of these findings. Occasionally, these lesions can be quite extensive, involving a large portion of the surface area of the stomach without invading beyond the submucosa. Type III early gastric cancers manifest as shallow ulcer craters with nodularity of the adjacent mucosa and clubbing or fusion of radiating folds due to infiltration of the adjoining folds by tumor. Advanced gastric carcinomas usually appear on barium studies as polypoid, ulcerative, or infiltrative lesions [22].

As with esophageal carcinoma, precise histologic diagnosis and highly accurate tumor staging of gastric cancer are prerequisites for selecting the most suitable treatment options. In early advanced gastric cancers, the outer border of the stomach is smooth. The probability of transmural extension of the tumor (T3) is directly correlated with mural thickness. In transmural extension, the serosal contour becomes blurred, and strand-like areas of increased attenuation may be seen extending into the perigastric fat. Tumor spread frequently occurs via ligamentous and peritoneal reflections to adjacent organs (T4). The liver may be invaded via the gastrohepatic ligament, the pancreas via the lesser sac, the spleen via the gastrosplenic ligament (Fig.), and the transverse colon via the gastrocolic ligament. The distal esophagus is directly involved by carcinoma of the cardia in about 60% of patients, whereas the duodenum is involved by carcinoma of the antrum in 13–18% of patients [22–24].

Lymphatic spread is found in 74–88% of patients with gastric carcinoma because of the abundant lymphatic vessels in the stomach. The frequency of lymphatic metastases is related to the size and depth of penetration of the tumor. N staging depends on the number of positive perigastric lymph nodes (N1 1–5, N2 6–15, and N3 >15 affected lymph nodes) [23, 24].

Hematogenous metastases from gastric carcinoma most commonly involve the liver because the stomach is drained by the portal vein. Less common sites include the lungs, adrenal glands, kidneys, bones, and brain. Lymph node involvement outside the perigastric location is considered M1 disease. Advanced cancers can develop peritoneal and ovarian (Krukenberg) metastases [24].

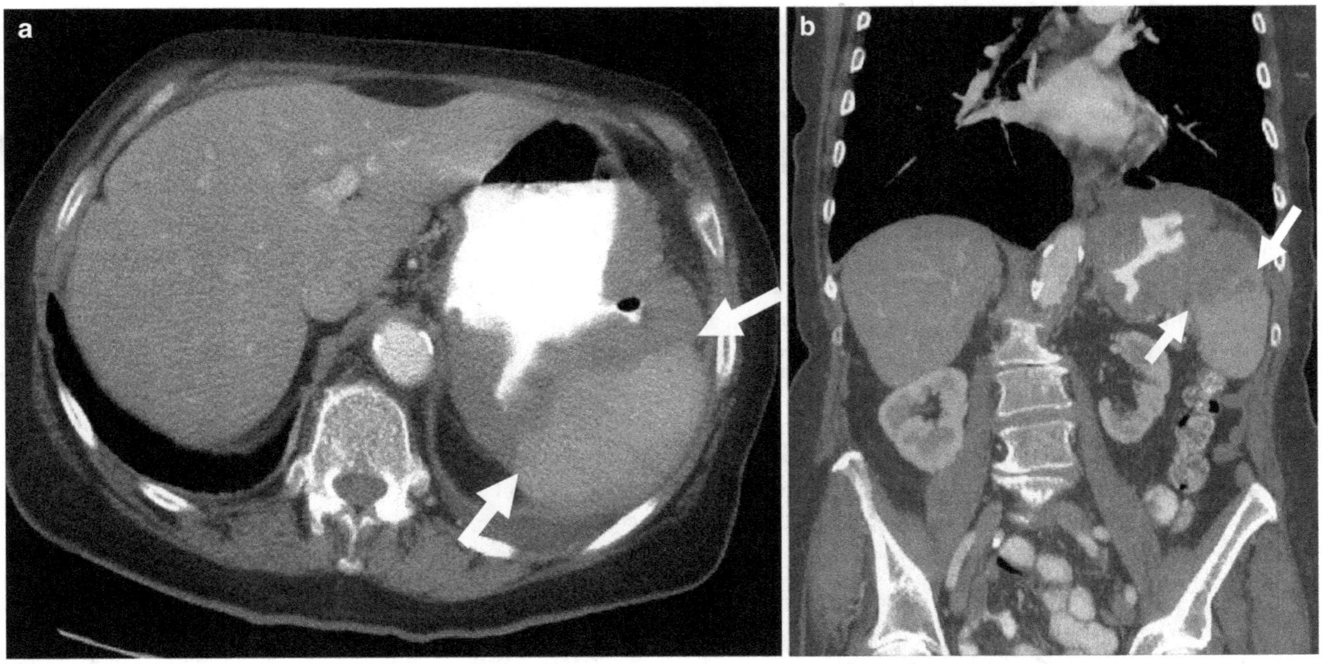

Fig. Adenocarcinoma of the stomach invading the gastrosplenic ligament and splenic hilum (arrows). This gastric neoplasm shows ulceration on the axial (**a**) and coronal (**b**) reformatted image

GastricLymphoma

Lymphoma involves the stomach more frequently than any other portion of the gastrointestinal tract. Primary gastric lymphomas are confined to the stomach and regional lymph nodes (about 35% of gastrointestinal lymphomas) and are predominantly non-Hodgkin lymphomas of B-cell origin. Lymphoma of mucosa-associated lymphoid tissue (MALT) is a distinct type of extranodal lymphoma that is characterized by a relatively indolent clinical course and has a much better prognosis than gastric carcinoma, with overall 5-year survival rates of 50–60%. Although the clinical symptoms in high-grade lymphoma and MALT lymphoma may be similar, they differ in several aspects [25, 26].

High-grade B-cell lymphoma has a relatively aggressive course as opposed to the more indolent and favorable outcome of MALT lymphoma. In high-grade gastric lymphomas, the extent of disease is usually greater at presentation, with involvement of adjacent organs and perigastric lymph nodes [25].

Lymphomas may involve any portion of the stomach. Transpyloric spread of tumor into the duodenum occurs in about 30% of patients. Despite extensive lymphomatous infiltration, the stomach usually remains pliable and distensible without significant luminal narrowing. Early gastric lymphoma is confined to the mucosa and submucosa, with an average size of only 3.5 cm at diagnosis. Gastric lymphomas are usually advanced lesions with a mean diameter of 10 cm. Most cases involve the antrum and body, although the entire stomach can be involved [24].

There are four gross pathologic types of gastric lymphoma [22]. Infiltrative gastric lymphomas manifest as focal or diffuse enlargement of gastric folds due to submucosal spread of tumor. One or more ulcerated lesions characterize ulcerative gastric lymphoma. Polypoid gastric lymphomas are characterized by intraluminal masses that may simulate polypoid carcinomas. Multiple submucosal nodules ranging in size between several millimeters and several centimeters characterize nodular gastric lymphoma.

CT is the primary imaging modality for pretreatment evaluation of abdominal lymphoma. In patients with suspected gastric lymphoma, CT provides depiction of gastric involvement and staging of generalized lymphoma in the abdomen and chest. Furthermore, CT may aid in early diagnosis of disease progression in patients undergoing therapy and follow-up for low-grade MALT lymphoma, which may progress to high-grade B-cell lymphoma. The CT appearances of lymphoma and gastric carcinoma may be very similar.

Gastrointestinal Stromal Tumor (GIST)

GISTs have recently been recognized as the most common mesenchymal neoplasm of the gastrointestinal tract. Many but not all mesenchymal tumors previously diagnosed as leiomyomas, leiomyoblastomas, and leiomyosarcomas on are now considered GISTs on the basis of specific immunohistochemical criteria- *c-kit* positivity. The malignant variety of GISTs represents only about 3% of all malignant gastrointestinal tumors. Approximately 60–70% are found in the stomach. It is known that 10–30% of GISTs are malignant, and the risk of malignancy increases with extragastric location, diameter greater than 5 cm, and extension into adjacent organ. Before and during surgery, in the absence of metastases, it is difficult to distinguish benign and malignant lesions. As with leiomyomas and leiomyosarcomas, intramural endogastric (Fig.) and exogastric lesions can be distinguished [27, 28] on cross-sectional imaging studies.

Carcinoid Tumors

Carcinoid tumors of the stomach are rare and have three subtypes, which have unique endoscopic and radiographic appearances. Type 1 gastric carcinoid tumors are associated with enterochromaffin-like cell hyperplasia, hypergastrinemia, and chronic atrophic gastritis, with or without pernicious anemia. Type 1 tumors generally represent benign disease. Nodal and hepatic metastases are very rare [29, 30]. Type 2 tumors are the least common type, representing 5–10% of gastric carcinoid tumors. They are seen in the hypergastrinemic state of Zollinger-Ellison syndrome in association with multiple endocrine neoplasia (MEN) type 1. Approximately 30% of patients with MEN 1 have gastric carcinoid tumors. Type 2 tumors also arise from enterochromaffin-like cells in the setting of hyperplasia. These tumors are multicentric and variable in size but are prone to developing local lymph node metastases. The appearance of these tumors on CT and radiographs of the upper gastrointestinal tract can be striking because there are multiple masses in the setting of diffuse gastric wall thickening [29, 30]. Type 3 gastric carcinoid tumors are sporadic tumors and are not associated with a hypergastrinemic state. They represent about 13% of gastric carcinoid tumors. Unlike type 1 and 2 tumors, type 3 tumors are large, solitary tumors that may show ulceration and are more likely to be invasive with distant metastases. The likelihood of metastasis is dependent on tumor size. Carcinoid syndrome may be seen in patients with hepatic metastases [29, 30].

When gastric carcinoid tumors are suspected, contrast material and water enhanced multidetector CT should be used to detect small mucosal masses. The discovery of polyps in a patient with chronic atrophic gastritis should alert the radiologist to the possibility of type 1 gastric carcinoid tumors. CT is necessary to properly assess type 2 (MEN 1 associated) and type 3 (sporadic) gastric carcinoid tumors, given the increased predisposition for nodal and hepatic metastases [29, 30].

Key Points

- In the presence of a hiatal hernia and reflux, a high esophageal stricture or reticular pattern should be strongly suggestive of Barrett's esophagus.
- Benign gastric ulcers classically appear en face as round or ovoid barium collections with a smooth, surrounding mound of edema and/or thin, straight folds radiating to the edge of the ulcer crater.
- Highly accurate tumor staging is a prerequisite for the selection of the most appropriate therapy of patients with upper gastrointestinal tract malignancies.
- Endoscopic ultrasound is more accurate for T staging than CT and MR in early upper gastrointestinal tract malignancies.
- PET/CT is recommended for staging locally advanced esophageal carcinoma.

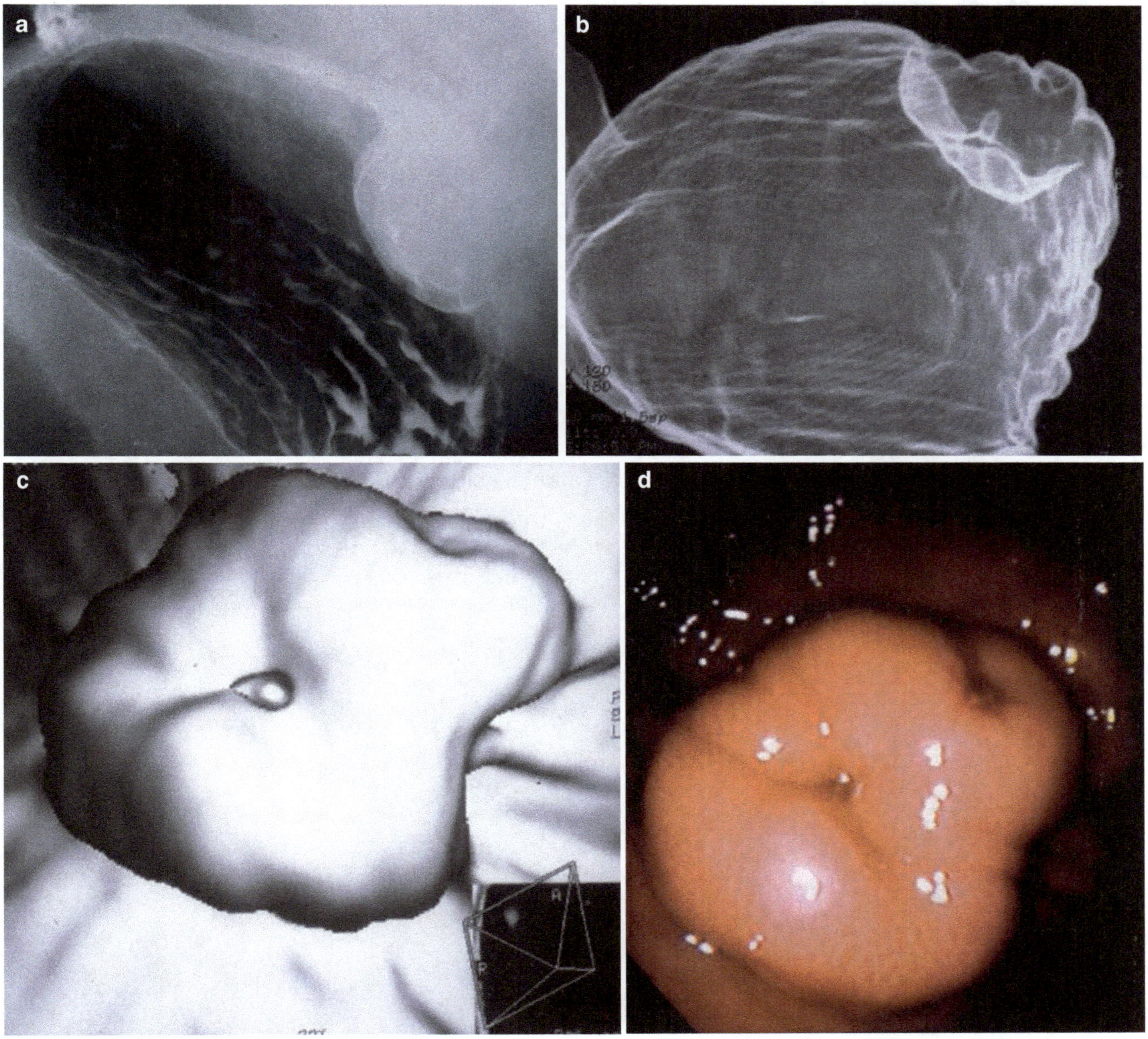

Fig. Gastric gastrointestinal stromal tumor. An ulcerating intramural mass is identified in the greater curvature aspect of the proximal gastric body. (**a**) Double-contrast upper GI series. (**b**) Shaded surface display from a CT gastrography study. (**c**) Endoluminal view from a CT gastrography study. (**d**) Upper GI endoscopic view of the lesion

References

1. Levine MS. Gastroesophageal reflux disease. In: Gore RM, Levine MS, editors. Textbook of gastrointestinal radiology. 4th ed. Philadelphia, PA: Elsevier; 2015. p. 291–311.
2. Levine MS, Kressel HY, Caroline DF, et al. Barrett esophagus: reticular pattern of the mucosa. Radiology. 1982;147:663–7.
3. Levine MS, Ahmad NA, Rubesin SE. Elevated Z line: a new sign of Barrett's esophagus on double-contrast barium esophagograms. Clin Imaging. 2015;39:1103–4.
4. Levine MS, Macones AJ, Laufer I. *Candida* esophagitis: accuracy of radiographic diagnosis. Radiology. 1985;154:581–7.
5. Levine MS, Woldenberg R, Herlinger H, et al. Opportunistic esophagitis in AIDS: radiographic diagnosis. Radiology. 1977;165: 815–20.
6. Levine MS, Loevner LA, Saul SH, et al. Herpes esophagitis: sensitivity of double-contrast esophagography. AJR. 1988;151:57–62.
7. Balthazar EJ, Megibow AJ, Hulnick DH. Cytomegalovirus esophagitis and gastritis in AIDS. AJR. 1985;144:1201–4.
8. Sor S, Levine MS, Kowalski TE, et al. Giant ulcers of the esophagus in patients with human immunodeficiency virus: clinical, radiographic, and pathologic findings. Radiology. 1995;194: 447–51.
9. Zimmerman SL, Levine MS, Rubesin SE, et al. Idiopathic eosinophilic esophagitis in adults: the ringed esophagus. Radiology. 2005;236:159–65.
10. White SB, Levine MS, Rubesin SE, et al. The small-caliber esophagus: radiographic sign of idiopathic eosinophilic esophagitis. Radiology. 2010;256:127–34.
11. Rauschecker AM, Levine MS, Whitson MJ, et al. Esophageal lichen planus: clinical and radiographic findings in eight patients. AJR. 2017;208:1–6.
12. Levine MS. Other esophagitides. In: Gore RM, Levine MS, editors. Textbook of gastrointestinal radiology. 4th ed. Philadelphia, PA: Elsevier; 2015. p. 326–49.
13. Levine MS. Inflammatory conditions of the stomach and duodenum. In: Gore RM, Levine MS, editors. Textbook of gastrointestinal radiology. 4th ed. Philadelphia, PA: Elsevier; 2015. p. 496–522.
14. Levine MS, Verstandig A, Laufer I. Serpiginous gastric erosions caused by aspirin and other nonsteroidal anti-inflammatory drugs. AJR Am J Roentgenol. 1986;146:31–4.
15. Sohn J, Levine MS, Furth EE, et al. *Helicobacter pylori* gastritis: radiographic findings. Radiology. 1995;195:763–7.
16. Levine MS. Peptic ulcers. In: Gore RM, Levine MS, editors. Textbook of gastrointestinal radiology. 4th ed. Philadelphia, PA: Elsevier; 2015. p. 467–95.
17. Levine MS, Kelly MR, Laufer I, et al. Gastrocolic fistulas: the increasing role of aspirin. Radiology. 1993;187:359–61.
18. Levine MS, Halvorsen RA. Carcinoma of the esophagus. In: Gore RM, Levine MS, editors. Textbook of gastrointestinal radiology. 4th ed. Philadelphia, PA: Elsevier; 2015. p. 366–93.
19. Shah MA. Future directions in improving outcomes for patients with gastric and esophageal cancer. Hematol Oncol Clin North Am. 2017;31(3):545–52.
20. Mehta K, Bianco V, Awais O, Luketich JD, Pennathur A. Minimally invasive staging of esophageal cancer. Ann Cardiothorac Surg. 2017;6(2):110–8.
21. Goel R, Subramaniam RM, Wachsmann JW. PET/computed tomography scanning and precision medicine: esophageal cancer. PET Clin. 2017;12(4):373–91.
22. Levine MS, Megibow AJ, Kochman ML. Carcinoma of the stomach and duodenum. In: Gore RM, Levine MS, editors. Textbook of gastrointestinal radiology. 4th ed. Philadelphia, PA: Elsevier; 2015. p. 546–70.
23. Hayes T, Smyth E, Riddell A, Allum W. Staging in esophageal and gastric cancers. Hematol Oncol Clin North Am. 2017;31(3):427–40.
24. Gore RM, Kim JH, Chen C-Y. MDCT, EUS, PET/CT, and MRI in the management of patients with gastric neoplasms. In: Gore RM, editor. Gastric cancer. Cambridge, UK: Cambridge University Press; 2010. p. 120–94.
25. Ikoma N, Badgwell BD, Mansfield PF. Multimodality treatment of gastric lymphoma. Surg Clin North Am. 2017;97(2):405–20.
26. Ma Z, Fang M, Huang Y, He L, et al. CT-based radiomics signature for differentiating Borrmann type IV gastric cancer from primary gastric lymphoma. Eur J Radiol. 2017;91:142–7.
27. Keung EZ, Raut CP. Management of gastrointestinal stromal tumors. Surg Clin North Am. 2017;97(2):437–52.
28. Scola D, Bahoura L, Copelan A, Shirkhoda A, Sokhandon F. Getting the GIST: a pictorial review of the various patterns of presentation of gastrointestinal stromal tumors on imaging. Abdom Radiol. 2017;42(5):1350–64.
29. Corey B, Chen H. Neuroendocrine tumors of the stomach. Surg Clin North Am. 2017;97(2):333–43.
30. Lin YM, Chiu NC, Li AF, Liu CA, Chou YH, Chiou YY. Unusual gastric tumors and tumor-like lesions: radiological with pathological correlation and literature review. World J Gastroenterol. 2017;23(14):2493–504.

9

Renal Tumors

Lejla Aganovic and Richard H. Cohan

Learning Objectives

- To be familiar with the Bosniak cystic renal mass classification system
- To learn when very small renal masses can be ignored and when they should be followed
- To be aware of ultrasound, CT, and MRI appearance of angiomyolipomas
- To learn about imaging features of non-macroscopic fat containing renal masses
- To be familiar with renal cancer staging and use of RENAL nephrometry
- To be knowledgeable of the normal imaging appearance of patients after treatment of renal cancer and the appearance of treated and untreated metastatic disease
- To be aware of unique features related to treatment of metastatic renal cancer with targeted chemotherapeutic agents, including immunotherapy

Introduction

In recent years, there have been dramatic developments in imaging assessment of renal tumors and their treatment, some of which will be provided in the paragraphs that follow.

L. Aganovic, M.D. (✉)
Department of Radiology, University of California, San Diego, Medical Center, San Diego, CA, USA

R. H. Cohan, M.D.
Department of Radiology, University of Michigan Hospital, Ann Arbor, MI, USA
e-mail: rcohan@umich.edu

Modalities for Imaging Renal Masses

Ultrasound

Although noncontrast ultrasound evaluates the internal morphology of cystic lesions with more detail than CT, it is not as sensitive in detecting or accurate in characterizing renal masses as CT or MRI. Most consider ultrasound to be diagnostically definitive only when it identifies a renal mass as a simple cyst.

CT and MRI

Renal tumors may be detected incidentally on CT or MRI examinations. On CT, it is quite common for only contrast-enhanced images to have been obtained, in which case assessment of mass enhancement is limited. When only contrast-enhanced CT images are available, it may be difficult to distinguish hyperdense cysts from solid hypoenhancing renal lesions. Renal cancers are unlikely to measure >70 HU on unenhanced CT and <40 HU on contrast-enhanced CT [1].

Key Point

- Patients referred to CT or MRI with known or suspected renal masses should be evaluated with unenhanced and at least one contrast-enhanced series (with the unenhanced MRI sequences including T1-weighted, fat-suppressed, T2-weighted, in- and out-of-phase gradient-echo, diffusion-weighted images).

Key Point

- Renal mass detection and characterization are maximized when delayed rather than early contrast-enhanced images are obtained (either in the nephrographic phase [NP], which begins 90–100 s after initiation of a contrast injection, or the excretory phase [EP], which begins when excreted contrast material is first detected in the renal collecting system, usually 120 s or more after initiation of contrast injection) [2].

Very Small Renal Masses (<1–1.5 cm)

Very small renal masses (<1.0–1.5 cm in maximal diameter) are detected on nearly half of all adult patients undergoing CT scans [3]. Many such renal masses detected with CT and MRI cannot be characterized due to their size. Accurate attenuation measurements in these lesions are problematic, due to volume averaging and pseudoenhancement. Fortunately, the likelihood of any one of these lesions being malignant is exceedingly low [3]. The overwhelming majority of these lesions will be benign renal cysts.

Because very small renal masses are so common, further assessment of all of these lesions is not feasible, even though a few will be cancers.

Key Point

- Follow-up imaging of tiny renal masses should be performed only when they subjectively appear to be complex with evidence of heterogeneity, internal septations, mural nodules, wall thickening, or heterogeneity.

Some homogeneous low attenuation lesions can be considered suspicious if they appear in high-risk patients, such as those with known or suspected hereditary cancer syndromes (such as von Hippel-Lindau, hereditary papillary renal cell cancer, Birt-Hogg-Dubé, or hereditary leiomyomatosis-renal cancer syndrome) [4]. When a very small renal mass is deemed suspicious, further evaluation should be performed within 6–12 months. Suspicious masses should be followed for at least 5 years. While follow-up can be obtained with CT or MRI, MRI is more accurate. Even tiny cysts have characteristic high T2 signal intensity. MRI is also much more sensitive to contrast enhancement than is CT, and it is not compromised by pseudoenhancement [5].

Key Point

- Most benign and malignant very small renal masses grow at comparable slow rates, with many of these masses enlarging at a rate of no more than 3–5 mm in maximal diameter per year [6]. As a result, interval enlargement of a renal mass cannot be used to predict that the mass being followed is malignant. Instead, masses should be assessed for changes in morphology. These changes include increasing heterogeneity or the progression of the other aforementioned complicating features [5].

Cystic Renal Masses

Many radiologists and urologists classify cystic renal lesions using the Bosniak classification system, which was first proposed in 1986 [7] and revised several times, including in 2005 [8]. This system classifies renal cystic masses into five categories, based upon their likelihood of being malignant. It is important to emphasize that the Bosniak system was designed for use with dedicated renal mass CT and not for ultrasound or MRI.

Category I lesions, which constitute the overwhelming majority of cystic renal masses, are simple renal cysts. They are homogeneous masses. They are anechoic on ultrasound and of water attenuation on CT or water signal intensity on MRI. They have imperceptible walls and do not contain nodules or calcifications. They do not enhance when contrast material is administered. Category I lesions are always benign and no follow-up is needed. *Category II lesions* are minimally complex. They may contain one to three septations or thin peripheral calcifications. Hyperdense renal cysts <3 cm in diameter are also Category II lesions. Category II lesions are essentially always benign and no follow-up is needed. *Category IIF lesions* contain multiple or thickened septa, thickened walls, or coarse calcifications. Hyperdense cysts measuring >3 cm in diameter are also Category IIF lesions.

Key Point

- Category IIF cysts have been found to represent cancers or progress to become cancers about 11% of the time [9] and, for this reason, must be followed, with repeat imaging studies performed at 6 months and then annually for at least 5 years. Cancer should be suspected, not when these lesions grow over time, but instead if they become increasingly complex.

Studies have indicated that such follow-up can be performed safely. In the series reported by Hindman et al. [9], none of 17 Category IIF renal cystic masses that were ultimately diagnosed as cancers developed locally recurrent or metastatic disease during the follow-up period. *Category III lesions* contain thickened irregular enhancing septa or walls. They are malignant about 50–60% of the time. When malignant, they tend to be less aggressive than other renal cancers. Treatment of these lesions is usually recommended due to the high risk of malignancy. *Category IV lesions* are cystic lesions that have irregular enhancing walls or enhancing nodules. These lesions are nearly always malignant, so treatment is warranted.

The Bosniak system has been adopted for use with ultrasound and MRI; however, the percentages of lesions of different categories that are malignant with these modalities are not well known. For example, on MRI, about 20% of cystic renal masses appear more complex and are assigned to higher categories than they would have been if imaged with CT [10]. This is largely due to MRI's ability to detect internal cyst features not visible with CT.

Angiomyolipomas (AMLs)

AMLs are the most common benign solid renal neoplasms. They are composed of angiomatous, myomatous, and fatty elements, in varying relative distribution. Eighty percent occur sporadically. The remainder are associated with syndromes (tuberous sclerosis or lymphangioleiomyomatosis) [11].

While nearly all AMLs are echogenic on ultrasound, so are some small renal cancers. It has been found, however, that the likelihood of a small echogenic renal case being a cancer is exceedingly low. In one recent study, only 1 of 161 small renal masses (measuring 1 cm or smaller) were subsequently found to be renal cancers [12]. Acoustic shadowing has been identified posterior to some echogenic AMLs, but not posterior to any echogenic renal cancers [13]. An echoic rim or intratumoral cysts have been observed around or in some renal cancers, but not any AMLs.

Echogenic masses detected on US are often further evaluated with CT or MRI to determine if macroscopic fat is present in the mass. If macroscopic fat is identified on CT or MRI, then the mass can be diagnosed definitely as an AML (with only case reportable exceptions).

Key Point

- On CT, visualization of at least some small areas within a renal mass measuring–(negative) 10 HU or less is considered diagnostic of macroscopic fat and of an AML [14].

Key Point

- On MRI, fat typically has high T1 and T2 signal and loses signal with fat suppression. On opposed-phase chemical shift imaging, there is a characteristic "India ink" artifact at fat-water interfaces in the AML and between the AML and adjacent renal tissue (Fig.) [15].

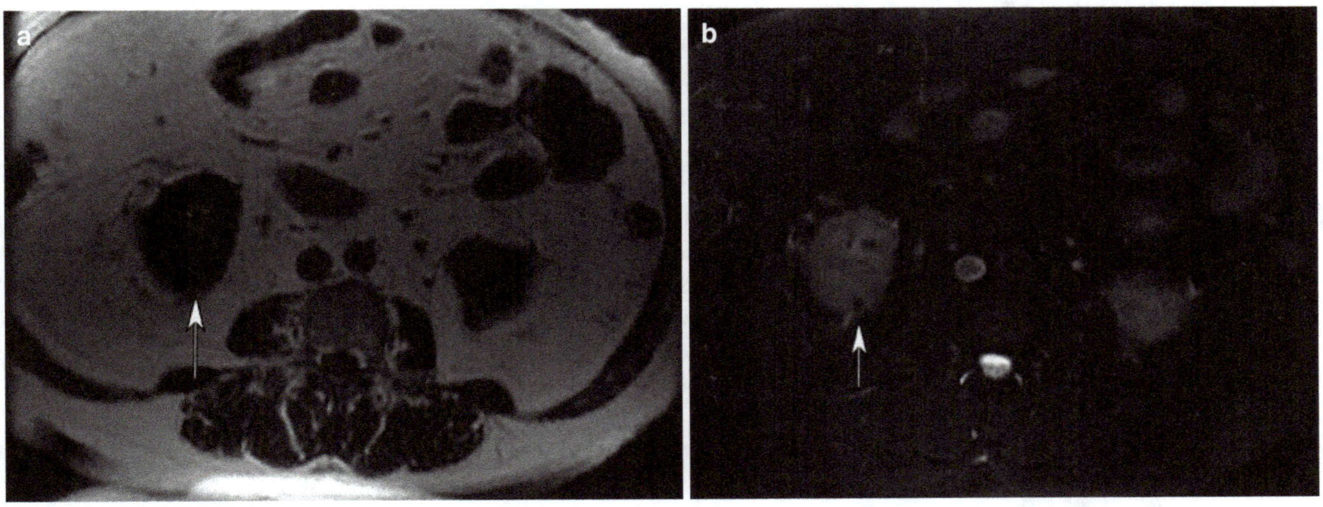

Fig. MRI of an AML. (**a**) Axial T1-weighted MR image shows a tiny hyperintense mass in the lower pole of the right kidney (arrow). (**b**) Axial T2-weighted MR image with fat suppression shows that the lesion has lost signal (arrow), confirming the diagnosis. (**c**) Opposed-phase MR image demonstrates India ink artifact at the interface of the renal mass with the kidney (arrow)

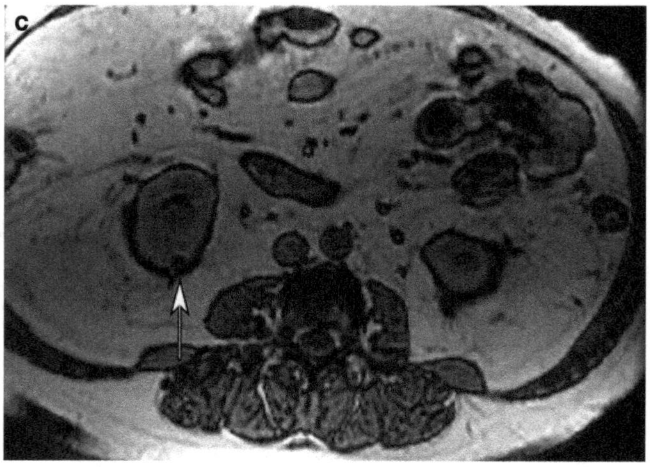

Fig. (continued)

Occasionally, exophytic AMLs can be difficult to differentiate from perinephric liposarcomas. Some imaging features can be used to facilitate differentiation. AMLs are more likely to invaginate into the kidneys and produce a focal parenchymal defect. Liposarcomas, in comparison, merely compress the kidney, without having an associated defect. AMLs are more likely to contain large vessels that extend to the renal cortex than are liposarcomas [16].

Some AMLs do not contain easily identifiable macroscopic fat. These AMLs are referred to as fat-poor AMLs (fpAMLs) and include fpAMLs that have the same or higher attenuation than normal renal parenchyma on unenhanced CT and AMLs with epithelial cysts (AMLEC), which can appear as solid masses with small cystic areas or multilocular cystic lesions [11].

Many studies have attempted to identify small foci of fat or other imaging features that might permit fpAMLs to be correctly distinguished from other solid renal neoplasms. These features have included assessing unenhanced CT mass attenuation, CT histograms, quantitatively assessed fat on MRI, and the degree and homogeneity of mass of enhancement [11, 17–19]. Results have been mixed. For example, some fpAMLs have higher unenhanced attenuation than normal renal parenchyma, but papillary renal cancers can also demonstrate this feature [20]. Some fpAMLs have low signal intensity on T2-weighted MR images, but papillary renal cancers may also demonstrate this behavior. Fortunately, fpAMLs usually demonstrate more MR contrast enhancement than do papillary renal neoplasms, so a hypervascular lesion that demonstrates a combination of high attenuation on unenhanced CT and/or low-T2 signal intensity on MRI is most likely to be an AML.

A rare type of AML is the epithelioid AML (eAML). Some epithelioid AMLs behave aggressively. They can spread locally to invade the renal vein or IVC, involve regional lymph nodes, or even metastasize distantly [11]. Epithelioid AMLs do not demonstrate imaging features that allow them to be differentiated from other AMLs. While many epithelioid AMLs do not contain identifiable macroscopic fat on imaging studies, some do [21]. Because this subtype of AML is so rare, AMLs that have a classic appearance on imaging studies should all be treated as benign lesions anyway. Exceptions should be considered to be case reportable.

Other Solid Renal Masses

Many solid renal masses do not contain identifiable fat. This includes oncocytomas and renal cancers. A large number of studies attempting to distinguish among the various nonfat- or minimal-fat-containing solid renal masses on CT and MRI have met with limited success; however, a few occasionally suggestive imaging features have been described.

Oncocytomas

Oncocytomas are benign renal tumors. They may contain central scars that can be detected on imaging studies; however, this feature is not diagnostic. Necrosis in renal cancers is indistinguishable from scars in oncocytomas. Further, most oncocytomas evaluated on CT do not contain visible central scars [22]. One feature that has been used by some to differentiate oncocytomas from renal cancers is segmental enhancement inversion, in which two differently enhancing components identified on CMP images reverse their attenuation on EP images, with the initially higher attenuation and briskly enhancing component becoming lower in attenuation than the initially lower attenuation and less intensely enhancing component [23]. This feature is not consistently detected in oncocytomas and is, therefore, frequently not helpful [24].

Renal Cancers

In the past, it was believed that there were only a few types of cancer; however, chromosomal analysis has demonstrated that there are at least 13 distinct types of renal cancer, with most being very rare. This includes clear cell (about 70–80%), papillary (10–15%), chromophobe (less than 10%), acquired renal cystic disease-associated, clear cell and papillary combined, collecting duct, renal medullary, mucinous tubular and spindle cell, succinate dehydrogenase-deficient, tubulocystic, and unclassified cancers, multilocular cystic neoplasms of low malignant potential, and MiT translocation cancers including Xp11.2 [25]. Sarcomatoid renal cancer is no longer believed to be a distinct cell type. Instead, any type of primary renal neoplasm can dedifferentiate and develop sarcomatoid features. While again imaging differentiation among most renal cancers is not possible, some cell types tend to demonstrate certain imaging features, as summarized below.

Clear Cell Renal Cancer

Clear cell renal cancers have the highest metastatic potential and poorest survival of the major histologic RCC subtypes. They are usually heterogeneous renal cortical masses. On unenhanced MRI, most clear cell cancers demonstrate hyperintensity on T2-weighted images. Due to abundant intracellular fat, clear cell cancers can lose signal on opposed-phase gradient-echo T1-weighted images. Clear cell carcinomas usually demonstrate heterogeneous enhancement, with peak enhancement occurring early, on CMP images [26] (Fig.).

Papillary Renal Cancer

Most papillary cancers behave less aggressively than do clear cell cancers. On contrast-enhanced CT or MRI, papillary cancers tend to be homogeneous. On unenhanced CT, they may have higher attenuation than adjacent renal parenchyma. On unenhanced MRI, they often are hypointense on T2-weighted images and can lose signal on in-phase T1-weighted images due to presence of hemosiderin [27]. They usually enhance homogeneously, more slowly, and to a lesser extent than do other renal cancers, with peak enhancement not occurring until the NP or even the EP [28] (Fig.).

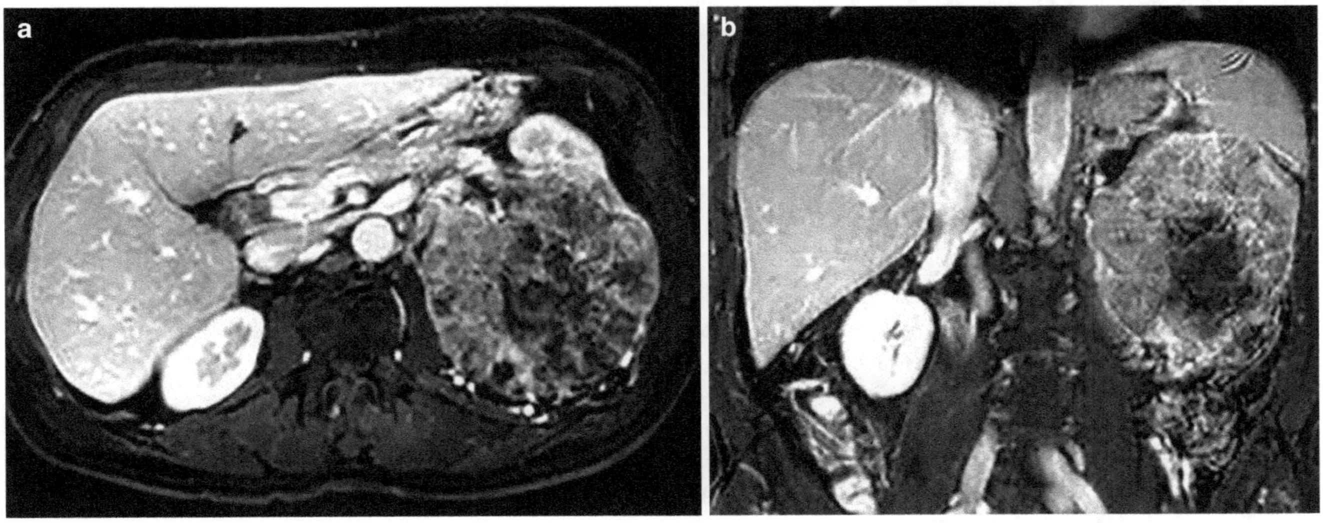

Fig. Clear cell renal cell carcinoma. Contrast-enhanced axial (**a**) and coronal (**b**) images obtained during the CMP demonstrate a heterogeneously and briskly enhancing left renal mass, subsequently confirmed to be a clear cell RCC

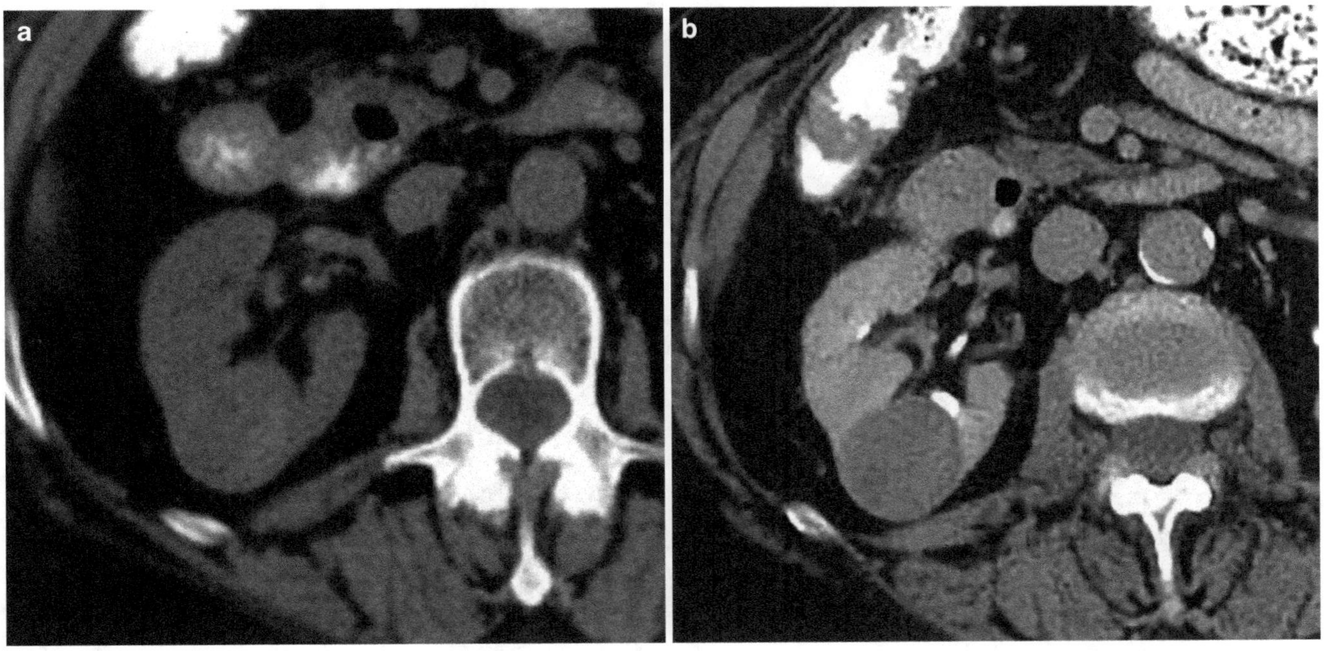

Fig. Papillary renal cell carcinoma. Unenhanced (**a**) and excretory phase (EP) contrast-enhanced (**b**) axial CT images demonstrate a mildly heterogeneous hypoenhancing papillary cancer in the posterior aspect of the mid right kidney

Chromophobe Renal Cancer

Chromophobe renal cancers are generally well-differentiated cancers and, provided that they do not have sarcomatoid degeneration, are slow growing and have an excellent prognosis. They do not have a unique appearance on imaging studies and cannot be reliably distinguished from other solid renal masses that do not contain macroscopic fat.

Uncommon Renal Cancer Cell Types

Many of the uncommon renal cancers do not have suggestive imaging appearances. A few specific comments about some of these cancers can be made, however. Renal medullary, collecting duct, and XP11.2 translocation cancers generally arise in the renal medulla. Collecting duct cancers frequently occur in older adults; renal medullary and XP11.2 cancers are usually encountered in young patients [25]. Renal medullary cancers typically develop in patients with sickle cell trait [29].

Urothelial Neoplasms, Lymphoma, and Renal Artery Aneurysms

It can occasionally be difficult to distinguish centrally located RCC from urothelial cancers; however, the correct etiology may be predicted in many instances. Unlike RCC, urothelial cancers have an epicenter in the renal collecting system, can produce renal pelvic filling defects, and tend to preserve the normal renal contour. They also rarely contain cystic/necrotic areas seen in many, but not all, RCCs [30]. Other centrally located renal masses that can be encountered and that can occasionally mimic urothelial cancers of RCC include renal lymphoma and renal artery aneurysms.

Solid Renal Mass Growth Rates

Both benign and malignant solid renal masses can remain stable in size or enlarge over time, with growth rates of both types of lesions usually being similarly slow [31]. It has been suggested that a small solid mass that has an average growth rate of <3 mm/year over at least a 5-year period and that has not changed in morphology should be considered stable. Such a lesion, even if malignant, is exceedingly unlikely to metastasize. Conversely, rapid growth of a mass (by more than 5 mm in 12 months) may indicate aggressiveness/malignancy [32].

Radiomics

In recent years, there has been increasing interest in the utility of computer-assisted diagnosis (CAD) in detecting and characterizing genitourinary abnormalities. With respect to renal masses, this has centered on the ability of computer-assisted techniques to differentiate among different types of renal masses. For example, studies using computer-assisted diagnosis have demonstrated clear cell renal cancers to have greater objective heterogeneity (pixel standard deviation, entropy, and uniformity) than papillary renal cancers or AMLs [33]. CAD detection of differences in peak lesion attenuation has also been used to differentiate clear cell renal cancers from other renal neoplasms with some success [34]. Renal mass perfusion parameters have been employed to distinguish some renal cancers of higher Fuhrman grade from those of lower grade [35]. These results are promising but preliminary.

Use of Imaging for Solid Renal Mass Differentiation

Key Point

- Due to overlap of many imaging findings detected subjectively and using CAD, at the present time, imaging differentiation of many malignant from benign nonfat-containing solid renal masses (or among the various types of malignant solid renal masses) is not possible.

Percutaneous Biopsy of Renal Masses

Given the substantial overlap in the imaging features of many renal lesions, percutaneous biopsy is necessary for determining the nature of many renal masses prior to treatment. Biopsy can be performed accurately and safely [36]. The risk of needle tract seeding of tumor is minimal. There are only isolated case reports of renal cancer seeding [37]. One potential pitfall of biopsy relates to the fact that only a few portions of a renal mass are sampled. Areas containing higher-grade cancer may not be sampled, leading to underestimation of tumor aggressiveness.

Pretreatment Assessment of Renal Cancer

Staging

CT and MRI (obtained during the portal venous phase of enhancement) are at least 90% accurate in renal cancer staging, with the TNM staging system as follows:

Stage	Feature
T1a	≤4 cm in greatest diameter and limited to the kidney
T1b	>4–7 cm and limited to the kidney
T2a	7–10 cm and limited to the kidney
T2b	>10 cm and limited to the kidney

Stage	Feature
T3a	Extension into the renal vein or its branches or invading perirenal or renal sinus fat
T3b	Extension into the IVC below the diaphragm
T3c	Extension into the IVC above the diaphragm or invading the IVC wall
T4	Invasion beyond perinephric fascia or into ipsilateral adrenal gland
N0	No lymph node involvement
N1	Regional lymph node involvement
M0	No distant metastases
M1	Distant metastases
Mx	Distant metastatic status not determined

The most substantial limitation of imaging in stage renal cancers results from the fact that both CT and MRI have difficulty in determining whether a renal cancer has invaded the renal capsule and spread into the perirenal or renal sinus fat (differentiating T2 from T3 cancer). Perinephric soft tissue stranding can be produced by tumor, edema, or blood vessels [38]. It is recommended that T3 disease be diagnosed on CT or MRI only when nodular tissue is identified in the perinephric space.

RENAL Nephrometry

Many urologists prefer that RENAL nephrometry scoring of suspected or known renal cancers also be obtained prior to surgery. Nephrometry scoring allows the urologist to predict the likelihood that partial nephrectomy can be performed effectively and safely [39]. With this system, a renal mass receives a score of 1–3 points for each of five features (**R**enal mass size, **E**xophyticity, **N**earness to the renal collecting system, **A**nterior or posterior location, and **L**ocation with respect to the upper and lower polar lines (see table immediately below). Tumors that have composite nephrometry scores of 4–6 are considered to be very amenable to partial nephrectomy, while those that have scores of 10–12 are poor candidates for partial nephrectomy. Complete nephrectomy should be considered in the latter group.

Feature	1 point	2 points	3 points
R = diameter	≤4 cm	>4 to <7 cm	≥7 cm
E = exophyticity	≥50%	<50%	Entirely endophytic
N = nearness to collecting system or renal sinus	≥7 mm	>4 to <7 mm	≤4 mm
A = anterior or posterior	No points given. Mass is listed as a, p, or neither (x)		
L = location relative to polar lines Add "h" if touches renal artery or vein	Above upper or lower pole line	Crosses polar line	>50% of mass crosses polar line or crosses midline or entirely interlobar

From Ref. [39]

Renal Cancer Management

Management of renal cancers that have not metastasized regionally or distantly now ranges from active surveillance (for small [<4 cm] indolent (low Fuhrman grade) tumors in elderly patients with significant comorbidities) to thermal ablation, partial nephrectomy, or complete nephrectomy [32, 37]. Patients on active surveillance should undergo subsequent imaging every 6 months for a year, followed by annual imaging for at least 5 years. Intervention in these patients is only considered when masses exceed 4 cm in size or grow by >5 mm per year [32].

Imaging After Renal Cancer Treatment

After Renal Mass Ablation or Resection

After successful renal mass radiofrequency or cryoablation, there is initial expansion of the ablation site. Initially, some enhancement may be detected normally in the ablation bed, particularly on MRI exams. This normal enhancement resolves over time [40]. In the months following ablation, the ablation bed typically decreases but rarely disappears completely. Other normal post-ablation findings include fat invagination between the ablation bed and normal renal parenchyma and a peri-lesional halo, changes that create an appearance that can be confused with an AML (Fig.). Ablation bed expansion is not typically seen after microwave ablation.

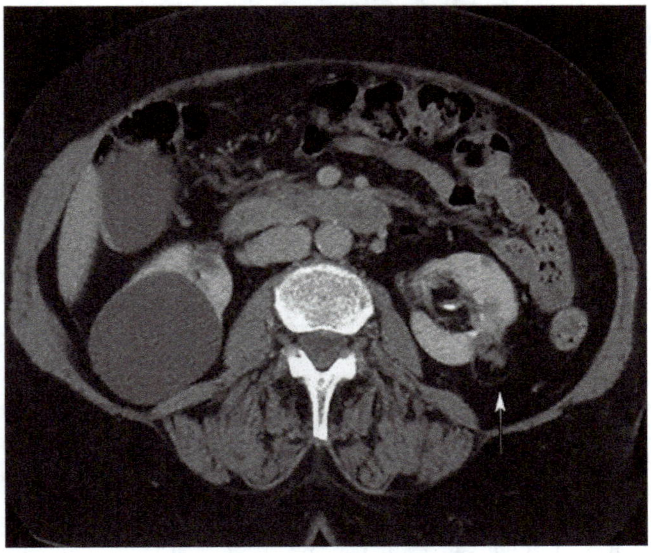

Fig. Normal post-thermal ablation appearance. An EP contrast-enhanced CT image on a patient, who had a left renal radiofrequency ablation 7 months earlier, demonstrates a normal post-ablation appearance. Soft tissue attenuation material is surrounded by invaginated perinephric fat, an appearance that can be confused with an AML

Key Point

- Frequent imaging should be performed after ablation (e.g., at 1, 3, 6, and 12 months). This is because residual or recurrent tumor is usually detectable within the first few months of ablation [41].

Persistent or recurrent tumor should be suspected after ablation if the ablation bed progressively increases (rather than decreases) in size, when there is increased perinephric nodularity, or when persistent or new areas of nodular or crescentic enhancement are detected, with these areas usually located at the interface of the ablation bed with adjacent renal parenchyma [41].

Imaging After Partial or Total Nephrectomy

After partial or total nephrectomy, it is common to see postoperative inflammatory or fibrotic changes in the surgical bed, along with deformity of the renal contour at the site of partial nephrectomy [42]. Gore-Tex mesh along the nephrectomy site appears as a linear area of high attenuation along the renal margin.

Key Point

- Frequently used hemostatic material can be mistaken for infection or tumor, since an occasional gas within the material and its low attenuation components can persist for months after surgery.

Complication rates after partial nephrectomy are typically higher than after total nephrectomy, with complications including pseudoaneurysm, urinoma, or abscess. If urinoma is a concern, delayed imaging >1–2 h after contrast administration might prove useful to document the urinary leak.

After partial or total nephrectomy, recurrent tumor may develop in the surgical bed and/or regionally or distantly. Surgical bed recurrences may initially be difficult to differentiate from postoperative scarring/fibrosis, although tumor often demonstrates detectable enhancement and enlarges over time. Renal cancer usually metastasizes to regional lymph nodes, the liver, the adrenal glands, the lungs, and the bones. Adrenal cancer metastases from clear cell renal cancer can be problematic, since they may contain large amounts of intracellular fat. As a result, similar to adenomas, adrenal metastases can demonstrate low signal intensity on opposed-phase MR images and can also demonstrate pronounced (>60%) washout on delayed enhanced CT. Renal cancer metastasizes to the pancreas more commonly than do other neoplasms [43].

Imaging After Treatment of Metastatic Disease

RECIST

Patients who present with or develop metastatic renal cancer must receive systemic treatment. Imaging is then performed regularly to determine whether or not patients are responding to their chemotherapy. Metastatic foci are then measured and compared, from one imaging study to the next. The most commonly used measurement system for assessing tumor response to chemotherapy has been the **r**esponse **e**valuation **c**riteria **i**n **s**olid **t**umors (RECIST) system [44]. The RECIST 1.1 system involves measurements of up to five metastatic lesions (no more than two per organ, with each measured lesion being at least 10 mm in length). Most metastases are measured in maximal dimensions; however, lymph nodes are measured in short axis diameter. Complete response is diagnosed when all metastases resolve on follow-up imaging. A partial response is diagnosed when the sum of all target lesions decreases by ≥30% from one study to the next. Progressive disease is diagnosed when the sum of all target lesions increases by ≥20% or more. Any change in between a 30% decrease and a 20% increase is considered stable disease.

Key Point

- While RECIST 1.1 has worked well for following metastatic disease treated by prior standard chemotherapy, there are problems with its use in patients treated with anti-angiogenesis drugs, including multikinase inhibitors. This is because multikinase inhibitors may produce necrosis (and resulting diminished attenuation on contrast-enhanced CT) in responding metastatic lesions without these lesions decreasing significantly in size. As a result, a patient who is a partial responder can be misidentified as not having responded to treatment, if only RECIST is used.

MultikinaseInhibitors

A number of alternative measuring systems have been devised, which take into account changes in lesion attenuation, as well as changes in size. This includes the Choi, modified Choi, and the morphology, attenuation, size, and structure (MASS) systems [45, 46]. With the Choi criteria, for example, a decrease in target lesion size of only 10% or more or a decrease in target attenuation of 15% or more indicates a partial response. With the modified Choi criteria, both of these features must be present at the same time.

Immunotherapy

In the last few years, patients with metastatic renal cancer have been treated with immunotherapy. These agents are antibodies targeted to attack receptors on lymphocytes or surface ligands on tumor cells. They work by interfering with a tumor's ability to inhibit an immune response. At the present time, the immune checkpoints which are being inhibited include those related to cytotoxic T-lymphocyte-associated antigen 4 (CTLA4) and the program cell death protein 1 receptor on T-cells (PD-1) or its related ligands on tumor cells (PDL1 and PDL2) [47].

Key Point

- A unique feature of metastases treated by immunotherapy is that some responding lesions may initially appear stable or even enlarge to such an extent that progressive disease would be diagnosed if RECIST 1.1 were to be used. An apparent initial increase in size should be considered to be unconfirmed progressive disease (UPD). UPD must be confirmed by another follow-up imaging study in no less than 4 weeks [48]. If metastases continue to enlarge, then progressive disease can be diagnosed. In some instances, however, a subsequent study will indicate tumor response (consisting of decreased size and/or attenuation), confirming that the initial change in size was merely "pseudoprogression" (Fig.). The system for assessing metastatic tumor in immunotherapy patients has been modified to take this issue into account (iRECIST criteria) [48].

Initial studies on the efficacy of immunotherapy in treating patients with metastatic renal cancer have been promising. Many patients have had sustained responses, which have even persisted after therapy was discontinued.

Complications of Multikinase Inhibitor Treatment and Immunotherapy

Complications encountered in patients undergoing new systemic treatments include hepatic steatosis, cholecystitis, pancreatitis, bowel perforation, and arterial thrombosis

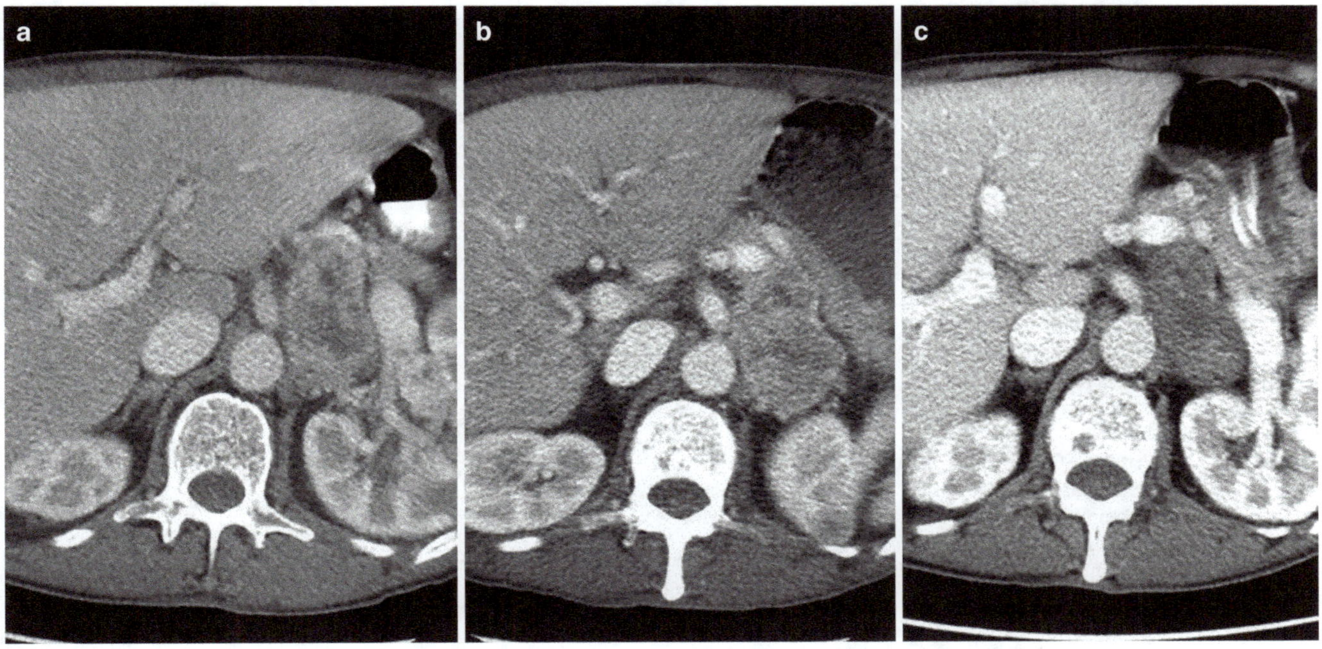

Fig. Adrenal metastasis treated with immunotherapy. (**a**) Initial contrast-enhanced CT image demonstrates a large left adrenal mass. (**b**) The mass remains heterogeneous and is larger on a follow-up CT obtained 6 weeks later. (**c**) A follow-up study obtained after another 4 weeks now shows the mass to be necrotic and smaller (after multikinase therapy) and colitis (segmental or diffuse), pneumonitis, and dermatitis and, less commonly, thyroiditis, hypophysitis, pancreatitis, and adrenal dysfunction (after immunotherapy) [49].

ConcludingRemarks

There have been many exciting recent developments with respect to the imaging, diagnosis, and treatment of solid renal masses in the past few years. This has included the identification of imaging features that can differentiate among some of the many cystic and solid renal masses. Unfortunately, in many patients, overlapping features still prevent distinction of renal cancers from benign renal lesions. For this reason, biopsy, which can be performed safely and without concern for tumor tract seeding, is often used for diagnosis. Imaging remains crucial for staging of renal cancer, as it is very accurate. In patients with organ-confined disease, imaging can be used to determine which patients are candidates for partial versus total nephrectomy. It has become increasingly clear that some patients with small malignant renal masses may never need to have the masses treated. Novel chemotherapeutic agents have greatly prolonged survival of patients with regional or distant metastatic disease. Tumor response after treatment with the new targeted agents can be sustained but can sometimes be delayed. Tumor necrosis without size reduction can be seen occasionally and should not be confused with a lack of response.

References

1. Agochukwu N, Huber S, Spektor M, et al. Differentiating renal neoplasms from simple cysts on contrast-enhanced CT on the basis of attenuation and homogeneity. AJR. 2017;208:801–4.
2. Cohan RH, Sherman LS, Korobkin M, et al. Renal masses: assessment of corticomedullary-phase and nephrographic-phase CT scans. Radiology. 1995;196:445–51.
3. Hindman NM. Approach to very small (<1.5 cm) cystic renal lesions: ignore, observe, or treat? AJR. 2015;204:1182–9.
4. Choyke PL. Imaging of hereditary renal cancer. Radiol Clin North Am. 2003;41:1037–51.
5. Herts BR, Silverman SG, Hindman NM, et al. Management of the incidental renal mass on CT: a white paper of the ACR incidental findings committee. J Am Coll Radiol. 2017. https://doi.org/10.1016/j.jacr.2017.04.028. [Epub ahead of print]
6. Bosniak MA, Birnbaum BA, Krinsky GA, et al. Small renal parenchymal neoplasms: further observations on growth. Radiology. 1995;197:589–97.
7. Bosniak MA. The current radiological approach to renal cysts. Radiology. 1986;158:1–10.
8. Israel GM, Bosniak MA. How I do it: evaluating renal masses. Radiology. 2005;236:441–50.
9. Hindman NM, Hecht EM, Bosniak MA. Follow-up for Bosniak category 2F cystic renal lesions. Radiology. 2014;272:757–66.
10. Israel GM, Hindman N, Bosniak MA. Evaluation of cystic renal masses: comparison of CT and MR imaging by using the Bosniak classification system. Radiology. 2004;231:365–71.
11. Jinzaki M, Silverman SG, Akita H, et al. Diagnosis of renal angiomyolipomas: classic, fat-poor, and epithelioid types. Semin Ultrasound CT MRI. 2017;38:37–46.
12. Doshi AM, Ayoola A, Rosenkrantz AB. Do incidental hyperechoic renal lesions measuring up to 1 cm warrant further imaging? Outcomes of 161 lesions. AJR. 2017;209:1–5.
13. Farrelly C, Delaney H, McDermott R, et al. Do all non-calcified echogenic renal lesions found on ultrasound need further evaluation with CT? Abdom Imaging. 2008;33:44–7.
14. Davenport MS, Neville AM, Ellis JH, et al. Diagnosis of renal angiomyolipoma with Hounsfield Unit thresholds: effect of size and region of interest and nephrographic phase imaging. Radiology. 2011;260:158–65.
15. Israel GM, Hindman N, Hecht E, et al. The use of opposed-phase chemical shift MRI in the diagnosis of renal angiomyolipomas. AJR. 2005;194:1868–72.
16. Israel GM, Bosniak MA, Slywotzky CM, et al. CT differentiation of large exophytic renal angiomyolipomas and perirenal liposarcomas. AJR. 2005;179:769–73.
17. Catalano OA, Samir AE, Sahani DV, et al. Pixel distribution analysis: can it be used to distinguish clear cell carcinomas from angiomyolipomas with minimal fat? Radiology. 2008;247:738–46.
18. Simpfendorfer C, Herts BR, Motta-Ramirez GA, et al. Angiomyolipoma with minimal fat on MDCT: can counts of negative attenuation pixels aid diagnosis? AJR. 2009;192:438–43.
19. Kim JK, Kim HS, Jang YJ, et al. Renal angiomyolipoma with minimal fat: differentiation from other neoplasms at double-echo chemical shift FLASH MR imaging. Radiology. 2006;239:274–80.
20. Zhang YY, Luo S, Liu Y, et al. Angiomyolipoma with minimal fat: differentiation from papillary renal cell carcinoma by helical CT. Clin Radiol. 2013;68:365–70.
21. Ryan MJ, Francis IR, Cohan RH, et al. Imaging appearance of renal epithelioid angiomyolipomas. J Comput Assist Tomogr. 2013;37:957–61.
22. Choudhary S, Rajesh A, Mayer NJ, et al. Renal oncocytoma: CT features cannot reliably distinguish oncocytoma from other renal neoplasms. Clin Radiol. 2009;64:517–22.
23. Woo S, Cho JY, Kim SY, et al. Segmental enhancement inversion of small renal oncocytoma: differences in prevalence according to tumor size. AJR. 2013;200:1054–9.
24. O'Malley MW, Tran P, Hanbidge A, et al. Small renal oncocytomas: is segmental enhancement inversion a characteristic finding at biphasic MDCT? AJR. 2012;199:1312–5.
25. Moch H, Cubilla AL, Humphrey PA, Reuter VE, Ulbright TM. The 2016 WHO classification of tumours of the urinary system and male genital organs – Part A: renal, penile, and testicular tumors. J Euro Urol. 2016;70:93–105.
26. Young JR, Margolis D, Sauk S, et al. Clear cell renal cell carcinoma: discrimination from other renal cell carcinoma subtypes and oncocytoma at multiphasic multidetector CT. Radiology. 2013;267:444–53.
27. Oliva MR, Glickman JN, Zou KH, et al. Renal cell carcinoma: T1 and T2 signal intensity characteristics of papillary and clear cell types correlated with pathology. AJR. 2009;192:1524–30.
28. Egbert ND, Caoili EM, Cohan RH, et al. Differentiation of papillary renal cell carcinoma subtypes on CT and MRI. AJR. 2013;201:347–55.
29. Zhu QQ, Wang ZQ, Zhu WR, et al. The multislice CT findings of renal carcinoma associated with XP11.2 translocation/TFE gene fusion and collecting duct carcinoma. Acta Radiol. 2013;54:355–62.
30. Raza SA, Sohaib SA, Sahdev A, et al. Centrally infiltrating renal masses on CT: differentiating intrarenal transitional cell carcinoma from centrally located renal cell carcinoma. AJR. 2012;198:846–53.
31. Choi SJ, Jim HS, Ahn SJ, et al. Differentiating radiological features of rapid- and slow-growing renal cell carcinoma using multidetector computed tomography. J Comput Assist Tomogr. 2012;36:313–8.

32. Pierorazio PM, Hyams ES, Mullens JK, et al. Active surveillance of small renal masses. Rev Urol. 2012;14:13–9.
33. Leng S, Takahashi N, Cardona DG, et al. Subjective and objective heterogeneity scores for differentiating small renal masses using contrast-enhanced CT. Abdom Radiol. 2017;42:1485–92.
34. Coy H, Young JR, Douek ML, et al. Quantitative computer-aided diagnostic algorithm for automated detection of peak lesion attenuation in differentiating clear cell from papillary and chromophobe renal cell carcinoma, oncocytoma, and fat-poor angiomyolipoma on multiphasic multidetector computed tomography. Abdom Radiol. 2017;42:1919–28.
35. Chen C, Kang Q, Wei Q, et al. Correlation between CT perfusion parameters and Fuhrman grade in pT1b renal cell carcinoma. Abdom Radiol. 2017;42:1464–71.
36. Halverson SJ, Kunju LP, Bhalla R, et al. Accuracy of determining small renal mass management with risk stratified biopsies: confirmation by final pathology. J Urol. 2013;189:441–6.
37. Park SH, Oh YT, Jung DC, et al. Abdominal seeding of renal cell carcinoma: radiologic, pathologic, and prognostic features. Abdom Radiol. 2017;42:1510–6.
38. Hedgire SS, Elmi A, Nadkarni ND, et al. Preoperative evaluation of perinephric fat invasion in patients with renal cell carcinoma: correlation with pathological findings. Clin Imaging. 2013;37:91–6.
39. Kutikov A, Uzzo RG. The RENAL nephrometry score: a comprehensive standardized system for quantitating renal tumor size, location and depth. J Urol. 2009;182:844–53.
40. Davenport M, Caoili EM, Cohan RH, et al. MR and CT characteristics of successfully ablated renal masses status-post radiofrequency ablation. AJR. 2009;192:1571–8.
41. Kawamoto S, Solomon SB, Bluemke DA, et al. Computed tomography and magnetic resonance imaging appearance of renal neoplasms after radiofrequency ablation and cryoablation. Semin Ultrasound CT MRI. 2009;30:67–77.
42. Lall CG, Patel HP, Fujimoto S, et al. Making sense of postoperative CT imaging following laparoscopic partial nephrectomy. Clin Radiol. 2012;67:675–86.
43. Corwin MT, Lamba R, Wilson M, et al. Renal cell carcinoma metastases to the pancreas: value of arterial imaging. Acta Radiol. 2013;54:349–54.
44. Nishino M, Jagannathan JP, Ramaiya NH, Van den Abbeele AD. Revised RECIST guideline version 1.1: what oncologists want to know and what radiologists need to know. AJR. 2010;195:281–9.
45. Smith AD, Shah SN, Rini BI, et al. Morphology, attenuation, size and structure (MASS) criteria: assessing response and predicting clinical outcome in metastatic renal cell carcinoma on antiangiogenic target therapy. AJR. 2010;194:1470–8.
46. Thian Y, Gutzeit A, Koh DM, et al. Revised Choi imaging criteria correlate with clinical outcomes in patients with metastatic renal cell carcinoma treated with sunitnib. Radiology. 2014;273:452–61.
47. Pardoll DM. The blockade of immune checkpoints in cancer immunotherapy. Nat Rev Cancer. 2012;12:252–64.
48. Seymour L, Bogaerts J, Perrone A, et al. iRECIST: guidelines for response criteria for use in trials testing immunotherapeutics. Lancet Oncol. 2017;18:e143–52.
49. Shinagare AB, Krajewski K, Braschi-Amirfarzan M, et al. Advanced renal cell carcinoma: role of the radiologist in the era of precision medicine. Radiology. 2017;284:333–51.

10

Adnexal Diseases

Andrea Rockall and Rosemarie Forstner

Learning Objectives

- To know the most common benign ovarian lesions
- To be aware of the indications for MRI of adnexal masses
- To know the sequences for basic and fully optimized MRI of adnexal masses
- To be able to use an algorithmic approach to characterize adnexal masses

Introduction

Adnexal masses are common and may present symptomatically with pelvic or abdominal pain or may be identified incidentally during the course of imaging for another indication. The majority of adnexal masses are benign, but a small number will be borderline tumors or invasive cancer. In the case of a benign lesion, the aim is to reassure the patient and manage according to the clinical need, without subjecting the patient to over-extensive or inappropriate surgery [1]. Conversely, in cases that demonstrate features with a higher likelihood of ovarian malignancy, referral to a specialist center will ensure the best possible outcome for the patient.

One major difficulty is that undertaking a biopsy to confirm the nature of an adnexal mass is not advised, if there is no peritoneal disease beyond the ovary. Biopsy could result in spillage of a potentially confined tumor and increase stage and risk for patient. Therefore, the clinical decision on how aggressively to manage the ovarian mass relies on the available clinical and image findings, rather than histology.

The clinical context at the time of presentation is relevant. The age and menopausal status of the patient and the presence of acute or chronic pain or fever may inform the interpretation of image findings. In premenopausal women with pain, a pregnancy test is indicated in order to rule out possible ectopic pregnancy as a cause of an adnexal mass.

Ultrasound is the first-line imaging modality, allowing the characterization of most adnexal masses. MRI is indicated in the characterization of sonographically indeterminate masses, whereas CT is indicated for further staging of a suspected ovarian cancer on US.

Imaging Modalities to Assess an Adnexal Mass

Ultrasound(US)

Optimally, transvaginal ultrasound (TVUS) and transabdominal ultrasound (TAUS) are combined to provide characterization of the adnexal mass and its differentiation from the uterus or other pelvic abnormalities. TAUS also provides information of ancillary findings that may be crucial for the diagnosis, e.g., presence of peritoneal implants, ascites, pleural effusion, and lymph node enlargement, and assessment of the kidneys and the bowels. For characterization of an adnexal mass, the following imaging features indicative of malignancy have been widely used: wall irregularity, thick septations (3 mm), papillary projections, solid components, and large size (4 cm) [1–3]. Unfortunately these features overlap with those of benign pathologies, e.g., tubo-ovarian abscess, corpus luteum cyst, endometriomas, and some rare benign tumors. Recently, the IOTA simple rules model has been introduced to preoperatively assess adnexal masses with US. Five sonographic imaging features each defining the B (benign) and M (malignant) categories are used to distinguish

A. Rockall
Consultant Radiologist, Department of Radiology, The Royal Marsden NHS Foundation Trust, London, UK

Professor of Radiology, Faculty of Medicine, Imperial College London, UK

R. Forstner (✉)
Faculty of Medicine, Imperial College London, London, UK
e-mail: R.Forstner@salk.at

between malignant and benign adnexal masses [4–6]. Thus, in expert hands approximately 78–80% of complex adnexal masses can be diagnosed with US alone. Limitations include mostly benign solid masses, e.g., endometriomas, fibromas, thecomas, and rare other ovarian tumors.

Magnetic Resonance Imaging (MRI)

MRI is recommended as a second-line imaging technique to evaluate adnexal masses that remain indeterminate on US [7]. MRI combines excellent contrast resolution and lack of nonionizing radiation, which is of utmost importance in children and in the reproductive age. It is most useful in women with a low pretest probability of malignancy of the adnexal mass. Studies show high diagnostic sensitivity (67–100%) and specificity (77–100%) [8–16].

Typical MRI protocols include T2-weighted imaging in two planes, usually the sagittal T2-weighted imaging providing overview of the uterus and the ovaries and a transaxial T1- and high-resolution fast spin echo (FSE) T2-weighted imaging sequence covering in thin slices the ovaries [7]. If the ovaries are not seen, oblique axial T2-weighted imaging taken along the long axis of the uterus will visualize the ovaries in atypical position along their ovarian axis. In equivocal cases, this plane or alternatively a coronal plane also serves in solving important differential diagnostic issues, e.g., the nonovarian origin of a parauterine mass (i.e., pedunculated uterine leiomyoma). Features of subserous uterine leiomyomas present presence of bridging vessels between the mass and the myometrium or the claw sign of the uterine myometrium. In contrast, demonstrations of follicles within or in the periphery of the mass and the ovarian beak sign are typical features of ovarian origin of a pelvic mass [7].

The majority of adnexal lesions can be characterized by their specific signal characteristics on T1- and T2-weighted imaging. Simple fluid has homogeneous low signal on T1-weighted imaging and high SI on T2-weighted imaging. Fat and hemorrhage have high SI on T1-weighted imaging. Fat suppression (FS) on T1-weighted imaging is used to differentiate fat-containing dermoids from hemorrhagic cystic lesions [7]. In solid and in cystic adnexal masses, characterization is best performed by complementing the basic sequences with DWI and intravenous administration of gadolinium [11, 15, 16]. For characterization of adnexal masses, the recommended high b value is between 800 and 1200 mm/s^2. Optimally, dynamic multiphase contrast-enhanced (DCE) MRI is used to characterize adnexal masses, as the time-intensity curve of a solid aspect of the mass in relation to the myometrium will provide important differential diagnostic information. Subtraction images are essential to evaluate enhancing aspects within hemorrhagic lesions, e.g., of nodules within endometriomas. Fasting for 4 h, application of antiperistaltic medication, and examination with a medium full bladder are used to optimize the image quality [7].

Computed Tomography(CT)

In clinical practice contrast-enhanced CT is widely used to assess abdominal pathologies, and usually this is accomplished by covering the abdomen and the pelvis. For characterization of a sonographically indeterminate mass, CT is not recommended, as it is inferior to both MRI and US to assess solid and hemorrhagic masses. CT is, however, the modality of choice to stage suspected ovarian cancer [17]. Another role of CT is in the emergency setting, where it is widely used to assess the acute abdomen, for both gynecological and non-gynecological causes [18].

PositronEmission Tomography/ Computed Tomography (PET/CT)

PET/CT using fluoro-2-deoxy-D-glucose (FDG) has currently no role in characterizing of adnexal lesions. Physiological uptake in premenopausal age in normal ovaries and in corpus luteum cysts is a well-known cause of misinterpretation [19]. FDG uptake can also be seen in benign ovarian tumors, such as dermoids, as well as in inflammatory and infectious processes. However, in postmenopausal age FDG avid uptake in the ovaries is typically associated with malignant disease. Currently the role of PET/CT includes assessment of suspected recurrence in two scenarios in patients with ovarian cancer: a) in biochemically suspected recurrence and no evidence of disease with other imaging techniques or b) to exclude systemic disease in surgical potential candidates with localized disease.

Adnexal Masses on MRI

Imaging characteristics of benign and malignant ovarian masses are summarized in Table .

Benign Cystic Ovarian Masses

OvarianCysts

In reproductive age physiological ovarian cysts constitute the vast majority of adnexal masses. Ovarian follicles and follicular cysts share the same imaging features of thin-walled lesions with watery contents, but per definition the term cyst should be reserved only to those larger than 3 cm in size [1]. Due to their high prevalence in premenopausal age, cysts ranging from 3 to 5 cm do not require further follow-up, unless they are symptomatic [1]. Ovarian cysts include either follicular cysts or corpus luteum cysts. The latter derive from failure of regression or hemorrhage into the corpus luteum. Corpus luteum and corpus luteum cysts typically have a well-vascularized thicker wall that may be crenulated and often contain blood products. Thus they display a lacelike appear-

Table . Imaging characteristics of benign and malignant ovarian masses

Mass	Age	Overall architecture	T2 SI of solid component	T1 SI	T1 Gd TIC (time-intens curve)	DWI ($b > 800$)	Side	Specific features
Ovarian follicular cyst	Fertile	Cystic		Low		Low		Regresses spontaneously
Serous cystadenoma	Pre-/postmenopausal	Cystic Uni- or multilocular		Low	TIC 1	Low	Bilateral	May mimic ovarian cyst, no regression
Mucinous cystadenoma	Pre-/postmenopausal	Cystic Multilocular	Low	Low/intermediate	TIC 1	Low	Unilateral	Large at diagnosis
Mature cystic teratoma	All ages, mostly young	Cystic Mixed	Intermediate	High	Variable	High, variable	Unilateral	Use FS Risk of torsion >5 cm
Fibroma/thecoma	Perimenopausal	Solid	Low	Intermediate	TIC 1, rarely 2	Low	Unilateral	Solid well circumscribed
Endometrioma	Fertile	Cystic Uni- or multilocular	Low	High	Low TIC 1 or 2	High	Often bilateral	Uniform wall enhancement No nodular enhancement CCP
Serous borderline tumor	Pre-/perimenopausal	Cystic Uni- or multilocular	Low/intermediate	Low	TIC 2	Low variable	Bilateral	Papillary projections >5 mm
Mucinous borderline tumor	Pre-/perimenopausal	Cystic Multiseptate	Intermediate	Intermediate	TIC 2	Low variable	Unilateral	Large at diagnosis, mural nodules
Metastases Cystic/solid	Perimenopausal	Mixed or solid	Intermediate	Intermediate	TIC 2 or 3	High	Often bilateral	Colon, GI tract cancer
Dysgerminoma	Young	Solid	Intermediate	Intermediate	TIC 2	High	Unilateral	Solid, multinodular
Serous ovarian cancer	Postmenopausal	Mixed or solid	Intermediate	Mixed	TIC 2 and 3	High	Often bilateral	Ascites
Tubo-ovarian abscess	Premenopausal	Mixed	Intermediate	High or intermediate	High	High	Bilateral	Pain, fever Peritonitis

ance in US and not watery contents but signal intensity of blood products on MRI (high SI on T1-weighted imaging and FS T1-weighted imaging or hemosiderin). Typical is unilaterality and regression in a 2-3 months interval.

Endometriomas

Endometriomas present endometriotic cysts of the ovaries and constitute the most common manifestation of endometriosis. Most commonly they present bilateral thick-walled uni- or multiloculated cystic lesions containing blood products. Pathognomonic features include high SI on T1-weighted imaging and FS T1-weighted imaging and low SI on T2-weighted imaging (shading) (Fig.) [ ]. The T2 dark spot sign presenting focal mural clot is another typical feature [21]. As in unilocular hemorrhagic cysts the distinction between endometriomas and hemorrhagic cysts may sometimes be difficult, follow-up US is recommended. Only functional cysts will resolve. Bilaterality and multicystic appearance favor endometrioma. Adhesions with low SI bands and distortion of the ovaries, the uterus, or the bowel are other typical findings in endometriosis. As deep endometriosis, particularly involving the posterior fornix or the rectosigmoid colon, is often associated with endometriomas, this area should also be scrutinized.

Benign Teratomas (Mature Cystic Teratomas or Dermoid Cysts)

The typical finding of a mature teratoma is that of a unilocular cystic lesion containing fatty elements. Often a mural nodule, the Rokitansky nodule or dermoid plug, projects into the lesion. It is composed of a variety of tissues and typically demonstrates fat and calcifications, representing teeth or bones. A minority (approx. 15%) of mature cystic teratomas will demonstrate no fat or only small foci of fat within the wall or the Rokitansky nodule [22].

As US features of dermoids may overlap with those of other entities, such as endometriomas or ovarian carcinomas, CT (Fig.) or MRI (Fig.) is performed in suspected dermoids, as they allow a specific diagnosis. In both

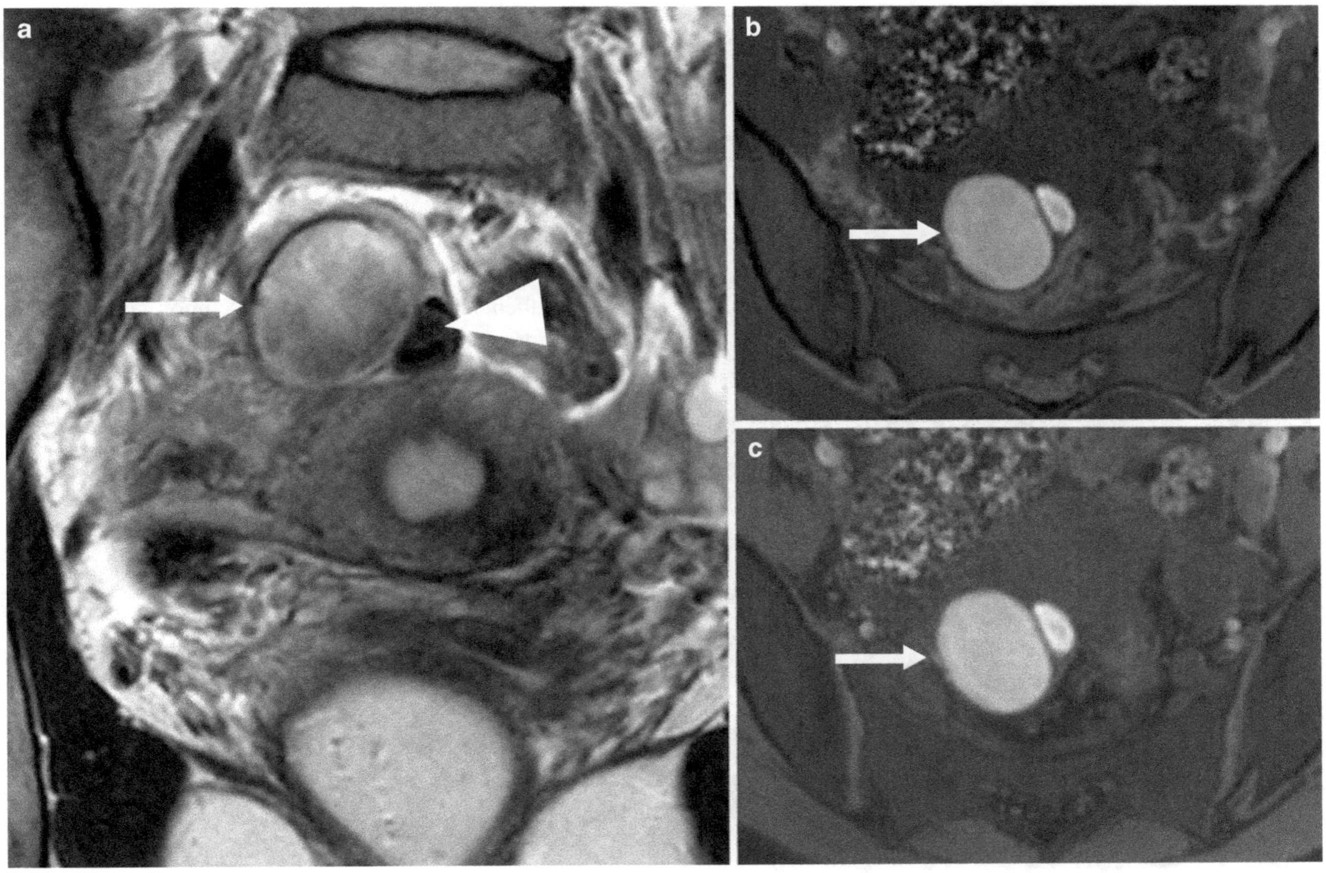

Fig. Right ovarian endometrioma. Coronal FSE T2-weighted imaging shows a septate right cystic ovarian lesion with thin walls (**a**) (arrow). It demonstrates diffuse moderate hypointensity and adjacent very low SI (shading effect) relating to chronic hemorrhage. (**b**) Transaxial T1-weighted imaging and (**c**) FS T1-weighted imaging (arrow) demonstrate high SI characteristic of internal blood products. There is no evidence of internal or mural nodularity of these techniques, identification of fat is the pivotal finding. On MRI, the fatty component will demonstrate high SI on both T1- and T2-weighted imaging, with the lipid-laden cyst fluid demonstrating a similar high SI on T1-weighted imaging and intermediate SI on T2-weighted imaging. Chemical shift artifact is often seen at the fat-fluid interface in dermoid cysts as bright or dark bands along the frequency-encoding gradient on T2-weighted imaging. Use of FS T1-weighted imaging enables dermoid cysts (which drop the SI) to be distinguished from hemorrhagic lesions or endometriomas (which retain high SI). In lipid poor dermoids chemical shift imaging techniques may assist in defining the correct diagnosis. Due to their very slow growth, surveillance is a treatment option in dermoids smaller than 5 cm in size.

Rarely, malignant transformation may develop within a dermoid cyst; most frequently this is squamous cell cancer in a woman of advanced age. Capsular penetration is the most reliable sign to establish this extremely rare complication [23].

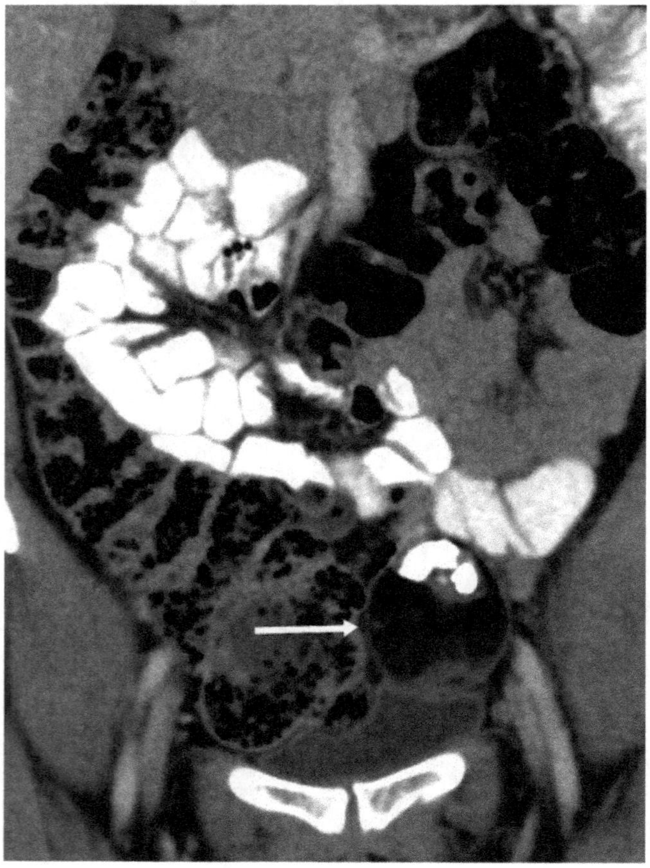

Fig. Benign teratoma. CT shows a well-defined cystic lesion with thin walls (arrow). Its fatty contents allow the specific diagnosis of a benign teratoma. Calcification presenting teeth within its superior aspect present another other common finding

Cystadenomas

Cystadenomas present common epithelial ovarian tumors, accounting for up to 50% of tumors in reproductive age and for up to 80% of benign ovarian tumors in postmenopausal age [24]. Both have now been recognized as precursors of ovarian cancer and may slowly transform to borderline tumors and to invasive ovarian cancer [25]. Serous cystadenomas are more common than mucinous cystadenomas. Although an overlap exists, imaging features aid in the differentiation of serous from mucinous cystadenomas [24]. In general, both entities are thin-walled cystic lesions (Fig.). Serous cystadenomas follow the pattern of a simple cyst or of a multiseptate mass, whereas a mucinous cystadenoma is typically a large multilocular lesion with locules of various fluid contents [26]. On MRI, cysts in mucinous tumors demonstrate various signal intensities on T1- and T2-weighted imaging, giving rise to the so-called "stained-glass" appearance. This is because on T1-weighted imaging locules with watery mucin generate lower SI than locules with thicker mucin. The opposite is generated on T2-weighted imaging. Cystadenomas can be differentiated from hydrosalpinx due to their complete septations on multiplanar imaging.

Benign Solid Ovarian Tumors

These present a rare subgroup of ovarian tumors mostly comprising fibromas, thecomas, and Brenner tumors. They are usually unilateral solid ovarian tumors found in perimenopausal age [27]. In clinical practice they have to be differentiated from their mimickers, the more common pedunculated uterine leiomyomas. Signs defining the ovarian origin are pivotal for the differentiation. Due to their composition of fibrous tissue, they usually display typical features of benign adnexal masses with solid elements displaying very low SI on T2-weighted imaging. In degenerative changes including edema, cystic changes, or torsion, their differentiation from malignant masses is challenging. However, when such a solid lesion demonstrates low SI on DWI using a high b value, malignancy can be ruled out [12, 16]. Mild and slow gadolinium (type 1) enhancement pattern is seen in the majority of cases. The triad of an ovarian fibroma, ascites, and pleural effusion constitutes the benign Meigs syndrome, which can be associated with elevated CA-125. Unlike fibromas, more than half of thecomas express estrogenes and may present with uterine bleeding, endometrial hyperplasia, or endometrial cancer [27]. Dense amorphous calcifications are a typically feature in Brenner tumors in CT.

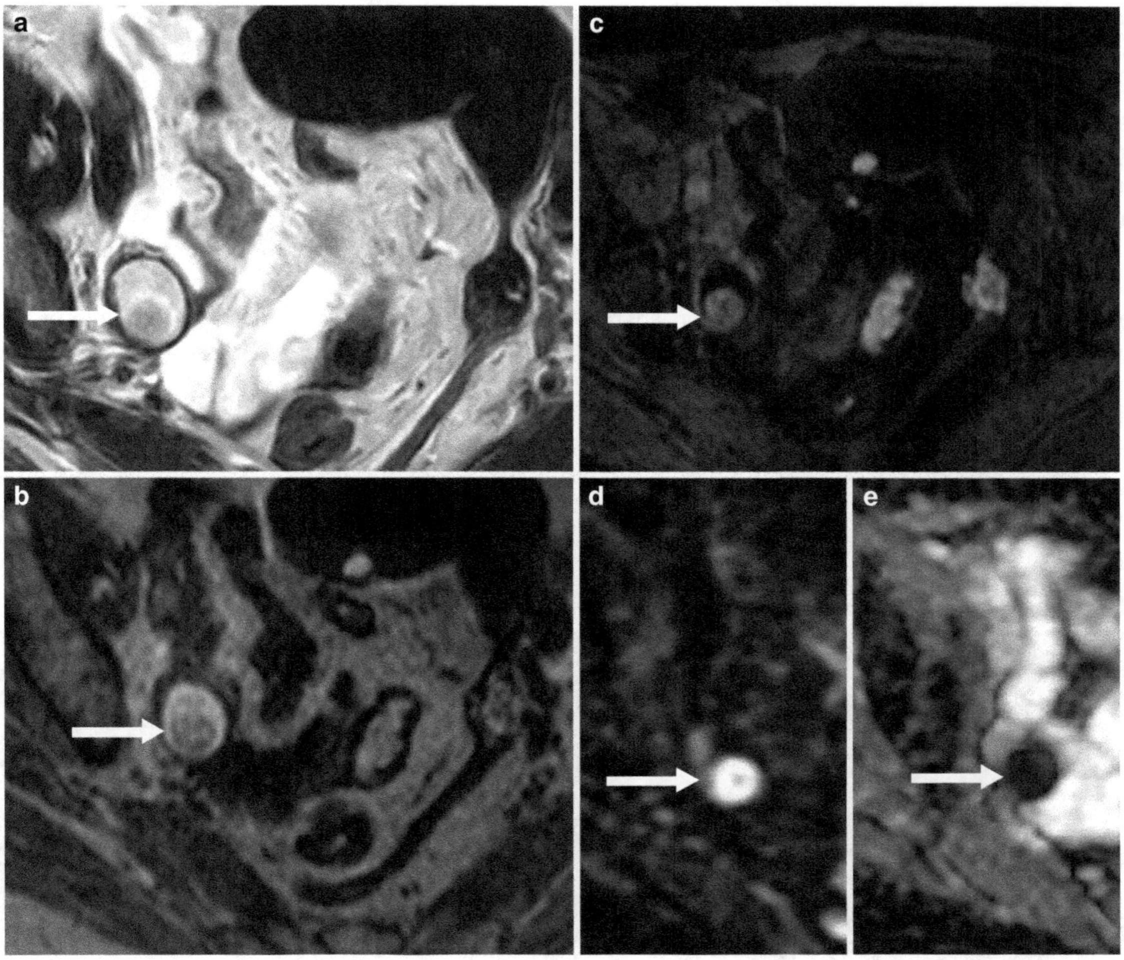

Fig. Benign teratoma. MRI shows a right adnexal mass of 2 cm in size (arrow). It displays high SI on transaxial FSE T2-weighted imaging (**a**) and internal chemical shift artifact. High SI on T1-weighted imaging (**b**) and loss of signal on FS T1-weighted imaging (**c**) are characteristic of fatty contents. A nodule, the Rokitansky nodule, is seen at its posterior aspect in **a–c**. On DWI using b1000 s/mm^2 (**d**) and on ADC (**e**), the lesion displays diffusion restriction that is due to its sebaceous contents and should not be misdiagnosed as sign of malignancy

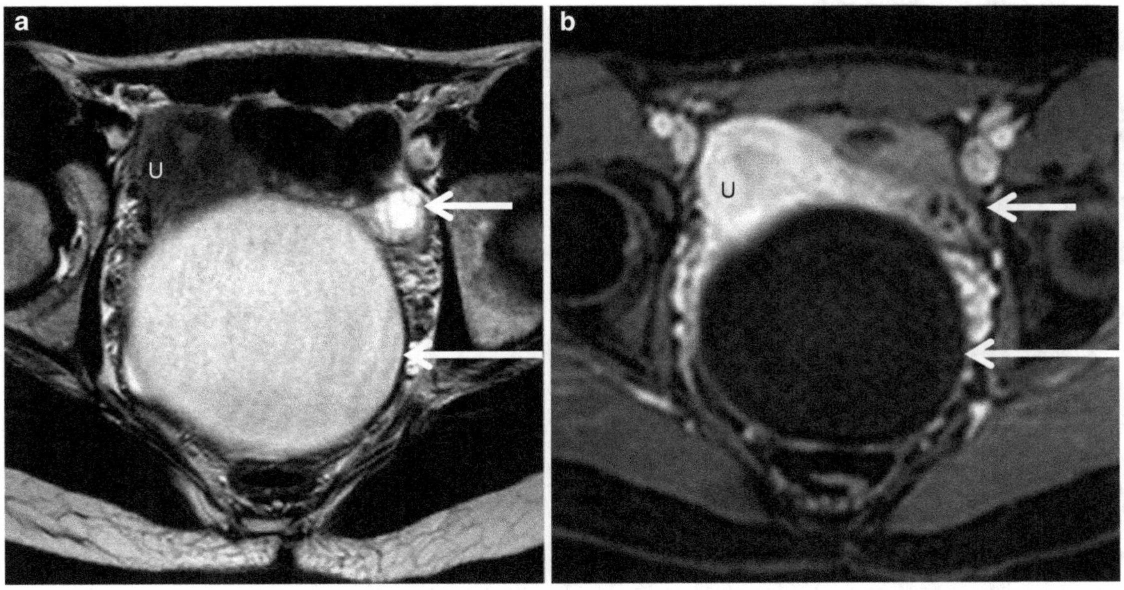

Fig. Benign ovarian cystadenoma. Axial T2 (**a**) and Axial T1 fat sat with contrast (**b**). There is a normal left ovary with follicles (short arrow). There is a unilocular thin-walled cyst with no solid tissue following contrast administration (long arrow). The uterus (U) enhances brightly. AdnexMR score is 2

Borderline and Malignant Ovarian Tumors

Borderline tumors account for approximately 15% of ovarian tumors. The vast majority of ovarian malignant lesions include invasive epithelial ovarian cancer and metastases. The latter constitute 15% of malignant ovarian masses and originate mostly from breast and the GI tract cancer. In contrast, sex cord-stromal tumors (granulosa cell and Sertoli-Leydig cell tumors) and malignant germ cell tumors are rare tumors, mostly found in young age.

Borderline tumors are now considered as precursor lesions that gradually progress to different subtypes of epithelial ovarian cancer type II. Serous high-grade ovarian cancer, the most common ovarian cancer, shares features of tubal and primary peritoneal cancer. It seems to develop de novo rapidly and is characterized by rapid dissemination into the peritoneal cavity and usually presents with tumor dissemination outside the pelvis and ascites at diagnosis [28].

Likelihood of malignancy increases with the presence of septations, mural nodules, and papillary projections (Fig.). MRI features suspicious for malignancy include mass 4 cm, cystic lesion with solid component, irregular wall thickness of 3 mm or more, septal thickness of 3 mm or more, presence of papillary projections or nodules, and presence of solid mass with necrosis and early, bright contrast enhancement [3, 16, 29]. In addition, ancillary criteria for suspected malignancy include direct local tissue invasion, peritoneal deposits, enlarged lymph nodes, and ascites. Dynamic CE (DCE)

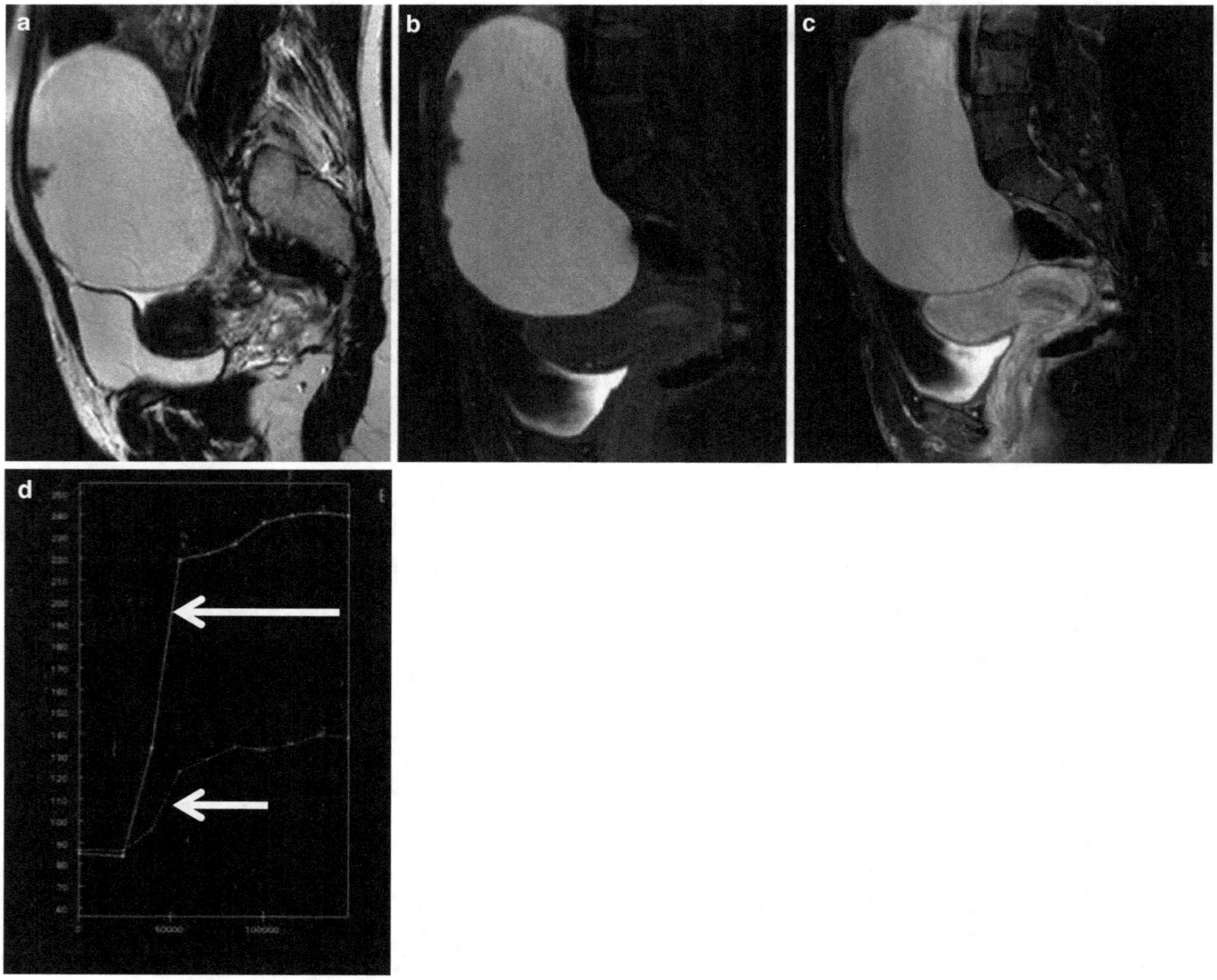

Fig. Serous borderline ovarian tumor. (**a**) T2-weighted image demonstrates a papillary formation arising from the anterior wall of a unilocular cyst. (**b**, **c**) T1 fat-saturated images before and after contrast demonstrate enhancement of multiple papillary structures at a different position in the cyst. (**d**) The time-intensity curve in the solid tissue is type 2 (short arrow is the enhancement curve of the papillary formation, and long arrow is the enhancement curve of the outer myometrium). AdnexMR score is 4

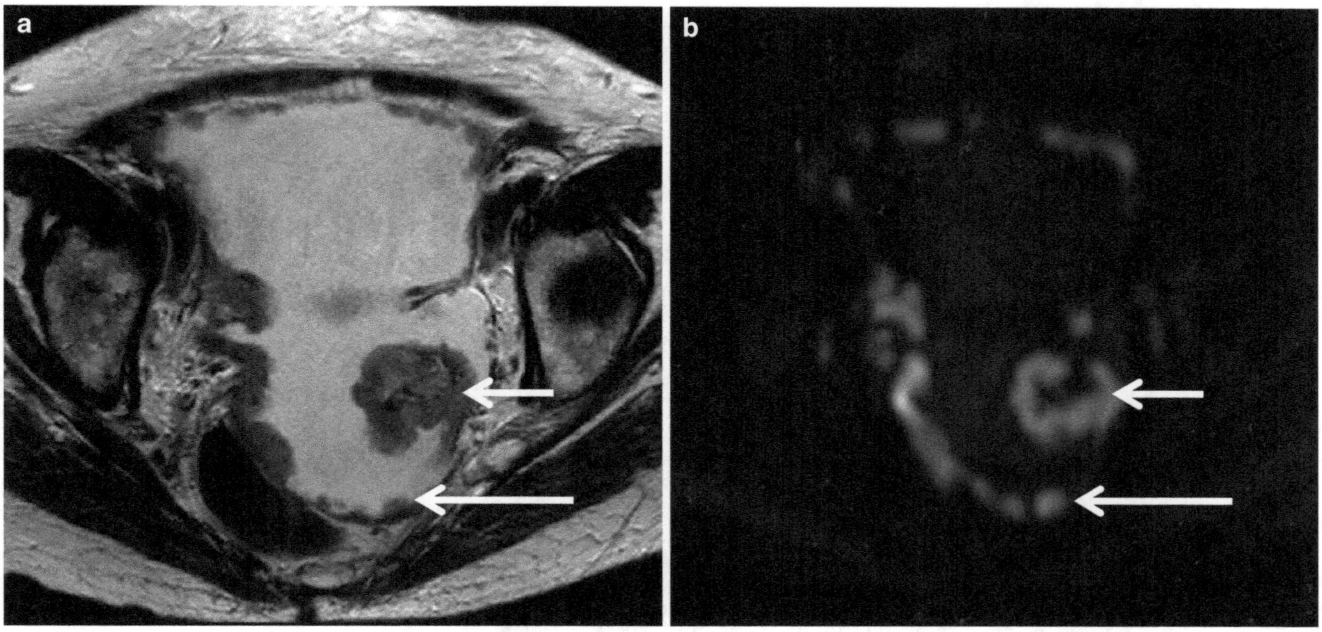

Fig. Disseminated peritoneal disease in tubo-ovarian cancer on MRI (**a**) axial T2 and (**b**) axial b1000 diffusion image. Left ovarian mass (short arrow) and peritoneal disease (long arrow). The solid tissue of the ovarian mass is intermediate in signal intensity. The ovarian solid tissue and the peritoneal disease are very bright on the diffusion image. AdnexMR score is 5 due to the presence of peritoneal disease

MRI is used for risk stratification in cystic and solid adnexal masses. Time-intensity curves types 1, 2, and 3 obtained from the solid aspects of such masses are associated with benign, borderline, and invasive tumors [16]. Gadolinium also improves peritoneal and omental implant detection in case of ovarian carcinoma. Due to the overlap of ADC values, DWI is less useful to characterize indeterminate adnexal masses, but it is pivotal to assess peritoneal carcinomatosis [14–17].

CE-CT remains the technique of choice for staging ovarian carcinoma [17] (Figs.).

Risk Stratification of Adnexal Masses Using the AdnexMR Score

When interpreting an adnexal mass on MRI, an algorithmic approach is strongly advocated. A risk stratification can also be applied (Table) [16].

1. The first step is to identify if indeed there is a pelvic mass, as occasionally a physiological ovarian mass may have resolved by the time of MRI. If there is a pelvic mass, then it is important to be sure whether it is arising from the ovary. Non-ovarian masses, such as leiomyomata, peritoneal inclusion cysts, or gastrointestinal stromal tumors, or some extraperitoneal lesions, such as Schwannoma, may be misinterpreted as adnexal on US. It is most important to check for the presence of normal ovaries, and this can also be challenging on MRI when a large mass fills the pelvis. It may be helpful to follow the

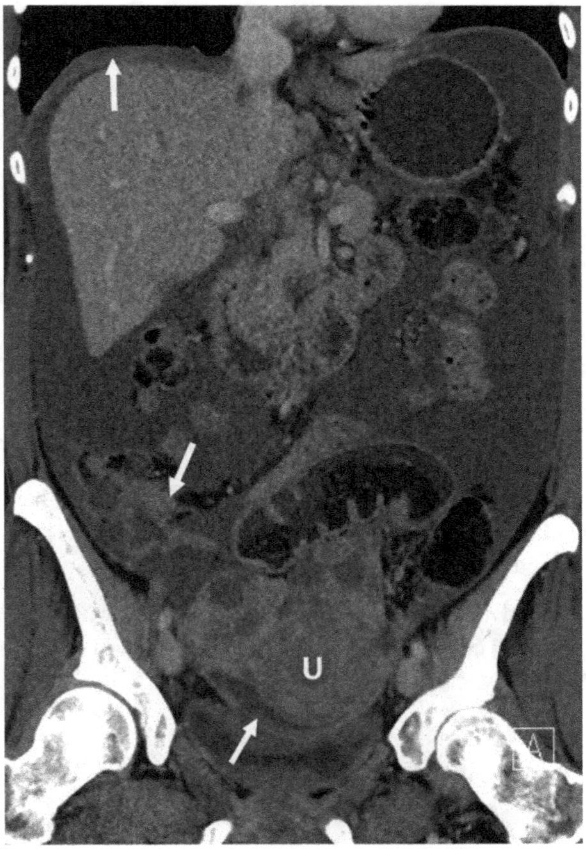

Fig. Ovarian cancer. CT demonstrates a solid and cystic ovarian mass adjacent to the uterus (u). Findings indicative of peritoneal dissemination in the pelvis and abdomen include large amounts of ascites and peritoneal deposits at the right diaphragm, bowel surface, and pelvic peritoneum (arrows)

Table AdnexMR scoring system [16]

AdnexMR score	Criteria
1. No ovarian mass	No mass
2. Benign ovarian mass	Purely cystic mass Purely endometriotic mass Purely fatty mass Absence of wall enhancement Low $b = 1000$ sec.mm^2 and low T2-weighted signal intensity within solid tissue
3. Probably benign mass	Absence of solid tissue Curve type 1 within solid tissue
4. Indeterminate MR mass	Curve type 2 within solid tissue
5. Probably malignant mass	Peritoneal disease Curve type 3 within solid tissue

gonadal vessels down into the pelvis, and the presence of follicles or a corpus luteum cyst, if present, is confirmatory. If two normal ovaries are identified, then the AdnexMR score is 1, and the MRI should focus on characterizing the non-ovarian mass.

2. If there is an ovarian lesion, then the next question is whether the cyst has benign features. This could include a unilocular cyst with no enhancing solid tissue, a typical endometrioma, or a mature cystic teratoma. Lesions with no wall enhancement or lesions with solid tissue that are homogeneously low signal intensity on both T2 and high b value DWI, with low enhancement, are almost certainly benign. These lesions all fall into an AdnexMR score of 2.

3. If an ovarian lesion does not comply with the above findings, then the presence and enhancement pattern of solid tissue is important. Solid tissue is defined as enhancing tissue in an irregular septation, papillary formation, or mural nodule or mass. The normal ovarian stroma, smooth wall or smooth septation, or non-enhancing internal debris is not defined as solid tissue. If solid tissue enhances with a low level type 1 time-intensity curve, the lesion is scored as AdnexMR score 3.

4. If solid tissue is present and it enhances with a time-intensity curve type 2, the lesion is considered indeterminate on MRI, AdnexMR score 4.

5. If solid tissue is present and it enhances with a time-intensity type 3 or if there is peritoneal disease, then the lesion is highly likely malignant and the AdnexMR score is 5.

By following this approach, most masses can be allocated a score according to the risk of malignancy, allowing the best clinical management for the patient.

Take-Home Messages

- Ultrasound is highly effective in the diagnosis of adnexal masses and can direct the treatment approach in most cases.
- It is important for radiologists to recognize the features of common benign and physiological findings.
- MRI is a second-line imaging modality which can be helpful in the characterization of sonographically indeterminate masses, acting as a problem-solving tool.
- For MRI, we recommend an algorithmic approach which includes DWI and contrast-enhanced sequences with DCE as the preferred contrast technique.

References

1. Levine D, Brown DL, Andreotti RF, et al. Management of asymptomatic ovarian and other adnexal cysts imaged at US: Society of Radiologists in Ultrasound Consensus Conference Statement. Radiology. 2010;256:943–54.
2. Buy JN, Ghossain MA, Hugol D, et al. Characterization of adnexal masses: combination of color Doppler and conventional sonography compared with spectral Doppler analysis alone and conventional sonography alone. AJR Am J Roentgenol. 1996;166:385–93.
3. Hricak H, Chen M, Coakley FV, et al. Complex adnexal masses: detection and characterization with MRI – multivariate analysis. Radiology. 2000;214:39–46.
4. Timmerman D, Valentin L, Bourne TH, International Ovarian Tumor Analysis (IOTA) Group, et al. Terms, definitions and measurements to describe the sonographic features of adnexal tumors: a consensus opinion from the International Ovarian Tumor Analysis (IOTA) Group. Ultrasound Obstet Gynecol. 2000;16:500–5.
5. Kaijser J, Vandecaveye V, Deroose CM, et al. Imaging techniques for the pre-surgical diagnosis of adnexal tumours. Best Pract Res Clin Obstet Gynaecol. 2014;28:683–95.
6. Timmerman D, Ameye L, Fischerova D, et al. Simple ultrasound rules to distinguish between benign and malignant adnexal masses before surgery: prospective validation by IOTA group. BMJ. 2010;341:c6839.
7. Forstner R, Thomassin-Naggara I, Cunha TM, et al. ESUR recommendations for MR imaging of the sonographically indeterminate adnexal mass: an update. Eur Radiol. 2017;27:2248–57.
8. Grab D, Flock F, Stohr I, et al. Classification of asymptomatic adnexal masses by ultrasound, magnetic resonance imaging, and positron emission tomography. Gynecol Oncol. 2000;77:454–9.
9. Huber S, Medl M, Baumann L, et al. Value of ultrasound and magnetic resonance imaging in the preoperative evaluation of suspected ovarian masses. Anticancer Res. 2002;22:2501–7.
10. Sohaib SA, Mills TD, Sahdev A, et al. The role of magnetic resonance imaging and ultrasound in patients with adnexal masses. Clin Radiol. 2005;60:340–8.
11. Bernardin L, Dilks P, Liyanage S. Effectiveness of semi-quantitative multiphase dynamic contrast-enhanced MRI as a predictor of malignancy in complex adnexal masses: radiological and pathological correlation. Eur Radiol. 2012;22:880–90.

12. Thomassin-Naggara I, Darai E, Cuenod CA, et al. Dynamic contrast-enhanced magnetic resonance imaging: a useful tool for characterizing ovarian epithelial tumors. J Magn Reson Imaging. 2008;28:111–20.
13. Thomassin-Naggara I, Bazot M, Darai E. Epithelial ovarian tumors: value of dynamic contrast-enhanced MR imaging and correlation with tumor angiogenesis. Radiology. 2008;248:148–59.
14. Thomassin-Naggara I, Daraï E, Cuenod CA, et al. Contribution of diffusion-weighted MR imaging for predicting benignity of complex adnexal masses. Eur Radiol. 2009;19:1544–52.
15. Thomassin-Naggara I, Toussaint I, Perrot N, et al. Characterization of complex adnexal masses: value of adding perfusion- and diffusion-weighted MR imaging to conventional MR imaging. Radiology. 2011;258:793–803.
16. Thomassin-Naggara I, Aubert E, Rockall A, et al. Adnexal masses: development and preliminary validation of an MR imaging scoring system. Radiology. 2013;267:432–43.
17. Forstner R, Sala E, Kinkel K, Spencer JA. ESUR guidelines: ovarian cancer staging and follow-up. Eur Radiol. 2010;20:2773–80.
18. Bhosale RP, Javitt CM, et al. ACR appropriateness criteria® acute pelvic pain in the reproductive age group. Ultrasound Q. 2016;32:108–15.
19. Prabhakar HB, Kraeft JJ, Schorge JO, et al. FDG PET–CT of gynecologic cancers: pearls and pitfalls. Abdom Imaging. 2015;40:2472.
20. Dias JL, Veloso Gomes F, Lucas R, Cunha TM. The shading sign: is it exclusive of endometriomas? Abdom Imaging. 2015;40:2566–72.
21. Corwin MT, Gerscovich EO, Lamba R, et al. Differentiation of ovarian endometriomas from hemorrhagic cysts at MR imaging: utility of the T2 dark spot sign. Radiology. 2014;271:126–32.
22. Yamashita Y, Hatanaka Y, Torashima M, Takahashi M, Miyazaki K, Okamura H. Mature cystic teratomas of the ovary without fat in the cystic cavity: MR features in 12 cases. AJR Am J Roentgenol. 1994;163:613–6.
23. Rha SE, Byun JY, Jung SE, et al. Atypical CT and MRI manifestations of mature ovarian cystic teratomas. AJR Am J Roentgenol. 2004;183:743–50.
24. Jung SE, Lee JM, Rha SE, Byun JY, Jung JI, Hahn ST. CT and MRI of ovarian tumors with emphasis on the differential diagnosis. Radiographics. 2002;22:1305–25.
25. Lengyel E. Ovarian cancer development and metastasis. Am J Pathol. 2010;177:1053–64.
26. Imaoka I, Wada A, Kaji Y, et al. Developing an MR imaging strategy for diagnosis of ovarian masses. Radiographics. 2006;26:1431–48.
27. Horta M, Cunha TM. Sex cord-stromal tumors of the ovary: a comprehensive review and update for radiologists. Diagn Interv Radiol. 2015;21:277–86.
28. Lalwani N, Prassad SR, Vikram R, Shanboghue AK, et al. Histologic, molecular, and cytogenetic features of ovarian cancers: implication for diagnosis and treatment. Radiographics. 2011;31:625–46.
29. Zhao SH, Quiang JW, Zhang GF, Wang SJ, Qiu HJ, Wang L. MRI in differentiating ovarian borderline from benign mucinous cystadenoma: pathologic correlation. J Magn Reson Imaging. 2014;39:162–6.

11

Diffuse Liver Disease: Cirrhosis, Focal Lesions in Cirrhosis, and Vascular Liver Disease

Khoschy Schawkat and Caecilia S. Reiner

Learning Objectives

- To know MR techniques useful to quantify liver steatosis and fibrosis
- To recognize the characteristic and atypical contrast-enhancement pattern of hepatocellular carcinoma
- To discuss the MR imaging appearance of focal lesions in the cirrhotic liver and the use of the standardized reporting system LI-RADS
- To learn about HCC mimics and diffuse vascular liver disease causing liver parenchyma alteration

Cirrhosis

Imaging of Pre-stages of Cirrhosis

With the growing epidemics of diabetes, obesity, and metabolic syndrome, the prevalence of nonalcoholic fatty liver disease (NAFLD) is rising worldwide. NAFLD has become one of the most common causes of chronic liver disease. It is commonly classified into two phenotypes, nonalcoholic fatty liver (NAFL) and nonalcoholic steatohepatitis (NASH). The need for noninvasive screening and monitoring protocols with imaging as an alternative to liver biopsy to define therapeutic targets and treatment end points in NASH is emerging with growing burden of NAFLD. Significant advances in magnetic resonance imaging (MRI) allow quantification of (PDFF) of MRI-visible protons bound to fat divided by all protons in the liver (bound to fat and water) with chemical shift imaging. The technique acquires multiple images at echo times optimally spaced for fat and water separation and T2* signal decay correction. Several studies proved that MRI-PDFF is a robust, quantitative, accurate, and reproducible noninvasive biomarker for the assessment of NAFLD [1–4].

The next step in the cascade of diffuse liver disease is the development of liver fibrosis commonly on the basis of steatohepatitis or hepatitis B or C. Quantification of hepatic fibrosis is either possible with ultrasound (US)-based or MR elastography (MRE). MRE can be accomplished with most MR scanners by adding hardware to generate mechanical waves. Increased rigidity caused by collagen deposition can be visualized by modified phase-contrast pulse sequences. The stiffness generated from the wave propagation information can be depicted on cross-sectional elastogram images. Several studies have demonstrated a high diagnostic accuracy of MRE (AUC 0.90–0.98, 95% CI 0.84–0.94) for identifying clinically significant fibrosis (stage 2 or higher) (Fig.) with advantages of MRE over US-based elastography [5–9].

Imaging of Cirrhosis

Cirrhosis as a common endpoint of chronic liver disease is characterized by progressive fibrosis of the liver parenchyma with ongoing regeneration. Cirrhosis is most commonly the result of hepatitis B and C or chronic alcoholism; other causes are metabolic, biliary, and cryptogenic diseases. At an early stage of cirrhosis, the liver may appear normal. With disease progression, heterogeneity and surface nodularity are observed. Because of the unique ability of the liver to regenerate in cirrhosis, the liver harbors a spectrum of hepatocellular nodules, most of which are regenerative. Due to

K. Schawkat · C. S. Reiner (✉)
Institute of Diagnostic and Interventional Radiology, University Hospital Zurich, Zurich, Switzerland
e-mail: khoschy.schawkat@usz.ch; caecilia.reiner@usz.ch

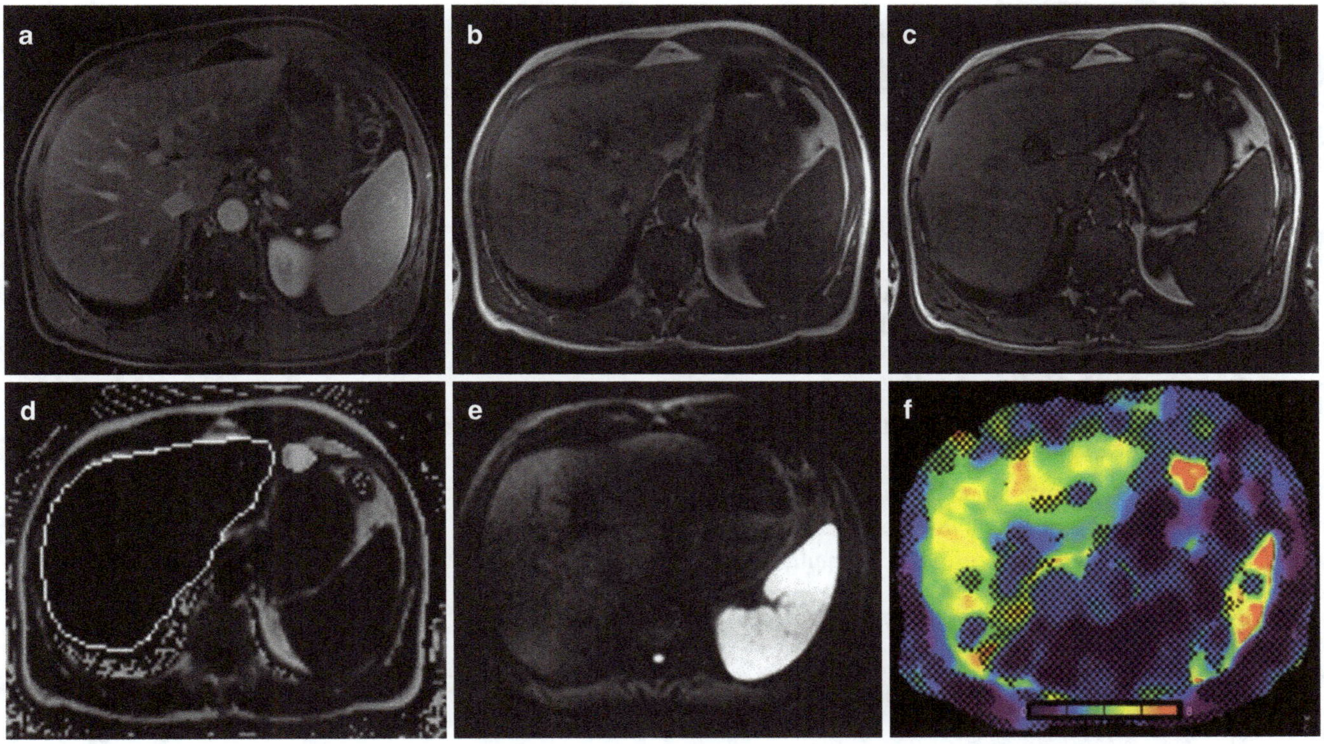

Fig. Imaging pre-stages of cirrhosis. 53-year-old male patient with chronic hepatitis C, genotype C. Histology proved moderate inflammatory activity (METAVIR A2) and portal fibrosis (METAVIR F3, Ishak 4). (**a**) Axial T1-weighted post-contrast magnetic resonance (MR) image in the portal venous phase does not show features of liver cirrhosis. No signal drop of the liver parenchyma is observed from the in-phase (**b**) to the out-of-phase gradient-dual-echo sequence (**c**). (**d**) Axial proton-density fat fraction map from a gradient multi-echo sequence with automated liver segmentation showed normal liver fat content (mean ± SD: 5.0 ± 0.8%). (**e**) Diffusion-weighted axial image with a b-value of 800 s/mm^2 shows increased signal of the liver parenchyma. (**f**) Stiffness map from MR elastography demonstrated increased stiffness of 4.9 ± 0.6 kPa corresponding to advanced fibrosis

the ongoing distortion of the liver parenchyma, the liver surface appears smooth, nodular, or lobular in most of the cases. Caudate lobe hypertrophy is the most characteristic morphologic feature of liver cirrhosis [10]. Alteration of blood flow results in typical morphologic abnormalities such as segmental hypertrophy involving the lateral segments of the left lobe (segment 2, 3) and segmental atrophy affecting the right lobe (segment 6, 7) and medial segment of the left lobe (segment 4). Other typical findings include enlargement of hilar periportal space, the right posterior notch sign, and generalized widening of the interlobar fissures. Less typical distribution of segmental atrophy and hypertrophy is seen in primary sclerosing cholangitis, where the distribution follows in part the distribution of the bile duct involvement, and, for example, atrophy of segments 2 and 3 or 5 and 7 may be seen. In 25% of cirrhosis, the liver shape and contour appears normal on CT or MRI.

Lymph adenopathy can appear in the liver hilum and peripancreatic region, which may mimic neoplastic lymph nodes, if the lymph nodes are large. Portal hypertension due to increased vascular resistance at the level of the hepatic sinusoids causes complications such as ascites and development of portosystemic shunts at the lower end of the esophagus and at the gastric fundus, via periumbilical veins and left gastric vein. Other shunts include splenorenal collaterals, hemorrhoidal veins, and abdominal wall and retroperitoneal collaterals [10]. These collateral veins are seen as enhancing tortuous vessels. The typical nodular liver contour and liver shape of cirrhosis as well as its vascular complications can be seen on ultrasound, CT, or MRI. MRI very well depicts fibrotic bands between regenerative nodules as T2 hyperintense and progressively or delayed enhancing structures.

Focal Lesions in Cirrhotic Liver

RegenerativeNodules

Regenerative nodules are present in a cirrhotic hepatic environment surrounded by fibrous septa and result from continuous injury to the liver parenchyma resulting usually in cirrhosis. They play a role in the stepwise carcinogenesis of HCC, most frequently through dedifferentiation, which occurs in the following order: regenerative nodule, low-grade dysplastic nodule, high-grade dysplastic nodule, and HCC. Most regenerative nodules do not progress in the dedifferentiation process. They are macronodular (≥9 mm) or micronodular (3–9 mm). MR imaging demonstrates regenerative nodules with greater sensitivity than other imaging modalities; these nodules are visualized in only 25% of unenhanced CT scans and approximately in 50% of MR images [11]. Regenerative nodules are usually iso- to hypointense on T2-weighted images. Variable signal intensity on T1-weighted images is due to lipid, protein, or copper content leading to a T1-weighted hyperintense appearance or iron deposition in the so-called siderotic nodules leading to a hypointense appearance on T1-weighted images. The most usual appearance on T1-weighted images is isointense. Using extracellular gadolinium-containing contrast agent, regenerative nodules appear hypointense in the arterial and portal venous phase and isointense during equilibrium and delayed phases. After administration of hepatobiliary-specific contrast material, regenerative nodules enhance to the same degree as adjacent liver because they have normal hepatocellular and phagocytic functions [12].

Dysplastic Nodules

Dysplastic nodules are regenerative nodules that contain atypical hepatocytes, measuring at least 1 mm, not meeting histologic criteria for malignancy. They are classified as low- or high-grade dysplastic nodules. High-grade dysplastic nodules are considered premalignant and are characterized by moderate cytologic and architectural atypia to a degree insufficient to render a diagnosis of HCC. The differentiation between a regenerative nodule and a low-grade dysplastic nodule is difficult due to similar appearance on MRI with iso- to hypointense appearance on T2-weighted images and iso- or hyperintense appearance on T1-weighted images. Dysplastic nodules are rarely detected on CT. Dysplastic nodules usually are hypovascular and do not show hyperenhancement with extracellular contrast agents. In high-grade dysplastic nodules, arterial vascularization can increase leading to arterial hyperenhancement on imaging. Using hepatocyte-specific MR contrast agents, dysplastic nodules show variable signal intensity in the hepatocyte-specific phase. With progressing dedifferentiation, the nodules lose their ability to take up the hepatocyte-specific contrast agent (Gd-EOB-DTPA) and appear hypointense in the hepatobiliary phase. These hepatobiliary hypointense dysplastic nodules may be mistaken for HCC. Dysplastic nodules may also instead lose the ability to excrete the hepatocyte-specific contrast agent and appear iso- or hyperintense on hepatobiliary phase images. Hypovascular cirrhotic nodules with hypointense appearance in the hepatobiliary phase carry a significant risk of transforming into hypervascular HCC with a pooled overall rate of 28% (95% CI, 22.7–33.6%). The size of the hypovascular nodule is a second risk factor for hypervascular transformation with nodules ≥9 mm in size showing a higher risk [13].

The earliest definitive sign of dysplastic nodule dedifferentiation is the "nodule within a nodule" appearance which is a dysplastic nodule harboring a focus of HCC, occurring in approximately 6% of patients with dysplastic nodules. However, it is believed that the majority of dysplastic nodules do not progresses to an HCC.

Hepatocellular Carcinoma

Hepatocellular carcinoma (HCC) is the fifth most common cancer worldwide, and its incidence is rising occurring most frequently in patients with cirrhosis or chronic viral hepatitis. HCC occurs as a solitary lesion (in half of the cases) and as multiple lesions or diffuse. It differs from most malignancies because it is commonly diagnosed on the basis of imaging features alone without histological confirmation in the setting of cirrhosis. A multiphasic contrast material-enhanced study is used (either CT or MR imaging) to set the radiologic diagnosis of HCC. The nodules that are suspicious for HCC during surveillance are new nodules that measure more than 1 cm or nodules that enlarge over a time interval. Following hepatocarcinogenesis, regenerative nodule dedifferentiates to dysplastic nodules and then to hepatocellular carcinoma. The vascular supply of HCC is mainly arterial though neoangiogenesis supplied by abnormal, unpaired hepatic arteries. Characteristically, HCC enhances during the arterial phase because of its blood supply. In the portal venous and equilibrium phase, the surrounding liver parenchyma becomes relatively hyperattenuated, and the lesion is perceived to be hypoattenuated because of its lack of portal venous supply corresponding to the so-called washout effect (Fig.). The third characteristic feature is pseudocapsule enhance-ment in the equilibrium phase. The diagnosis of HCC can be made from a single imaging study when this characteristic enhancement patterns—that is, arterial phase hyperenhance-ment and venous or delayed phase washout—are present. These noninvasive criteria can only be applied to cirrhotic patients [14]. About 70% of HCCs show these characteristic enhancement features of hypervascular HCCs, while the other 30% either do not show washout appearance or are hypovascular HCCs. When looking at HCCs 1 cm in size or less, only about 47% show typical enhancement features. When using Gd-EOB-DTPA, about 90% demonstrate hypointensity on hepatobiliary phase images and 10% dem-onstrate iso- or hyperintensity. Especially in hypovascular HCCs, which are difficult to diagnose with extracellular con-trast agents, the hepatocyte-specific contrast agent (Gd-EOB- DTPA) is useful. Among the hypovascular HCCs,

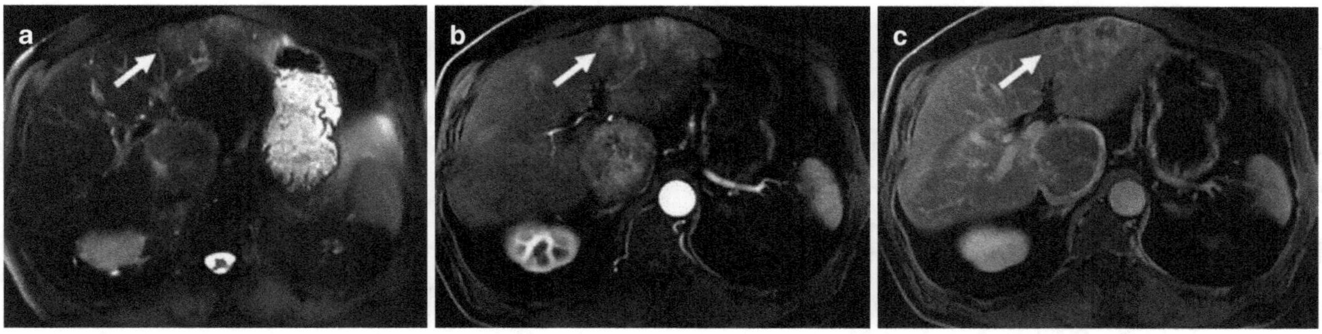

Fig. Multifocal HCC. 69-year-old patient with biopsy-proven metabolic toxic liver cirrhosis. (**a**) Axial T2-weighted magnetic resonance image demonstrates an iso- to slightly hyperintense lesion in the caudate lobe and multiple confluent lesions in the left liver lobe (white arrow) with early enhancement in the arterial phase (**b**) and washout with peripheral enhancement (pseudocapsule appearance) in the equilibrium phase (**c**). With the typical appearance, the lesions can be categorized as LI-RADS 5 lesions

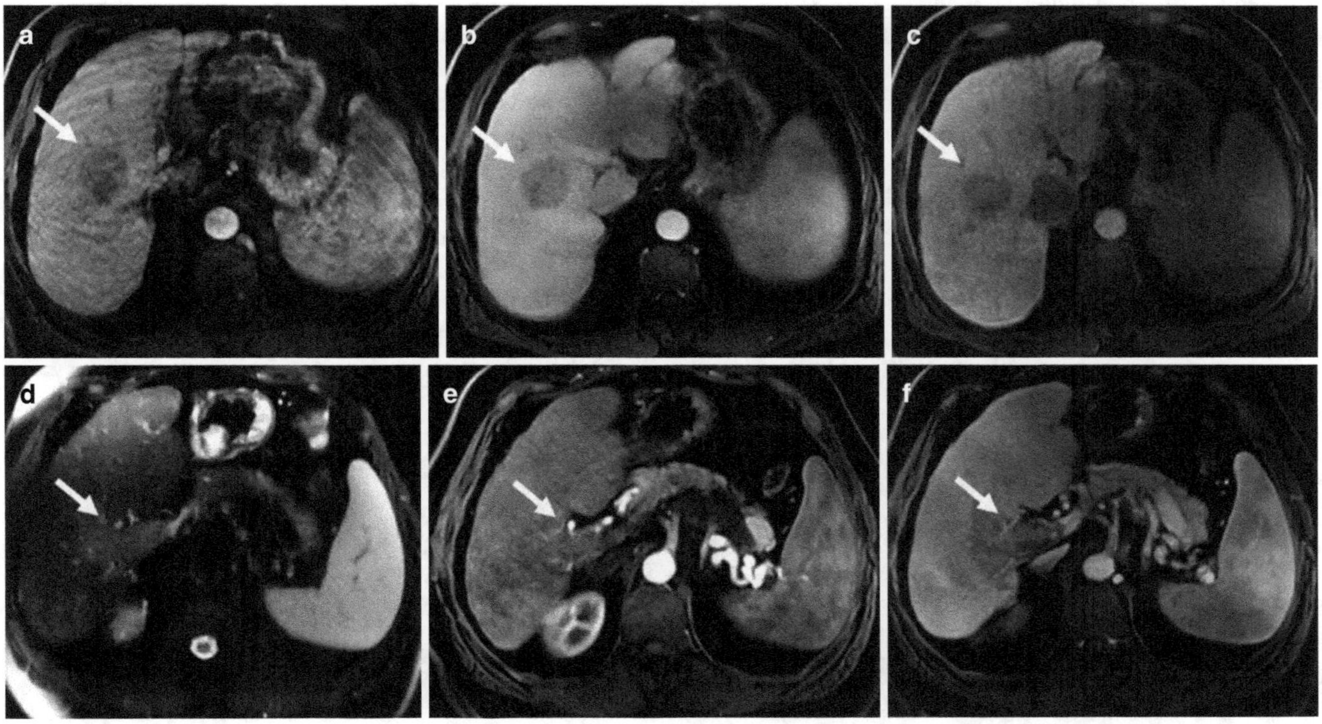

Fig. Hypovascular HCC. 60-year-old male patient with chronic hepatitis B and Child C cirrhosis. Initial imaging study (**a–c**) showed a focal hypovascular lesion (arrow) in liver segment 5 and 8 without contrast enhancement (Gd-EOB-DTPA) in the arterial (**a**), portal venous (**b**), and hepatocyte-specific phase (**c**) consistent with an atypical hypovascular HCC. No treatment was performed, and the follow-up study 3 months later (**d–f**) shows progression of the tumor (arrow) with invasion into the portal vein

97% demonstrate hypointensity on hepatobiliary phase images (Fig.) [15]. In dynamic phases the contrast enhancement of typical, hypervascular HCCs with hepatocyte- specific contrast agent is comparable to extracel-lular contrast agents. In delayed phase (2–4 min after con-trast administration), the washout may appear more pronounced because the surrounding liver parenchyma pro-gressively takes up the contrast agent. The pseudocapsule appearance may be less visible due to background liver enhancement.

Cholangiocellular Carcinoma

Intrahepatic cholangiocellular carcinoma (ICC) is the second most common primary hepatic tumor and accounts for 10–20% of all primary hepatic tumors. Recently, cirrhosis and viral hepatitis C and B have been recognized as risk factors for cholangiocarcinoma, especially for the intrahepatic type [16]. Radiologic features of cholangiocarcinoma such as progressive contrast enhancement from arterial to venous and late phase and arterial or both arterial and venous rim enhancement can help differentiate ICC from HCC in the cirrhotic liver [17] (Fig.). Mixed hepatocellular cholangiocarcinoma has emerged as a distinct subtype of primary liver cancer [16, 18]. A strong enhancing rim and irregular shape on gadoxetic acid-enhanced MRI favors mixed hepatocellular-cholangiocellular carcinoma, and lobulated shape, weak rim and targeted appearance favors a mass-forming intrahepatic cholangiocarcinoma [16, 19].

Standardized Reporting Approach

Given the spectrum of focal liver lesions in stepwise hepatocarcinogenesis ranging from regenerative nodules to poorly differentiated HCC and the overlap in imaging features between the different steps, a definite diagnosis of a benign or malignant lesion in the cirrhotic liver is often not possible. Furthermore, a great variety in nomenclature of imaging features of cirrhotic nodules is used. To overcome these difficulties, the Liver Imaging Reporting and Data System (LI-RADS) has recently been developed, which is a comprehensive system for standardized interpretation and reporting of computed tomography (CT) and magnetic resonance (MR) examinations performed in patients at risk for HCC. It uses a standardized nomenclature and provides a diagnostic algorithm that uses imaging features to categorize the observations seen in patients at risk for HCC along a spectrum from benign to malignant. Liver lesions in these patients are rated for their risk of being an HCC. LI-RADS 1 category observations are those that demonstrate imaging features diagnostic of a benign entity, e.g., cyst and hemangioma. LI-RADS 2 category observations are those that are probably benign, such as a hemangioma with an atypical enhancement pattern or a probably benign cirrhotic nodule. Major features including arterial-phase enhancement, lesion diameter, washout appearance, capsule appearance, and threshold growth are imaging features used to categorize LI-RADS 3 (indeterminate probability of HCC), LI-RADS 4 (probably HCC), and LI-RADS 5 (definitely HCC) lesions. LI-RADS 5 lesions have typical imaging features diagnostic for HCC (Fig.) [20].

Diffuse Vascular Liver Disease

Arteriovenous Shunts

Intrahepatic arterioportal shunts are communications between the hepatic arterial system and a portal vein or between hepatic arteries and hepatic veins which can be either at the level of the trunk, sinusoids, or peribiliary venules. In a cirrhotic liver, they can occur spontaneously, represent pseudolesions, and subsequently resolve. Secondary shunts may be posttraumatic, postbiopsy, or

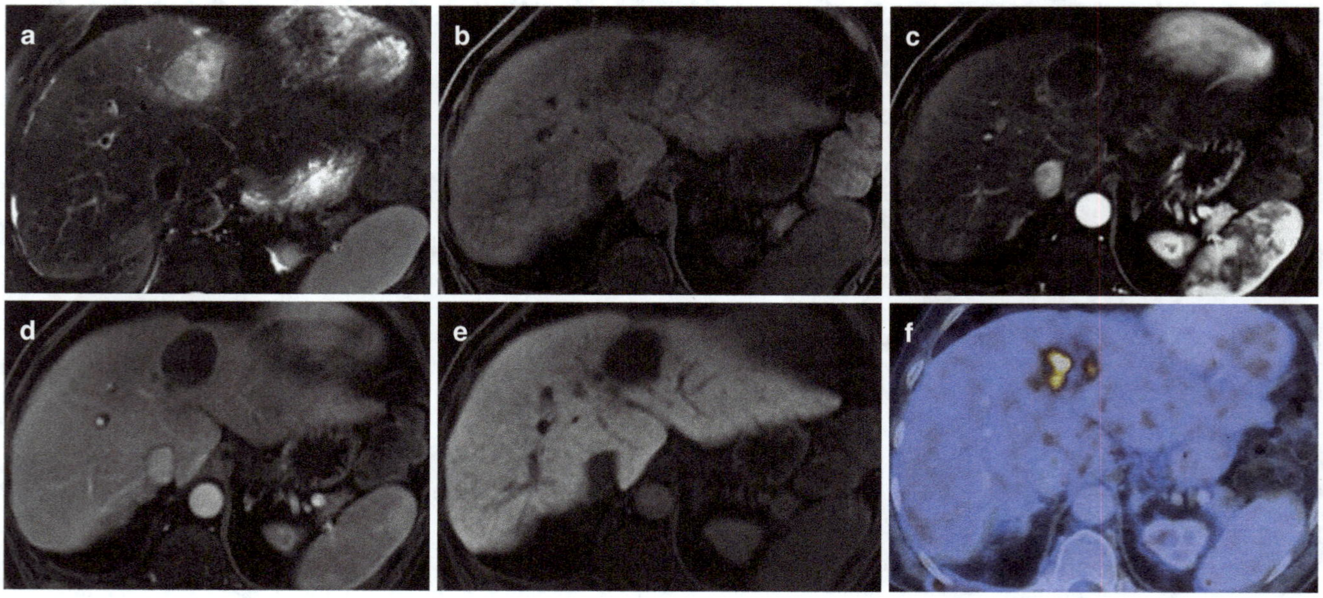

Fig. Cholangiocellular carcinoma in cirrhosis. 63-year-old male patient with chronic hepatitis C and Child A cirrhosis. (**a**) Axial T2-weighted magnetic resonance (MR) image shows features of cirrhosis with a focal hyperintense mass in the liver segment 2/4a with inhomogeneous signal intensity. (**b–e**) Corresponding axial gradient-echo T1-weighted images acquired before and after administration of hepatocyte-specific contrast agent (Gd-EOB-DTPA): (**b**) on pre-contrast image, the lesion is hypointense; (**c**) in the arterial phase, the lesions shows rim enhancement, which persists in the portal venous phase (**d**); (**e**) in hepatocyte-specific phase, the lesion is hypointense. (**f**) Axial-fused image of fluoro-18-deoxyglucose (FDG) positron-emission tomography and computed tomography shows peripheral FDG uptake favoring cholangiocellular carcinoma over hepatocellular carcinoma, which was histologically confirmed instrumentation. On imaging they appear as small, peripheral, nonspherical enhancing foci, which become isoattenuating to the liver in the portal venous phase. It may be difficult to distinguish an arterioportal shunt from a small hepatocellular carcinoma. Repeating imaging after 6 months usually helps distinguishing these entities and demonstrates resolution or stability of an arterioportal shunt or growth of an HCC.

Portal Venous Thrombosis

A thrombus in the portal vein can be either bland or through venous invasion from adjacent malignancies. Several causes lead to thrombosis of the portal vein system such as cirrhosis, hypercoagulable states, trauma, or abdominal tumors [21]. Disruption of the portal venous endothelium can occur in intra-abdominal inflammatory processes such as chronic inflammatory bowel disease, schistosomiasis, and pylephlebitis leading to portal venous thrombosis [11]. After acute occlusion numerous periportal collaterals can develop within 6–20 days even if partial recanalization of the thrombus develops, representing cavernous transformation of the portal vein [22] (Fig.), also known as portal cavernoma (PC). At ultrasound it appears as a mass of veins in the porta hepatis with hepatopetal flow that lacks the normal respira-tory variation of the portal vein [21, 22]. PC represents a portoportal collateral pathway that substitutes for a throm-bosed portal vein. The veins are usually insufficient to bypass the entire splenomesenteric inflow, and signs of por-tal hypertension such as splenomegaly frequently coexist [23]. On contrast-enhanced CT or MR scans, inhomogeneous, peripheral, patchy areas of high attenuation can be seen during the hepatic arterial phase. This pattern of perfusion occurs because the central regions of the liver are better supplied by the cavernous portal vein than are the peripheral regions; therefore, a peripheral increase in arterial inflow develops [23]. Portal biliopathy (PB) is defined as the presence of biliary abnormalities in patients with non-cirrhotic/nonneoplastic extrahepatic portal vein obstruction (EHPVO) and PC (Fig.). The pathogenesis of PB is due to the compression of bile ducts by PC and/or to ischemic damage secondary to an altered biliary vascularization in EHPVO and PC [24].

Budd-Chiari Syndrome

Budd-Chiari syndrome is defined as lobar or segmental hepatic venous outflow obstruction at the level of the inferior vena cava (IVC, type 1) or at the level of the hepatic veins (type 2) or occlusion of small centrilobular veins (type 3). Primary causes include congenital causes such as webs and diaphragms, outflow obstruction at the level of the right atrium, injury, and infection. Rarely the outflow obstruction may be due to mass effects from hepatic mass-forming malignancies. Secondary causes most commonly are thrombotic including obstruction after chemotherapy or radiation and hypercoagulability state due to oral contraceptive use, pregnancy, or polycythemia. The imaging findings are variable and depend on the disease state. Characteristic findings include hepatic venous outflow obstruction. In the acute state, the IVC and/or hepatic veins may appear hyperattenuating on unenhanced CT images because of the increased attenuation

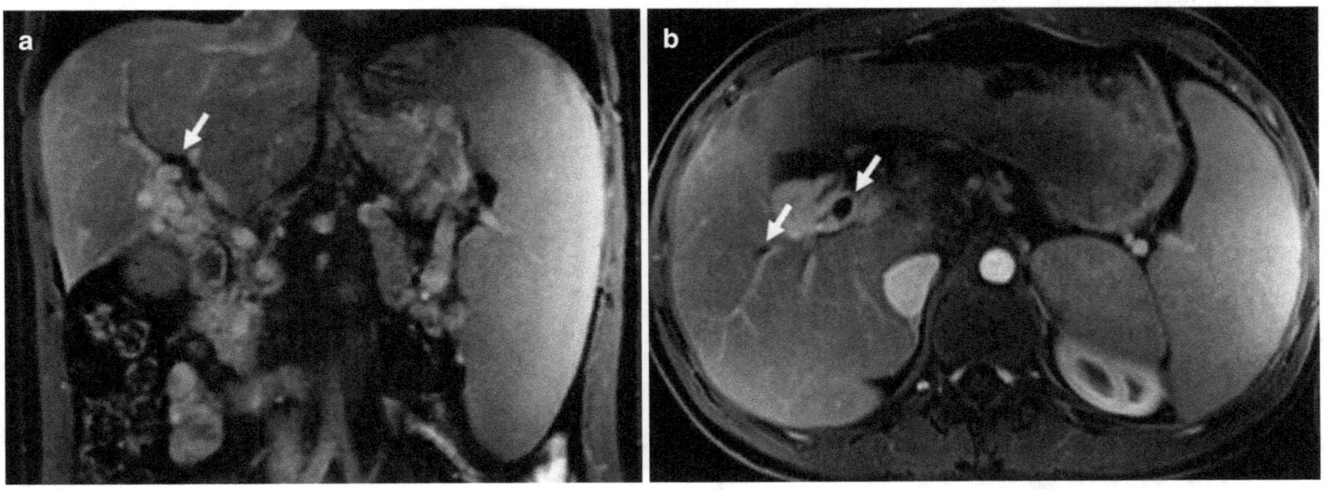

Fig. Chronic portal venous thrombosis with cavernous transformation. 16-year-old male patient with Faktor-V-Leiden mutation and history of omphalitis with portal vein thrombosis since infancy. Coronal (**a**) and axial (**b**) T1-weighted contrast-enhanced magnetic resonance (MR) images in the portal venous phase demonstrate cavernous transformation of the portal vein with serpentine-like vessels in the porta hepatis and splenomegaly. In addition, dilated intra- and extrahepatic bile ducts (arrows) are noted caused by stenosis of the distal hepatocholedochal duct probably due to the varices in the porta hepatis (the so-called portal biliopathy)

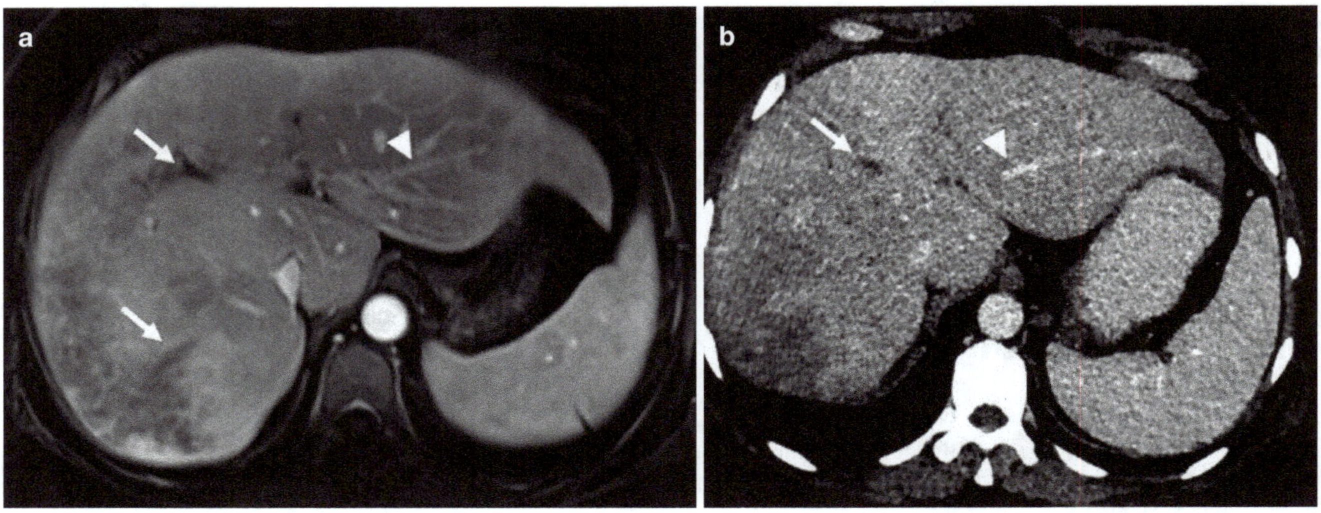

Fig. Budd-Chiari syndrome. 48-year-old female patient with chronic primary immunothrombocytopenia. (**a**) Axial T1-weighted magnetic resonance image in portal venous phase and (**b**) axial CT image in portal venous phase show a filling defect in the thrombosed middle and right hepatic vein (arrow) and normal left hepatic vein (arrow head). (**a, b**) Diminished peripheral contrast enhancement is seen in the right liver lobe due to acute venous occlusion

of a thrombus. On contrast-enhanced CT or MRI, a vascular filling defects due to thrombotic material, reduction of hepatic vein caliber, missing connection between hepatic veins, and IVC can be present, or hepatic veins may not be visible at all. In the acute phase, diminished enhancement of the liver periphery and accentuated enhancement of central liver parts and caudate lobe are seen. Later on peripheral liver enhancement becomes heterogeneous as disorganized, comma-shaped intrahepatic collateral veins and systemic collateral veins develop. Large regenerative nodules in a dysmorphic liver are frequent findings in longer-standing venous outflow obstruction. These regenerative nodules appear hyperintense on hepatobiliary phase images after administration of a hepatocyte-specific c ontrast a gent. H ypertrophy o f t he c audate lobe with variation in attenuation due to separate venous drainage should not be interpreted as a tumor [25]. Figure shows an example of acute Budd- Chiari syndrome.

Passive Hepatic Congestion

Passive hepatic congestion is due to chronic right-sided heart failure which leads to stasis of blood within the liver parenchyma. An enlarged, heterogeneous liver may be seen as a manifestation of acute or early cardiac disease. Early arterial enhancement of the dilated IVC and central hepatic veins is caused by reflux of contrast material from the right atrium into the IVC. A heterogeneous, mottled mosaic pattern of enhancement is present in the parenchymal phase, a condition also known as "nutmeg" liver. In long-standing disease, progressive cellular necrosis results in a small cirrhotic liver.

Key Points

- MR elastography can accurately diagnose clinically significant hepatic fibrosis.
- Hypovascular cirrhotic nodules with hypointense appearance on hepatobiliary phase images carry a significant risk of transformation into a hypervascular HCC.
- The diagnosis of HCC in cirrhotic patients can be made from a single imaging study when characteristic enhancement patterns—that is, arterial phase hyperenhancement and venous or delayed phase washout—are present.
- The presence of arterial or both arterial and venous rim enhancement can help differentiate intrahepatic cholangiocarcinoma from HCC in the cirrhotic liver.
- LI-RADS provides a diagnostic algorithm that uses imaging features to categorize the observations seen in patients at risk for HCC along a spectrum from benign to malignant.
- It may be difficult to distinguish an arterioportal shunt from a small hepatocellular carcinoma. Repeating imaging after 6 months usually helps distinguishing these entities.
- Budd-Chiari syndrome is a heterogeneous group of disorders characterized by hepatic venous outflow obstruction at the level of the hepatic veins, the inferior vena cava (IVC), or the right atrium [26].

References

1. Dulai PS, Sirlin CB, Loomba R. MRI and MRE for non-invasive quantitative assessment of hepatic steatosis and fibrosis in NAFLD and NASH: clinical trials to clinical practice. J Hepatol. 2016;65(5):1006–16.
2. Permutt Z, Le TA, Peterson MR, et al. Correlation between liver histology and novel magnetic resonance imaging in adult patients with non-alcoholic fatty liver disease—MRI accurately quantifies hepatic steatosis in NAFLD. Aliment Pharmacol Ther. 2012;36(1):22–9.
3. Tang A, Tan J, Sun M, et al. Nonalcoholic fatty liver disease: MR imaging of liver proton density fat fraction to assess hepatic steatosis. Radiology. 2013;267(2):422–31.
4. Idilman IS, Aniktar H, Idilman R, et al. Hepatic steatosis: quantification by proton density fat fraction with MR imaging versus liver biopsy. Radiology. 2013;267(3):767–75.
5. Singh S, Venkatesh SK, Wang Z, et al. Diagnostic performance of magnetic resonance elastography in staging liver fibrosis: a systematic review and meta-analysis of individual participant data. Clin Gastroenterol Hepatol. 2015;13(3):440.e6–51.e6.
6. Loomba R, Wolfson T, Ang B, et al. Magnetic resonance elastography predicts advanced fibrosis in patients with nonalcoholic fatty liver disease: a prospective study. Hepatology. 2014;60(6):1920–8.
7. Kim D, Kim WR, Talwalkar JA, Kim HJ, Ehman RL. Advanced fibrosis in nonalcoholic fatty liver disease: noninvasive assessment with MR elastography. Radiology. 2013;268(2):411–9.
8. Yoon JH, Lee JM, Joo I, et al. Hepatic fibrosis: prospective comparison of MR elastography and US shear-wave elastography for evaluation. Radiology. 2014;273(3):772–82.
9. Ichikawa S, Motosugi U, Morisaka H, et al. Comparison of the diagnostic accuracies of magnetic resonance elastography and transient elastography for hepatic fibrosis. Magn Reson Imaging. 2015;33(1):26–30.
10. Brancatelli G, Federle MP, Ambrosini R, et al. Cirrhosis: CT and MR imaging evaluation. Eur J Radiol. 2007;61(1):57–69.
11. Hodler JK-HR, von Schulthess GK, Zolliker CL. Diseases of the abdomen and pelvis 2014–2017. Milan: Springer; 2014.
12. Parente DB, Perez RM, Eiras-Araujo A, et al. MR imaging of hypervascular lesions in the cirrhotic liver: a diagnostic dilemma. Radiographics. 2012;32(3):767–87.
13. Suh CH, Kim KW, Pyo J, Lee J, Kim SY, Park SH. Hypervascular transformation of Hypovascular Hypointense nodules in the Hepatobiliary phase of Gadoxetic acid-enhanced MRI: a systematic review and meta-analysis. AJR Am J Roentgenol. 2017;209(4):781–9.
14. McEvoy SH, McCarthy CJ, Lavelle LP, et al. Hepatocellular carcinoma: illustrated guide to systematic radiologic diagnosis and staging according to guidelines of the American Association for the Study of Liver Diseases. Radiographics. 2013;33(6):1653–68.
15. Choi JW, Lee JM, Kim SJ, et al. Hepatocellular carcinoma: imaging patterns on gadoxetic acid-enhanced MR images and their value as an imaging biomarker. Radiology. 2013;267(3):776–86.
16. Razumilava N, Gores GJ. Cholangiocarcinoma. Lancet. 2014;383(9935):2168–79.
17. Huang B, Wu L, Lu XY, et al. Small intrahepatic Cholangiocarcinoma and hepatocellular carcinoma in cirrhotic livers may share similar enhancement patterns at multiphase dynamic MR imaging. Radiology. 2016;281(1):150–7.
18. Komuta M, Govaere O, Vandecaveye V, et al. Histological diversity in cholangiocellular carcinoma reflects the different cholangiocyte phenotypes. Hepatology. 2012;55(6):1876–88.
19. Chong YS, Kim YK, Lee MW, et al. Differentiating mass-forming intrahepatic cholangiocarcinoma from atypical hepatocellular carcinoma using gadoxetic acid-enhanced MRI. Clin Radiol. 2012;67(8):766–73.
20. Santillan CS, Tang A, Cruite I, Shah A, Sirlin CB. Understanding LI-RADS: a primer for practical use. Magn Reson Imaging Clin N Am. 2014;22(3):337–52.
21. Elsayes KM, Shaaban AM, Rothan SM, et al. A comprehensive approach to hepatic vascular disease. Radiographics. 2017;37(3):813–36.
22. De Gaetano AM, Lafortune M, Patriquin H, De Franco A, Aubin B, Paradis K. Cavernous transformation of the portal vein: patterns of intrahepatic and splanchnic collateral circulation detected with Doppler sonography. AJR Am J Roentgenol. 1995;165(5):1151–5.
23. Gallego C, Velasco M, Marcuello P, Tejedor D, De Campo L, Friera A. Congenital and acquired anomalies of the portal venous system. Radiographics. 2002;22(1):141–59.
24. Franceschet I, Zanetto A, Ferrarese A, Burra P, Senzolo M. Therapeutic approaches for portal biliopathy: a systematic review. World J Gastroenterol. 2016;22(45):9909.
25. Torabi M, Hosseinzadeh K, Federle MP. CT of nonneoplastic hepatic vascular and perfusion disorders. Radiographics. 2008;28(7):1967–82.
26. Ludwig J, Hashimoto E, McGILL DB, van HEERDEN JA. Classification of hepatic venous outflow obstruction: ambiguous terminology of the Budd-Chiari syndrome. Mayo Clinic Proceedings: Elsevier; 1990. p. 51–5.

12

Small Bowel Disease

Andrea Laghi and Amy K. Hara

> **Learning Objectives**
> - To understand the role of different imaging modalities in small bowel diseases
> - To learn the most common CT findings in the emergency setting, including small bowel obstruction and ischemia
> - To learn the relevant CT and MR findings in the diagnosis of Crohn's disease, according to different disease phenotypes
> - To be aware of small bowel injury induced by non-steroidal anti-inflammatory drugs (NSAID)
> - To learn imaging findings in celiac disease
> - To learn how to perform a differential diagnosis among different small bowel tumors

Techniques (US, CTE, MRE)

Ultrasonography (US), magnetic resonance (MR), and computed tomography (CT) have a complementary role in the evaluation of small bowel disorders [1].

US is a powerful tool for bowel assessment in patients with known or suspected gut-related disease, especially in combination with oral (SICUS) [2] and intravenous (CEUS) contrast agents [3]. It is often the first imaging modality used in patients with undiagnosed abdominal pain [4]. Initial US evaluation of the gut should be performed in all four quadrants using curvilinear probe (3.5–5 MHz). The goal is to identify thickened bowel and/or ancillary findings of inflammation (fluid collections, lymphadenopathy). Higher-frequency probe (7–12 MHz) provides better resolution of the bowel wall layers and surrounding tissues and can be subsequently used to evaluate regions of suspected bowel disease. Color Doppler US provides additional information regarding mural vascularity [5].

CT and MR evaluations of the small bowel require lumen distention, achievable by fluid administration after nasojejunal intubation (CT/MR enteroclysis, CTE) or per os (CT/MR enterography, MRE). Enterography should be preferred, in the setting of inflammatory bowel disorders, due to less invasiveness and similar diagnostic accuracy compared to enteroclysis. Usually for an average-size adult, the dose is around 1500–2000 mL of enteral contrast agent, divided into three aliquots administered starting around 60 min before CT scanning to reduce patient's discomfort [1, 6]. Spasmolytic agents should be administered intravenously immediately before the examination, in order to minimize motion artefacts [1]. Intravenous injection of contrast media is mandatory to depict mural enhancement pattern [1].

Advantages of MR imaging over computed tomography (CT) include high contrast resolution, lack of radiation exposure, and use of intravenous contrast media with better safety profiles. MRE also allows dynamic assessment of small bowel peristalsis and distensibility of lumen narrowing, providing functional information [1].

Limitations of MR imaging include costs and variability in examination quality (related to patient cooperation and breath-holding ability), and its role in the emergency setting is still limited [6].

NormalAnatomy

The small bowel has an average length of 6 m (ranging between 3 and 10 m) and includes the duodenum, jejunum (proximal), and ileum (distal). It is attached at the posterior

A. Laghi
Department of Radiological, Oncological and Pathological Sciences, Sapienza— University of Rome, ICOT Hospital, Latina, Italy

A. K. Hara (✉)
Department of Radiology, Mayo Clinic Arizona, Phoenix, AZ, USA
e-mail: Hara.amy@mayo.edu

abdominal wall thought the mesentery formed by the double fold of peritoneum. Its root extends from the left of L2 to the right sacroiliac joint and it is 15 cm long.

The duodenum is the first and shortest segment of the small intestine (20–30 cm) and continues into the jejunum at the duodenojejunal flexure, fixed to the retroperitoneum by ligament of Treitz. The jejunum occupies the left upper abdomen and constitutes about one third of the small bowel. One of the typical morphological finding in jejunum are the circular mucosal folds, known as valvulae conniventes or plicae semilunaris, more prominent than in the ileum and easily depicted during an MRE or CTE. The ileum occupies the central and right lower part of the abdomen, and the ileocecal valve separates the small from large intestine.

Two main normal anatomical aspects should be considered during the evaluation of small bowel: wall thickness and caliber. The normal caliber of jejunal and ileal lumen, without the administration of spasmolytic agents, must be <30 mm, and the wall thickness <3 mm [1].

Pathology

Emergency

US is often the first imaging method for undiagnosed abdominal pain [4]. However, CT is considered the gold standard, offering a more comprehensive evaluation of emergency conditions. Small bowel obstruction (SBO), bowel hemorrhage, and ischemia are easily detected with CT.

SBO continues to be a substantial cause of morbidity and mortality. Adhesions, hernias, and malignancies account for more than 80% of all SBOs. The task of the radiologist is to determine its site, cause, and the presence or absence of complications such as ischemia or perforation. The hallmark of SBO is dilated small bowel (>3 cm) proximal to the site of obstruction with decompressed distal bowel. Air-fluid levels and string of beads sign (fluid-filled loops of bowel with a small amount of remaining gas trapped in folds between valvulae conniventes) may be identified. In high-grade obstruction, stasis and mixing of small bowel contents with gas creates the so-called "small bowel feces" sign, an appearance analogous to feces in colon [7] (Fig.).

The three main causes of mesenteric ischemia are arterial occlusion, venous occlusion, and poor cardiac output or hypovolemia. CT findings associated with ischemic bowel include bowel with thickening, mesenteric edema and fluid adjacent to bowel loops, abnormal decreased bowel wall enhancement, and pneumatosis with or without associated gas in mesenteric or portal veins.

Bleeding in the GI tract has many possible causes, including ulcers, vascular malformations, and tumors. Active small bowel bleeding at multiphase CTE is observed as a gradual accumulation of contrast material within the bowel lumen [8].

Inflammatory

Crohn's Disease (CD)

One of the most common inflammatory diseases of the small bowel is Crohn's disease (CD) which can involve the entire gastrointestinal tract from the mouth to the anus, most commonly affecting the ileocecal region (approximately 50% of cases), followed by the ileum (30%) and colon (20%) [9]. Perianal disease is present in 20% of CD patients at initial presentation. CD exhibits skip lesions with transmural inflammation of the bowel wall, deep ulcerations at endoscopy [10], granulomas, and focal crypt irregularity on histology [9].

Cross-sectional imaging of the small bowel with CTE or MRE is performed to identity the presence, length, and severity of inflammation as well as to identify complications such as fistulas, abscesses, and obstruction [11]. CTE and MRE have similar performance for diagnosing CD [12]. CT is more widely available and less time consuming than MR, but MR spares radiation exposure which can be considerable over time [11].

CD phenotypes include quiescent, active inflammatory, stricturing, and penetrating. Due to the chronic and relapsing nature of CD, these phenotypes often coexist (Fig.). A primary responsibility of the radiologist is to communicate if there are signs of active inflammation such as mural enhancement, perienteric inflammation, bowel wall thickening/edema, dilated vasa recta, ulcerations, and restricted diffusion [13]. As these findings are nonspecific and can be seen with a wide variety of other disease processes, the pattern of bowel wall involvement can be helpful. Asymmetric bowel wall involvement that prefers the mesenteric side of the bowel wall predominantly is a pattern that is specific for CD and not in other disease processes.

Chronic changes of CD include bowel wall fibrosis, strictures, obstruction, and chronic mesenteric venous occlusion. Thus, in addition to identifying signs of active inflammation that could lead to medical therapy, the radiologist must report findings that could result in surgical intervention such as strictures with upstream bowel dilations >3 cm, fistulas, frank perforation, and abscesses [13].

NSAID Enteropathy

Nonsteroidal anti-inflammatory drugs (NSAID) [14] can induce small bowel injury, primarily through direct mucosal injury, resulting in ulcers and eventually characteristic circumferential strictures/diaphragms. Clinically, patients can present with obscure GI bleeding with iron deficiency

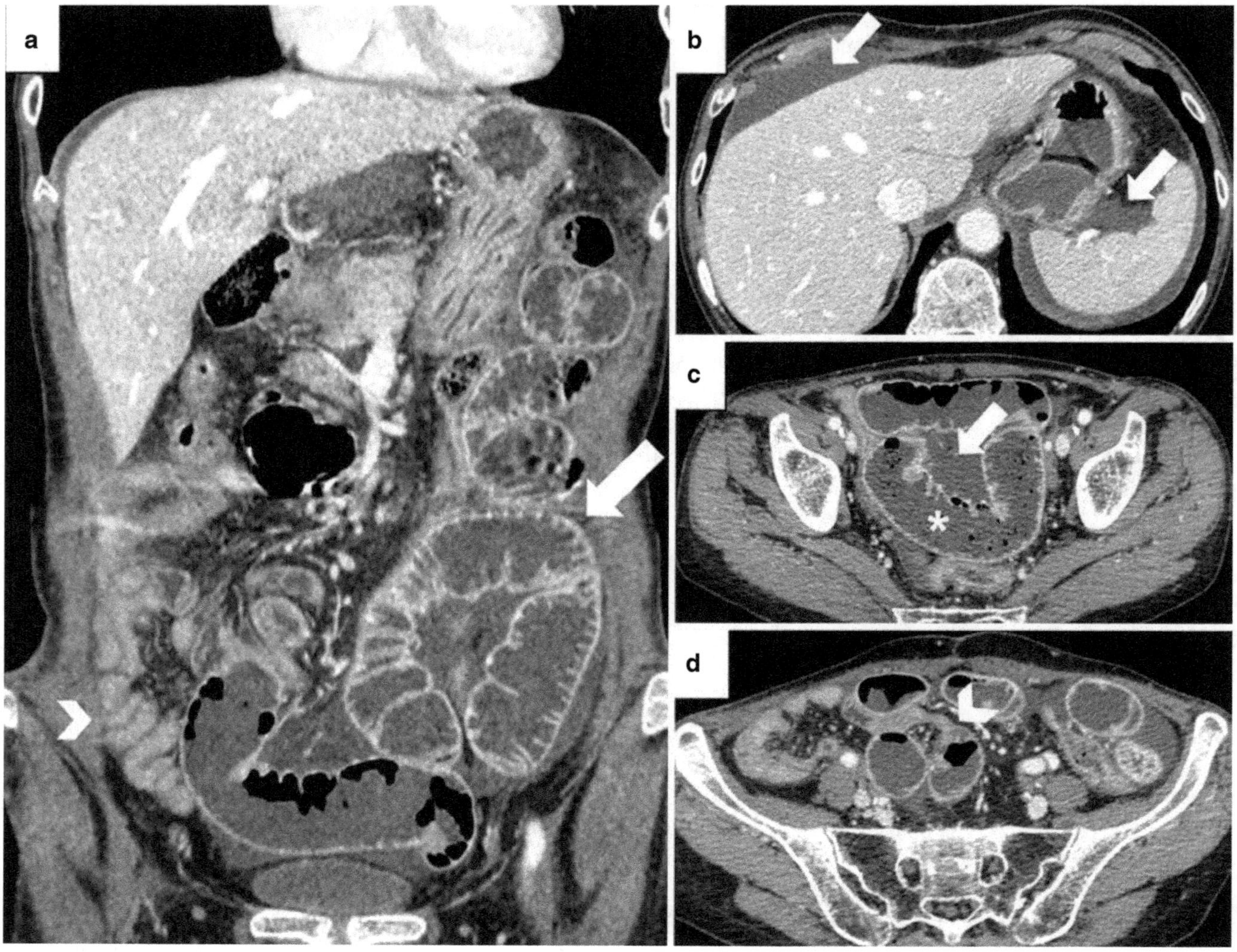

Fig. A 55-year-old man with SBO caused by adhesive bands secondary to a prior laparotomy. Contrast enhanced coronal CT reformation shows dilated fluid-filled small bowel (arrow in **a**) with decompressed distal small bowel (arrowhead) consistent with obstruction. Peritoneal fluid is identified in axial images (arrow in **b** and **c**) both in upper and lower abdomen. Obstruction point (arrowhead in **d**) is identified at the point of transition, immediately below a dilated bowel segment filled with gas bubbles mixed with particulate matter (asterisk in **c**) (feces sign)

anemia, abdominal pain, and bowel obstruction. The gold standard for detecting NSAID enteropathy is capsule endoscopy and balloon enteroscopy. Treatment includes endoscopic dilatation, stricturoplasty, or resection.

These strictures can be challenging to detect at CTE, MRE, and barium exams as they are typically short segment and weblike (Fig.) rather than longitudinal strictures seen with CD. Unlike CD, the bowel wall involvement is typically circumferential and does not prefer the terminal ileum. These strictures are commonly multifocal and, depending on the presence of active inflammation, may or may not present with bowel thickening and increased mural enhancement. Without increased mural enhancement and upstream bowel dilatation, a small bowel diaphragm can be difficult to differentiate from a peristaltic contraction or underdistention. In these cases, multiphasic imaging and optimized bowel distention is useful.

Diagnoses that can simulate NSAID enteropathy at imaging are strictures due to radiation, CD, potassium chloride tablets, and eosinophilic gastroenteritis. The diagnosis can be narrowed by the clinical history, bowel location, and other associated radiologic features. For example, fistulas or fatty deposition would favor CD or involvement of pelvic small bowel loops only favor radiation injury in a patient with that clinical history.

CeliacDisease

Celiac disease [15] is an inflammatory s mall b owel d isease triggered by gluten ingestion and typically resulting in diarrhea predominant symptoms but can be asymptomatic and detected by screening for antibodies against tissue transglutaminase.

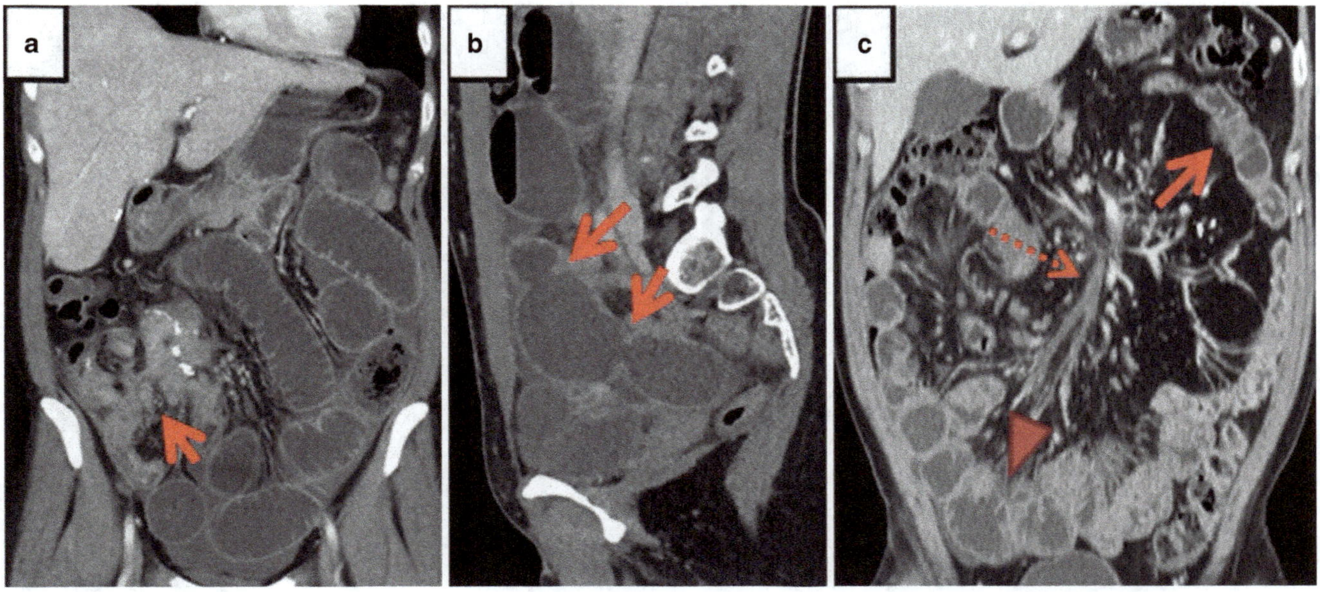

Fig. Inflammatory bowel diseases. (**a**) Crohn's disease showing complex enteroenteric fistula involving the terminal ileum (arrow), active inflammation of involved bowel loops, and strictures with small bowel dilatation. (**b**) NSAID enteropathy with multiple weblike strictures (arrows) and small bowel dilatation. (**c**) Celiac disease with decreased jejunal folds (arrow), increased ileal folds (arrowhead), and superior mesenteric vein thrombosis (dotted arrow)

The diagnosis is confirmed by biopsy which shows intraepithelial lymphocytes, crypt hyperplasia, and villous atrophy. A subset of patients may have persistent symptoms even with gluten avoidance leading to a diagnosis of refractory celiac disease (RCD). Type 2 RCD is associated with enteropathy associated T-cell lymphoma (EATL) leading to higher mortality.

Imaging features of celiac disease at cross-sectional imaging and barium exams include reversal of the jejunal-ileal fold pattern (decreased jejunal folds and increased ileal folds) (Fig.), intussusception, dilated small bowel, and bowel lymphoma. Additional associated findings at CT/MR are mesenteric/retroperitoneal adenopathy and hyposplenism. Findings of active inflammation as seen in CD can also be present with celiac disease including mural enhancement, bowel wall thickening, and dilated vasa recta.

Small Bowel Tumors

Small bowel tumors account for 3–6% of all GI neoplasms and 1–3% of all GI malignancies [16]. The most common subtypes are adenocarcinoma (30–45%), neuroendocrine tumors (20–40%), lymphoma (10–20%), and sarcomas (10–15%) [17] (Fig.). Small bowel tumor incidence has been rising for unclear reasons, although the mortality rate is stable and 5-year survival has been improving [18].

Adenocarcinoma (ACA) is the most common primary malignancy of the small bowel, follows the adenoma-carcinoma sequence and typically arises in the proximal small bowel. Risk factors for ACA include conditions associated with chronic inflammation such as CD, celiac disease, ileostomy or duodenal/jejunal bypass surgery, as well as syndromes such as Peutz-Jeghers and familial polyposis. At imaging, ACA classically has an apple-core appearance associated with bowel obstruction and adenopathy. If it is an intraluminal polypoid mass, it can predispose to intussusception. It typically enhances more than lymphoma but less avidly compared to carcinoid and GI stromal tumors [19].

Carcinoid neuroendocrine tumors (NET) are the second most common primary small bowel malignancy. Unlike ACA, NET most commonly arise in the ileum, are multifocal in 15–35% of cases and hypervascular. These tumors commonly metastasize to mesenteric lymph nodes resulting in the classic calcified mesenteric mass with associated desmoplastic response, tethering and obstructing adjacent bowel loops, and causing vascular engorgement. Nuclear studies with 68Gallium Dotatate or Indium −111 octreotide, somatostatin analogues, can be used to detect the primary tumor as well as metastatic disease [20].

Lymphoma is the third most common small bowel malignancy and can be the primary site or a site of secondary involvement. The distal ileum is the most common location because it has the most lymphoid tissue. Most cases are non-Hodgkin B-cell lymphoma although T-cell lymphoma is more common in celiac disease and occurs in the jejunum. At imaging, lymphoma can have a wide variety of presentations from mucosal nodules to circumferential bowel wall thickening with aneurysmal dilatation to a large exocentric mass [19].

GI stromal tumors arise from the interstitial cells of Cajal, intestinal pacemaker cells that line the GI tract [21]. They are initiated by mutations in KIT, a tyrosine kinase growth factor receptor, which allows the cells to grow and divide

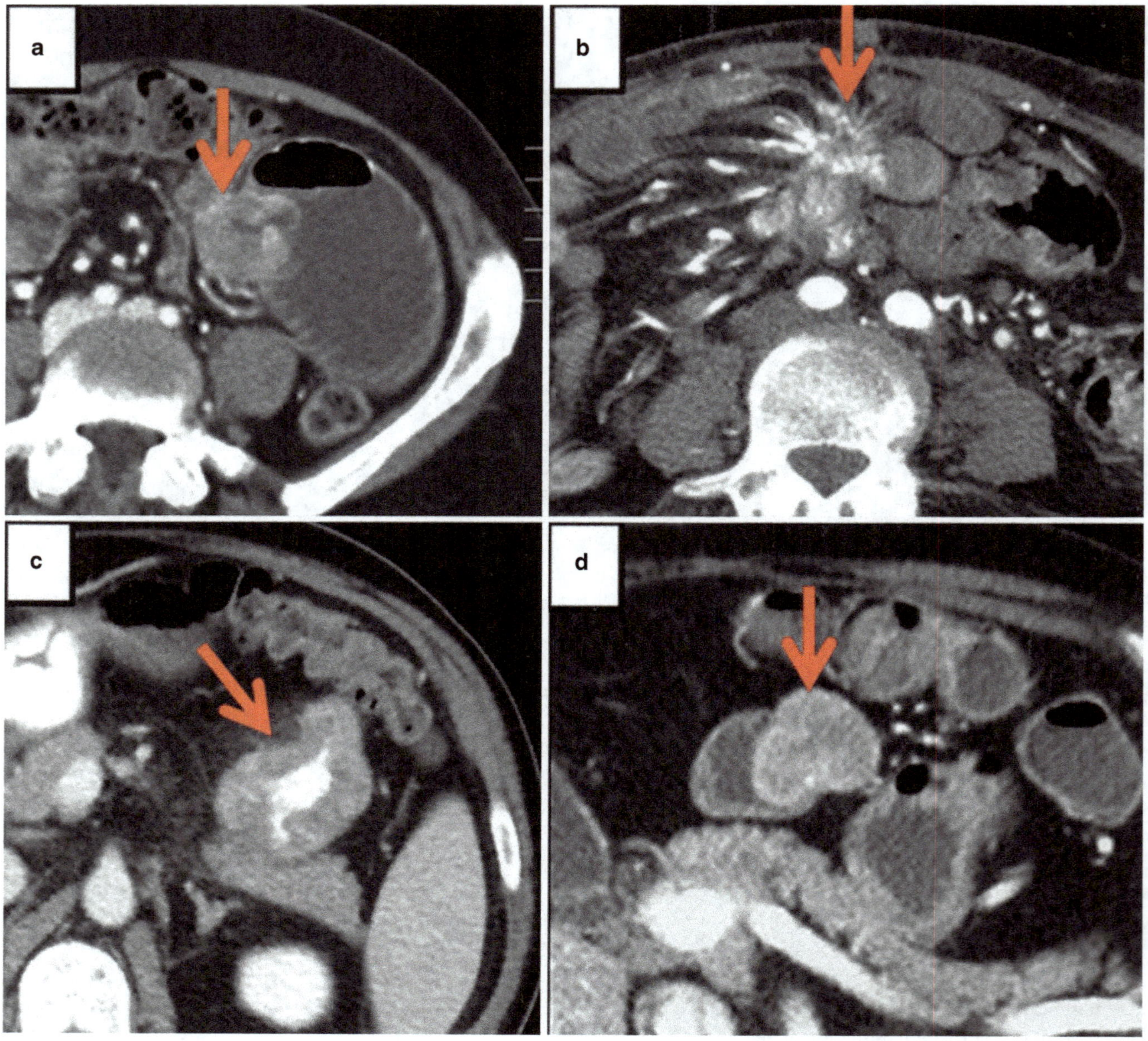

Fig. Small bowel tumors at CT. (**a**) Adenocarcinoma (arrow) with mild enhancement and associated small bowel obstruction. (**b**) Carcinoid (arrow) with mesenteric mass, associated bowel obstruction, desmoplastic response, and vascular engorgement. (**c**) Jejunal lymphoma (arrow) with bowel wall thickening and preservation of the lumen (aneurysmal dilatation). (**d**) GI stromal tumor (arrow) with typical lobulated, homogenous hypervascular appearance without bowel obstruction

abnormally. Thus, they can be treated by tyrosine kinase inhibitors such as imatinib mesylate. These tumors can have a wide variety of imaging appearances, presenting as a homogeneously hypervascular enhancing small bowel mass to a large hypoenhancing exophytic cavitary mass. They are typically large at presentation as they don't commonly cause bowel obstruction, unlike ACA and NET. Surgical resection is typically the treatment of choice. Target therapies with tyrosine kinase inhibitors are used if not surgically resectable or to prevent recurrence/metastases. PET/CT can be used to evaluate treatment response as size criteria alone can underestimate response.

Concluding Remarks

Diagnostic imaging and in particular cross-sectional modalities (US, CT, and MR) have a critical and complementary role in diagnosis and management of small bowel diseases. Radiologists should be aware of advantages and disadvantages of each imaging test in order to choose the best option, considering the specific small bowel disease and the patient's characteristics (age, gender, clinical status). A deep knowledge of the different entities involving the small bowel is also critical in order to reach a correct diagnosis and to provide the necessary information for patient management.

Take-Home Messages

- A small bowel loop is considered normal when caliber is <30 mm and wall thickness <3 mm.
- US is a powerful diagnostic test for bowel assessment in patients with known or suspected gut-related disease, especially in combination with the administration of oral and/or intravenous contrast agents.
- CT is the imaging modality of choice in the emergency setting (i.e., small bowel occlusion, ischemia, and, in some circumstances, bleeding).
- MR is the preferred imaging modality in inflammatory bowel diseases (IBD) because of multiparametric approach, evaluation of bowel motility, and lack of radiation exposure.
- In IBD, cross-sectional imaging is performed to identity the presence, length, and severity of inflammation as well as to assess complications such as fistulas, abscesses, and obstruction.
- Imaging features of celiac disease at cross-sectional imaging and barium exams include reversal of the jejunal-ileal fold pattern (decreased jejunal folds and increased ileal folds), intussusception, dilated small bowel, and bowel lymphoma.
- Small bowel tumors account for 3–6% of all GI neoplasms and 1–3% of all GI malignancies; in order of frequency, they are adenocarcinoma (30–45%), neuroendocrine tumors (20–40%), lymphoma (10–20%), and sarcomas (10–15%).

References

1. Taylor SA, Avni F, Cronin CG, et al. The first joint ESGAR/ ESPR consensus statement on the technical performance of cross-sectional small bowel and colonic imaging. Eur Radiol. 2017;27:2570–82.
2. Calabrese E, Zorzi F, Onali S, et al. Accuracy of small-intestine contrast ultrasonography, compared with computed tomography enteroclysis, in characterizing lesions in patients with Crohn's disease. Clin Gastroenterol Hepatol. 2013;11:950–5.
3. Serafin Z, Białecki M, Białecka A, Sconfienza LM, Kłopocka M. Contrast-enhanced ultrasound for detection of Crohn's disease activity: systematic review and meta-analysis. J Crohns Colitis. 2016;10:354–62.
4. Laméris W, van Randen A, van Es HW, et al. Imaging strategies for detection of urgent conditions in patients with acute abdominal pain: diagnostic accuracy study. BMJ. 2009;338:b2431.
5. Muradali D, Goldberg DR. US of gastrointestinal tract disease. Radiographics. 2015;35:50–68.
6. Murphy KP, McLaughlin PD, O'Connor OJ, Maher MM. Imaging the small bowel. Curr Opin Gastroenterol. 2014;30:134–40.
7. Paulson EK, Thompson WM. Review of small-bowel obstruction: the diagnosis and when to worry. Radiology. 2015;275:332–42.
8. Nakashima K, Ishimaru H, Fujimoto T, et al. Diagnostic performance of CT findings for bowel ischemia and necrosis in closed-loop small-bowel obstruction. Abdom Imaging. 2015;40:1097–103.
9. Hart A, Ng SC. Crohn's disease. Medicine. 2011;39:229–36.
10. Shergill AK, Lightdale JR, Bruining DH, et al. The role of endoscopy in inflammatory bowel disease. Gastrointest Endosc. 2015;81:1101-21.e1–1101-21.e13.
11. Panes J, Bouhnik Y, Reinisch W, et al. Imaging techniques for assessment of inflammatory bowel disease: joint ECCO and ESGAR evidence-based consensus guidelines. J Crohns Colitis. 2013;7:556–85.
12. Horsthuis K, Stokkers PC, Stoker J. Detection of inflammatory bowel disease: diagnostic performance of cross-sectional imaging modalities. Abdom Imaging. 2008;33:407–16.
13. Deepak P, Park SH, Ehman EC, et al. Crohn's disease diagnosis, treatment approach, and management paradigm: what the radiologist needs to know. Abdom Radiol. 2017;42:1068–86.
14. Frye JM, Hansel SL, Dolan SG, et al. NSAID enteropathy: appearance at CT and MR enterography in the age of multi-modality imaging and treatment. Abdom Imaging. 2015;40:1011–25.
15. Tennyson CA, Semrad CE. Small bowel imaging in celiac disease. Gastrointest Endosc Clin N Am. 2012;22:735–46.
16. Pan SY, Morrison H. Epidemiology of cancer of the small intestine. World J Gastroint Onc. 2011;3:33–42.
17. Sokhandon F, Al-Katib S, Bahoura L, et al. Multidetector CT enterography of focal small bowel lesions: a radiological-pathological correlation. Abdom Radiol. 2017;42:1319–41.
18. National Cancer Institute. SEER stat fact sheets: small intestine cancer. Available at: http://seer.cancer.gov/statfacts/html/smint.html.
19. Buckley JA, Fishman EK. CT evaluation of small bowel neoplasms: spectrum of disease. Radiographics. 1998;18:379–92.
20. Yu R, Wachsman A. Imaging of neuroendocrine tumors: indications, interpretations, limits, and pitfalls. Endocrinol Metab Clin N Am. 2017;46:795–814.
21. Scola D, Bahoura L, Copelan A, et al. Getting the GIST: a pictorial review of the various patterns of presentation of gastrointestinal stromal tumors on imaging. Abdom Radiol. 2017;42:1350–64.

13

Pathways for the Spread of Disease in the Abdomen and Pelvis

James A. Brink and Brent J. Wagner

Learning Objectives

- To discuss the ligamentous anatomy of the upper abdomen and how it can inform the spread of disease by direct invasion and lymphatic extension
- To learn about the anatomy of the peritoneal spaces and how it can inform the spread of disease by intraperitoneal seeding

Introduction

Disease may spread through the abdomen and pelvis by a variety of mechanisms. For example, intra-abdominal malignancies may metastasize through hematologic routes, and tumors may spread by directly invading adjacent tissues and organs or via the lymphatic system. When tumors break through the visceral peritoneum, they may also spread via intraperitoneal seeding. While hematologic spread of disease is beyond the scope of this chapter, direct invasion, lymphatic extension, and intraperitoneal seeding will be discussed relative to the anatomy that guides these pathways for the spread of disease in the abdomen and pelvis [1].

Direct invasion and lymphatic extension occur through the peritoneal ligaments and mesenteries that interconnect the abdominal viscera with other organs in the abdomen and pelvis, the retroperitoneum, and the body wall. Moreover, these structures guide the flow of peritoneal fluid through the abdomen and pelvis, thereby dictating the routes of spread through intraperitoneal seeding. In short, understanding these pathways for the spread of disease ties closely to a clear understanding of a ligamentous anatomy of the abdomen and pelvis.

J. A. Brink, M.D. (✉)
Department of Radiology, Massachusetts General Hospital, Boston, MA, USA
e-mail: jabrink@partners.org

B. J. Wagner, M.D.
West Reading Radiology Associates, West Reading, PA, USA
e-mail: Brent.Wagner@towerhealth.org

Peritoneal Ligaments as Conduits for the Spread of Disease

The upper abdominal viscera is interconnected by three pairs of ligaments: the gastrohepatic and hepatoduodenal ligaments (that together comprise the lesser omentum), the gastrosplenic and splenorenal ligaments, and the gastrocolic ligament and transverse mesocolon. Each of these ligamentous pairs contains one ligament that bridges to the retroperitoneum: the hepatoduodenal ligament, the splenorenal ligament, and the transverse mesocolon. Thus, disease from the abdominal viscera may spread to the retroperitoneum and vice versa through these ligamentous pairs.

Gastrohepatic and Hepatoduodenal Ligaments

The gastrohepatic and hepatoduodenal ligaments form an important pathway of disease from the lesser curvature of the stomach to the porta hepatis and retroperitoneum. The gastrohepatic ligament extends from the lesser curvature of the stomach to the porta hepatis, inserting into the fissure for the ligamentum venosum. Containing the left gastric artery, the left gastric vein or coronary vein, and associated lymphatics, the gastrohepatic ligament may be recognized on cross-sectional imaging as the fatty plane connecting the lesser curvature of the stomach to the left lobe of the liver and containing these vessels (Fig.). Nodes in the gastrohepatic ligament are typically 8 mm or less in diameter, somewhat smaller than elsewhere in the abdomen [2]. Care must be taken to avoid misidentifying unopacified loops of bowel, the pancreatic neck, or the papillary process of the caudate lobe as enlarged nodes in the gastrohepatic ligament [3, 4].

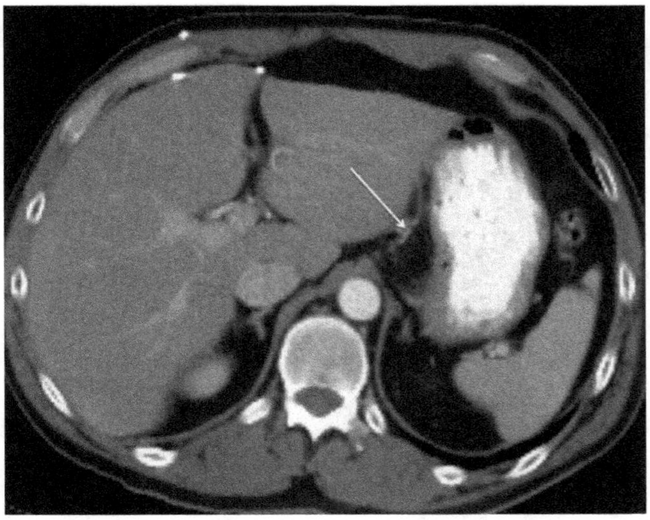

Fig. Transaxial CT image demonstrates the gastrohepatic ligament (GHL), seen as a fatty plane interposed between the lesser curvature of the stomach and the lobe of the liver. The GHL contains the left gastric artery (arrow), the left gastric vein (coronary vein), and associated lymphatics

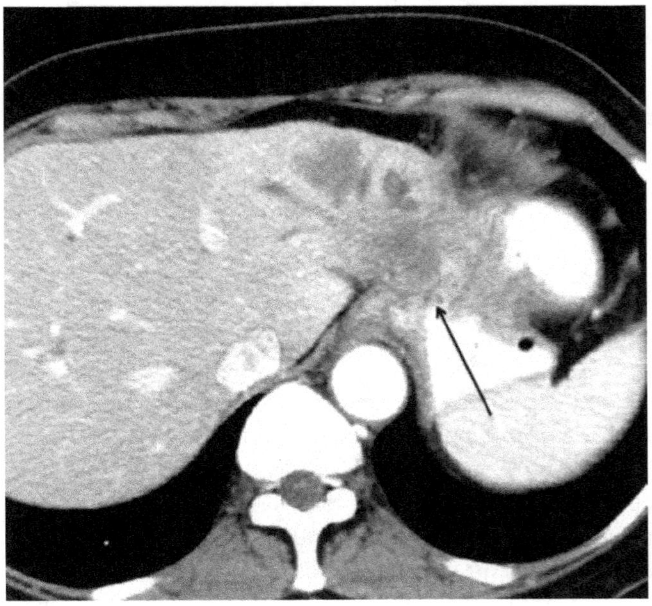

Fig. Transaxial CT image demonstrates a heterogenous mass (arrow) centered in the gastrohepatic ligament (GHL), with invasion of the left hepatic lobe and the stomach. Prospectively, it was unclear as to the organ of origin, but it proved to be a hepatoma extending through the GHL to involve the stomach

A unique feature of the gastrohepatic ligament is continuity of its subperitoneal areolar tissue with the perivascular fibrous capsule of the liver (Glisson capsule). This anatomic continuity provides a direct pathway for the spread of disease from the gastric lesser curvature into the left hepatic lobe via the gastrohepatic ligament and vice versa. Both neoplastic and inflammatory conditions can spread in this fashion (Fig.). Gastric and esophageal cancer commonly spread via lymphatic extension and direct invasion through the gastrohepatic ligament, allowing these tumors to spread to the liver, and conversely hepatoma and cholangiocarcinoma may spread to the stomach through these pathways as well.

The free edge of the gastrohepatic ligament is the hepatoduodenal ligament, and together, the gastrohepatic and hepatoduodenal ligaments comprise the lesser omentum. The hepatoduodenal ligament is the thickest ligament in the upper abdomen owing to the portal structures that it contains: the portal vein, the hepatic artery, the common bile duct, and associated lymphatics. The hepatoduodenal ligament extends from the porta hepatis to the flexure between the first and second duodenum forming a tent-like structure that extends from superior to inferior as it courses from anterior to posterior. The foramen of Winslow, or epiploic foramen, lies immediately posterior to the ligament connecting the right posterior perihepatic space with the lesser sac [5]. Here, nodes at the base of the hepatoduodenal ligament at the epiploic foramen (in the portocaval space) can be quite prominent in size and still normal. These nodes can be up to 2.0 cm in transverse dimension and up to 1.5 cm in anteroposterior dimension and still be normal. Pathology within these nodes may be difficult to identify but may be suggested when the nodes assume a more spherical shape or have central necrosis [6, 7].

A host of neoplastic and inflammatory conditions spread commonly via the hepatoduodenal ligament from the porta hepatis to the retroperitoneum, following antegrade flow of lymphatic fluid from the liver and biliary tree to nodes surrounding the duodenum and pancreas. However, lymphatic extension can also occur in a retrograde fashion through these lymphatics, originating from disease in nodes surrounding the superior mesenteric artery, as may occur in pancreatic and colon cancer, and spreading up the lymphatic channels in the hepatoduodenal ligament to the liver (Fig.).

Structures intimately related to the hepatoduodenal ligament may also spread via direct invasion through the ligament, as occurs commonly with gastric cancer arising in the lesser curvature and spreading to peripancreatic and periduodenal lymph nodes via the gastrohepatic and hepatoduodenal ligaments. Many inflammatory conditions also spread commonly through the hepatoduodenal ligament including inflammatory processes within the gall bladder and biliary tree. Pancreatitis may also spread via this pathway as well. Occasionally, vascular complications may be seen in the hepatoduodenal ligament related to both malignant and inflammatory conditions coursing through it. These include portal vein thrombosis as well as hepatic arterial pseudoaneurysms [1, 5].

Gastrosplenic and Splenorenal Ligaments

An important highway of disease is provided in the left upper abdomen by the gastrosplenic and splenorenal ligaments, connecting the gastric greater curvature to the splenic hilum and the retroperitoneum, respectively (Fig.). The gastrosplenic

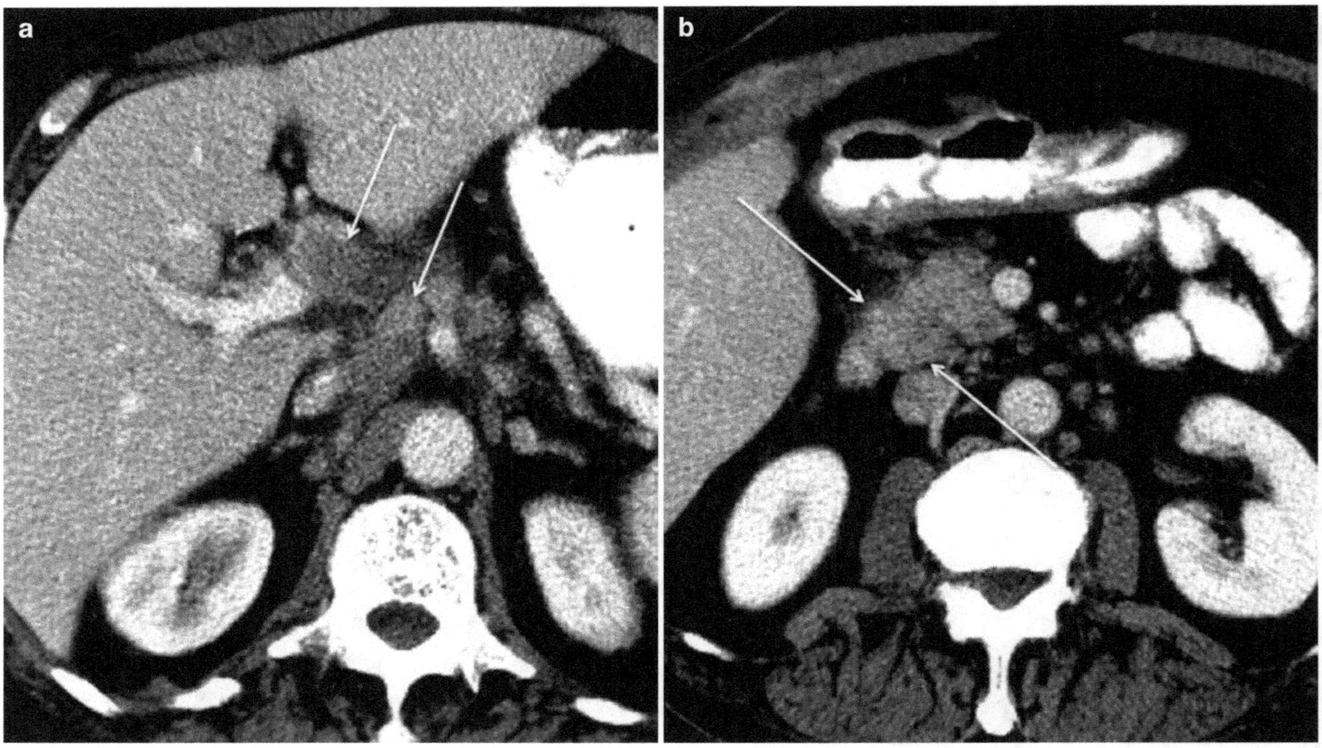

Fig. Transaxial CT images through the porta hepatis (**a**) and the uncinate process (**b**) demonstrate bulky lymphadenopathy (arrows) in the hepatoduodenal ligament (HDL) in a patient with gallbladder carcinoma. Tumor has spread bidirectionally within the HDL proximally (**a**) and distally to the insertion of the HDL on the second portion of the duodenum

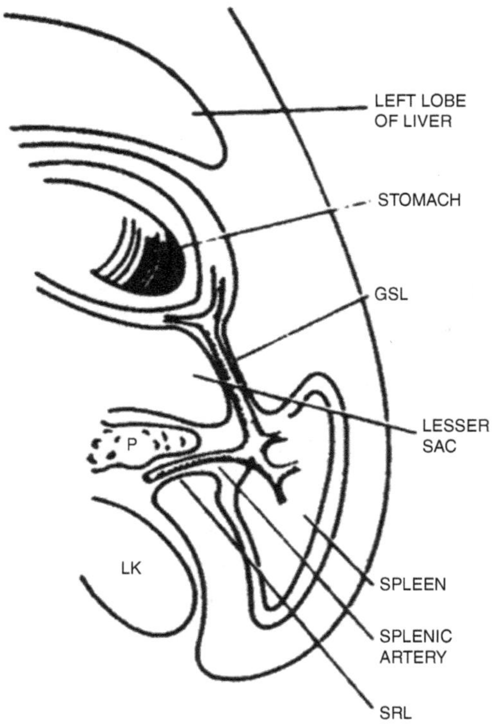

Fig. The gastrosplenic ligament (GSL) and splenorenal ligament (SRL) comprise the left wall of the lesser sac and provide a conduit for the spread of metastatic disease from the greater curvature of the stomach to the retroperitoneum and vice versa (Reprinted with permission from Myers MA. Dynamic Radiology of the Abdomen: Normal and Pathologic Anatomy, New York: Springer, 1994)

ligament is a rather thin delicate structure that connects the superior third of the greater curvature of the stomach to the splenic hilum. This ligament contains the left gastroepiploic and short gastric vessels and their associated lymphatics. The gastrosplenic ligament can direct diseases arising in the stomach to the splenic hilum, and both neoplastic and inflammatory disease may invade the spleen via this pathway.

Posteriorly and medially, the gastrosplenic ligament is continuous with the splenorenal ligament. Once disease reaches the splenic hilum from the stomach via the gastrosplenic ligament, it may turn and extend to the retroperitoneum via the splenorenal ligament. Here, disease may surround and invade the pancreatic tail and compromise the splenic artery and splenic vein (Fig.) [ ]. Just as gastric disease can spread to the retroperitoneum via this ligamentous pair, both inflammatory and neoplastic disease of the pancreas may spread in the opposite direction to the splenic hilum and greater curvature via the splenorenal and gastrosplenic ligaments, respectively [1].

Gastrocolic Ligament and Transverse Mesocolon

As the gastrohepatic and hepatoduodenal ligaments in the right abdomen and the gastrosplenic and splenorenal ligaments in the left abdomen form important pathways of

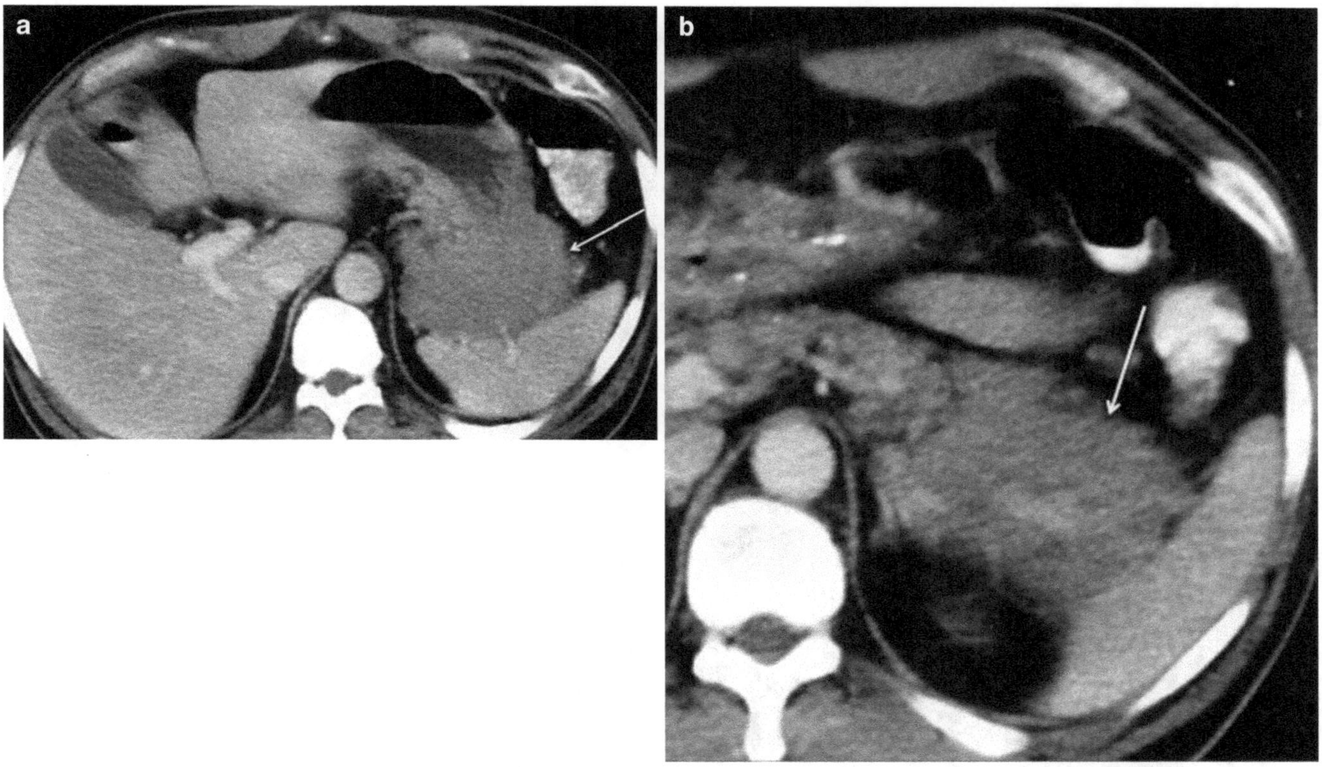

Fig. Transaxial CT images through the gastrosplenic ligament (GSL) (**a**) and the splenorenal ligament (SRL) (**b**), in a patient with lymphoma. Tumor is seen within the GSL, interposed between the gastric greater curvature and the spleen (**a**), and within the SRL, encasing the splenic vasculature (**b**)

disease from the upper abdominal viscera to the retroperitoneum, the gastrocolic ligament and transverse mesocolon form a similar pathway in the mid-abdomen. The gastrocolic ligament (greater omentum) connects the inferior two thirds of the greater curvature of the stomach to the transverse colon (Fig.). On the left, the gastrocolic ligament is continuous with the gastrosplenic ligament, and on the right, it ends at the gastroduodenal junction near the hepatoduodenal ligament. Embryologically, the gastrosplenic ligament gives rise to the gastrocolic ligament and the transverse mesocolon in the adult, with fusion of the anterior and posterior leaves of the embryonic gastrosplenic ligament. In consequence, the gastrocolic ligament has a potential space within it that can fill with fluid when tense ascites in the lesser sac dissects open this potential space. This can result in a cyst-like appearance within the gastrocolic ligament/greater omentum.

The gastrocolic ligament contains the gastroepiploic vessels and associated lymphatics which can help identify the ligament as the fatty plane connecting the stomach to the transverse colon. Both benign and malignant diseases from the inferior two thirds of the greater curvature of the stomach may spread to the transverse colon via this pathway, and vice versa (Fig.). The transverse mesocolon completes the pathway from the stomach to the retroperitoneum in the mid-abdomen; disease involving the stomach and transverse colon are connected via the gastrocolic ligament, and disease involving the transverse colon and pancreas/retroperitoneum

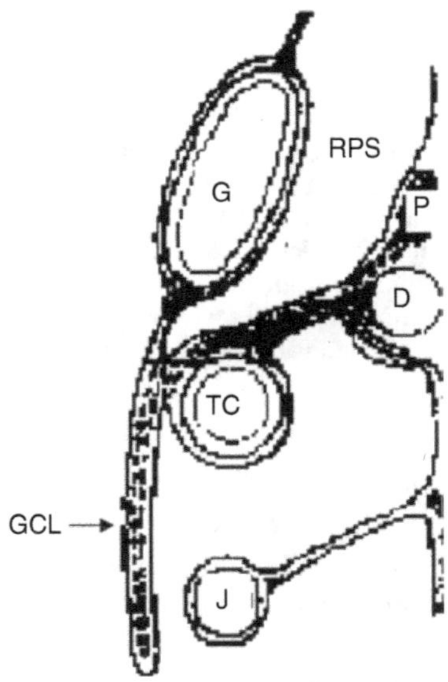

Fig. The gastrocolic ligament (GCL) joins the greater curvature of the stomach (G) to the transverse colon (TC). In concert with the transverse mesocolon, a pathway of disease is formed between retroperitoneal structures such as the pancreas (P) and the duodenum (D) to the anterior aspect of the intraperitoneal cavity (Modified from Langman J., Medical Embriology, New York: Saunders, 1971)

are connected by the transverse mesocolon. In addition, the greater omentum continues inferior to the transverse colon as a fatty veil that forms an important nidus for carcinomatosis, as commonly occurs with ovarian, gastric, colon, and pancre-

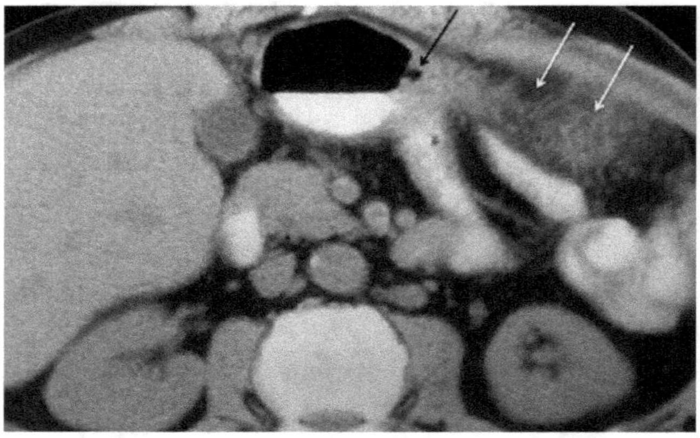

Fig. . Transaxial CT image through the gastrocolic ligament (GCL) demonstrates a gastric ulcer extending into the GCL (black arrow) with associated inflammation in the greater omentum (white arrows)

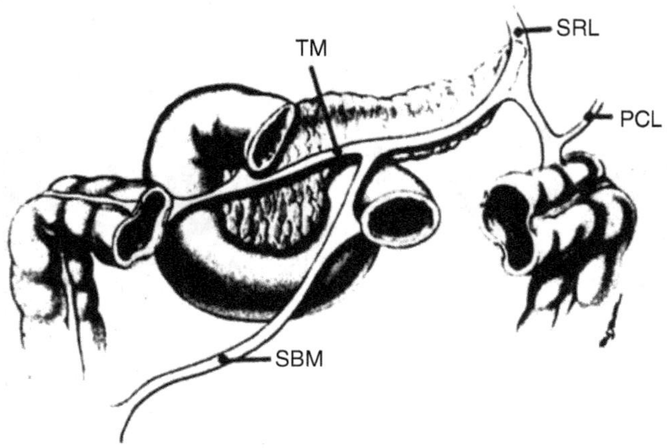

Fig. The transverse mesocolon (TM) provides an important conduit for the spread of disease across the mid-abdomen. It is continuous with the splenorenal ligament (SRL) and phrenicocolic ligament (PCL) on the left and with the duodenocolic ligament on the right. In its midportion, it is continuous with the small bowel mesentery (SBM) (Reprinted with permission from Myers MA. Dynamic Radiology of the Abdomen: Normal and Pathologic Anatomy, New York: Springer, 1994)

atic cancers [10, 11]. Sometimes, gastroepiploic collaterals may be recognized in the gastrocolic ligament which should raise concern about the possibility of splenic venous compromise as what commonly occurs in pancreatic carcinoma.

The transverse mesocolon connects the transverse colon to the retroperitoneum but also forms a broad conduit for disease across the mid-abdomen; bare areas link the pancreas to the transverse colon, spleen, and small bowel (Fig.). The transverse mesocolon is continuous with the phrenicocolic ligament and the splenorenal ligaments in the left abdomen, with the small bowel mesentery in the mid-abdomen, and with the duodenocolic ligament in the right abdomen. The transverse mesocolon may be recognized as the fatty plane that connects the transverse colon to the retroperitoneum at the level of the uncinate process of the pancreas. As this structure lies commonly in a paracoronal orientation, recognition of the middle colic vessels and associated lymphatics within the mesocolon can aid in its identification. Pancreatic disease, both benign and malignant, often spreads ventrally into the transverse mesocolon and then on to the transverse colon (Fig.). Pancreatitis often results in adjacent fluid collections that can dissect open the potential space within the transverse mesocolon formed by fusion of the anterior and posterior leaves of the embryonic gastrosplenic ligament. Free fluid in the lesser sac is often confused with contained fluid collections within the transverse mesocolon.

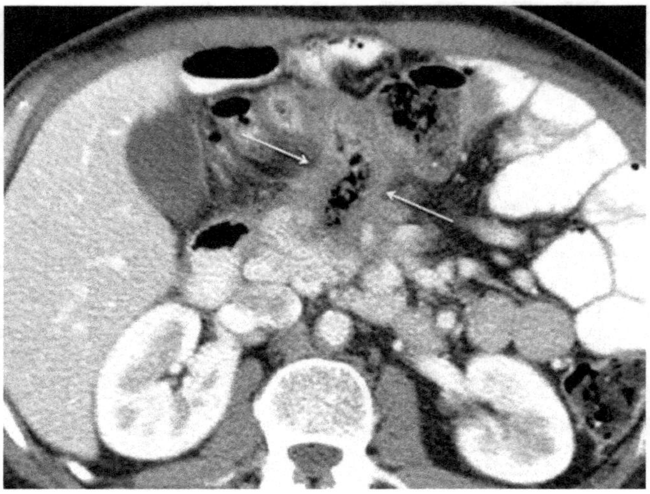

Fig. Transaxial CT image through the transverse mesocolon (TMC) in a patient with pancreatic adenocarcinoma demonstrates invasion of the TMC with necrotic tumor (arrows). The tumor in the TMC has fistulized with the transverse colon resulting in gas accumulating within the necrotic debris

The duodenocolic ligament, the right edge of the transverse mesocolon, forms an important pathway for the spread of right colon cancers via lymphatic drainage from the right colon passing through this ligament. Tumors of the right colon may spread via these lymphatics to deposit in nodes around the duodenum and pancreas [1]. Gastric outlet obstruction may occur once this adenopathy becomes sufficiently severe to obstruct the second duodenum explaining how cancers of the right colon may result in upper gastrointestinal obstruction on rare occasion.

Peritoneal Spaces as Pathways for the Spread of Disease

Peritoneal fluid flows naturally through the peritoneal spaces that are defined by the peritoneal ligaments and mesenteries in the abdomen and pelvis. However, certain neoplastic and inflammatory conditions within the peritoneal cavity may leverage this natural flow of peritoneal fluid to spread throughout the peritoneal spaces. Tumors that arise from the peritoneal lining or break through the visceral peritoneum may shed their cells directly into the peritoneal fluid. Similarly, inflammatory processes within the peritoneal cavity may also leverage this natural flow of ascitic fluid and spread throughout the peritoneal spaces of the abdomen and pelvis. A thorough knowledge and understanding of this anatomy can help narrow the differential diagnosis for intra-abdominal pathologies and may help radiologists better predict the organ of origin and likely route of spread for certain conditions (Fig.).

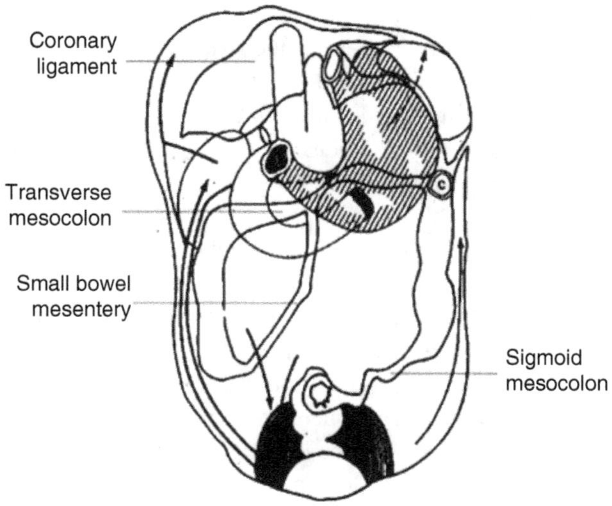

Fig. Posterior peritoneal reflections and recesses. Intraperitoneal fluid flows naturally from the pelvis to the upper abdomen. Flow occurs preferentially through the right rather than left paracolic gutters owing to the broader diameter of the right gutter. In addition, flow in the left paracolic gutter is cut off from reaching the left subphrenic space by the phrenicocolic ligament. The transverse mesocolon divides the abdomen into supra- and inframesocolic spaces. In the right inframesocolic space, fluid is impeded from draining into the pelvis via the small bowel mesentery. Owing to natural holdup of fluid at the root of the small bowel mesentery and sigmoid mesocolon, these structures are naturally predisposed to involvement with serosal-based metastases in the setting of peritoneal carcinomatosis (Reprinted with permission from Myers MA. Dynamic Radiology of the Abdomen: Normal and Pathologic Anatomy, New York: Springer, 1994)

Left Peritoneal Space

The left peritoneal space is comprised of four compartments: the left anterior perihepatic space, the left posterior perihepatic space (gastrohepatic recess), the left anterior subphrenic space, and the left posterior subphrenic space (perisplenic space).

Anteriorly, the left peritoneal space extends to the right as the left anterior perihepatic space, ventral to the left lobe of the liver. It is bounded laterally on the right by the falciform ligament and on the left by the anterior wall of the stomach. Posteriorly, it extends along the diaphragm and is limited by the left coronary ligament, the left superior extension of the bare area of the liver (Fig.).

Along the medial margin of the left hepatic lobe, the left anterior perihepatic space turns to form the left posterior perihepatic space as it extends along the inferior margin of the left hepatic lobe posteriorly, deep into the fissure for the

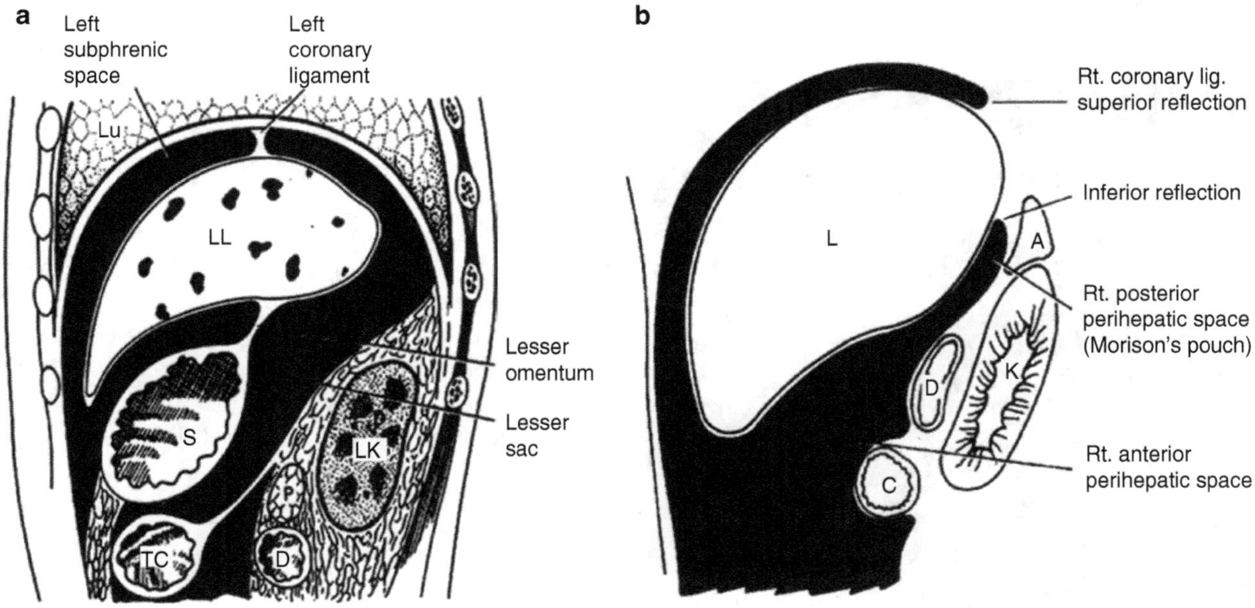

Fig. Left (**a**) and right (**b**) perihepatic spaces. The left and right perihepatic spaces are bounded posteriorly by the coronary ligaments. The reflections of the coronary ligaments mark the site of the nonperitonealized "bare area" of the liver (*LL* left lobe of the liver, *LK* left kidney, *S* stomach, *TC* transverse colon, *P* pancreas, *D* duodenum, *Lu* lung, *L* liver [right lobe], *A* adrenal, *K* kidney, *C* colon) (Reprinted with permission from Myers MA. Dynamic Radiology of the Abdomen: Normal and Pathologic Anatomy, New York: Springer, 1994)

ligamentum venosum. Also known as the gastrohepatic recess, the left posterior perihepatic space is bounded on the left by the lateral wall of the stomach and is juxtaposed to the anterior wall of the duodenal bulb, the anterior wall of the gallbladder, and the porta hepatis [8]. Fluid in the gastrohepatic recess is separated from fluid in the superior recess of the lesser sac by the lesser omentum as it inserts into the fissure for the ligamentum venosum. Fluid collections in the gastrohepatic recess are relatively easy to drain owing to the lack of intervening structures between this space and the body wall, along the medial margin of the left hepatic lobe. Conversely, fluid collections in the lesser sac may be more difficult to approach percutaneously owing to the presence of intervening vasculature in the lesser omentum.

Laterally in the left abdomen, the left anterior subphrenic space connects with the left anterior perihepatic space across the mid-abdomen. This space is cut off from the left paracolic gutter by the phrenicocolic ligament, unlike the right subphrenic space which communicates freely with the right paracolic gutter. Thus, fluid can accumulate within the left anterior subphrenic space by passing ventral to the stomach, but once it enters this space, it is relatively static owing to the phrenicocolic ligament. Thus, fluid in the left anterior subphrenic space is a common site for peritoneal carcinomatosis and abscess formation consequent to peritonitis [12].

The posterior extension of the left anterior subphrenic space is the left posterior subphrenic space also known as the perisplenic space (Fig.). The bare areas of the spleen that result from insertion of the gastrosplenic and splenorenal ligaments into the splenic hilum may be highlighted by fluid that surrounds the spleen within the perisplenic space [13–15]. Superiorly, the perisplenic space surrounds completely the upper margin of the spleen [16].

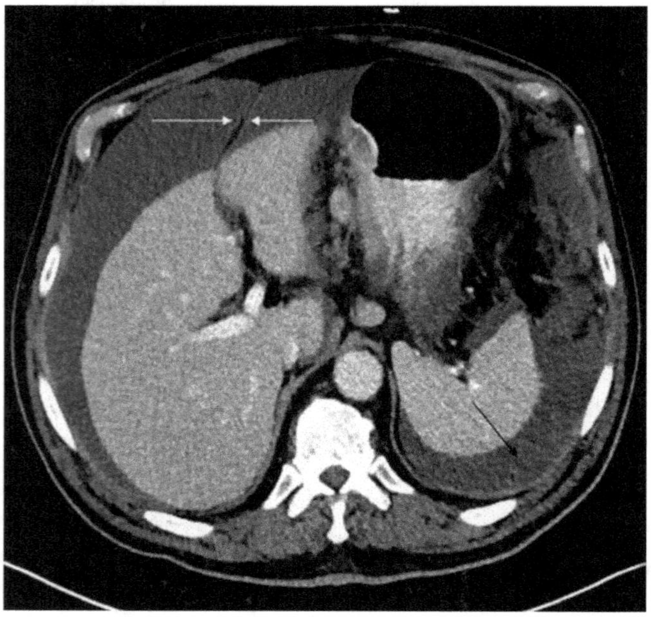

Fig. Transaxial CT image from a patient with carcinomatosis secondary to gastric cancer demonstrates fluid in the left posterior subphrenic space (black arrow) and fluid in the right and left anterior perihepatic spaces, separated by the falciform ligament (white arrows)

Right Peritoneal Space

The right peritoneal space is comprised of three compartments: the right subphrenic space/right anterior perihepatic space, the right posterior perihepatic space (hepatorenal recess/Morison's pouch), and the lesser sac.

The right subphrenic space surrounds the upper margin of the liver, separating it from the right hemidiaphragm (Figs.). Posteriorly and medially, the right coronary ligament (bare area of the liver) forms the posteromedial border of the right subphrenic space [17] (Fig.).

Inferior to the right coronary ligament, the hepatorenal recess (Morison's pouch) is the medial extension of the right subphrenic space, located between the right lobe of the liver and the anterior border of the kidney.

The lesser sac is the leftward extension of the right posterior perihepatic space/hepatorenal recess/Morison's pouch as it extends through the foramen of Winslow. The lesser sac is comprised of superior and inferior recesses [9, 18]. Fluid in the superior recess of the lesser sac surrounds the caudate lobe producing a reverse C-shaped configuration as it surrounds this structure (Figs.). A raised peritoneal reflection along the posterior aspect of the lesser sac serves as an anatomic boundary that separates the superior from the inferior recesses. This gastropancreatic plicae contains the proximal left gastric artery and may be recognized, particularly when surrounded by ascitic fluid in the superior and inferior recesses.

The inferior recess of the lesser sac is bounded laterally by the gastrosplenic and splenorenal ligaments, inferoposteriorly by the transverse mesocolon, and anteriorly by the stomach. Percutaneous drainage of fluid in lesser sac collections is problematic owing to the presence of abdominal organs, ligaments, and mesenteries that surround both superior and inferior recesses completely [19].

Concluding Remarks

Upper abdominal disease may spread from the upper abdominal organs to the retroperitoneum and vice versa via the gastrohepatic and hepatoduodenal ligaments in the right abdomen, the gastrosplenic and splenorenal ligaments in the left abdomen, and the gastrocolic ligament and transverse mesocolon in the mid-abdomen. Disease in any of these ligamentous pairs can suggest the organ of origin and, in

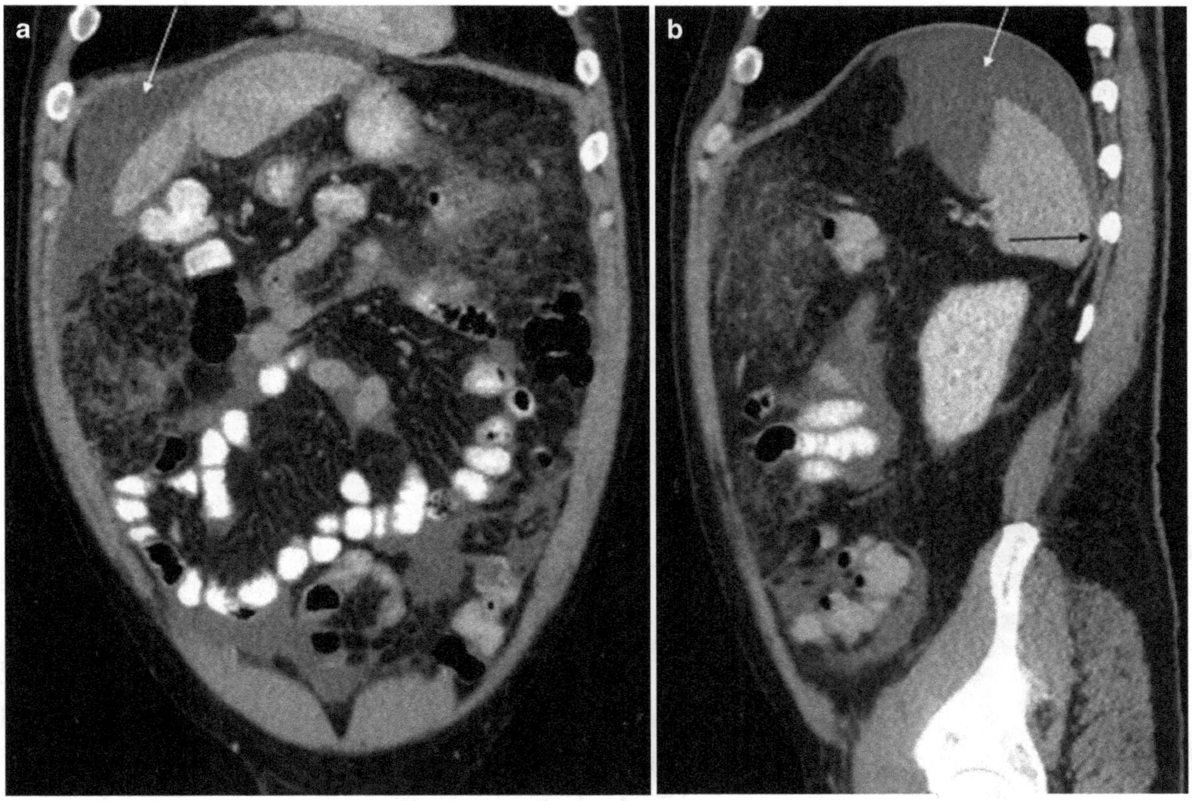

Fig. Coronal (**a**) and sagittal (**b**) reformatted CT images from a patient with peritoneal mesothelioma demonstrate fluid in the right subphrenic space (white arrows) bounded posteriorly by the right coronary ligament (black arrow)

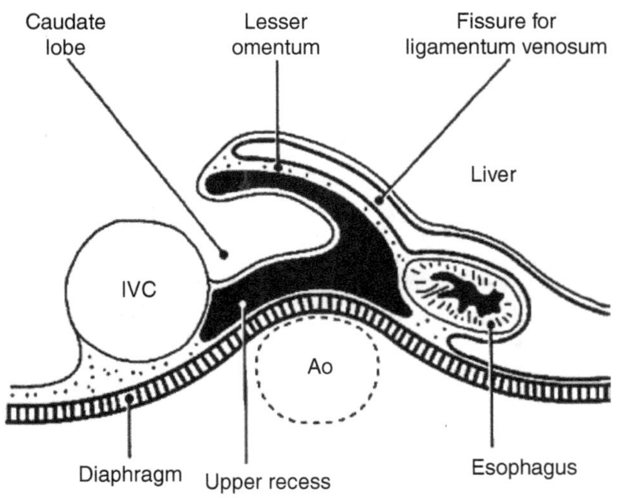

Fig. The boundaries of the superior recess of the lesser sac may be recognized when fluid engulfs the caudate lobe. The lesser omentum separates this fluid from fluid in fissure for the ligamentum venosum which is in continuity with the left posterior perihepatic space (gastrohepatic recess) (*IVC* inferior vena cava, *Ao* aorta) (Reprinted with permission from Myers MA. Dynamic Radiology of the Abdomen: Normal and Pathologic Anatomy, New York: Springer, 1994)

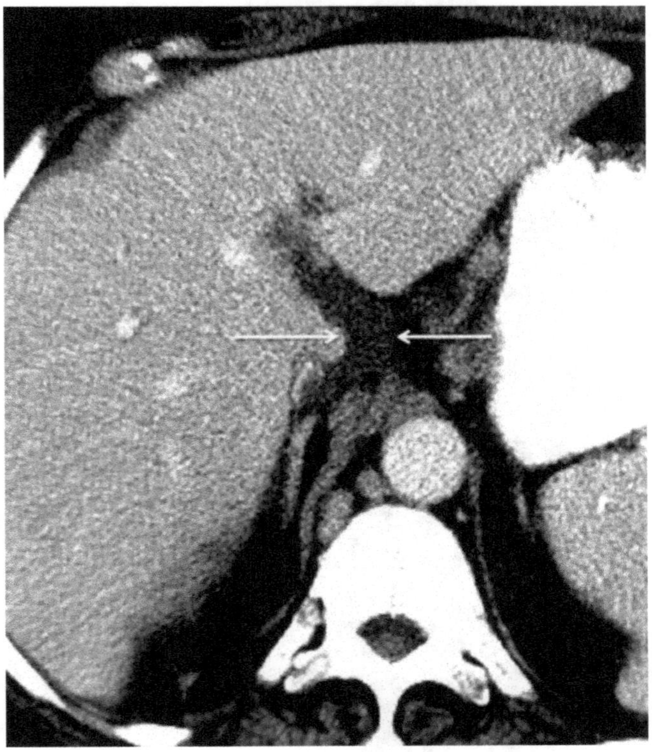

Fig. . Transaxial CT image through the superior recess of the lesser sac in a patient with gallbladder cancer (same patient as is illustrated in Fig.). Malignant ascites has accumulated in the superior recess of the lesser sac (arrows), seen with a characteristic reverse C-shaped configuration surrounding the caudate lobe

some cases, the location of the disease within the organ. Peritoneal ligaments and mesenteries also guide the flow of intraperitoneal fluid throughout the peritoneal spaces that they define. Neoplastic and inflammatory diseases that arise de novo or extend into the peritoneal cavity may spread through these spaces and deposit in predictable areas within the peritoneal cavity.

Key Points

- Disease may spread through the abdomen and pelvis by the following mechanisms:
  via the bloodstream
  via lymphatic extension
  via direct invasion
  via intraperitoneal seeding
- Direct invasion and lymphatic extension occur commonly through the peritoneal ligaments and mesenteries that interconnect the abdominal viscera
- Intraperitoneal spread occurs by seeding the peritoneal cavity with cells that spread via the natural flow of peritoneal fluid via the peritoneal spaces

Take-Home Message

A thorough understanding of the peritoneal ligaments and mesenteries as well as the peritoneal spaces that they define can inform the pathways by which inflammatory and neoplastic diseases may spread throughout the abdomen and pelvis.

References

1. Meyers MA, Oliphant M, Berne AS, Feldberg MAM. The peritoneal ligaments and mesenteries: pathways of intraabdominal spread of disease. Radiology. 1987;163:593–604.
2. Balfe DM, Mauro MA, Koehler RE, Lee JKT, Weyman PJ, Picus D, Peterson RR. Gastrohepatic ligament: normal and pathologic CT anatomy. Radiology. 1984;150:485–90.
3. Auh YH, Rosen A, Rubenstein WA, Engel IA, Whalen JP, Kazam E. CT of the papillary process of the caudate lobe of the liver. AJR. 1984;142:535–8.
4. Donoso L, Martinez-Noguera A, Zidan A, Lora F. Papillary process of the caudate lobe of the liver: sonographic appearance. Radiology. 1989;173:631–3.
5. Weinstein JB, Heiken JP, Lee JKT, DiSantis DJ, Balfe DM, Weyman PJ, Peterson RR. High resolution CT of the porta hepatis and hepatoduodenal ligament. Radiographics. 1986;6:55–74.
6. Zirinsky K, Auh YH, Rubenstein WA, Kneeland JB, Whalen JP, Kazam E. The portacaval space: CT with MR correlation. Radiology. 1985;156:453–60.
7. Ito K, Choji T, Fujita T, Kuramitsu T, Nakaki H, Kurokawa F, Fujita N, Nakanishi T. Imaging of the portacaval space. AJR. 1993;161:329–34.
8. Vincent LM, Mauro MA, Mittelstaedt CA. The lesser sac and gastrohepatic recess: sonographic appearance and differentiation of fluid collections. Radiology. 1984;150:515–9.
9. Dodds WJ, Foley WD, Lawson TL, Stewart ET, Taylor A. Anatomy and imaging of the lesser peritoneal sac. AJR. 1985;144:567–75.
10. Cooper C, Jeffrey RB, Silverman PM, Federle MP, Chun GH. Computed tomography of omental pathology. J Comput Assist Tomogr. 1986;10(1):62–6.
11. Rubesin SE, Levine MS, Glick SN. Gastric involvement by omental cakes: radiographic findings. Gastrointest Radiol. 1986;11:223–8.
12. Halvorsen RA, Jones MA, Rice RP, Thompson WM. Anterior left subphrenic abscess: characteristic plain film and CT appearance. AJR. 1982;139:283–9.
13. Vibhakar SD, Bellon EM. The bare area of the spleen: a constant CT feature of the ascitic abdomen. AJR. 1984;141:953–5.
14. Rubenstein WA, Auh YH, Zirinsky K, Kneeland JB, Whalen JP, Kazam E. Posterior peritoneal recesses: assessment using CT. Radiology. 1985;156:461–8.
15. Love L, Demos TC, Posniak H. CT of retrorenal fluid collections. AJR. 1985;145:87–91.
16. Crass JR, Maile CW, Frick MP. Catheter drainage of the left posterior subphrenic space: a reliable percutaneous approach. Gastrointest Radiol. 1985;10:397–8.
17. Rubenstein WA, Auh TH, Whalen JP, Kazem E. The perihepatic spaces: computed tomographic and ultrasound imaging. Radiology. 1983;149:231–9.
18. Jeffrey RB, Federle MP, Goodman PC. Computed tomography of the lesser peritoneal sac. Radiology. 1981;141:117–22.
19. Meyers MA. Dynamic radiology of the abdomen: normal and pathologic anatomy. 4th ed. New York: Springer; 1994.

14

Malignant Diseases of the Uterus

Yulia Lakhman and Caroline Reinhold

Learning Objectives

- To describe the role of MRI and PET/CT for initial treatment selection, planning, and response assessment in uterine malignancies
- To explain eligibility criteria for fertility preservation in cervical cancer
- To highlight combined MR features that may distinguish uterine sarcoma from atypical leiomyoma (LM)

CervicalCancer

Epidemiology and Diagnosis

Cervical cancer is the fourth most common malignancy among women worldwide [1, 2]. Most cases and deaths occur in developing countries, whereas in developed countries widespread cytology-based screening has led to a sharp decline in incidence [1, 3].

The main risk factor is chronic human papillomavirus (HPV) infection [1, 3]. Thus, cervical cancer can be effectively prevented with HPV vaccines and HPV DNA-based screening [1]. Abnormal cytology or positive high-risk HPV test should prompt colposcopy and cervical biopsy. Squamous cell carcinoma comprises 70–80% and adenocarcinoma 20–25% of cases [1].

Y. Lakhman (✉)
Department of Radiology, Memorial Sloan Kettering Cancer Center, New York, NY, USA
e-mail: lakhmany@mskcc.org

C. Reinhold (✉)
Department of Radiology, McGill University Health Centre, Montreal, QC, Canada
e-mail: caroline.reinhold@mcgill.ca

Initial Staging and Management

Cervical cancer is staged using the International Federation of Gynecology and Obstetrics (FIGO) classification [4]. It is the only gynecologic malignancy staged clinically owing to high prevalence in developing countries. Lymph node (LN) status, a major prognostic factor, is excluded from FIGO staging as clinical detection is not possible [1]. Cross-sectional imaging is not accepted for formal assignment of FIGO stage but is used routinely in developed countries to guide treatment decisions [1, 5]. Treatment selection is determined by tumor stage and presence/location of LN metastases (Fig.).

MRI and Initial Staging

MRI is the method of choice to evaluate locoregional extent (Table) [6, 7]. Small field-of-view T2-weighted imag-ing in the sagittal and short-axis planes is the mainstay of staging MRI (Fig.) [6]. Diffusion-weighted imaging (DWI) in conjunction with T2-weighted imaging improves delineation of tumor margins. Dynamic contrast-enhanced imaging (DCE) is used largely in research for prognosis and response assessment.

Stage I: Cervix-Confined Disease

Stage IA is microscopic in size. Stage IB is visible clinically and is divided based on size into IB1 (≤4 cm) and IB2 (>4 cm). The tumor has intermediate signal intensity (SI) on T2-weighted imaging and shows diffusion restriction. Intact rim of low-SI fibrous cervical stroma around the tumor indicates cervix-confined disease (Fig.) [6]. Fertility preservation (LN assessment + cone/trachelectomy) is possible for patients with ≤Stage IB1 (Table) [8, 9].

Fig. Diagram (adapted from [6]) highlights the role of MRI and PET/CT to assess disease extent and guide treatment decisions in patients with new diagnosis of cervical cancer

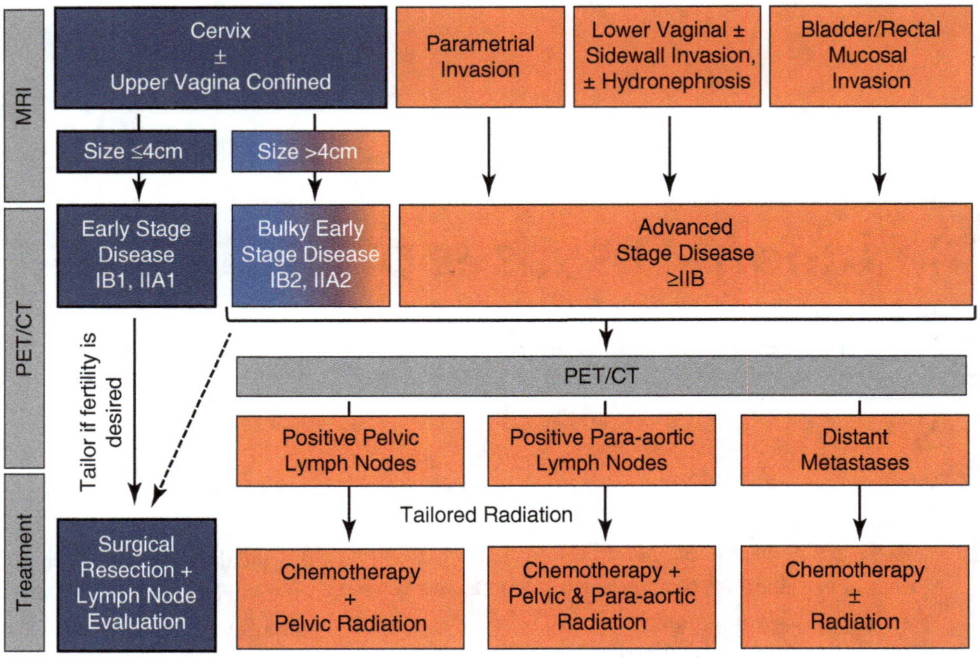

Table Suggested MRI protocol to stage cervical and endometrial cancer [7]

Sequences	Planes	Field of view (FOV)	Assessment/detection of
T1-weighted imaging	Axial	Large FOV, Kidneys to pubic symphysis	• Pelvic and para-aortic LNs • Bones
T2-weighted imaging	Axial	Pelvis, small FOV	• Hydronephrosis • Pelvic sidewall invasion • Adnexal involvement
	Sagittal	Pelvis, small FOV	Cervical cancer • Endocervical extent Endometrial cancer • Depth of myometrial invasion Both • Cervical stromal invasion • Vaginal involvement
	Short-axis plane perpendicular to cervix (cervical cancer) or endometrium (endometrial cancer)	Pelvis, small FOV	Endometrial cancer • Depth of myometrial invasion Both • Cervical stromal invasion • Parametrial invasion
DWI $B = 0, \geq 800$	Sagittal	Pelvis, small FOV	• Adjunct to T2-weighted imaging to assess tumor extent
	Short-axis plane (as above)	Pelvis, small FOV	• Adjunct to T2-weighted imaging to assess tumor extent • Increase in LN conspicuity
Optional for cervical cancer	• Vaginal gel: Upper vaginal invasion • Endovaginal coil: Small tumors prior to fertility preservation • Long-axis plane T2-weighted imaging + DWI (parallel to cervix) – Endocervical extent – Cervical stromal invasion – Parametrial invasion		
Optional for endometrial cancer	• Long-axis plane T2-weighted imaging + DWI (parallel to endometrium) – Depth of myometrial invasion – Cervical stromal invasion		

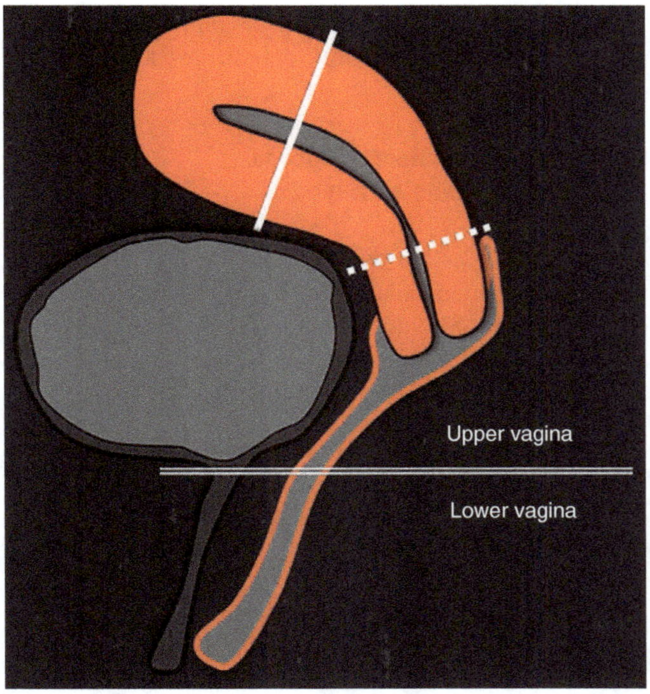

Fig. Drawing illustrates orientations of short-axis planes to stage endometrial cancer (solid line oriented perpendicular to endometrium) and cervical cancer (dashed line oriented perpendicular to endocervical canal). Double line is drawn at the bladder base/urethral junction and divides the vagina into upper and lower portions

Stage II: Cervical + Upper Vaginal Disease ± Parametrial Invasion

Stage IIA invades the upper vagina (upper two-thirds) but not the parametrium. Similar to Stage IB, it is divided into IIA1 (≤4 cm) and IIA2 (>4 cm). Vaginal invasion is diagnosed when intermediate-SI tumor disrupts low-SI vagina on T2-weighted imaging. A horizontal line drawn at the bladder base on sagittal T2-weighted imaging divides the vagina into upper and lower portions (Fig.).

Stage IIB invades the parametrium. Complete loss of low-T2 SI stromal ring does not always indicate parametrial invasion. Parametrial invasion is present if tumor disrupts low-SI stroma *AND* causes spiculated/nodular tumor-parametrial interface ± encases parametrial vessels (Fig.) [6]. DWI + T2-weighted imaging improve specificity for detecting parametrial invasion [10]. Accurate diagnosis is important as parametrial invasion indicates concurrent chemotherapy and radiation (CCRT) as treatment of choice (Fig.).

Stage III: Pelvic Sidewall Invasion, Lower Vaginal Involvement, Hydronephrosis, or Nonfunctional Kidney

Stage IIIA invades the lower vagina. Stage IIIB extends to the pelvic sidewall ± causes hydronephrosis. Tumor

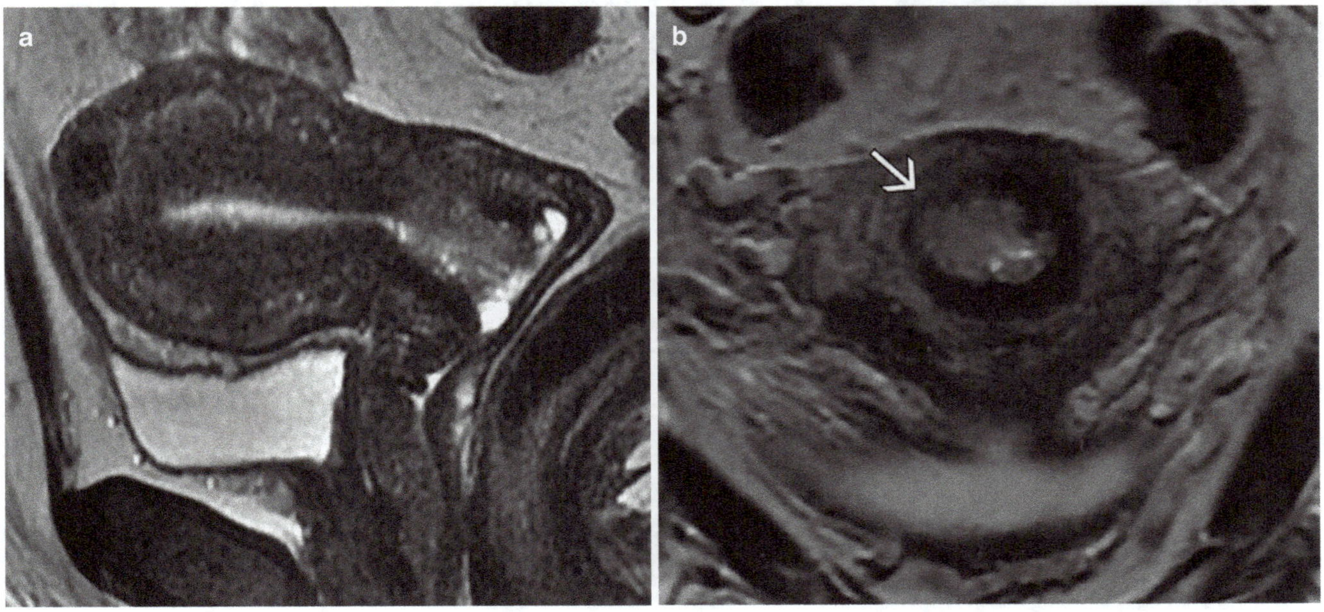

Fig. 52-year-old woman with Stage IB1 cervical adenocarci-noma. Sagittal T2-weighted imaging (**a**) and short-axis T2-weighted imaging (**b**) demonstrate 1.8 cm tumor with intermediate SI on T2-weighted imaging. Tumor involves partial thickness of cervical stroma with intact low-SI stromal ring (arrow) ruling out parametrial invasion

Table Selection criteria for conservative management of women with ≤ Stage IB1 lesions and desire for fertility

Eligibility criteria
• Squamous cell carcinoma, adenocarcinoma, or adenosquamous carcinoma
• Tumor size ≤2 cm
– Some centers ≤4 cm
• Tumor-to-internal os distance ≥1 cm
– Some centers ≥0.5 cm
• Cervical stromal invasion <50%
– Some centers, any depth
• Cervix-confined disease
– Absence of parametrial invasion or LN metastases

within 3 mm of iliac vessels or obturator internus, piriformis, or levator ani muscles indicates sidewall invasion [6].

Stage IV: Bladder/Rectal Mucosal Invasion or Extension Beyond the Pelvis

Stage IVA invades the bladder/rectal mucosa; invasion is present when intermediate-SI tumor disrupts low-SI muscle wall and extends into the mucosa on T2-weighted imaging. Bullous edema alone (high-SI mucosa) does not mean Stage IVA [6]. Stage IVB is indicated by the presence of

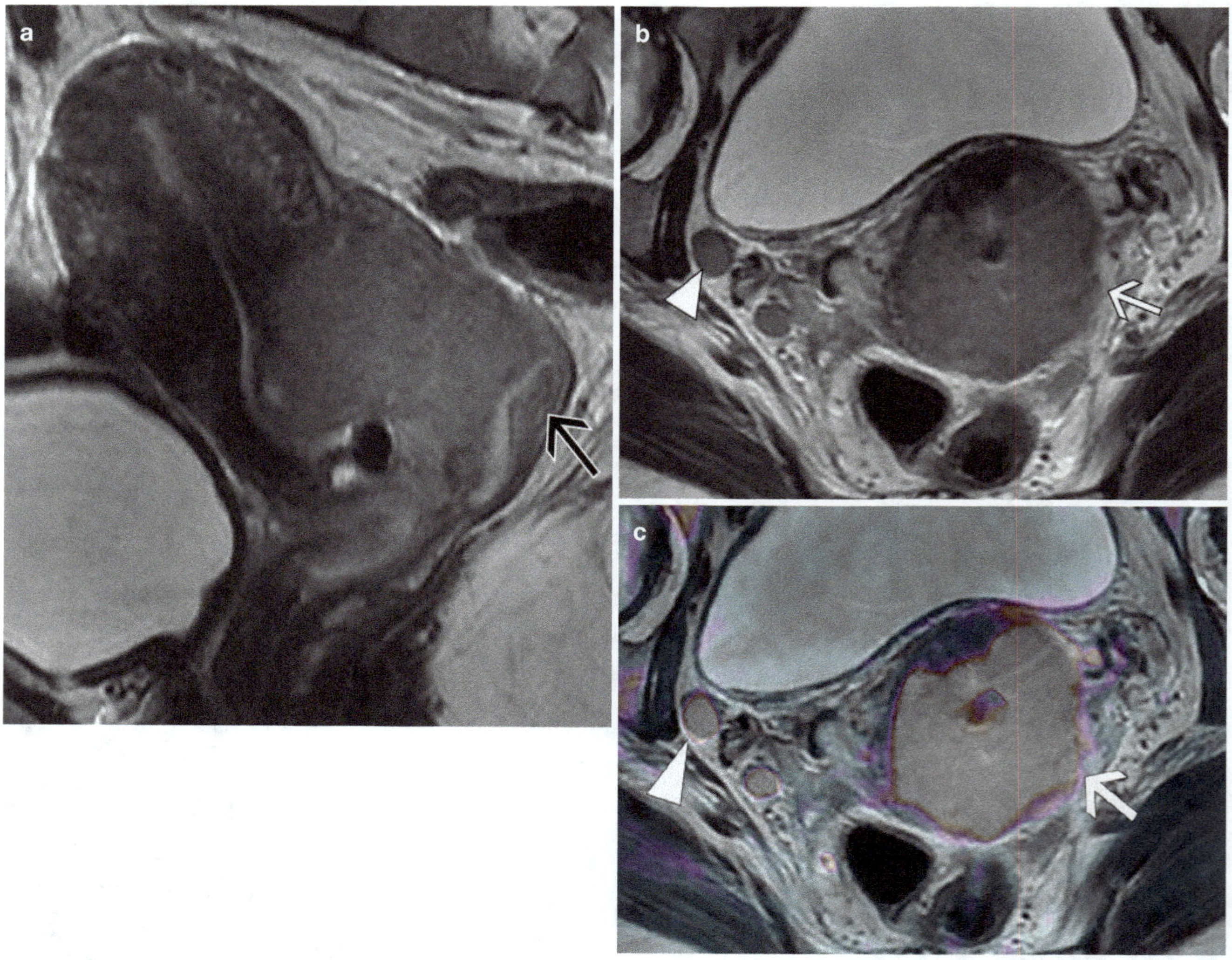

Fig. 35-year-old woman with Stage IIB cervical squamous cell carcinoma. Sagittal T2-weighted imaging (**a**), short-axis T2-weighted imaging (**b**), and fused T2-weighted imaging + DWI (**c**) demonstrate 5.2 cm tumor involving the lower uterus, upper vagina (arrow), and parametrial regions. There is nodular interface between the tumor and parametrium (arrow). Also note right internal iliac LNs (arrowhead)

distant metastases (including LN metastases beyond the pelvis).

PET/CT and Initial Staging

LN metastases impact prognosis and treatment. On MRI (and CT) short-axis diameter ≥ 1 cm is a main diagnostic criterion but yields low-to-moderate sensitivity because metastases to normal-sized LNs remain undetected (Fig.) [11]. LNs show high SI on DWI, increasing their conspicuity (Fig.); however, DWI is not used to distinguish benign from malignant LNs due to overlap in ADC values [10]. PET/CT improves N and M staging and is recommended for Stage ≥ IB2 disease (Fig.) [5, 12].

Evaluation During and After Initial Treatment

After radical hysterectomy, imaging is obtained if recurrence is suspected clinically [1, 5]. After fertility-sparing surgery, MRI is recommended at 6 months and annually thereafter [5].

MRI and PET/CT are useful for radiotherapy (RT) planning. For example, RT field is extended to para-aortic regions if para-aortic LN metastases are present on pretreatment PET/CT (Figs.) [1, 5], and mid-treatment MRI allows adjustment of brachytherapy dose based on volume/location of residual tumor [13, 14].

Low-SI stroma on T2-weighted imaging indicates tumor-free cervix, but an abnormal signal may persist up to

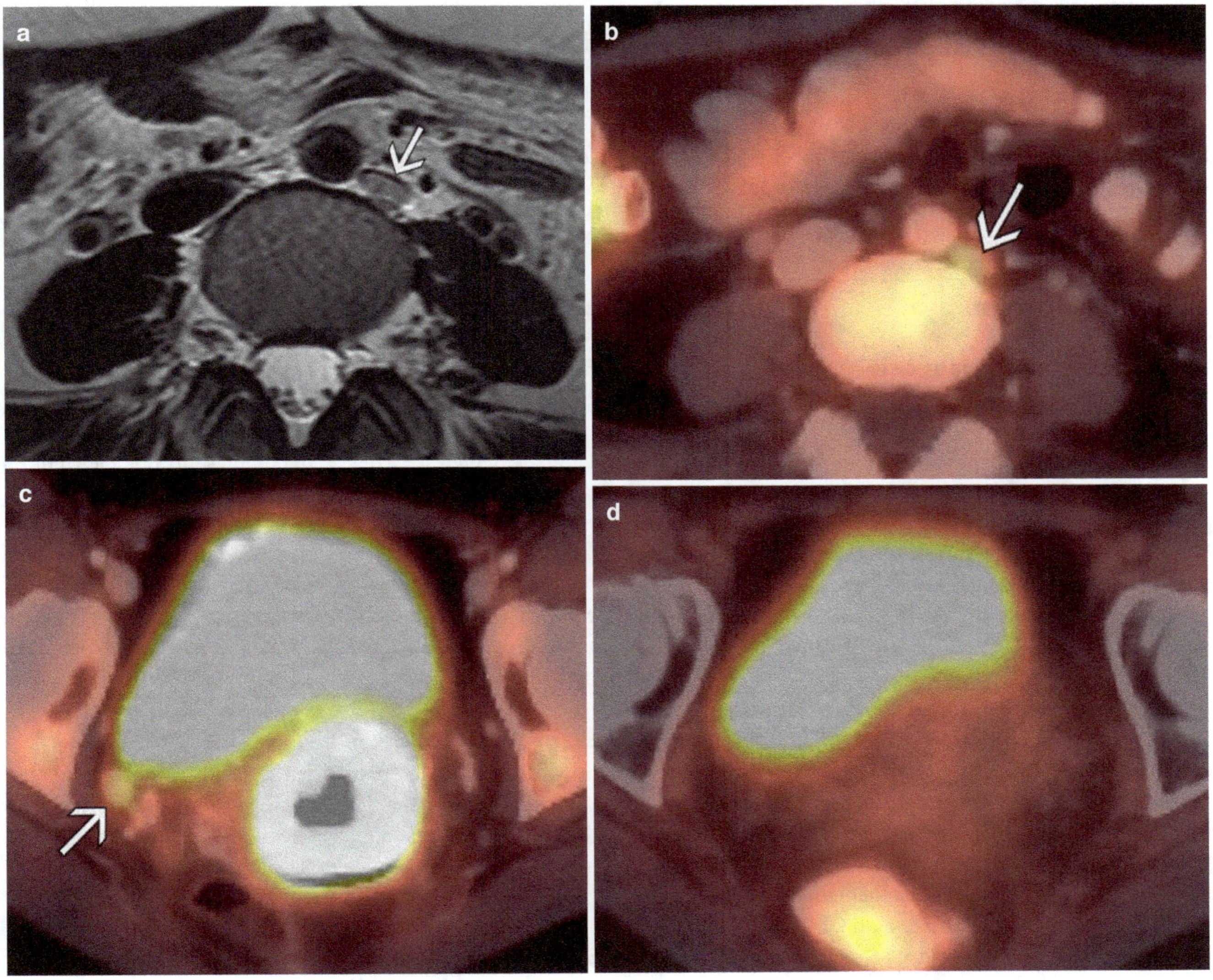

Fig. Same patient as in Fig.. Axial T2-weighted imaging and PET/CT images show 0.5 cm short-axis FDG-avid left para-aortic LN (**a**, **b**). (**c**) Baseline axial PET/CT image through the pelvis demonstrates FDG-avid cervical tumor and right internal iliac LN (arrow). (**d**) Complete resolution of FDG avidity after CCRT

6 months after CCRT [6]. Thus, PET/CT obtained 3–6 months after CCRT is useful. Absent FDG avidity indicates low risk of recurrence; diminished FDG avidity signifies moderate risk; and unchanged, increased, or new FDG-avid foci indicate persistent disease (Fig.) [15]. The role of DWI and DCE to assess response is an area of active research [10, 13].

Evaluation of Recurrence

Recurrent cervical cancer has similar imaging features as primary lesions [6]. In the absence of prior pelvic RT, localized recurrence may be approached with CCRT. Radical surgery is the only potential cure in previously irradiated pelvis. MRI and PET/CT are essential to determine eligibility and tailor the extent of surgery [16].

FutureDirections

PET/MRI may offer a “one-stop-shop” approach to the evaluation of cervical cancer in both primary and recurrent settings [17].

EndometrialCancer

Epidemiology and Diagnosis

Endometrial cancer is the sixth most common malignancy among women worldwide and the most common gynecological cancer in developed countries [2]. Incidence has steadily increased, primarily due to increased longevity and obesity in developed countries. Approximately 75% of cases occur in postmenopausal women and >90% present with postmenopausal bleeding. As such, most patients are diagnosed at an early stage with 5-year survival rates >90% in this subgroup [18].

Initial evaluation includes pelvic ultrasound (US) and pipelle endometrial biopsy or dilatation and curettage. Thresholds of endometrial thickness of 4–5 mm in postmenopausal women detect endometrial cancer with a sensitivity of up to 95% and a specificity of 77% [19]. Endometrial cancer is traditionally subdivided into two types based on biological behavior: *type 1* tumors are estrogen-dependent and include FIGO grades 1 and 2 endometrioid adenocarcinomas, while *type 2* tumors include serous papillary carcinomas, clear cell adenocarcinomas, carcinosarcomas, and FIGO grade 3 endometrioid adenocarcinomas [18]. *Type 2* tumors are not estrogen dependent, present at a higher stage, and behave more aggressively.

Initial Staging and Management

Endometrial cancer is staged surgically using the FIGO system [4]. The standard surgical staging procedure consists of total abdominal hysterectomy, bilateral salpingo-oophorectomy, LN dissection, peritoneal washing, and omental biopsies. FIGO stage correlates well with prognosis, but preoperative staging remains important, since early-stage/low-grade tumors may be treated with minimally invasive surgery and may not require LN dissection [20, 21].

MRI and Initial Staging

MR imaging is the modality of choice to determine the depth of myometrial invasion, which correlates with tumor grade, LN metastases, and 5-year survival (Table) [22]. Small field-of-view high-resolution imaging in the sagittal and short-axis planes is the mainstay of MRI staging (Fig.) [6]. The combination of T2-weighted imaging, DCE, and DWI offers the best diagnostic accuracy with, its high-spatial resolution and larger field of view has a particular advantage over endovaginal US in the setting of bulky tumors, advanced stage, and concomitant benign disease, i.e., adenomyosis and LMs.

Stage I: Uterine-Confined Disease

Stage IA is confined to the endometrium or inner half of the myometrium, i.e., <50% myometrial thickness involvement (Fig.). Stage IB extends to the outer half of the myometrium (≥50%) (Fig.). The tumor has intermediate-to- low SI on T2-weighted imaging, is hypointense to myometrium on later phases of DCE, and shows restricted diffusion. However, small tumors may be iso- or only mini-mally hypointense relative to the normal endometrium and may be hypervascular relative to the endometrium early on after contrast administration. A partially intact, low-SI junc-tional zone around the tumor indicates the absence of deep myometrial invasion.

Stage II: Cervical Stromal Invasion

Stage II invades and disrupts the low-SI cervical stroma on T2-weighted imaging. Polypoid extension of the tumor into the endocervical canal or endocervical mucosal invasion is not sufficient to assign Stage II. Tumor extension beyond the cervix into the parametrium requires a radical hysterectomy.

Stage III: Invasion of Uterine Serosa, Adnexa, Vagina, and/or Pelvic or Para-Aortic Lymph Nodes

Stage IIIA invades the uterine serosa appearing as an area of intermediate SI on T2-weighted imaging with loss of normal rim enhancement of the outer myometrium on DCE. Direct

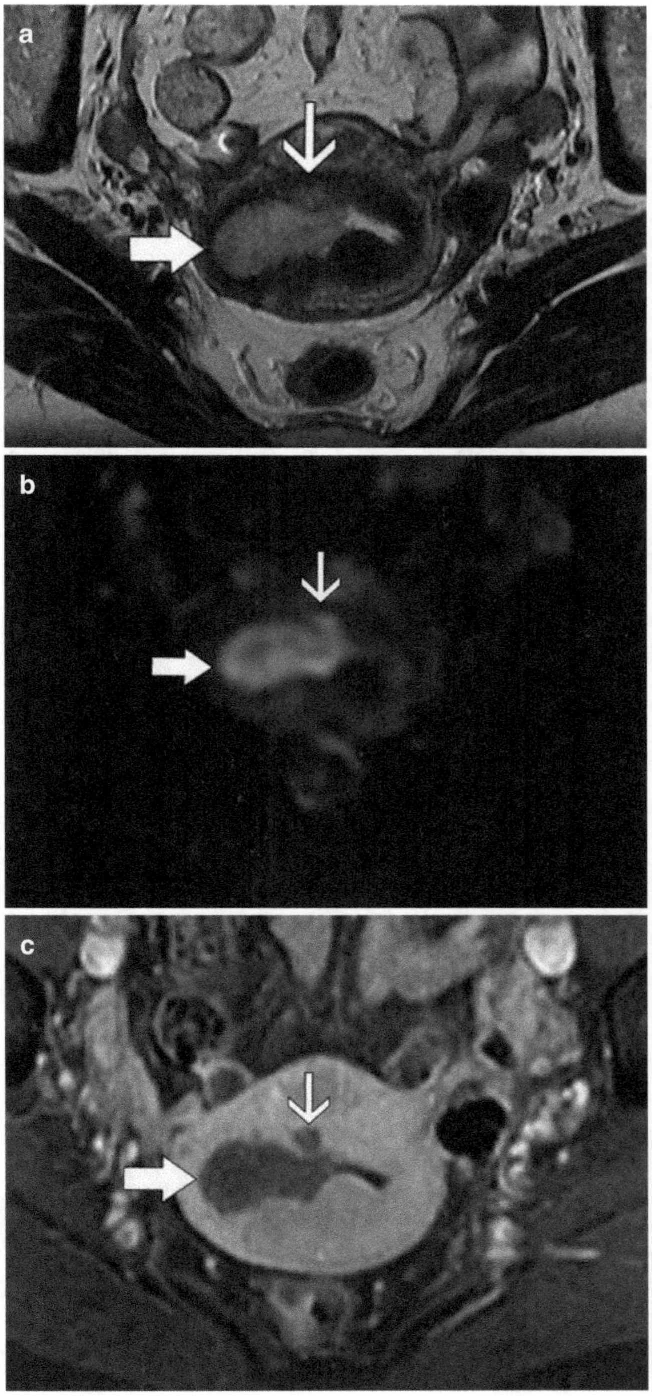

Fig. 62-year-old woman with Stage IA endometrioid adenocarci-noma (grade 2) of the endometrium. Short-axis (**a**) T2-weighted imag-ing, (**b**) B1000 DWI, and (**c**) delayed post gadolinium 3D T1-weighted imaging demonstrate an endometrial-based tumor (thick arrow) at the level of the fundus and right cornua. There is partial invasion of the inner half of the myometrium with a thin rim of junctional zone (thin arrow) remaining intact

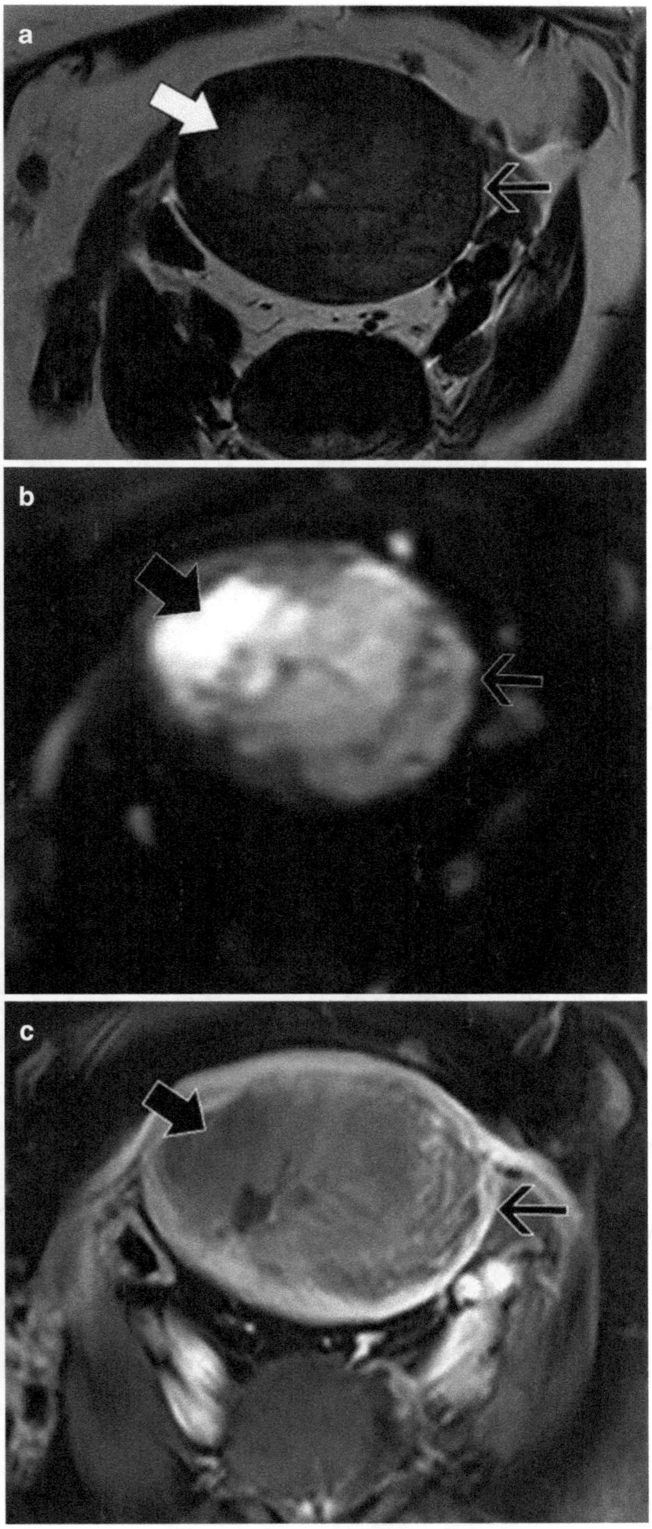

Fig. 76-year-old woman with Stage IB endometrioid adenocarci-noma (grade 3) of the endometrium. Short-axis (**a**) T2-weighted imag-ing, (**b**) B1000 DWI, and (**c**) delayed post gadolinium 3D T1-weighted imaging demonstrate a large tumor (thick arrow) invading the deep myometrium. There is a thin rim of intact outer myometrium (thin arrow) along the left aspect of the uterus excluding serosal involvement tumor spread to the adnexa or ovarian metastases is considered Stage IIIA disease. It is important but challenging to differentiate synchronous ovarian lesions from metastases to the ovaries. *Type 2* tumors have a higher pretest probability of advanced disease, and therefore a meticulous search for advanced tumor extent is required in this subgroup.

Stage IIIB involves the vagina either by contiguous spread or metastatic involvement.

Stage IIIC is diagnosed when there is pelvic (Stage IIIC1) and/or para-aortic (Stage IIIC2) LN metastatic involvement. The use of a 1 cm short-axis cutoff value results in a high specificity but poor sensitivity (range, 36–89.5%) for predicting LN metastases [6]. A cutoff value of 0.8 cm increases the sensitivity albeit at the cost of specificity. In practice, given that endometrial carcinoma is staged surgically, it is important to provide the size and detail the location of LNs exceeding 0.5–0.6 cm in short-axis. The role of DWI and ADC to assess LNs is the same as described for cervical cancer [10]. PET/CT improves N and M staging; however, PET/CT is currently not part of standard of care for initial staging of endometrial cancer.

Stage IV: Bladder/Rectal Mucosal Invasion or Extension Beyond the Pelvis

Please refer to section "MRI and Initial Staging of Cervical Carcinoma," as the findings are the same for endometrial and cervical carcinoma.

Evaluation of Recurrence

Recurrent endometrial cancer has a similar imaging appearance as the primary tumor. Risk factors for recurrence include advanced stage at presentation, high-grade disease, and lymphovascular invasion. More than 80% of recurrences occur within 3 years of initial treatment with LNs (46%) and the vaginal vault (42%) being the most common sites. MRI is useful to evaluate surgical resectability of pelvis-confined recurrent disease, while PET/CT is helpful to exclude distant and LN metastases [6, 16].

Uterine Sarcomas

Epidemiology and Presentation

Uterine sarcomas are rare aggressive tumors originating from mesenchyme and comprising <3% of uterine corpus tumors [6, 21]. Leiomyosarcoma (LMS) is the most common histologic subtype, followed by endometrial stromal sarcoma (ESS) and undifferentiated uterine sarcoma. ESS is subdivided into low- and high-grade ESS based on differences in histopathology and clinical outcomes [21]. Carcinosarcoma was previously categorized as uterine sarcoma but is now classified as high-grade endometrial carcinoma [6, 21].

Uterine sarcomas arise de novo and have no biologic link to LM [25]. Prompt radical surgery is the standard of care for uterine sarcomas [21]. In contrast, symptomatic LM can be approached with traditional surgery (hysterectomy, myomectomy) or newer minimally/noninvasive strategies (embolization, ablation, medical therapy). The latter do not yield histologic diagnosis, highlighting the need for precise initial diagnosis [26].

Uterine sarcoma and LM manifest with similar symptoms. Large size and rapid growth are unreliable signs of malignancy [25]. Growth of uterine mass after menopause and elevated LDH, particularly LDH isozyme type 3, should be viewed as suspicious for LMS [25]. Endometrial sampling may aid diagnosis of uterine sarcoma, but sensitivity is limited due to myometrial origin [21, 25].

Role of Imaging

MRI is the imaging method of choice if uterine sarcoma is suspected clinically or if intervention is planned for symptomatic LM (to map tumors and exclude sarcoma) [26].

No single MR feature can reliably distinguish uterine sarcoma (including LMS) from atypical LM (degeneration or histologic variants). Combined MR features may suggest correct diagnosis including a single large uterine mass with hemorrhage (high SI on T1-weighted imaging), heterogeneous high SI on T2-weighted imaging, infiltrative/nodular borders on T2-weighted imaging, and central necrosis [27]. Uterine sarcoma also demonstrates rapid early enhancement of solid components on DCE and restricted diffusion (Fig.) [27]. Diffusion restriction alone is insufficient for diagnosis because it may be observed with LM, especially cellular LM [27].

ESS often demonstrates distinct MR features that aid diagnosis including an ill-defined myometrial mass with endometrial component, wormlike low-SI bands on T2-weighted imaging (normal myometrium compressed by tumor), and contiguous extension along the fallopian tubes, periuterine vessels, and pelvic ligaments [6].

Key Points

- MRI excels at locoregional staging of cervical and endometrial cancer for treatment stratification, while PET/CT improves N and M staging in uterine malignancies.
- MRI facilitates patient selection prior to fertility preservation for early stage cervical and endometrial cancers.
- MRI aids the characterization of clinically suspected uterine sarcoma.

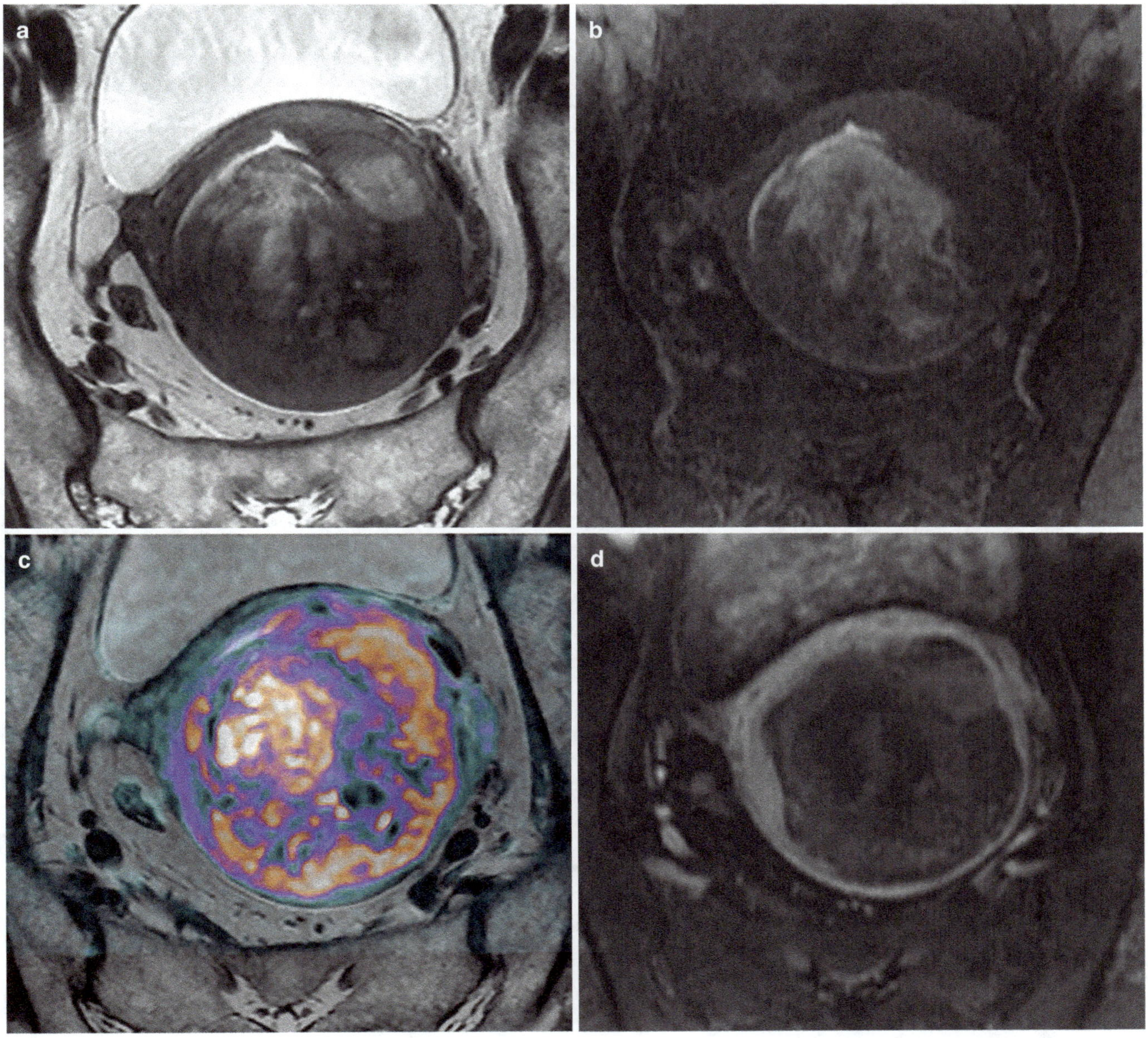

Fig. 69-year-old woman with uterine sarcoma. Short-axis images show ill-defined myometrial mass with heterogeneous high SI on T2-weighted imaging (**a**), hemorrhage on fat-saturated T1-weighted imaging (**b**), diffusion restriction on fused T2-weighted imaging +DWI (**c**), and central necrosis on DCE (**d**)

References

1. Marth C, Landoni F, Mahner S, McCormack M, Gonzalez-Martin A, Colombo N. Cervical cancer: ESMO clinical practice guidelines for diagnosis, treatment and follow-up. Ann Oncol. 2017;28:iv72–83.
2. Ferlay J, Soerjomataram I, Dikshit R, et al. Cancer incidence and mortality worldwide: sources, methods and major patterns in GLOBOCAN 2012. Int J Cancer. 2015;136:E359–86.
3. Ginsburg O, Bray F, Coleman MP, et al. The global burden of women's cancers: a grand challenge in global health. Lancet. 2017;389:847–60.
4. Pecorelli S. Revised FIGO staging for carcinoma of the vulva, cervix, and endometrium. Int J Gynaecol Obstet. 2009;105:103–4.
5. National Comprehensive Cancer Network Clinical Practice Guidelines in Oncology. Cervical Cancer. Version 1.2017. https://www.nccn.org/professionals/physician_gls/pdf/cervical.pdf. Accessed 1 July 2017.
6. Sala E, Rockall AG, Freeman SJ, Mitchell DG, Reinhold C. The added role of MR imaging in treatment stratification of patients with gynecologic malignancies: what the radiologist needs to know. Radiology. 2013;266:717–40.
7. Raithatha A, Papadopoulou I, Stewart V, Barwick TD, Rockall AG, Bharwani N. Cervical cancer staging: a Resident's primer: Women's imaging. Radiographics. 2016;36:933–4.
8. Bentivegna E, Gouy S, Maulard A, Chargari C, Leary A, Morice P. Oncological outcomes after fertility-sparing surgery for cervical cancer: a systematic review. Lancet Oncol. 2016;17:e240–53.

9. Rockall AG, Qureshi M, Papadopoulou I, et al. Role of imaging in fertility-sparing treatment of gynecologic malignancies. Radiographics. 2016;36:2214–33.
10. deSouza NM, Rockall A, Freeman S. Functional MR imaging in gynecologic cancer. Magn Reson Imaging Clin N Am. 2016;24:205–22.
11. Choi HJ, Ju W, Myung SK, Kim Y. Diagnostic performance of computer tomography, magnetic resonance imaging, and positron emission tomography or positron emission tomography/computer tomography for detection of metastatic lymph nodes in patients with cervical cancer: meta-analysis. Cancer Sci. 2010;101:1471–9.
12. Signorelli M, Guerra L, Montanelli L, et al. Preoperative staging of cervical cancer: is 18-FDG-PET/CT really effective in patients with early stage disease? Gynecol Oncol. 2011;123:236–40.
13. Khan SR, Rockall AG, Barwick TD. Molecular imaging in cervical cancer. Q J Nucl Med Mol Imaging. 2016;60:77–92.
14. Potter R, Georg P, Dimopoulos JC, et al. Clinical outcome of protocol based image (MRI) guided adaptive brachytherapy combined with 3D conformal radiotherapy with or without chemotherapy in patients with locally advanced cervical cancer. Radiother Oncol. 2011;100:116–23.
15. Schwarz JK, Siegel BA, Dehdashti F, Grigsby PW. Association of posttherapy positron emission tomography with tumor response and survival in cervical carcinoma. JAMA. 2007;298:2289–95.
16. Lakhman Y, Nougaret S, Micco M, et al. Role of MR imaging and FDG PET/CT in selection and follow-up of patients treated with pelvic Exenteration for gynecologic malignancies. Radiographics. 2015;35:1295–313.
17. Bagade S, Fowler KJ, Schwarz JK, Grigsby PW, Dehdashti F. PET/MRI evaluation of gynecologic malignancies and prostate cancer. Semin Nucl Med. 2015;45:293–303.
18. Morice P, Leary A, Creutzberg C, Abu-Rustum N, Darai E. Endometrial cancer. Lancet. 2016;387:1094–108.
19. Smith-Bindman R, Kerlikowske K, Feldstein VA, et al. Endovaginal ultrasound to exclude endometrial cancer and other endometrial abnormalities. JAMA. 1998;280:1510–7.
20. Colombo N, Creutzberg C, Amant F, et al. ESMO-ESGO-ESTRO consensus conference on endometrial cancer: diagnosis, treatment and follow-up. Int J Gynecol Cancer. 2016;26:2–30.
21. National Comprehensive Cancer Network Clinical Practice Guidelines in Oncology. Uterine Neoplasms. Version 3.2017. https://www.nccn.org/professionals/physician_gls/pdf/uterine.pdf. Accessed 15 Oct 2017.
22. Kinkel K, Forstner R, Danza FM, et al. Staging of endometrial cancer with MRI: guidelines of the European Society of Urogenital Imaging. Eur Radiol. 2009;19:1565–74.
23. Andreano A, Rechichi G, Rebora P, Sironi S, Valsecchi MG, Galimberti S. MR diffusion imaging for preoperative staging of myometrial invasion in patients with endometrial cancer: a systematic review and meta-analysis. Eur Radiol. 2014;24:1327–38.
24. Deng L, Wang QP, Chen X, Duan XY, Wang W, Guo YM. The combination of diffusion- and T2-weighted imaging in predicting deep Myometrial invasion of endometrial cancer: a systematic review and meta-analysis. J Comput Assist Tomogr. 2015;39:661–73.
25. Ricci S, Stone RL, Fader AN. Uterine leiomyosarcoma: epidemiology, contemporary treatment strategies and the impact of uterine morcellation. Gynecol Oncol. 2017;145:208–16.
26. Silberzweig JE, Powell DK, Matsumoto AH, Spies JB. Management of Uterine Fibroids: a focus on uterine-sparing interventional techniques. Radiology. 2016;280:675–92.
27. Bolan C, Caserta MP. MR imaging of atypical fibroids. Abdom Radiol. 2016;41:2332–49.

15

The Pediatric Gastrointestinal Tract: What Every Radiologist Needs to Know

Emily A. Dunn, Øystein E. Olsen, and Thierry A. G. M. Huisman

Learning Objectives
- To compare imaging modalities commonly used in the assessment of pediatric gastrointestinal disease.
- To understand gastrointestinal pathology affecting children of different age groups.
- To recognize classic imaging features of gastrointestinal diseases commonly encountered in infants and children.

Imaging Techniques

Plain Film Radiography and Fluoroscopy

Conventional radiography remains the first-line imaging in most hospitals for infants and children presenting with suspected gastrointestinal pathology.

Fluoroscopy is particularly useful when evaluating dynamic processes such as gastrointestinal motility. Fluoroscopy can also be used for guiding procedures/interventions such as foreign body removal and intussusception reduction.

E. A. Dunn (✉) · Thierry A. G. M. Huisman
Division of Pediatric Radiology, Russell H. Morgan Department of Radiology and Radiological Science, Johns Hopkins University School of Medicine, Charlotte R. Bloomberg Children's Center, Baltimore, MD, USA
e-mail: Edunn18@jhmi.edu; Thuisma1@jhmi.edu

Ø. E. Olsen
Radiology Department, Great Ormond Street Hospital for Children NHS Foundation Trust, London, UK
e-mail: oystein.olsen@gosh.nhs.uk

Ultrasound

Ultrasound (US) is one of the most valuable imaging tools for the initial evaluation of gastrointestinal disease, due to its high-resolution, real-time capability, wide availability and acceptance, and lack of ionizing radiation and because it rarely requires sedation. There are two key factors for success: (1) knowing how to deal with children of all ages and (2) using high-end US equipment/high-frequency probes.

Computed Tomography

In children, CT should be used with caution and is usually reserved for troubleshooting equivocal findings made in the initial diagnostic workup of acutely and critically sick children. CT is consequently often performed as first-line imaging for emergent indications, such as blunt and penetrating trauma. As a general rule, only one acquisition is needed, and multiphase contrast enhanced sequences should be avoided.

Magnetic Resonance Imaging

MRI is rarely used in the first-line evaluation of gastrointestinal pathology; however, it may serve as an adjunct in challenging/unequivocal cases. In children, MRI is typically performed in the assessment of intestinal pathology such as inflammatory bowel disease and appendicitis, focal and diffuse disease of the abdominal viscera, and diseases of the biliary tree.

Intestinal Obstruction

In neonates and young children, there is no radiographic "signature" for the large and small bowel. Plain film radiographs of the normal newborn demonstrate swallowed air reaching the rectum by 24 h of life. In a clinically obstructed newborn, the number of dilated loops ("dilated" meaning roughly wider than the vertebral interpedicular space) may be more helpful. Whether there is one gas bubble (gastric outlet obstruction), a double bubble (duodenal obstruction), 3–4 bubbles/loops (other high small bowel obstruction), or more (low obstruction), the bowel gas pattern can help decide which contrast study is appropriate. A bowel gas pattern suspicious for a high obstruction may be assessed further with an upper GI contrast study. A bowel gas pattern suggesting a low obstruction should be followed by a contrast enema.

Neonatal Obstruction

Neonatal intestinal obstruction can be classified by location, with "high" obstructions occurring through the level of the proximal jejunum and "low" obstructions occurring after the proximal jejunum. Etiologies of neonatal intestinal obstruction are commonly congenital. In most cases, a fluoroscopic contrast study is required.

The differential diagnosis for high intestinal obstruction includes atresia of the esophagus, stomach, duodenum and jejunum, duodenal stenosis from annular pancreas, duodenal web, and malrotation possibly complicated by midgut volvulus.

The differential diagnoses for low intestinal obstruction include ileal and colonic atresia, anorectal malformation, meconium ileus, colonic dysmotility syndromes, and Hirschsprung's disease. Congenital abdominopelvic cysts or masses can cause both high and low (usually partial) obstruction.

An understanding of clinical presentation as well as the expected postnatal bowel gas progression throughout the abdomen on radiographs can help to detect the level of obstruction [1].

Esophageal atresia (Fig.) is a clinical diagnosis. If the diagnosis is established, then any gas in the gastrointesti-nal system distal to the esophagus on plain radiographs means there is also a tracheoesophageal fistula. Radiology has a greater role in the follow-up of these children. Fistulae may recur, and the contrast esophagogram is the imaging test of choice for diagnosis of recurrence; this is performed by trained operators as there is a considerable aspiration risk.

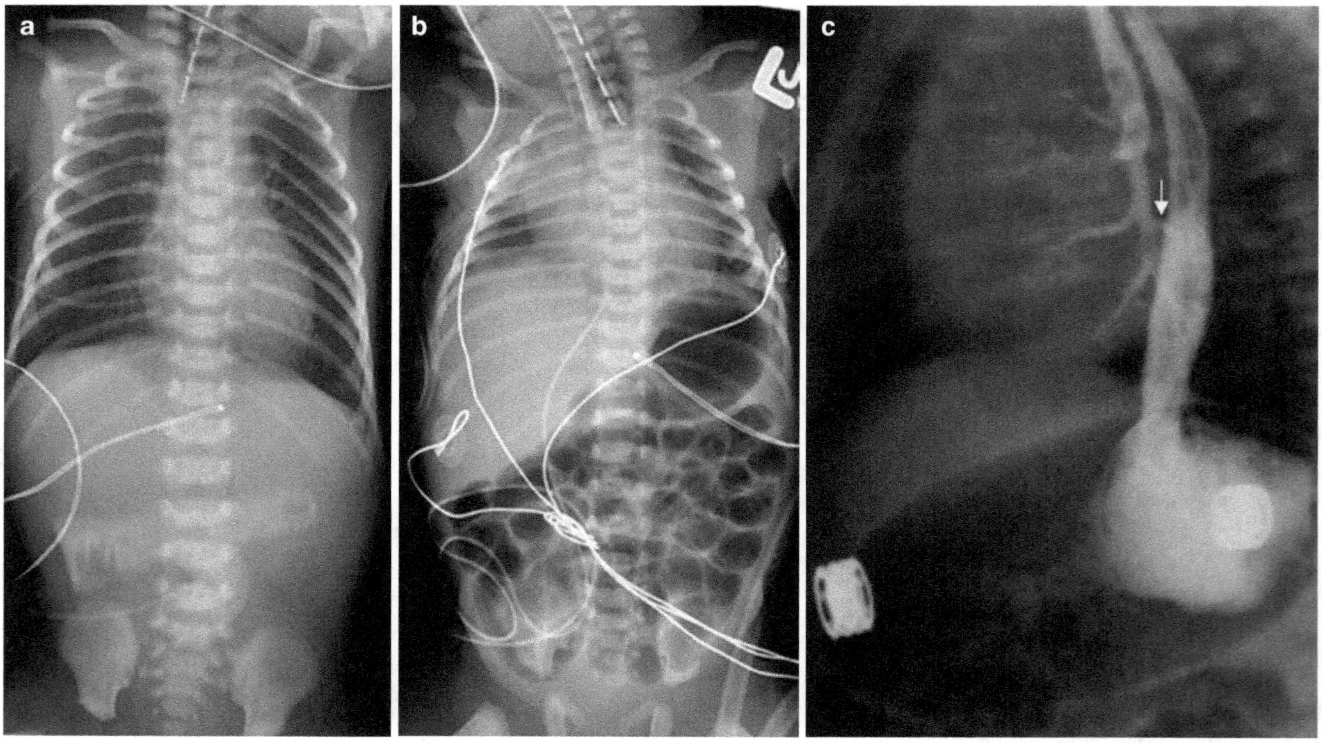

Fig. Esophageal atresia and tracheoesophageal fistula represent a spectrum of anomalies believed to result from abnormal formation and separation of the embryological foregut. These anomalies range from isolated EA to isolated TEF. Classification of congenital tracheoesophageal anomalies depends on the presence and location of the fistulous communication between both structures. (**a**) Radiograph of a newborn with isolated esophageal atresia (no fistula) shows no bowel gas distally. Those with isolated EA may have polyhydramnios in utero, and at birth, there is failure of passage of the orogastric tube beyond the level of the atresia. (**b**) Radiograph of a newborn with esophageal atresia and a fistula between the airway and the distal atretic segment demonstrates gas in the gastrointestinal tract despite failure to pass a feeding tube. (**c**) Fluoroscopic image in an infant with isolated tracheoesophageal fistula (arrow) following instillation of water-soluble contrast medium in the esophagus

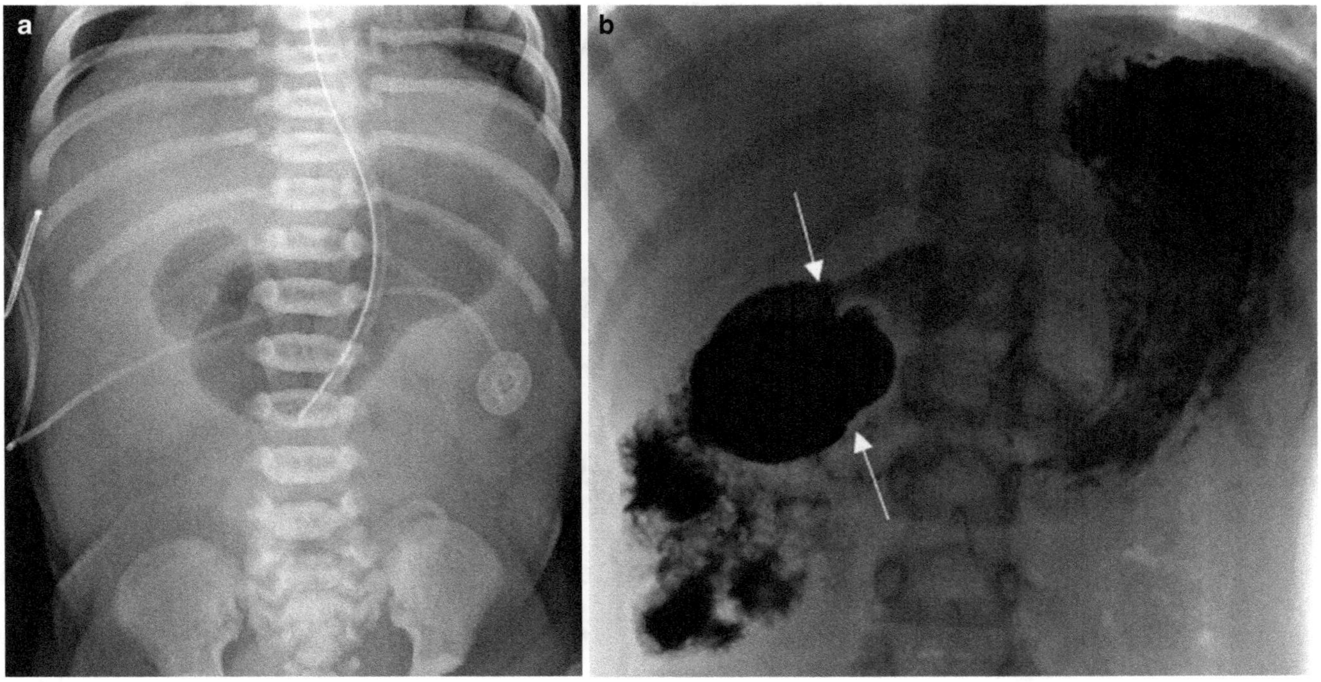

Fig. Duodenal obstruction (complete or partial) is commonly caused by duodenal atresia, duodenal stenosis, duodenal web, annular pancreas, and midgut volvulus. (**a**) Radiograph of a 12-hour-old newborn with prenatally diagnosed duodenal atresia. Abdominal radiograph shows the "double bubble" appearance of the air-distended stomach and proximal duodenum and no gas distally. These findings suggest duodenal obstruction. It should be noted that annular pancreas and midgut volvulus may produce a similar radiographic appearance. (**b**) Newborn with vomiting. The first and second portions of the duodenum are distended. A curvilinear filling defect is observed at the transition point (arrows), representing the "windsock" appearance of the duodenal web

For suspected anastomotic stricture, contrast swallow is performed. There is almost always relative narrowing at the anastomosis, so it is a functional holdup which suggests a potential need for dilatation [2, 3]. Esophageal atresia may be observed as part of the VACTERL association. Additional anomalies should be actively searched for.

Duodenal obstruction (Fig.) may have several causes. In duodenal atresia the classic radiographic findings are a double bubble and no distal intestinal gas. Duodenal atresia is thought to result from failure or incomplete recanalization of the intestine in utero.

Annular pancreas is caused by failed migration of the anlagen, and it may be evident sonographically (or with CT/MRI). Duodenal stenosis and duodenal web cause partial obstruction and may be difficult to distinguish. The classic sign of a web on a contrast study is the "windsock sign" [4, 5].

Malrotation with midgut volvulus (Fig.) is a surgical emergency in the neonate as well as in infants and children. The failed intestinal rotation manifests as a right-sided/midline low duodenojejunal flexure and a high cecum. This is associated with a short mesenteric root, which predisposes for volvulus. The normal position of the duodenojejunal flexure is at the height of the pylorus and to the left of the midline, at least as far as the left vertebral pedicles. Volvulus is suggested by bilious vomiting and is verified by the finding of a spiraling outline of a malrotated duodenum/proximal jejunum on the contrast study [6, 7]. On US a whirlpool of vessels is typically seen.

Small bowel atresia and stenosis (Fig.) are relatively common causes of complete and incomplete obstruction in the neonate. Multiple atresias may coexist; the etiology is thought to be in utero mesenteric vascular accidents. Accurate diagnosis is critical, since early surgical invention is usually performed. Bilious vomiting may be observed in those with obstruction beyond the level of the pancreatic ampulla. The typical findings of atresia on contrast enema are a small-caliber (unused) colon and distal small bowel and the inability to reflux contrast into dilated small bowel loops (distinguishing it from meconium ileus; see below) [4, 5].

Meconium ileus (Fig.) has a very high association (>80%) with cystic fibrosis. The distal ileum is impacted with sticky meconium. The findings on contrast enema are similar to those in small bowel atresia except that when contrast refluxes into the ileum, it outlines pellets of meconium, and it is usually possible to eventually fill dilated small bowel loops. In uncomplicated cases, (repeated) contrast enemas using water soluble contrast material are used therapeutically to soften and wash out meconium pellets. Both meconium ileus and intestinal atresias may be complicated by in utero bowel necrosis/perforation and meconium peritonitis [8, 9].

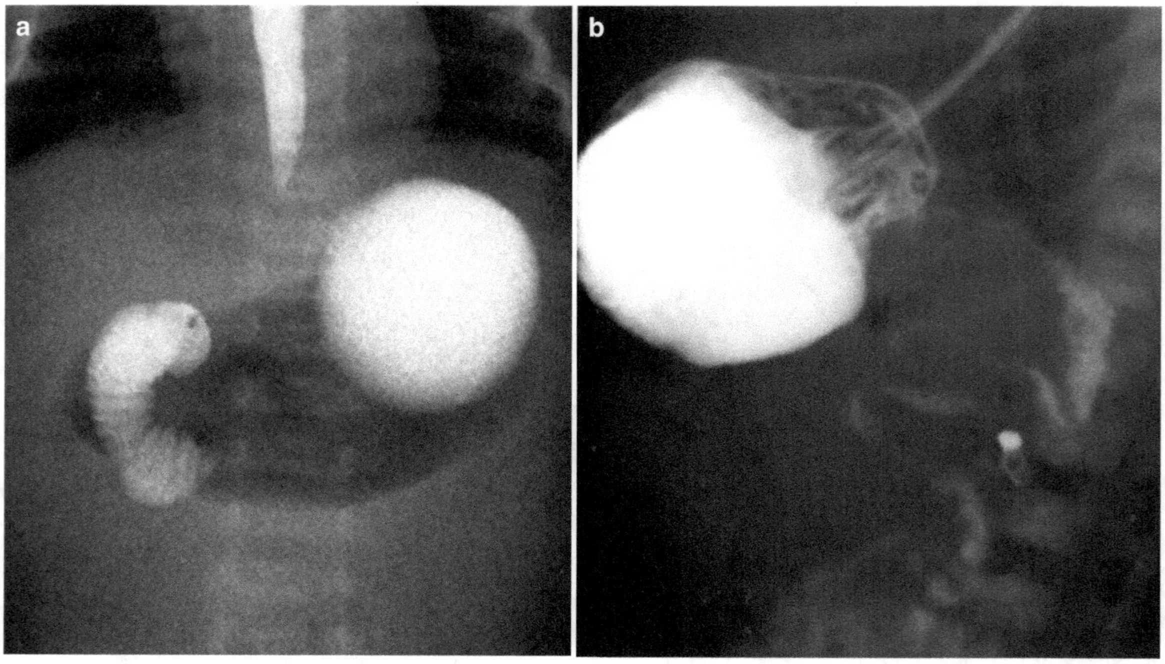

Fig. Intestinal malrotation results from incomplete rotation and fixation of the bowel in utero, with the duodenojejunal junction and cecum lying closer. This shortening of the mesenteric pedicle predisposes to midgut volvulus, in which the abnormally fixed bowel loops twist about the axis of the superior mesenteric artery and may obstruct the duodenum. While malrotation with midgut volvulus may occur at any age, the great majority present within their first month and many within their first week. Midgut volvulus can lead to intestinal ischemia necessitating bowel resection. Emergent and accurate imaging diagnosis is therefore critical. Bilious vomiting and abdominal distention in a newborn infant should raise the suspicion for an obstruction distal to the ampulla of Vater, and imaging should be pursued. Radiographs are normal in many cases of malrotation, and a fluoroscopic upper gastrointestinal series, which is considered the gold standard for diagnosis, should be performed in highly suspect cases. (**a**) Malrotation with midgut volvulus. In the case of malrotation with midgut volvulus, contrast material fails to pass beyond the obstructed third portion of the duodenum. (**b**) Malrotation with midgut volvulus in the setting of an incomplete obstruction. There is corkscrew configuration of contrast within the twisted midgut bowel loops

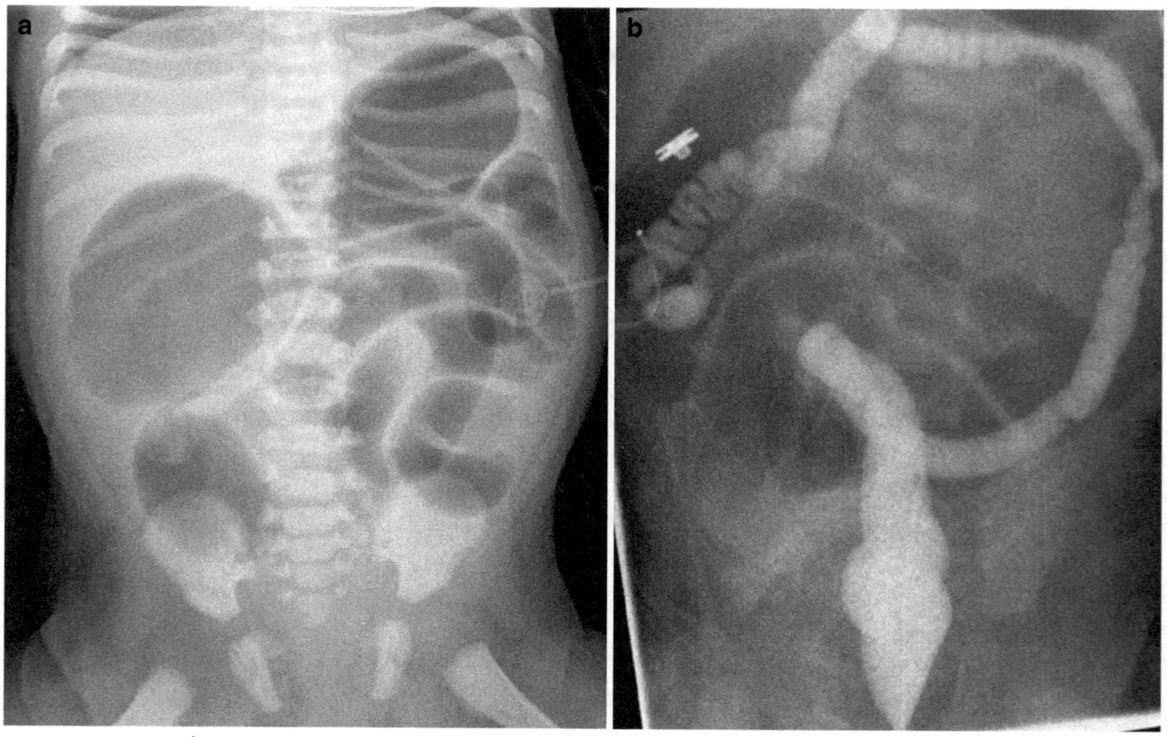

Fig. Ileal atresia is thought to result from mesenteric vascular events in utero. (**a**) Radiograph of a newborn infant with ileal atresia shows distention of multiple bowel loops throughout the abdomen, suggesting a low obstruction. (**b**) Fluoroscopic contrast enema in the same child demonstrates a typical "microcolon" (unused colon) and retrograde filling of non-dilated distal ileum to the level of the atresia (arrow). More proximal bowel loops are distended and air filled

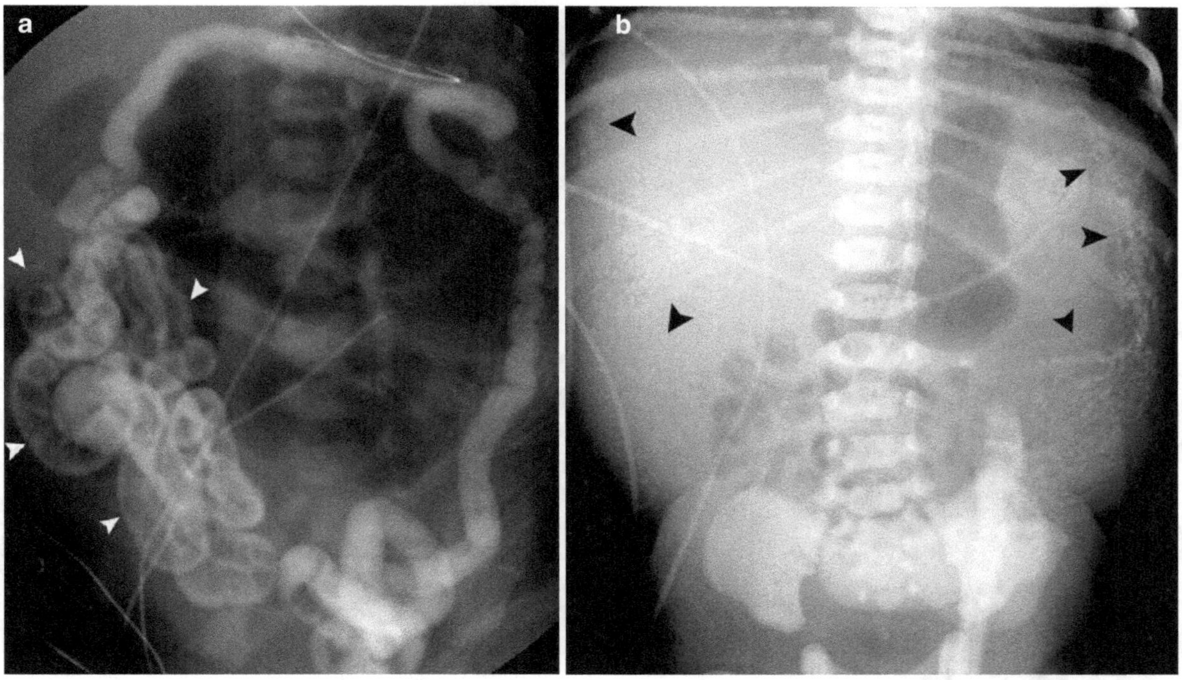

Fig. Meconium ileus represents obstruction of the distal ileum by viscous, impacted meconium pellets. There is a high association with cystic fibrosis (presenting symptom in 15% of neonates with CF). (**a**) Fluoroscopic contrast enema demonstrates contrast opacification o f a " microcolon" (unused colon due to proximal obstruction). Contrast has refluxed into the distal ileum (arrowheads) and outlines numerous impacted meconium pellets. (**b**) Abdominal radiograph demonstrates punctate calcifications scattered throughout the abdomen, suggestive of meconium peritonitis which can occur with intestinal atresias as well as meconium ileus, and results from perforation of meconium-containing bowel

Colonic atresia is exceedingly rare, and the diagnosis is often made clinically (vomiting and failure to pass meconium) on plain radiographs (no gas in the rectum). Contrast enema reveals failed reflux of contrast proximal to the level of the colonic atresia [10].

In Hirschsprung's disease (Fig. , intermuscular and submucosal nerve plexuses are absent due to arrested migration of intestinal ganglion cells, producing a functional intestinal obstruction. Since this migration occurs from proximal to distal large bowel, the aganglionic segment extends proximally from the anus. The typical clinical presentation is delayed passage of meconium in the neonate beyond 24 h of age.

Most affected patients demonstrate short-segment involvement, in which the transition point between normal and aganglionic bowel is located in the rectosigmoid colon. Rarely, the entire colon may be involved. Meconium/fecal impaction, a zone of transition from dilated to non-dilated bowel, and abnormal peristalsis of the affected colon segment with "sawtooth" appearance of the wall are classical findings at contrast enema. Very short-segment aganglionosis lacks a clear transition zone and is therefore difficult to diagnose radiologically. Hirschsprung's disease can only be definitively diagnosed by rectal (suction) biopsy [4, 11].

Functional immaturity of the colon, small left colon, and meconium plug syndrome (Fig.) are entities with con-siderable overlap. The risk is greater in babies of diabetic mothers. Radiologically there is a relatively smaller left colon and proximal meconium impaction. It is difficult to make a categorical diagnosis as similar findings may be seen in Hirschsprung's disease [12, 13].

Anorectal malformation is a clinical diagnosis. These malformations are classified as "high" or "low" depending on the location of the distal-most bowel segment relative to the puborectalis sling, with high lesions terminating above and low lesions terminating below this level. The role of radiology is to assess the length of the atretic anorectal segment and to map the fistula(e) [14].

Intestinal Obstruction in the Older Neonate and Infant

In older infants and children, obstruction may be related to other etiologies, such as adhesions, hypertrophic pyloric stenosis, intussusception, incarcerated intestinal hernia, appendicitis, sigmoid volvulus, and Meckel's diverticulum. Plain film radiographs can occasionally suggest the level of obstruction in older infants and children. In many cases, however, ultrasound and, occasionally, CT or MRI may be necessary to reach the diagnosis.

Hypertrophic pyloric stenosis (Fig.) classically pres-ents with forceful "projectile" vomiting and failure to gain weight in an infant. The diagnosis is made sonographically

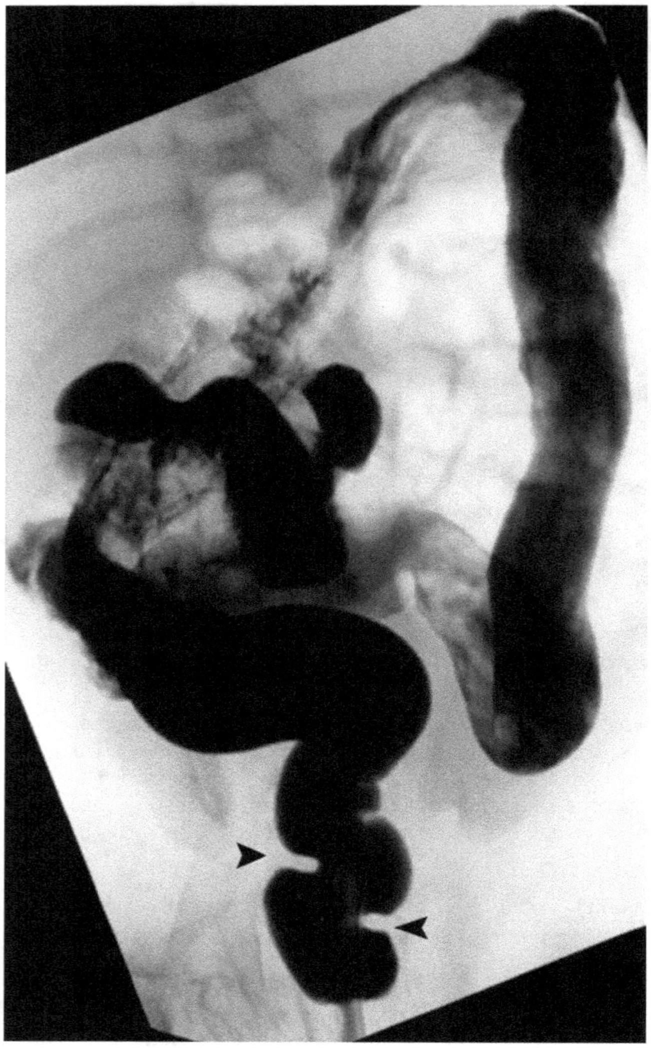

Fig. A fluoroscopic contrast enema in a 2-day-old with biopsy-proven Hirschsprung's disease shows a small-caliber rectum with mild distention of more proximal large bowel loops. Note the "sawtooth" appearance of the aganglionic segment (arrowheads), which reflects irregular contractions

where the typical findings are (1) thickened muscularis (>4 mm); (2) elongated pylorus (>15 mm), with redundant mucosa occasionally protruding into the antrum of the stomach; (3) gastric hyperperistalsis; and (4) persistent closed pyloric channel after a test feed. A contrast meal is rarely indicated except in a few equivocal cases [15].

Incarcerated intestinal hernia is a surgical emergency. The presentation and imaging findings are similar to those in adults.

Congenital abdominopelvic masses (Fig.) comprise a spectrum of abnormalities where gastrointestinal obstruction is relatively unusual. Sacrococcygeal masses (e.g., germ cell tumors, such as teratomas, or anterior meningoceles) may cause rectal obstruction. A cystic obstructive mass should raise suspicion for meconium pseudocyst or enteric duplication cyst. Duplication cysts may occur anywhere along the gastrointestinal tract and may have a relatively thick layered wall (akin to bowel) and a mucus-fluid level.

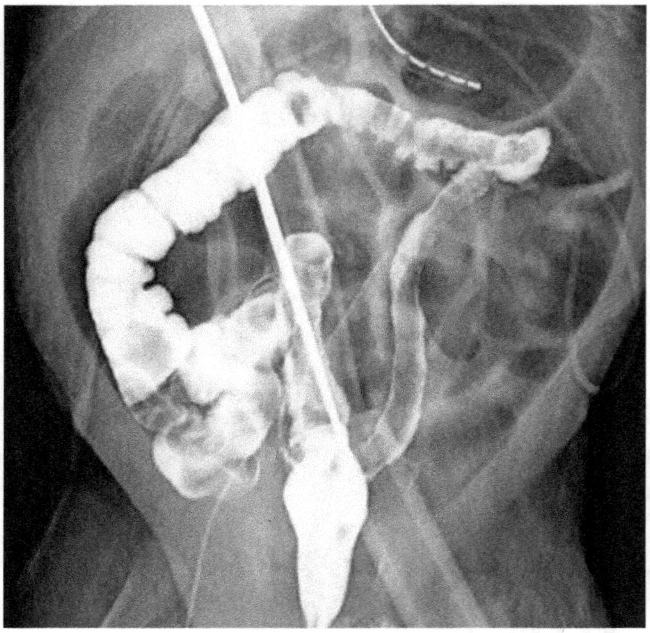

Fig. Functional immaturity of the colon, along with meconium plug and small left colon, represent syndromes of colonic dysmotility. Those affected typically present with delayed passage of meconium. There is a reported increased incidence in babies with mothers who are diabetic or who have received magnesium sulfate during pregnancy for preeclampsia. This image from a contrast enema reveals a small caliber of the descending and sigmoid colon, which are filled with meconium, proximal dilatation, and a normal-caliber rectum

Differential diagnoses for abdominal cystic lesions that are rarely obstructive include choledochal, mesenteric, and ovarian cysts, renal cystic dysplasia, and hydroureter [16].

Intestinal Obstruction in the Infant and Older Child

Ileocolic intussusception (Fig.) is a surgical emergency, usually occurring in infants and toddlers with maximum incidence at just under 1 year of age. The typical presentation is with abdominal pain, bloody stools, and a palpable mass. A clear cause (i.e., a "lead point," such as a mesenteric lymph node, lymphoid hyperplasia, duplication cyst, mural inflammation caused by Henoch-Schonlein purpura, or Meckel's diverticulum) may or may not be established. The sonographic diagnosis is fairly straightforward with the finding of a concentric doughnut shape in the transverse plane and sandwiching of the involved bowel segments (the "pseudokidney" sign) in the longitudinal plane [17].

Long-standing intussusception, trapped fluid in the involved segments, and trapped lymph nodes are thought to be associated with lower success rates for reduction with pressurized gas or fluid.

Colonic volvulus results from twisting of the colon around its mesenteric root and is a rare cause of obstruction in children. In children, cecal volvulus is more common compared with volvuli occurring in the sigmoid and transverse colon.

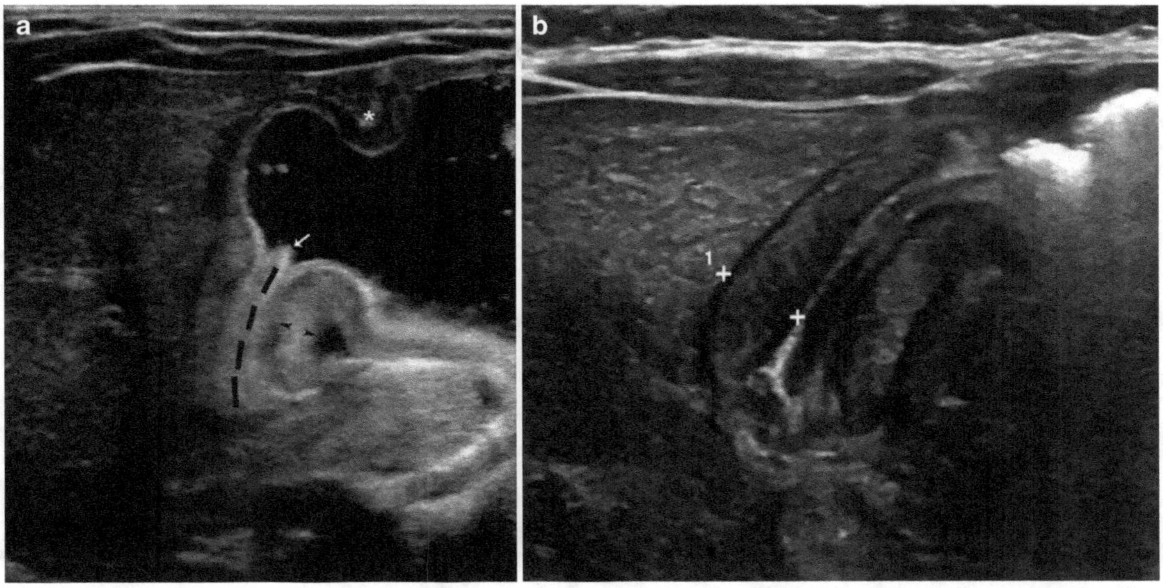

Fig. Hypertrophic pyloric stenosis is an acquired obstruction of the gastric outlet, characterized by elongation of the antropyloric chan-nel and thickening of the pyloric muscularis with varying degrees of mucosal hypertrophy. Infants typically present with non-bilious, projectile vomiting and occasionally a palpable hypertrophied pyloric "olive." Hypertrophic pyloric stenosis is usually not present at birth. Infants usually present with symptoms at 2–12 weeks of age. The diagnosis is made sonographically. (**a**) High-frequency ultrasound examination of the antropyloric region shows thickening of the muscularis layer to more than 3 mm (arrowheads) and elongation of the pyloric channel to more than 15 mm in length (dashed line). Dynamic imaging can detect the presence or absence of transit through the pyloric channel and may also identify hyperperistaltic gastric waves (asterisk) in the presence of a gastric outlet obstruction. Redundant pyloric mucosa may protrude into the gastric lumen (arrow), producing the "antral nipple sign." (**b**) High-frequency detailed ultrasound often demonstrates striation within the thickened muscularis (*between calipers*)

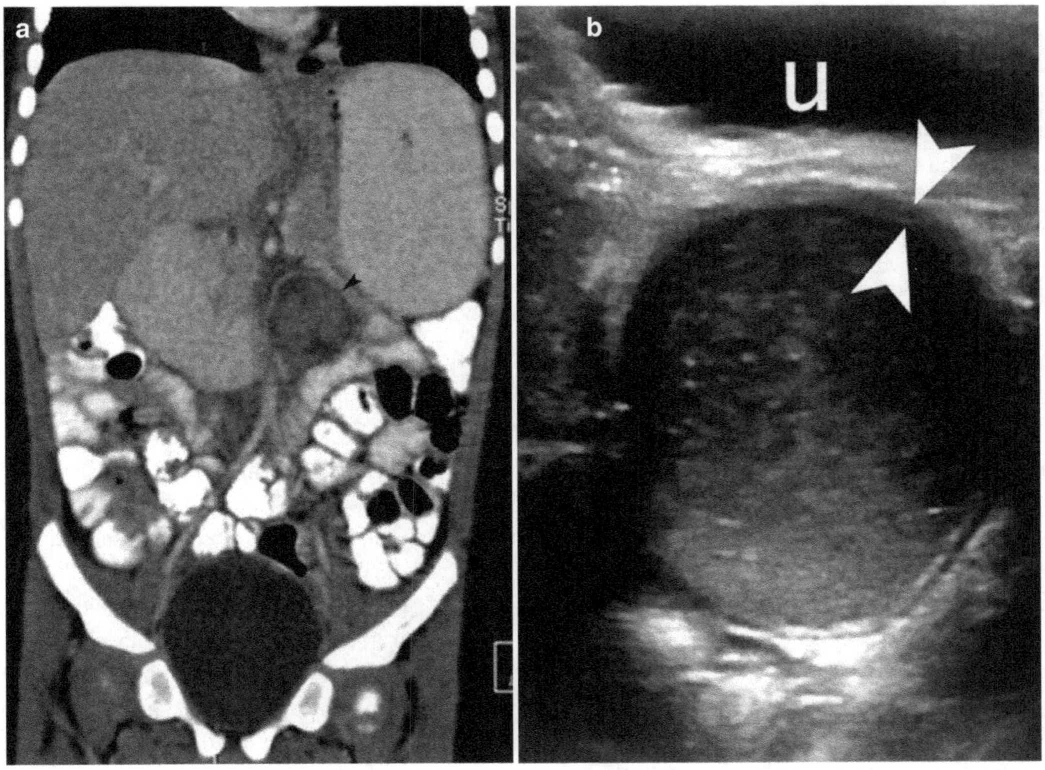

Fig. Duplication cysts represent closed congenital duplicated segments of any part of the gastrointestinal tract and may be diagnosed incidentally or as a result of obstruction. (**a**) Coronal reformat of computed tomography scan following oral and intravenous contrast medium administration demonstrates a small bowel duplication cyst (arrowhead). (**b**) Sagittal sonogram shows a cyst posterior to the urinary bladder (*u*). The diagnosis of a rectal duplication cyst is readily made by demonstrating a bowel wall appearance of the cyst wall (arrowheads)

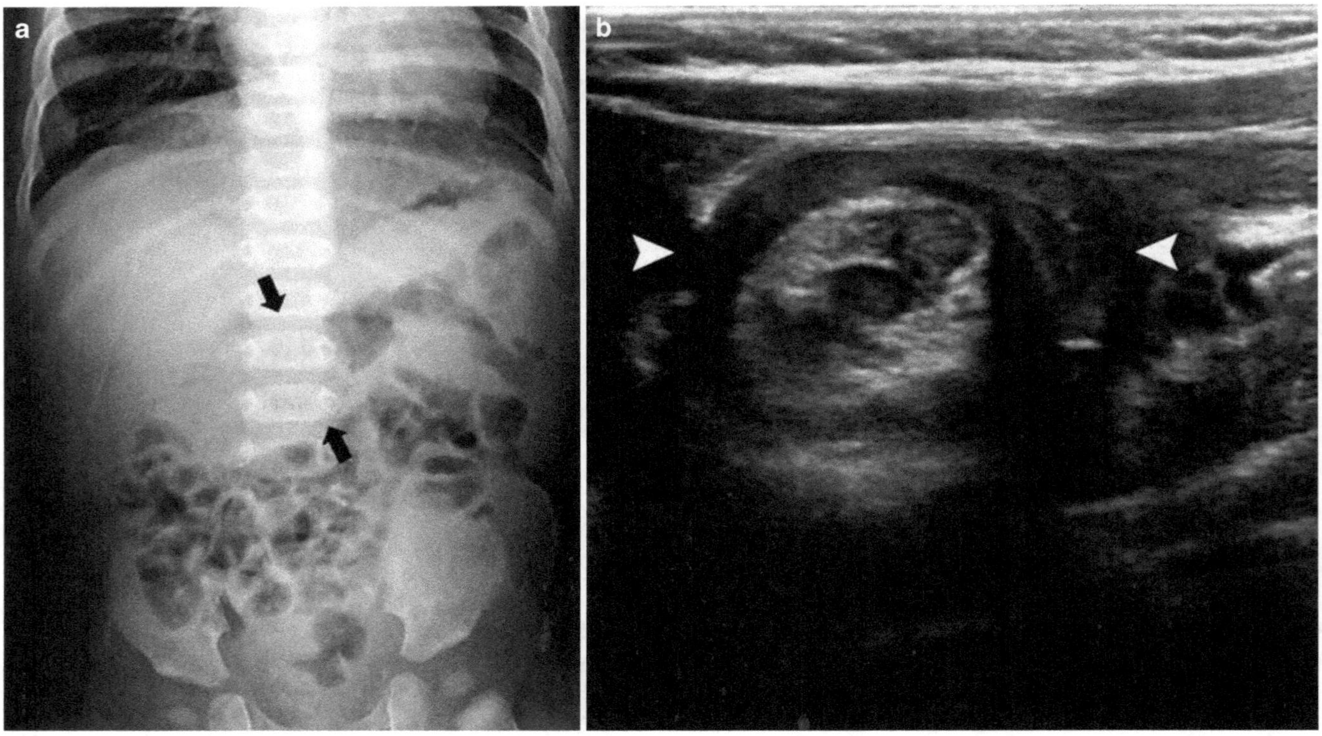

Fig. Intussusception, most commonly ileocolic, has peak inci-dence in late infancy and presents with abdominal distention and bloody stools. (**a**) Radiographs may show, as in this example, a well-defined opacity (arrows) representing the invaginate. (**b**) Ultrasound is diagnostic showing a typical doughnut configuration (arrowheads) of the telescoping bowel segments with trapped mesenteric fat (hyperechoic content)

Clinical presentation includes abdominal pain, vomiting, and distention. Depending on the type of twist, plain films may demonstrate marked distention of the colon and/or air-fluid levels resembling either a "bird's beak" or "coffee bean." CT demonstrates the "swirling" appearance of the sigmoid mesentery and its vasculature. While clinical and imaging findings are suggestive, sigmoid volvulus remains an often missed diagnosis which can be complicated by bowel ischemia, gangrene, perforation, shock, and even death [18–20].

Henoch-Schonlein purpura is an acute small-vessel vasculitis in young children typically involving the skin, kidneys, synovium, and bowel. Sonographically there is nonspecific mural inflammation [21].

Infectious, Ischemic, and Inflammatory Intestinal Pathology

Necrotizing enterocolitis (Fig.) is the most common gastrointestinal emergency in the newborn. The etiology of NEC is incompletely understood and is thought to involve multiple factors, including immaturity of the blood-gut barrier, early feeding, and bacterial colonization which ultimately lead to hemorrhagic and ischemic necrosis of the intestines. NEC typically occurs in preterm neonates especially with very low birthweight and less commonly term or late preterm neonates with congenital cardiac disease or Hirschsprung's disease. Although somewhat insensitive, plain films may demonstrate intestinal pneumatosis, portal venous air, and pneumoperitoneum. Intestinal ultrasound has proven useful in the diagnosis of NEC and may demonstrate the presence of free fluid and abnormal bowel peristalsis, increased wall thickness, echogenicity, and vascularity and may suggest impending complications such as perforation. Additionally, US has been shown to detect small amounts of intramural and portal venous "air bubbles" not demonstrated on plain film [22, 23].

Acute appendicitis is the most common surgical indication in children. Appendicitis results from obstruction of the appendix which leads to distention, mucosal ischemia, bacterial overgrowth, inflammation, and potentially wall compromise and perforation. Early diagnosis is therefore essential in order to avoid such complications. US is the initial test of choice due to its lack of ionizing radiation and is optimal for imaging children. With an experienced sonographer and use of graded compression technique, US is highly sensitive and specific for the diagnosis of appendicitis and its complications and approaches the accuracy of CT. Use of MRI in the diagnosis of appendicitis is increasing, particularly for children with equivocal ultrasound [24, 25].

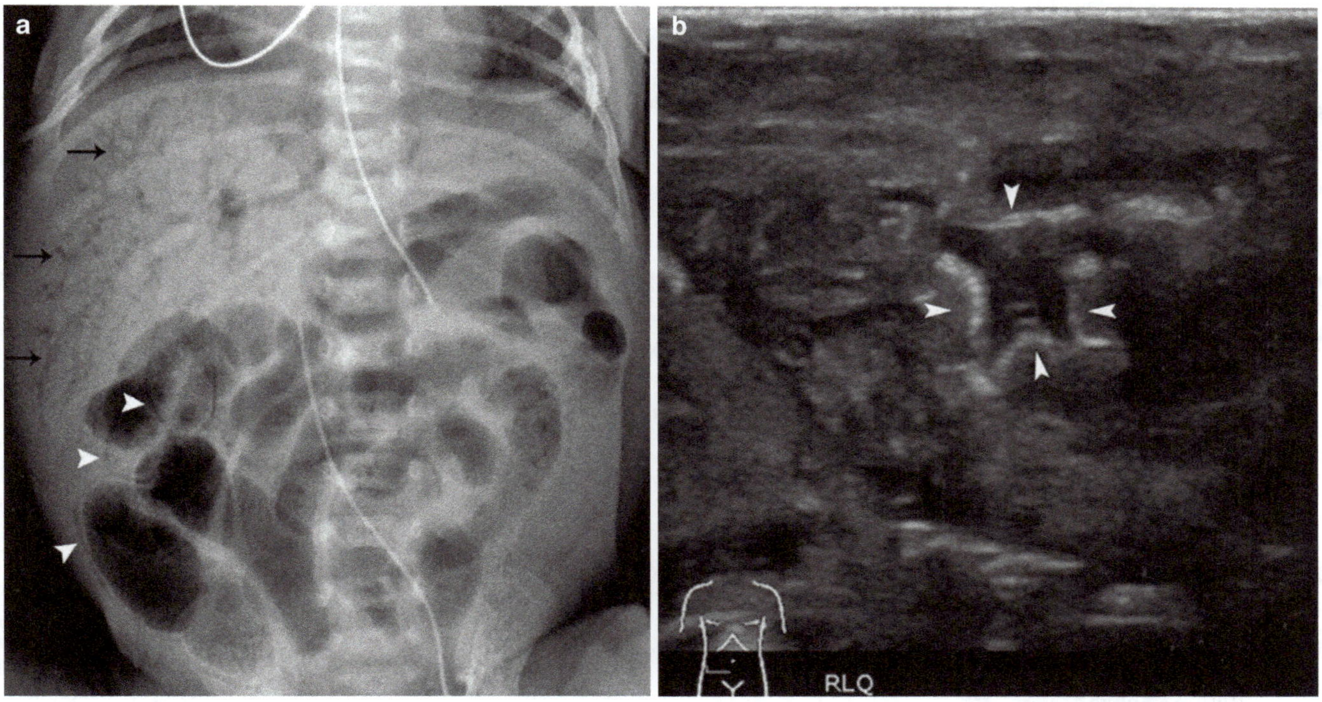

Fig. Necrotizing enterocolitis is a clinical diagnosis but may nevertheless have typical radiological features. (**a**) Abdominal radiograph demonstrates thick-walled gas-distended bowel loops with intramural gas seen as linear lucencies (arrowheads) and portal venous gas (arrows). (**b**) Intramural gas demonstrated sonographically as a string of hyperechoic "pearls" (arrowheads) in the bowel wall

Inflammatory bowel disease may be seen at any age, but early-onset disease is often more complex with associated immunological disorders. In older children and adolescents, the clinical picture and the imaging characteristics are more similar to those in adults. Conventional fluoroscopic contrast follow-through is rarely indicated. Both ultrasound and MR enterography are excellent for assessing the macroscopic disease: bowel wall thickening, mesenteric inflammation, mesenteric lymphadenopathy, hyperemia, and fistulation [26].

Meckel's diverticulitis is inflammation of a Meckel's diverticulum, an omphalomesenteric remnant containing gastric/pancreatic mucosa. Abdominal pain and melena are typical symptoms. The diagnosis is extremely difficult to make with radiographs and cross-sectional imaging alone, which are often insensitive. 99mTc-pertechnetate scintigraphy is typically diagnostic [27].

Gastrointestinal Trauma

Accidental and non-accidental traumas, particularly blunt trauma, are common causes of morbidity and mortality in children. Clinical and laboratory findings may suggest injury to the hollow and solid abdominal viscera, necessitating imaging follow-up. CT performed with intravenous contrast provides superb detail of vascular, solid organ, intestinal, and musculoskeletal anatomy, thus making it the imaging of choice in stable children presenting with trauma. US may be used in unstable patients and is especially helpful in the detection of hemoperitoneum. The liver, spleen, and kidneys are among the most common solid organ injuries observed in accidental trauma. In non-accidental trauma, the liver and pancreas are the most commonly injured solid organs. Intestinal injury is uncommon overall, yet occurs with more frequency in non-accidental versus accidental trauma.

Children with compensated shock following initial resuscitation efforts may demonstrate characteristic abdominal CT findings known as the hypoperfusion complex, which includes collapse of the aorta and inferior vena cava and hyperenhancement of the adrenals, kidneys, mesentery, and bowel walls. These findings signal impending hemodynamic collapse, and their immediate recognition is critical [28–30].

Take-Home Messages

- The differential diagnosis for neonatal high intestinal obstruction includes atresia of the esophagus, stomach, duodenum and jejunum, duodenal stenosis from annular pancreas, duodenal web, and malrotation with midgut volvulus.

- The differential diagnoses for neonatal low intestinal obstruction include ileal and colonic atresia, anorectal malformation, meconium ileus, colonic dysmotility syndromes, and Hirschsprung's disease.
- Congenital abdominopelvic cysts may lead to high or low intestinal obstruction.
- In older infants and children, intestinal obstruction may be related to adhesions, pyloric stenosis, intussusception, incarcerated intestinal hernia, appendicitis, sigmoid volvulus, and Meckel's diverticulum.
- Radiographic findings of NEC including free, intramural, and portal venous air are classic yet infrequently observed. Ultrasound improves sensitivity.
- In the hands of an experienced sonographer and with use of graded compression technique, sensitivity and specificity of intestinal ultrasound for acute appendicitis approaches that of CT.
- Contrast enhanced CT is the imaging standard in the evaluation of stable children with blunt or penetrating trauma.

References

1. Grob M. Intestinal obstruction in the newborn infant. Arch Dis Child. 1960;35:40–50.
2. Harmon C, Coran A. Congenital anomalies of the esophagus. In: Coran A, editor. Pediatric surgery. Philadelphia: Elsevier; 2012. p. 893–918.
3. Cumming WA. Neonatal radiology. Esophageal atresia and tracheoesophageal fistula. Radiol Clin N Am. 1975;13(2):277–95.
4. Hernanz-Schulman M. Imaging of neonatal gastrointestinal obstruction. Radiol Clin N Am. 1999;37(6):1163–86, vi–vii.
5. Berrocal T, Torres I, Gutierrez J, Prieto C, del Hoyo ML, Lamas M. Congenital anomalies of the upper gastrointestinal tract. Radiographics. 1999;19(4):855–72.
6. Millar AJ, Rode H, Cywes S. Malrotation and volvulus in infancy and childhood. Semin Pediatr Surg. 2003;12(4):229–36.
7. Torres AM, Ziegler MM. Malrotation of the intestine. World J Surg. 1993;17(3):326–31.
8. DeLorimier AA, Fonkalsrud EW, Hays DM. Congenital atresia and stenosis of the jejunum and ileum. Surgery. 1969;65(5):819–27.
9. Allan JL, Robbie M, Phelan PD, Danks DM. Familial occurrence of meconium ileus. Eur J Pediatr. 1981;135(3):291–2.
10. Etensel B, Temir G, Karkiner A, Melek M, Edirne Y, Karaca I, et al. Atresia of the colon. J Pediatr Surg. 2005;40(8):1258–68.
11. Stranzinger E, DiPietro MA, Teitelbaum DH, Strouse PJ. Imaging of total colonic Hirschsprung disease. Pediatr Radiol. 2008;38(11):1162–70.
12. Siddiqui MM, Drewett M, Burge DM. Meconium obstruction of prematurity. Arch Dis Child Fetal Neonatal Ed. 2012;97(2):F147–50.
13. Ellis H, Kumar R, Kostyrka B. Neonatal small left colon syndrome in the offspring of diabetic mothers-an analysis of 105 children. J Pediatr Surg. 2009;44(12):2343–6.
14. Berrocal T, Lamas M, Gutieerrez J, Torres I, Prieto C, del Hoyo ML. Congenital anomalies of the small intestine, colon, and rectum. Radiographics. 1999;19(5):1219–36.
15. MacMahon B. The continuing enigma of pyloric stenosis of infancy: a review. Epidemiology. 2006;17(2):195–201.
16. Khong PL, Cheung SC, Leong LL, Ooi CG. Ultrasonography of intra-abdominal cystic lesions in the newborn. Clin Radiol. 2003;58(6):449–54.
17. Applegate KE. Intussusception in children: evidence-based diagnosis and treatment. Pediatr Radiol. 2009;39(Suppl 2):S140–3.
18. Andersen JF, Eklof O, Thomasson B. Large bowel volvulus in children. Review of a case material and the literature. Pediatr Radiol. 1981;11(3):129–38.
19. Atamanalp SS, Yildirgan MI, Basoglu M, Kantarci M, Yilmaz I. Sigmoid colon volvulus in children: review of 19 cases. Pediatr Surg Int. 2004;20(7):492–5.
20. Moore CJ, Corl FM, Fishman EK. CT of cecal volvulus: unraveling the image. AJR Am J Roentgenol. 2001;177(1):95–8.
21. McCarthy HJ, Tizard EJ. Clinical practice: diagnosis and management of Henoch-Schonlein purpura. Eur J Pediatr. 2010;169(6):643–50.
22. Epelman M, Daneman A, Navarro OM, Morag I, Moore AM, Kim JH, et al. Necrotizing enterocolitis: review of state-of-the-art imaging findings with pathologic correlation. Radiographics. 2007;27(2):285–305.
23. Esposito F, Mamone R, Di Serafino M, Mercogliano C, Vitale V, Vallone G, et al. Diagnostic imaging features of necrotizing enterocolitis: a narrative review. Quant Imaging Med Surg. 2017;7(3):336–44.
24. Krishnamoorthi R, Ramarajan N, Wang NE, Newman B, Rubesova E, Mueller CM, et al. Effectiveness of a staged US and CT protocol for the diagnosis of pediatric appendicitis: reducing radiation exposure in the age of ALARA. Radiology. 2011;259(1):231–9.
25. Wan MJ, Krahn M, Ungar WJ, Caku E, Sung L, Medina LS, et al. Acute appendicitis in young children: cost-effectiveness of US versus CT in diagnosis—a Markov decision analytic model. Radiology. 2009;250(2):378–86.
26. Anupindi SA, Podberesky DJ, Towbin AJ, Courtier J, Gee MS, Darge K, et al. Pediatric inflammatory bowel disease: imaging issues with targeted solutions. Abdom Imaging. 2015;40(5):975–92.
27. Kotecha M, Bellah R, Pena AH, Jaimes C, Mattei P. Multimodality imaging manifestations of the Meckel diverticulum in children. Pediatr Radiol. 2012;42(1):95–103.
28. Sivit CJ. Imaging children with abdominal trauma. AJR Am J Roentgenol. 2009;192(5):1179–89.
29. Trout AT, Strouse PJ, Mohr BA, Khalatbari S, Myles JD. Abdominal and pelvic CT in cases of suspected abuse: can clinical and laboratory findings guide its use? Pediatr Radiol. 2011;41(1):92–8.
30. Sivit CJ, Taylor GA, Bulas DI, Kushner DC, Potter BM, Eichelberger MR. Posttraumatic shock in children: CT findings associated with hemodynamic instability. Radiology. 1992;182(3):723–6.

16

Benign Disease of the Uterus

Karen Kinkel, Susan M. Ascher, and Caroline Reinhold

Learning Objectives

- To be able to identify and classify Müllerian anomalies and leiomyomas with ultrasound and MRI
- To diagnose adenomyosis, deep endometriosis, and complicated leiomyomas
- To differentiate endometrial polyps from submucosal leiomyoma

Key Points

- The diagnosis of Müllerian anomalies takes into account the uterine shape, external contour, and width of internal indentation compared to the uterine wall thickness. Associated anomalies of the cervix or vagina are classified separately.
- Classification of leiomyomas indicates how far the myometrial anomalies traverse the interface between the endometrial/myometrial interface and the myometrial/serosal interface. Analysis of T2-, T1-, and diffusion-weighted signal intensity and contrast enhancement helps in determining treatment strategies in symptomatic patients.

K. Kinkel (✉)
Institut de radiologie, Clinique des Grangettes, Chêne-Bougeries, Geneva, Switzerland
e-mail: Karen.kinkel@grangettes.ch

S. M. Ascher
Department of Radiology, Georgetown University School of Medicine, Washington, DC, USA
e-mail: aschers@gunet.georgetown.edu

C. Reinhold
Department of Radiology, McGill University Health Center, Montreal, QC, Canada
e-mail: Caroline.reinhold@mcgill.ca

Introduction

Endovaginal sonography (EVS) is the procedure of choice for the initial evaluation of benign diseases of the female genital tract. When EVS findings are indeterminate, further evaluation is often performed with magnetic resonance imaging (MRI) due to its excellent soft tissue differentiation, multiplanar capabilities, and absence of ionizing radiation. MRI is used as a problem-solving tool in benign uterine diseases, for example, uterine malformations, adenomyosis, and deep endometriosis, and to select appropriate candidates for therapies such as myomectomy or different types of hysterectomy. The role of computed tomography (CT) is limited in the evaluation of benign disease of the female pelvis particularly due to its lack of soft tissue differentiation. CT is primarily employed in an emergency situation, such as in an acute abdomen caused by ovarian torsion or pelvic inflammatory disease.

Normal Anatomy of the Uterus

In women of reproductive age, the uterus is approximately 6–9 cm in length and varies in appearance according to the menstrual cycle. On EVS, the thickness of the endometrium in premenopausal women increases progressively during the menstrual cycle: from 3 to 8 mm in the proliferative phase to 8–12 mm or more in the secretory phase. The echotexture of the endometrium also varies. The endometrium is hypo- to isoechoic in the mid-proliferative phase and becomes trilaminar in the periovulatory phase. In the secretory phase, the endometrium becomes echogenic and may have a nodular appearance. In the inner myometrium, subjacent to the endometrium, a thin hypoechoic line is visible called the subendometrial halo. This line does not correspond anatomically to the junctional zone on MRI and is typically thinner. The remainder of the myometrium is of intermediate echogenicity. Sonographic studies of endometrial thickness in postmenopausal women have suggested an upper limit of 5 mm in patients not on hormone replacement and 8 mm for patients receiving hormonal therapy. EVS is highly sensitive for detecting endometrial pathology when these cutoff values are used as guidelines, to determine which patients would benefit from endometrial sampling [1]. The presence of endometrial thickening on EVS is nonspecific and may be due to endometrial hyperplasia, polyps, or carcinoma. The uterine zonal anatomy on MRI is best depicted using sagittal T2-weighted images (Fig.).

In the premenopausal woman, the high signal intensity endometrium varies in thickness, depending on the menstrual cycle. In postmenopausal patients, the uterine corpus, but not the cervix, decreases in size. On dynamic gadolinium-enhanced images, the endometrium is hypovascular relative to the myometrium and becomes iso- or hyperintense on delayed scans.

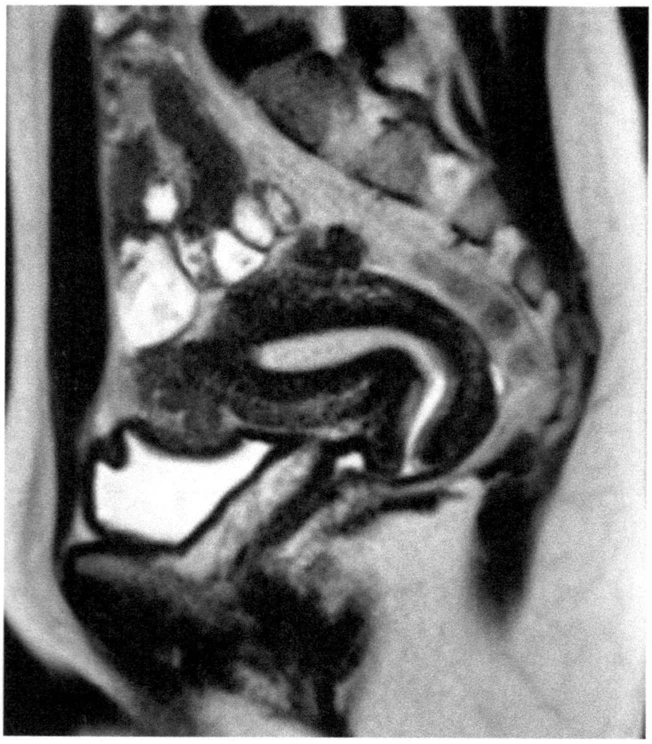

Fig. Normal MRI Uterine Anatomy Sagittal 3D T2-weighted multiplanar reconstruction of the uterus and cervix demonstrates normal zonal anatomy. There are three zones identifiable in the uterus: the hyperintense endometrium, the hypointense junctional zone and the intermediate signal intensity of the outer myometrium. Four zones are distinguished in the cervix: the hyperintense mucous within the endocervical canal, the intermediate signal intensity of the cervical mucosa, the hypointense cervical stroma, and the intermediate signal intensity of the outer smooth muscle

MRI Technique

Patient preparation is an important step to obtain optimal image quality. To minimize motion artifacts due to bowel motion, patients are asked to fast 6 h prior to imaging. Unless contraindicated, intravenous or intramuscular injection of peristaltic inhibitors, i.e., glucagon or butyl-scopolamine, is recommended to further decrease peristalsis artifacts. According to the clinical question, additional preparation might include bowel cleansing and/or vaginal opacification for chronic pelvic pain. Sonographic gel is used to opacify the vagina and to allow visualization of vaginal duplication or communication. An intravenous line is often required to inject contrast agent to determine vascularity of myometrial or endocavitary abnormalities. Examinations are usually performed in supine position using a body-flex phased-array MR surface coil. Imaging of the uterus should be performed using the smallest possible field of view (20–24 cm), thin sections of 3.5–4 mm, and the largest possible matrix size appropriate to each individual sequence. These imaging parameters provide important anatomic detail, which becomes critical when imaging uterine anomalies and endometrial pathology. When imaging large leiomyomas, the section thickness and field of view (FOV) may need to be adjusted accordingly. However, when establishing the myometrial origin of a subserosal leiomyoma, thin sections at the level of the pedicle are frequently helpful.

The most important sequence is a T2-weighted sequence nicely demonstrating the zonal anatomy of the uterus. Sagittal sections are best suited to image the uterus. Oblique coronal and axial slice orientation according to the long and short axis of the endometrial cavity should be applied for the assessment of uterine and cervical pathologies. It is important to train MR technologists on how to acquire these oblique sequences if physician supervision is not possible. The short-axis coronal oblique sequence (perpendicular to the long axis of the endometrial cavity) is particularly valuable for assessing localized endometrial pathology and for evaluating the thickness of the junctional zone. It is also valuable for determining the extent of a uterine septum. A T2-weighted sequence performed parallel to the long axis of the endometrial cavity is critical to characterize the external uterine contour in patients with Müllerian duct anomalies. Since this series is so important in the classification of uterine anomalies, it is best performed earlier in the examination, prior to bladder filling, which often displaces the uterus as it becomes increasingly distended. If the fundal contour is inadequately characterized by the T2-weighted images, T1-weighted images parallel to the long axis can facilitate characterization of the external contour due to increased contrast between the myometrial fundal contour and the overlying fat. Recent software advances allow for a 3D T2-weighted acquisition—allowing post-processing of the uterus in any plane and potentially obviating the need to acquire individual orthogonal 2D T2-weighted sequences.

In addition to T2-weighted sequences, T1-weighted sequences with and without fat suppression are helpful to distinguish bloody components in adenomyosis or potential sarcomas from fat or mucinous components. A T1-weighted 3D Dixon gradient echo sequence allows for T1-weighted in-phase, T1-weighted out-of-phase, T1-weighted water excitation, and T1-weighted fat excitation images within a single breath-hold. Routine use of this sequence helps standardize imaging protocols without additional exam time. In patients with congenital anomalies, a quick breath-hold T1-weighted sequence covering both kidneys is helpful to exclude renal agenesis or hydronephrosis.

An axial echo-planar diffusion-weighted imaging (DWI) sequence is an increasingly helpful functional imaging technique whose contrast derives from the random motion of water molecules within the extracellular tissue. In specific situation, such as patients with a leiomyoma of intermediate T2-weighted signal intensity, the high signal intensity of the DWI sequence combined with low or heterogeneous T1 signal intensity has the potential to differentiate leiomyomas from sarcomas or indeterminate myometrial masses with the use of an apparent diffusion coefficient (ADC) [2]. However measuring ADCs in all leiomyoma regardless T2 or DWI signal intensity is of no value and wrongly increases the rate of suspicion.

Gadolinium-enhanced imaging is not needed for most benign conditions, but can be useful in selected pathologies. We routinely perform contrast-enhanced imaging in patients referred for evaluation of endometrial pathology. In addition, contrast-enhanced imaging is also performed in patients with symptomatic leiomyomas scheduled for laparoscopic surgery or uterine artery embolization, in the latter case with additional MR angiography of the iliac arteries. Vascularity can help to predict response to treatment, and the enhancement may help distinguish a benign fibroid from a malignant leiomyosarcoma.

Congenital Anomalies

Between the 6th and 11th weeks of gestation, the paired Müllerian ducts undergo descent, fusion, and septum resorption to form the uterus, fallopian tubes, cervix, and upper 2/3 of the vagina [3]. Müllerian duct anomalies (MDAs) result when this process either fails or is interrupted. Depending on the anomaly, patients may be asymptomatic with normal fertility and obstetric outcomes, while others may have primary amenorrhea, menstrual irregularities, infertility, obstetric complications, and/or endometriosis. The reported prevalence of MDAs varies widely: 1–5% in the general population and 13–25% in women with recurrent fetal loss [4]. The ovaries and external genitalia/distal 1/3 of the vagina are spared because they originate from the primitive yolk sac and sinovaginal bud, respectively. Renal anomalies however are present in 30–50% of women with MDAs [5].

Appropriate classification is critical to ensure proper treatment. Buttram and Gibbons classified MDAs in 1979, and a revised classification by the American Society for Reproductive Medicine (formerly the American Fertility Society) was published in 1988 [6, 7]. While widely accepted, the AFS system had limitations "in terms of effective characterization of anomalies, clinical usefulness, simplicity and friendliness" [8]. To address these limitations, the European Society of Human Reproduction and Embryology (ESHRE) and the European Society for Gynaecological Endoscopy (ESHE) established a working group to develop a new updated classification system that would be more clinically oriented and based on anatomy. The group published their consensus classification of female genital tract congenital anomalies in 2013. The ESHRE/ESGE system sorts anomalies into classes and subclasses based on increasing severity of anatomical deviation, from normal (U0) to unclassified cases (U6) (Fig.).

Use of absolute numbers to define an anomaly was discarded; rather, the new system defines uterine deformity in relation to anatomical landmarks, for example, uterine wall thickness (UWT) which is defined as the distance between the interostial line and a parallel line on the top of the fundus [9].

When a MDA is suspected, US is the most commonly performed exam and may be diagnostic, especially if a 3D US is performed (Fig.). However, MRI remains the preferred imaging technique in patients where TVS is not possible due to vaginal agenesis, in patients with complex uterine anomalies, or in diagnostic dilemmas [9]. MRI has been shown in multiple studies to have excellent agreement with MDA subtype classifications [10].

Class 0 (Normal Uterus)

The normal uterus is defined as having either a straight or curved interostial line with an internal indentation ≤ 50% of the UWT at the fundal midline (Figs.).

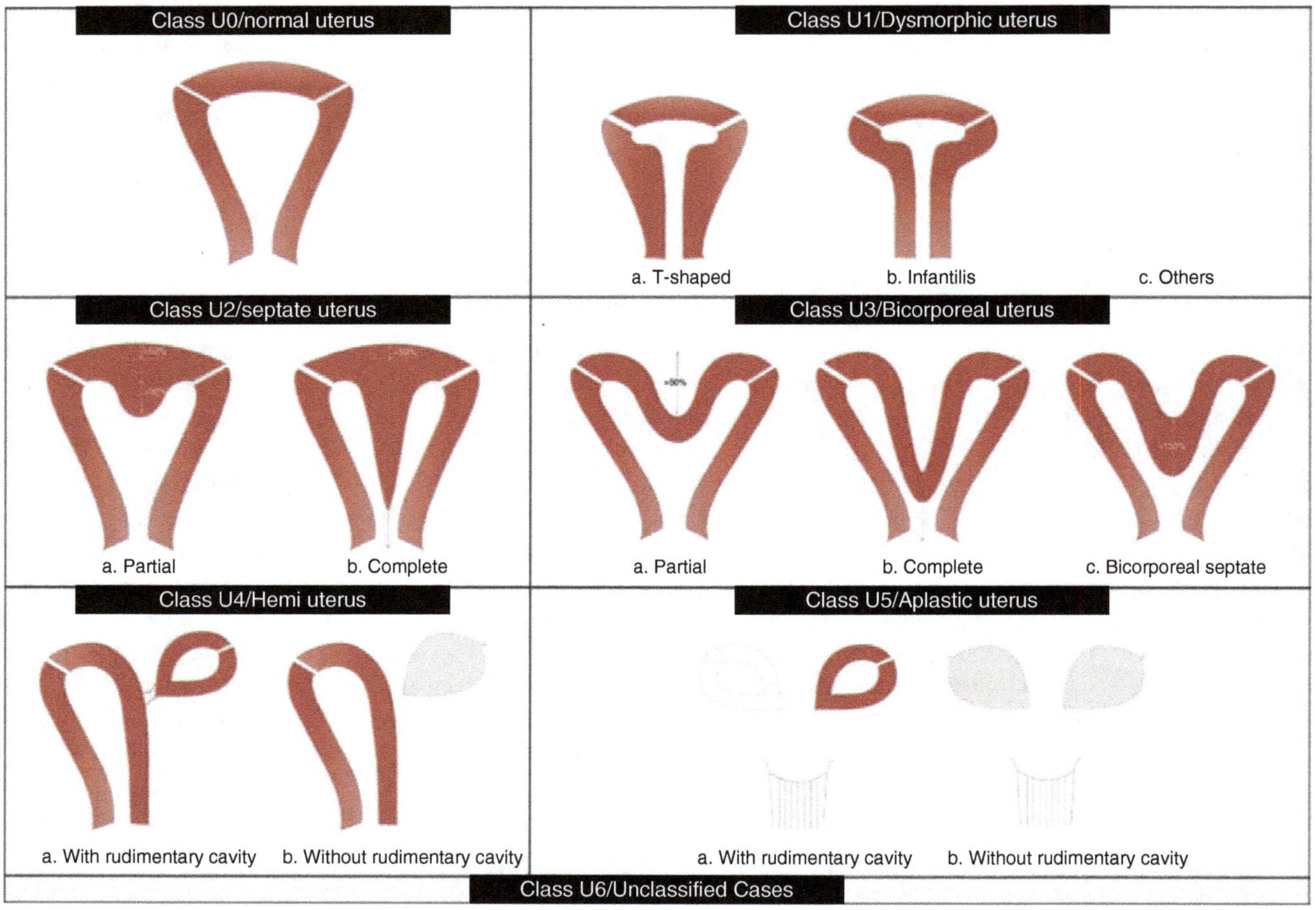

Fig. Schematic drawing of the ESHRE/ESGE classification system of uterine congenital anomalies from Ref. [8], dividing uterine anomalies in six classes

Class U1 (Dysmorphic Uterus)

This category encompasses uteri with a normal uterine outline that have an abnormal cavity excluding septa. U1 anomalies have three subtypes:

1. U1a (T-Shaped Uterus)—narrow uterine cavity with thickened lateral walls with a normal corpus-to-cervix ratio
2. U1b (Uterus Infantilis)—narrow uterine cavity with normal lateral walls with an abnormal corpus-to-cervix ratio
3. U1c (Others)—all other minor deformities of the uterine cavity with a midline, fundal, inner indentation <50% UWT

Class U2 (Septate Uterus) (Fig.)

This category reflects abnormal resorption of the midline septum following normal Müllerian duct fusion. The uterus has a normal outer contour, but the midline, fundal, inner indentation is >50% of the UWT. U2 anomalies have two subtypes:

1. U2a (Partial Septate)—midline fundal inner septum divides the uterine cavity above the internal os.
2. U2b (Complete Septate)—midline fundal inner septum divides the uterine cavity up to the internal os. There may be associated cervical or vaginal anomalies. Fig. . MRI of the pelvis: T2-weighted axial-oblique image (coronal plane of the uterine cavity) demonstrates a complete hypointense septum through the entire length of the hyperintense uterine cavity.

The composition of the septum is variable and is often myometrial proximally and more fibrous distally [11, 12]. Fetal wastage is common in these women with a spontaneous abortion rate of 65%. Treatment reflects the makeup of the septum. If the septum is primarily fibrous, a hysteroscopic septoplasty can be performed with good results. If, however, the septum is primarily myometrial, a combined laparoscopic-hysteroscopic surgical approach is warranted [13].

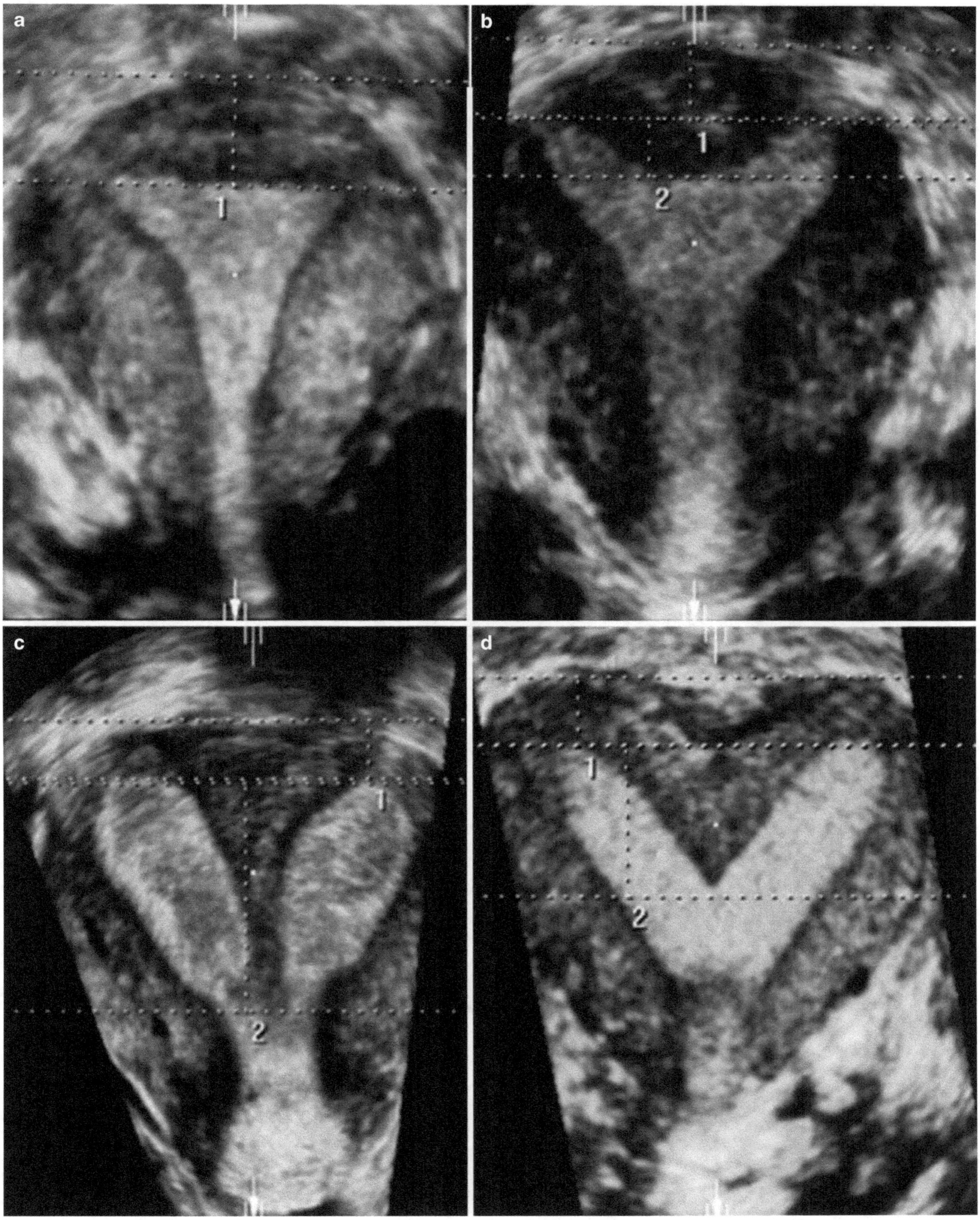

Fig. Ultrasound images of the uterus in a coronal plane of the uterine cavity (modified from Ref. [9], demonstrate how to measure the uterine wall thickness (1) as well as the length of the internal midline indentation (2) for a normal uterus (**a**), a partial septate uterus (**b**), a complete septate uterus (**c**) and a bicorporal uterus (**d**)

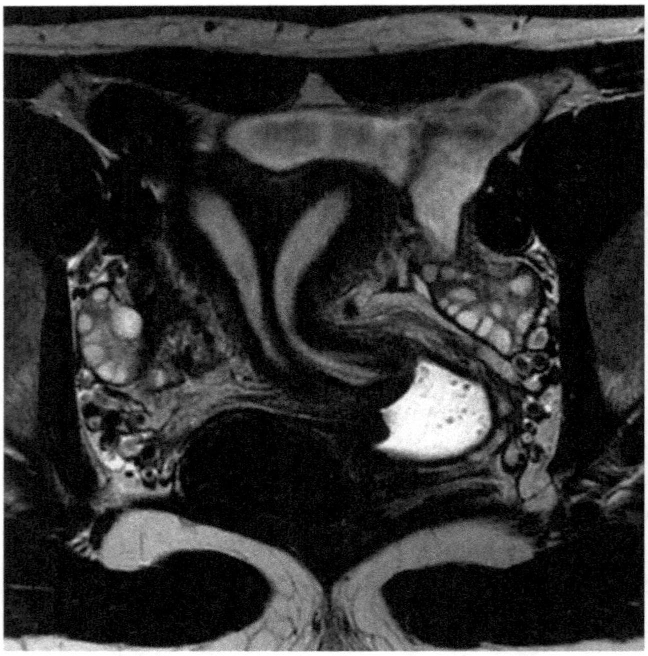

Fig. MRI of the pelvis: T2-weighted axial-oblique image (coronal plane of the uterine cavity) demonstrates a complete hypointense septum through the entire length of the hyperintense uterine cavity

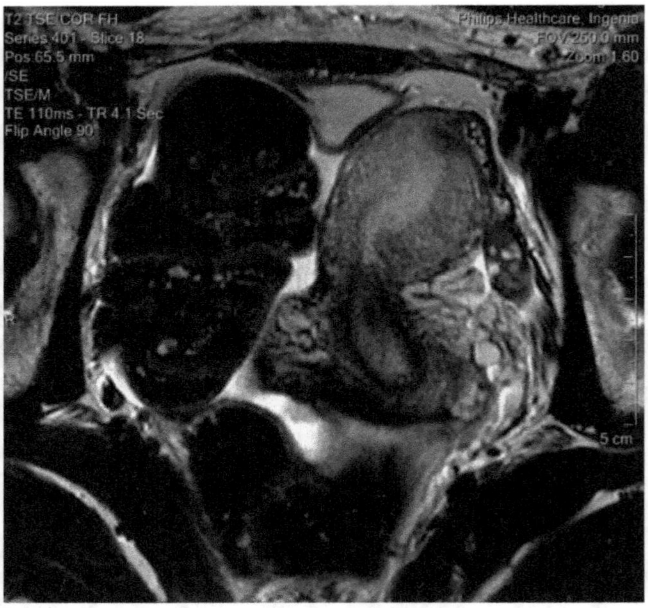

Fig. MRI of the pelvis: T2-weighted axial image through the coronal plane of a "banana"—shaped left hemi-uterus without evidence of a rudimentary remnant uterine horn

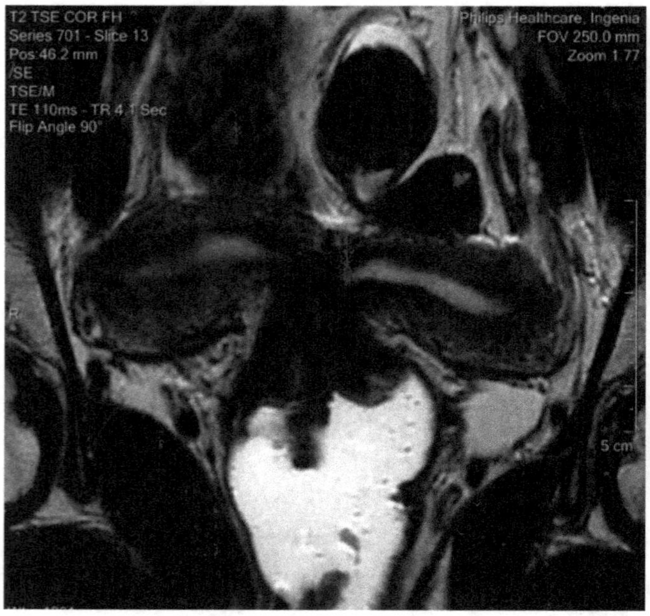

Fig. MRI of the pelvis: T2-weighted coronal image through the coronal plane of the uterine cavity of the bicorporeal complete uterus with an associated double normal cervix (C2). Opacification of the vagina with sonographic gel helps to exclude vaginal septa

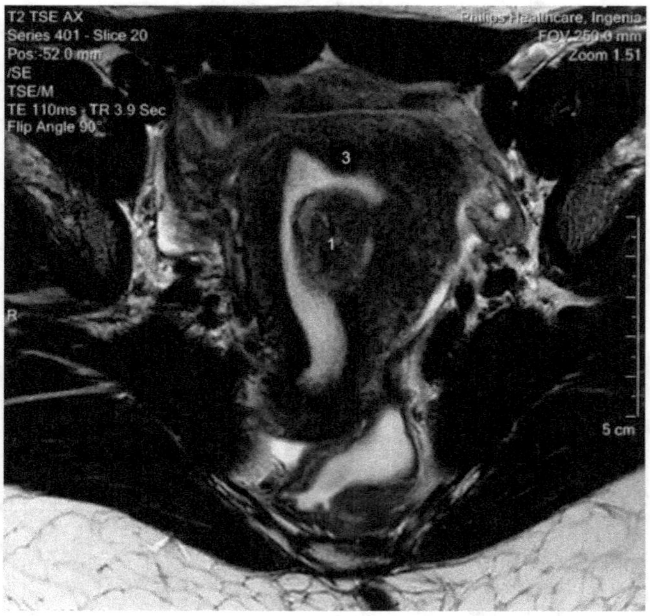

Fig. MRI of the pelvis: T2-weighted coronal oblique view of the uterine cavity shows a type 1 submucosal leiomyoma with more than 50% of the volume inside the uterine cavity. A second leiomyoma lies in close contact to the endometrium (class 3 of an intra-mural leiomyoma)

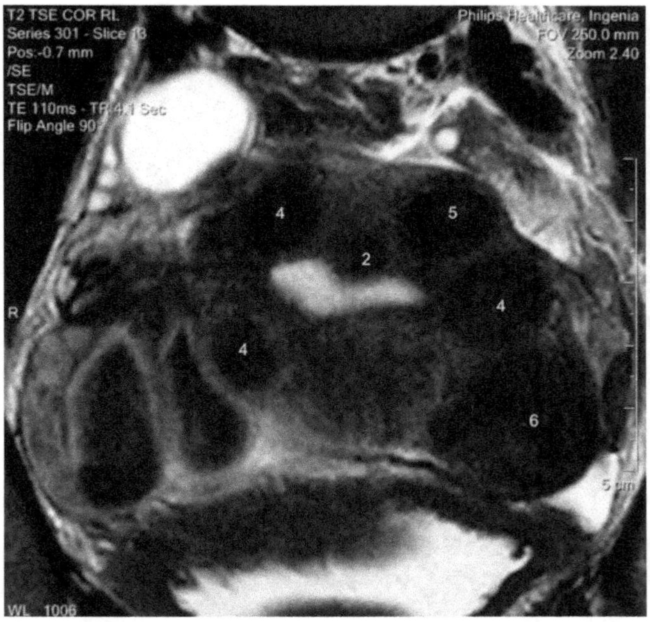

Fig. MRI of the pelvis T2-weighted coronal image (axial oblique orientation of the uterus) with type 3, 4, 5 and 6 leiomyomoma

Class U3 (Bicorporeal Uterus, syn: Bicornuate Uterus) (Fig.)

This category is a result of abnormal fusion of Müllerian ducts. The uterus will have an abnormal fundal contour with an external indentation at the fundal midline >50% of the UWT. U3 anomalies have three subtypes:

1. U3a (Partial Bicorporeal Uterus)—external fundal indentation divides the uterus above the internal os.
2. U3b (Complete Bicorporeal Uterus)—external fundal indentation divides the uterus to the internal os. There may be associated cervical and/or vaginal anomalies.
3. U3c (Bicorporeal Septate Uterus)—the width of the midline inner fundal indentation >150% of the UWT.

Vaginal or hysteroscopic septoplasty is reserved for patients with an obstructing vaginal septum (U3b) or septate form of the anomaly (U3c), respectively.

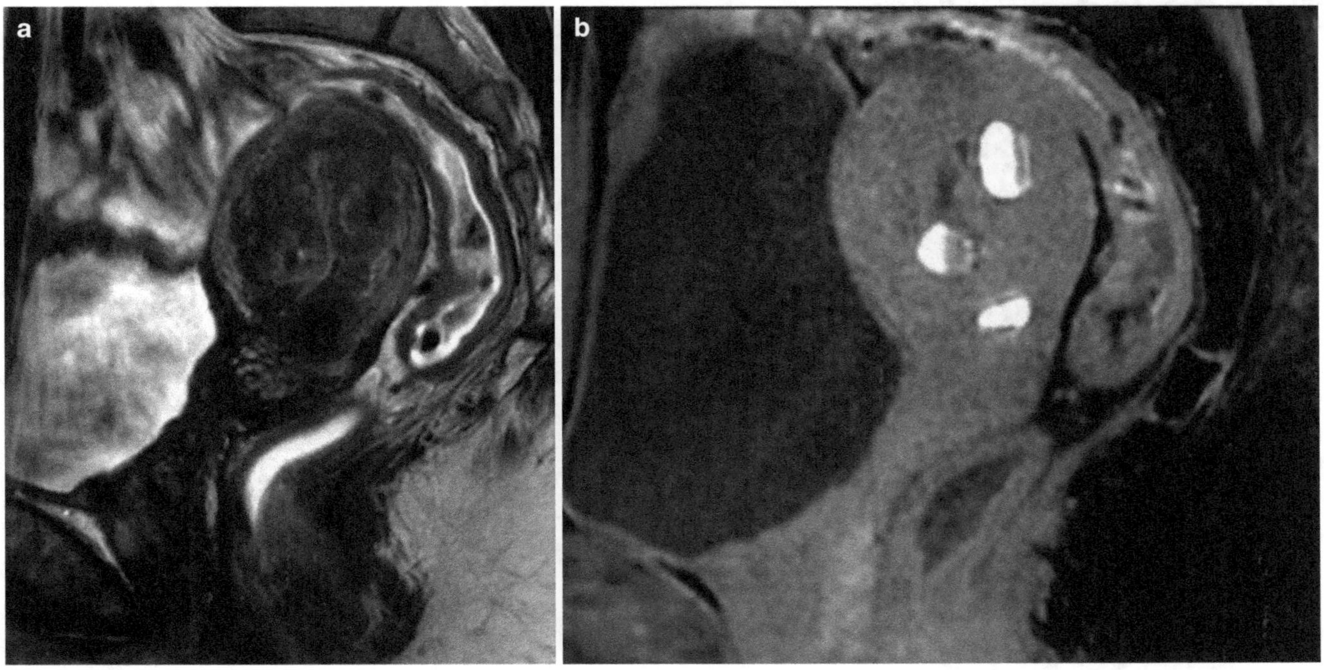

Fig. (**a**) MRI of the pelvis T2-weighted sagittal image through the mid uterine body: a thickened junctional zone is associated with two cystic structures containing blood products of various ages. (**b**) MRI of the pelvis T1-weighted fat saturated sagittal image through the mid uterine body (same patient and level than in Fig.): The hyperintense bloody component of the myometrial cysts makes their identification easier in T1 fat suppressed images than in T2 (Fig.)

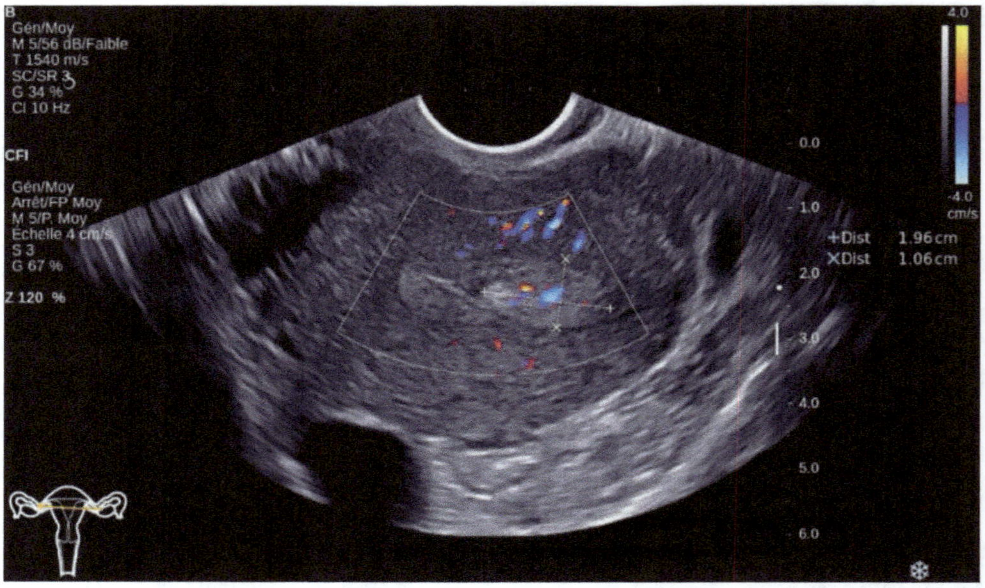

Fig. Endovaginal ultrasound of the uterus in an axial orientation with Color Doppler shows the hyperechoic polyp with a central feeding vessel

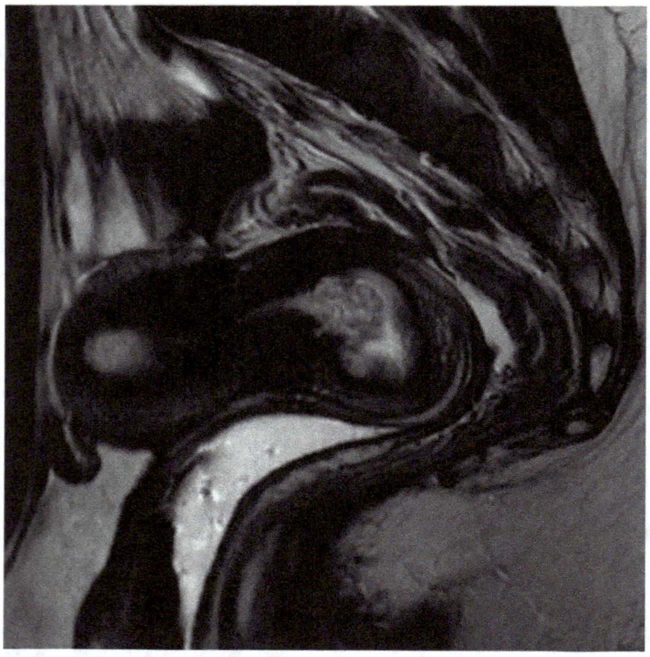

Fig. MRI of the pelvis Sagittal T2-weighted image of the uterus with a polyp located at the internal os of the endocervical channel of a the signal intensity that is slightly hypointense compared to the normal endometrium

Class U4 (Hemi-uterus) (Fig.)

This anomaly is a formation defect resulting in unilateral uterine development. The contralateral part ranges from absent to incomplete formation (uterine horn remnant). U4 anomalies have two subtypes:

1. U4a (Hemi-uterus with a contralateral rudimentary (functional) cavity)—the contralateral horn has a functioning endometrial cavity that may or may not communicate with the hemi-uterus.
2. U4b (Hemi-uterus without a contralateral rudimentary (functional) cavity)—the contralateral horn is either nonfunctional or aplastic.

There is a high association with renal anomalies in these patients, especially renal agenesis, ipsilateral to the contralateral rudimentary horn or remnant (40%). Patients with rudimentary horns, Class U4a, require laparoscopic surgical excision. This is done to prevent hematometra and/or obstetric complications to include uterine rupture [14].

At imaging, the hemi-uterus is deviated to one side of the pelvis, and the endometrial morphology is described as "banana-" or "bullet-shaped." Uterine zonal anatomy is preserved, as is the endometrial-to-myometrial width and ratio [11]. When present, a rudimentary functional horn will have normal zonal anatomy. If it is noncommunicating, the endometrial cavity may be distended with blood, and/or there may be imaging manifestations of endometriosis. In cases without a rudimentary functional horn, the contralateral uterine horn remnant, when present, images as diffuse low to intermediate signal intensity.

Class U5 (Aplastic Uterus)

This anomaly is a formation defect incorporating all types of uterine aplasia. It occurs early in gestation. Affected females have no unilaterally developed or fully developed uterine cavity. U5 anomalies have two subtypes depending on

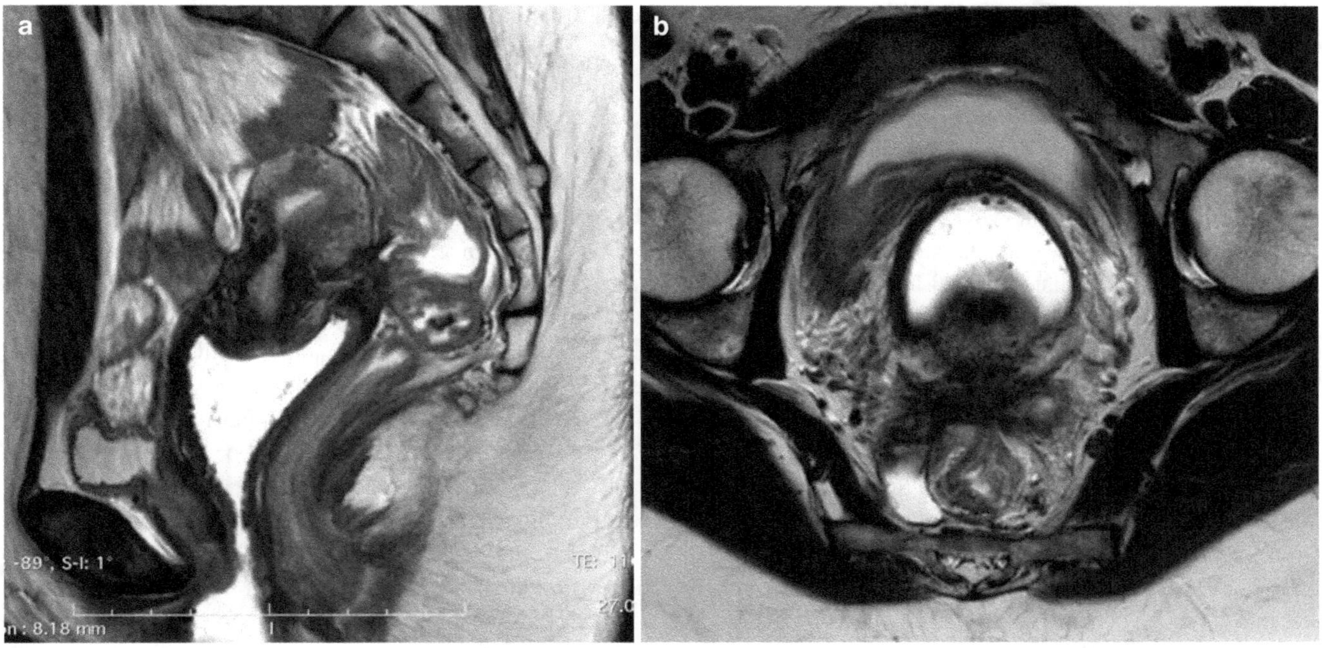

Fig. . (**a**) MRI of the pelvis Sagitall T2-weighted image through the uterine midline demonstrate a hypointense mass obliterating the posterior vaginal cuff and the retro-cervical region. Dark bandlike hypointense structures stretch towards the anterior rectal wall. (**b**) MRI of the pelvis: Corresponding axial T2-weighted image through the upper vaginal cuff shows lateral extension to both uterosacral ligaments and posterior extensions to the anterior rectal wall. Some fluid lies in the right para-rectal space delineating the posterior part of the normal distal right uterosacral ligament

whether or not there is a functional cavity in a uterine remnant if present:

1. U5a (Aplastic uterus with a rudimentary (functional) cavity)—uni- or bilateral functional uterine horn is present.
2. U5b (Aplastic uterus without rudimentary (functional) cavity)—full uterine aplasia or a non-cavitary uterine horn remnant may be present.

Cases of aplastic uterus may have coexisting defects. For example, the Mayer-Rokitansky-Küster-Hauser (MRKH) syndrome is characterized by agenesis of the vagina, cervix, and uterus.

Treatment for Class U5 patients with a rudimentary cavitary horn is not well worked out. For patients with MRKH syndrome, treatment is focused on enabling sexual function via creation of a neovagina.

On MRI, a uni- or bilateral cavitary rudimentary horn is characterized by increased T2-weighted signal intensity in the cavity, whereas a uni- or bilateral uterine horn remnant without a cavity images as diffuse low to intermediate signal intensity on T2-weighted images. For females with MRKH syndrome, fatty and connective tissue is seen in the expected location of the upper 2/3 of the vagina. No normal cervix or uterus is present. A truncated vagina may be seen between the urethra anteriorly and the rectum posteriorly.

Class U6 (Unclassified Cases)

A sixth class was established for cases of "infrequent anomalies, subtle changes or combined pathologies that could not be allocated correctly to one of the six groups," Classes 0–5 [8].

Classification of Congenital Anomalies of the Cervix and the Vagina

Coexisting anomalies of the cervix are classified from C0 to C4 according to the presence of a normal cervix (C0), a septate cervix (C1), a double "normal" cervix (C2), and a unilateral (C3) or complete cervical aplasia (C4) [8] (see Fig.). The classification of coexisting vaginal anomalies ranges from V0 (normal vagina) to V4 (vaginal aplasia) and distinguishes three types of vaginal septum: V1 is longitudinal nonobstructing, V2 longitudinal obstructing, and V3 transverse septum or imperforate hymen [8].

Leiomyoma (Figs.

Ordinary leiomyomas, also called fibroid or myoma, represent benign smooth muscle tumors that can be nondegenerated or degenerated with five subcategories according to the type of degeneration (cystic, hemorrhagic, fatty, hyaline, or myxoid). The presentation at MRI shows various T2 and T1 signal intensities according to the subcategory. Variants of leiomyoma are intermediate types of leiomyoma that can be either mitotically active, cellular, atypical, or smooth muscle tumors of uncertain malignant potential (STUMP) [15]. There is currently no clinical or imaging characteristic to distinguish efficiently between ordinary leiomyoma, a very frequent gynecological tumor, and their intermediate variants. Leiomyosarcoma is an uncommon malignant smooth muscle tumor that is difficult to differentiate from ordinary leiomyoma.

On EVU leiomyomas classically represent as well-circumscribed hypoechoic masses, often associated with posterior shadowing due to calcification or at the interface with the normal myometrium. Depending on the site of development, leiomyomas are further subdivided into submucosal, intramural, or subserosal according to the FIGO classification of causes of abnormal uterine bleeding [16]. Submucosal fibroids can be either pedunculated (type 0) or of more (type 1) or less (type 2) than 50% within the cavity.

A type 3 leiomyoma contacts the endometrium. The type 4 leiomyoma is purely intramural without contact with the endometrium or the serosa.

Type 5 contacts the serosa, is subserosal, and has more than 50% intramural, and type 6 is subserosal with less than 50% intramural.

Type 7 is subserosal and pedunculated and type 8 other (e.g., cervical or broad ligament).

MRI is useful for distinguishing leiomyomas from other myometrial pathology and solid pelvic masses, especially in patients with nondiagnostic or equivocal ultrasound findings. The presence of feeding vessels originating in the myometrium further supports the uterine origin of the mass. However, if a mass is adjacent to the uterus and is of intermediate or high signal intensity relative to the myometrium on T2-weighted images, the differential diagnosis includes both degenerated leiomyoma and extrauterine tumors (benign and malignant). In these patients, the diagnosis of leiomyoma should be reserved only for cases where the uterine origin of the mass is firmly established. Occasionally, it may be difficult to distinguish a pedunculated subserosal leiomyoma from an ovarian fibroma, since both lesions may be hypointense on T2-weighted images. This distinction is likely not significant as the latter is rarely malignant.

The risk of development of a leiomyosarcoma increases with age and in black woman. The previously held view of rapid growth being at greater suspicion for sarcomas is no longer maintained as benign leiomyomas can grow rapidly and sarcomas slowly [17]. Although studies focusing on the differential diagnosis between leiomyomas and sarcomas introduce new criteria at MRI, surgical procedures have been modified because morcellation of an unsuspected leiomyosarcoma increases dissemination [18]. According to a retrospective study using MRI to differentiate 26 benign and 25 uncertain or malignant leiomyomas, the performance of MRI reached an accuracy of 92.4% using a combination of T2-weighted, B1000, and ADC features [2]. The diagnosis of malignancy could be excluded for leiomyomas that had either low (ordinary) or high T2 signal intensities (myxoid), as well as intermediate T2 and low B1000 signal intensities (cystic). For leiomyomas with intermediate T2 and high B1000, further characterization required the use of T1 signal intensities. If T1 signal intensity was high, the leiomyoma had hemorrhagic or fatty degeneration and was benign. If T1 signal intensity was low or heterogeneous, ADC values obtained at B1000 at 1.5 T were useful and only in this specific situation. A cut-off value of 0.8 was predictive of a sarcoma, above 1.2 of a benign leiomyoma, and from 0.8 to 1.2 of a leiomyoma of uncertain malignancy.

Symptomatic leiomyoma are a burden for the women affected, as well as society. In the USA, symptomatic leiomyoma remains the number one cause of hysterectomies per year and costs up to 34.4 billion dollars annually—reflecting both the direct costs of providing care to women and the indirect costs associated with lost work days and pregnancy-related issues [19]. These statistics have led to an increase in uterine-conserving therapies for affected women [20]. MRI provides a comprehensive evaluation for women who are potential uterine artery embolization (UAE) candidates. It accurately displays leiomyoma size, number, and location [21]. Additionally, in at least 20% of cases, MRI identifies autoinfarcted, comorbid, or alternative conditions that preclude UAE as primary therapy [22]. Following UAE, MRI is able to assess treatment response and identify complications such as leiomyoma delivery and pyomyoma [22–25].

Adenomyosis (Fig.

Adenomyosis is defined as ectopic endometrial cells surrounded by stromal tissue within the myometrium and must be differentiated from leiomyoma, although these conditions frequently coexist. Differentiating the two entities may be critical because uterine-conserving therapy is established for leiomyomas, whereas hysterectomy remains the definitive treatment for debilitating adenomyosis. MRI is extremely accurate in making this distinction, especially in patients with diffuse adenomyosis with junctional zone widening >12 mm and foci of increased signal on T2-W sequences [26].

The hyperintense foci correspond to the heterotopic endometrial tissue. The surrounding muscular hyperplasia results in the low-signal myometrial lesion or widening of the junctional zone.

Hemorrhagic foci can be seen on T1-weighted sequences in approximately 20% of patients due to the presence of progesterone receptors. However, the imaging features of focal adenomyosis can overlap with those of leiomyomas [26–28]. Imaging characteristics that favor the diagnosis of focal adenomyosis include a lesion with poorly defined margins, a lesion that is elliptical in shape extending along the endometrium, a lesion that has little mass effect upon the endometrium relative to its size, and a lesion with high signal intensity striations [radiating from the endometrium into the myometrium]. Cystic adenomyosis needs to be differentiated from a leiomyoma with central hemorrhagic degeneration or a unicornuate uterus with an obstructed noncommunicating rudimentary horn.

Myometrial Contractions

Myometrial contractions can mimic leiomyoma or adenomyosis. They usually change or resolve over the course of the exam. Contractions correspond to transient low signal intensity lesions within the myometrium that deform the endometrium while sparing the outer uterine contour. Kinematic sequences using a single-shot fast spin-echo T2-weighted technique (HASTE, SSFSE) can differentiate true widening related to adenomyosis from apparent widening of the junctional zone due to myometrial contractions or uterine peristalsis, a physiologic rhythmic form of myometrial contraction most marked during the menstrual and periovulatory phase that can present as diffuse widening of the junctional zone.

Endometrial Pathology

Endometrial polyps are among the most common pathologic lesions of the uterine corpus. Patients with postmenopausal bleeding and endometrial polyps usually undergo endometrial sampling and removal of the polyps. Endometrial polyps have a variable appearance at EVS but are typically echogenic with an intact overlying endometrium or subendometrial halo. A vascular pedicle is usually identified at color/power Doppler imaging (Fig.

Figure MRI of the pelvis Sagittal T2-weighted images of the uterus: A polyp is located at the internal os of the endocervical canal with signal intensity that is slightly hypointense compared to normal endometrium.

Large polyps are frequently heterogeneous in signal intensity [29]. On T2-weighted sequences, the fibrous core is seen as a hypointense area within a polyp. The addition of gadolinium-enhanced sequences significantly improves the detection rate of endometrial polyps. Endometrial polyps show a variable degree of enhancement after gadolinium administration. Small polyps enhance early and are well delineated against the hypointense endometrial complex on early dynamic scans. In addition, a vascular stalk can frequently be identified during the arterial phase.

Endometrial synechia results from traumatic injury to the endometrium and may be demonstrated both with EVS and MRI. Sonohysterography improves the detection of endometrial synechiae. In severe cases of Asherman's syndrome resulting in an obliterated uterine cavity, synechiae may result in infertility, recurrent pregnancy loss, and amenorrhea. On EVS, synechiae present as echogenic or hypoechoic bands traversing the endometrial cavity. These bands can be thick and broad or thin and easily disrupted. On MRI, these bands are hypointense on T2-weighted sequences and usually show enhancement after gadolinium administration.

Benign Pathology of the Cervix and Vagina

Bartholin's cysts are caused by retained secretions within the vulvovaginal glands, mostly as a result of chronic inflammation or trauma. They are located in the posterolateral parts of the lower vagina and vulva, whereas nabothian cysts are retention cysts of the cervical glands and clefts.

Gartner duct cysts represent remnants of the caudal end of the Wolffian or mesonephric ducts and are typically located in the anterolateral wall of the vagina above the inferior margin of the symphysis pubis.

Müllerian cysts, representing embryologic remnants of Müllerian (paramesonephric) ducts, are the most common congenital cysts of the female genital tract and can be found from the introitus to the level of the cornua. They are typically lined by mucinous, columnar epithelium. At the level of the vagina, they are most commonly located anterolaterally and are indistinguishable from Gartner duct cysts. The majority of Müllerian cysts are small and asymptomatic. Large, symptomatic cysts require excision.

DeepEndometriosis

Endometriosis is a common gynecological disease, defined by functional ectopic endometrial glands and stroma outside the uterus. When located elsewhere than in the ovary or on the superficial peritoneum, endometriosis is often referred to as being deep usually lying 5 mm below the peritoneum within the bladder, vaginal, or bowel wall. Other localizations include the area behind the cervix, the upper vaginal cuff, the ureter, the round ligament, the parameter, the utero-sacral ligaments, the presacral nerves, the anterior abdominal wall, and/or the diaphragm. According to the European Society of Urogenital Radiology (ESUR), guidelines for imaging endometriosis with MRI agreed that the diagnosis of deep pelvic endometriosis requires the joint presence of morphological and signal intensity anomalies [30]: tissue areas corresponding to fibrosis with a signal close to that of pelvic muscle on T1-weighted and T2-weighted images; hyperintense foci on T1-weighted and/or fat-suppressed T1-weighted MR images, corresponding to hemorrhagic foci; and small hyperintense cavities on T2-weighted images. Morphological anomalies depend on the localization of deep endometriosis. Within the frame of this chapter, only retro-cervical, uterosacral ligaments and vaginal localization are specified (Fig.). Retrocervical endometriosis is also called endometriosis of the torus uterinus and corresponds at MRI to a T2 hypointense band in the upper midportion of the posterior cervix. Endometriosis of the uterosacral ligament demonstrates as an irregular nodule or thickening compared to the normal ligament. When bilateral it usually includes the torus uterinus and presents as an arciform anomaly. Vaginal endometriosis obliterates the posterior vaginal cuff with a T2 hypointense mass behind the posterior wall of the cervix. The nodule or mass may contain foci of high T2- and T1-weighted signal intensities. Vaginal endometriosis and endometriosis of the uterosacral ligaments are often associated with rectosigmoid endometriosis.

Concluding Remarks

Ultrasound is the first-line diagnostic tool for most benign uterine condition. MRI is an extremely useful complement in symptomatic patients with indeterminate or complex uterine presentation, particularly before surgery.

> **Take-Home Message**
> Ultrasound is the first-line imaging technique to localize an anomaly of the uterus to either the myometrium or the endometrium. MRI has ideal capabilities in tissue characterization and requires careful comparison between T2- and T1-weighted sequences. Image orientation perpendicular to the axis of the uterine corpus helps to assess the impact of an anomaly on the uterine cavity.

References

1. Smith-Bindman R, Kerlikowske K, Feldstein VA, et al. Endovaginal ultrasound to exclude endometrial cancer and other endometrial abnormalities. JAMA. 1998;280:1510–7.
2. Thomassin-Naggara DS, Bonneau C, et al. How to differentiate benign from malignant myometrial tumors using MR imaging. Eur Radiol. 2013;23:2306–14.
3. Troiano RN, McCarthy SM. Müllerian duct anomalies: imaging and clinical issues. Radiology. 2004;233:19–34.
4. Behr SC, Coutier JL, Qayyum A. Imaging of Müllerian Duct Anomalies. Radiographics. 2012;32:1619–20.
5. Li S, Qayyum A, Coakley FV, Hricak H. Association of renal agenesis and Müllerian duct anomalies. J Comput Assist Tomogr. 2000;24:829–34.
6. Buttram VC Jr, Gibbons WE. Müllerian anomalies: a proposed classification. (An analysis of 144 cases). Fertil Steril. 1979; 32:40–6.
7. The American Fertility Society classifications of adnexal adhesions, distal tubal occlusion, tubal occlusion secondary to tubal ligation, tubal pregnancies, Müllerian anomalies and intrauterine adhesions. Fertil Steril. 1988;49:944–55.
8. Grimbizis GF, Gordts S, Di Spiezio Sardo A, et al. The ESHRE/ESGE consensus on the classification of female genital tract congenital anomalies. Hum Reprod. 2013;28:2032–44.
9. Grimbizis GF, Di Spiezio SA, et al. The Thessaloniki ESHRE/ESGE consensus on diagnosis of female genital anomalies. Hum Reprod. 2016;31(1):2–7.
10. Mueller GC, Hussain HK, Smith YR, et al. Müllerian duct anomalies: Comparison of MRI diagnosis and clinical diagnosis. AJR Am J Roentgenol. 2007;189:1294–302.
11. Pellerito JS, McCarthy SM, Doyle MB, et al. Diagnosis of uterine anomalies: relative accuracy of MR imaging, endovaginal sonography, and hysterosalpingography. Radiology. 1992;183: 795–800.
12. Zreik TG, Troiano RN, Ghoussoub RA, et al. Myometrial tissue in uterine septa. J Am Assoc Gynecol Laparosc. 1998;5: 155–60.
13. Chandler TM, Machan LS, Cooperberg PL, et al. Müllerian duct anomalies: from diagnosis to intervention. Br J Radiol. 2009;82:1034–42.
14. Jayasinghe Y, Rane A, Stalewski H, Grover S. The presentation and early diagnosis of the rudimentary uterine horn. Obstet Gynecol. 2005;105:1456–67.
15. Arleo EK, Schwartz PE, Hui P, et al. Review of leiomyoma variants. AJR. 2015;205:912–21.
16. Munro MG, Crithcley HOD, Fraser IS, for the FIGO Working Group on Menstrual Disorders. The FIGO classification of causes of abnormal uterine bleeding. Int J Gynaecol Obstet. 2011; 113(1):1–2.
17. Peddada SD, Laughlin SK, Miner K. Growth of uterine leiomyomata among premenopausal black and white women. Proc Natl Acad Sci U S A. 2008;105(19):887–19,892.
18. FDA. UPDATED Laparoscopic Uterine Power Morcellation in Hysterectomy and Myomectomy: FDA Safety Communication 2014. Available at: http://www.fda.gov/MedicalDevices/Safety/AlertsandNotices/ucm424443.htm.
19. Cardozo ER, Clark D, Banks NK, et al. The estimated annual cost of uterine leiomyomata in the United States. Am J Obstet Gynecol. 2012;206:21.e1–9.

20. Jacobson GF, Shaber RE, Armstrong MA, Hung Y-Y. Changes in rates of hysterectomy and uterine conserving procedures for treatment of uterine leiomyoma. Am J Obstet Gynecol. 2007;196(6): 601.e1.
21. Jha RC, Ascher SM, Imaoka I, Spies JB. Symptomatic fibroleiomyomata: MR imaging of the uterus before and after uterine artery embolization. Radiology. 2000;217:228–35.
22. Nikolaidis PN, Siddiqi AH, Carr JC, et al. Incidence of nonviable leiomyomas on contrast material enhanced pelvic MR imaging in patients referred for uterine artery embolization. J Vasc Interv Radiol. 2005;16:1465–147.
23. Kroencke TJ, Scheurig C, Poellinger A, et al. Uterine artery embolization for leiomyomas: percentage of infarction predicts clinical outcome. Radiology. 2010;255:834–41.
24. Kitamura Y, Ascher SM, Cooper C, et al. Imaging manifestations of complications associated with uterine artery embolization. Radiographics. 2005;25:S119–32.
25. Radeleff B, Eiers M, Bellemann N, et al. Expulsion of dominant submucosal fibroids after uterine artery embolization. Eur J Radiol. 2010;75:e57–63.
26. Reinhold C, McCarthy S, Bret PM, et al. Diffuse adenomyosis: comparison of endovaginal US and MR imaging with histopathologic correlation. Radiology. 1996;199:151–8.
27. Togashi K, Ozasa H, Konishi I, et al. Enlarged uterus: differentiation between adenomyosis and leiomyoma with MR imaging. Radiology. 1989;171:531–4.
28. Mark AS, Hricak H, Heinrichs LW, et al. Adenomyosis and leiomyoma: differential diagnosis with MR imaging. Radiology. 1987;163:527–9.
29. Grasel RP, Outwater EK, Siegelman ES, et al. Endometrial polyps: MR imaging features and distinction from endometrial carcinoma. Radiology. 2000;214:47–52.
30. Bazot M, Bharwani N, Huchon C, et al. European society of urogenital radiology (ESUR) guidelines: MR imaging of pelvic endometriosis. Eur Radiol. 2017;27(7):2765–75.

17

Therapy Monitoring of Oncologic Disease in the Abdomen (Including PET/CT)

Irene A. Burger and Regina G. H. Beets-Tan

Learning Objectives

- To understand the opportunities and limitations of the different modalities for therapy monitoring based on anatomical and physiological imaging
- To know the pearls and pitfalls in therapy monitoring of gastrointestinal stromal tumors, neuroendocrine tumors, and metastasized prostate cancer
- To learn about the evidence, pearls, and pitfalls of imaging for the local assessment of response to neoadjuvant (chemo)radiotherapy in locally advanced rectal tumors

Introduction

The importance and the volume of scans for therapy monitoring are steadily increasing for oncologic diseases. Numerous reasons account for that. Most important is the occurrence of an increasing number of new and more specific therapies requiring early outcome measures preceding first results on survival benefits. Furthermore, the specific therapeutic approaches concomitant with longer therapy windows lead to an increase in mixed response results, requiring reliable evaluation by imaging approaches.

Therefore, an increasing need emerged, and focus has been put on how to best evaluate such early onset of therapeutic efficacy. In this chapter we will provide a brief overview on the most commonly used imaging modalities, their benefits and their pitfalls focusing on the evaluation of therapeutic efficacy with CT, MRI, and molecular imaging (PET/CT) of several abdominal tumors such as GIST, neuroendocrine tumors, and metastatic prostate cancer.

Furthermore, the increase of neoadjuvant therapy for high-risk tumors significantly improved outcome in various tumor entities. Here imaging is essential not only for overall response assessment but also to determine resectability. Therefore we will address the importance of endorectal ultrasonography (ERUS) and MRI in locally advanced rectal tumors treated with neoadjuvant (chemo)radiotherapy.

I. A. Burger (✉)
Department of Nuclear Medicine, UniversitätsSpital Zürich, Zürich, Switzerland
e-mail: Irene.burger@usz.ch

R. G. H. Beets-Tan
Department of Radiology, The Netherlands Cancer Institute, Amsterdam, The Netherlands
e-mail: r.beetstan@nki.nl

Assessment of Local Response to Neoadjuvant Treatment in Rectal Cancer

The local recurrence rate after rectal cancer surgery has significantly decreased from 40% three decades ago to 3% with current multimodality imaging and therapy. Three major steps have been taken forward: the introduction of the total mesorectal excision (TME) surgery, preoperative radiotherapy with or without chemotherapy, and imaging. The risk factors associated with local recurrence are the T stage, N stage, distance of the tumor to the mesorectal fascia, extramural vascular invasion, perineural invasion, lymph vessel invasion, and histological grade. Rectal cancer patients are now treated according to their risk for local recurrence with a differentiated treatment—immediate TME surgery for the low-risk tumors and preoperative neoadjuvant chemoradiotherapy for the very high risks. The decisions on preoperative treatment are based on risk assessment not only by digital rectal examination and endoscopy but also by imaging. Endorectal ultrasonography (ERUS) and MRI are considered as the two best locoregional imaging methods to assess the risk factors at primary staging and to evaluate local response to neoadjuvant treatment, while CT is restricted to distant staging. Here we'll focus on local response evaluation with MR and ERUS.

Selection of Patients for Neoadjuvant Therapy

The importance of the involvement of the mesorectal fascia as a prognostic factor and as a parameter of surgical quality has been recognized and confirmed in the last 30 years [1]. The ideal plane of resection in a total mesorectal excision is just outside the mesorectal fascia, and a positive circumferential resection margin can be the result of inadequate TME surgery. Preoperative assessment of involvement of the mesorectal fascia is crucial. An involved mesorectal fascia can be reliably determined on MRI and is defined as a closest distance of ≤1 mm between the tumor and the mesorectal fascia. These tumors should be treated with a preoperative (chemo)radiation regimen providing an opportunity for downsizing. Regardless of the choice for neoadjuvant treatment strategies, it is however important for the surgeon to know the exact anatomical relation of the tumor to the mesorectal fascia and the surrounding structures in order to obtain a complete resection, and MRI can provide this information. A number of studies in the past decades demonstrated that MRI could reliably identify the mesorectal fascia and predict its involvement [2, 3]. In a European multicenter study, the depth of extramural tumor invasion was compared between preoperative MRI and histology in 311 patients undergoing primary surgery; accuracy to within 0.5 mm was achieved in 95% of cases [4]. It is now widely adopted that MRI is the most accurate method for the assessment of an involved or threatened mesorectal fascia (Fig.).

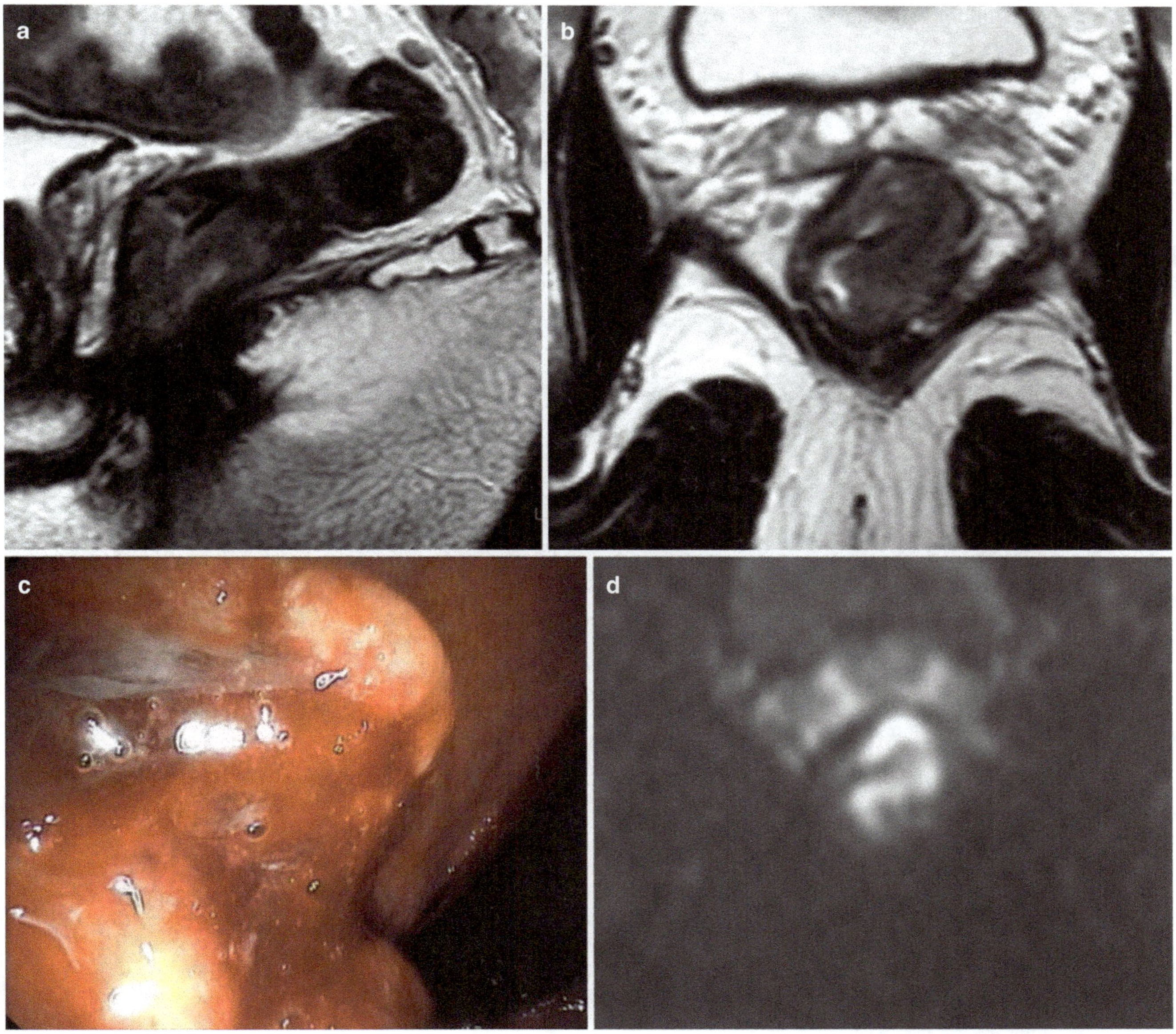

Fig. cT2N2 low rectal tumor before neoadjuvant chemoradiotherapy. Endoscopy shows a sessile semicircular mass anteriorly located just above the anal canal (**a–d**). T2-weighted MRI shows a semicircular tumor low anterior which is limited to the bowel wall. There is a suspicious large node in the mesorectum, visualized on the sagittal T2-weighted MR image. DWI (b1000) image confirms a rectal cancer with a restricted diffusion

Assessment of Local Tumor Response and Resectability

Assessment of local tumor response is generally performed by digital rectal examination, endoscopy, and MRI 6–8 weeks after completion of neoadjuvant chemoradiotherapy [5]. MRI can indicate tumor volume shrinkage. Reported negative predictive values (NPVs) as high as 90% for the detection of an involved mesorectal fascia suggest that MRI can accurately identify clearance of an initially suspicious invaded mesorectal resection margin. The high NPV is at the expense of a PPV as low as 50%. As a result of the irradiation, the initial tumor mass often becomes fibrotic, and it may be very difficult to distinguish on T2-weighted MRI between fibrosis with and without minimal residual tumor. This holds true also for fibrotic masses adjacent to the mesorectal fascia, the reason why in such a setting one should be cautious to overcall persistent involvement of a mesorectal fascia after chemoradiotherapy (Fig.) [ ].

Restaging MRI can therefore be valuable as a road map for surgeons and to decide whether tumor regression visualized on MRI justifies alteration of the initial resection plan. The obvious prerequisite for the value of a restaging MRI is that both the surgeon and the patient must be willing to change the initial plan.

Assessment of Complete Response After Chemoradiotherapy

Rectal cancer patients with clinical complete or near complete response after chemoradiotherapy have shown to have a good oncological outcome with a nonoperative management with survival figures as good as when these patients would have undergone a resection. This treatment shows an improved functional outcome without compromising oncological outcome. Habr-Gama et al. and the group of Beets et al. were pioneers of these so-called watch and wait policy [8, 9]. Today more and more patients with clinical complete response are considered a watch and wait policy.

A watch and wait treatment for the clinical complete or near complete responders requires accurate assessment of response to chemoradiotherapy and accurate monitoring of response. Although this is generally done by digital rectal examination, imaging has shown its benefit. The two important questions are whether there is still a significant volume of residual tumor within the fibrotic tumor bed and whether there are still involved nodes after CRT. When it comes to primary T staging, MRI is the preferred staging method for large advanced tumors, while ERUS remains the best method to image the superficial tumors limited to the submucosa (T1) [10].

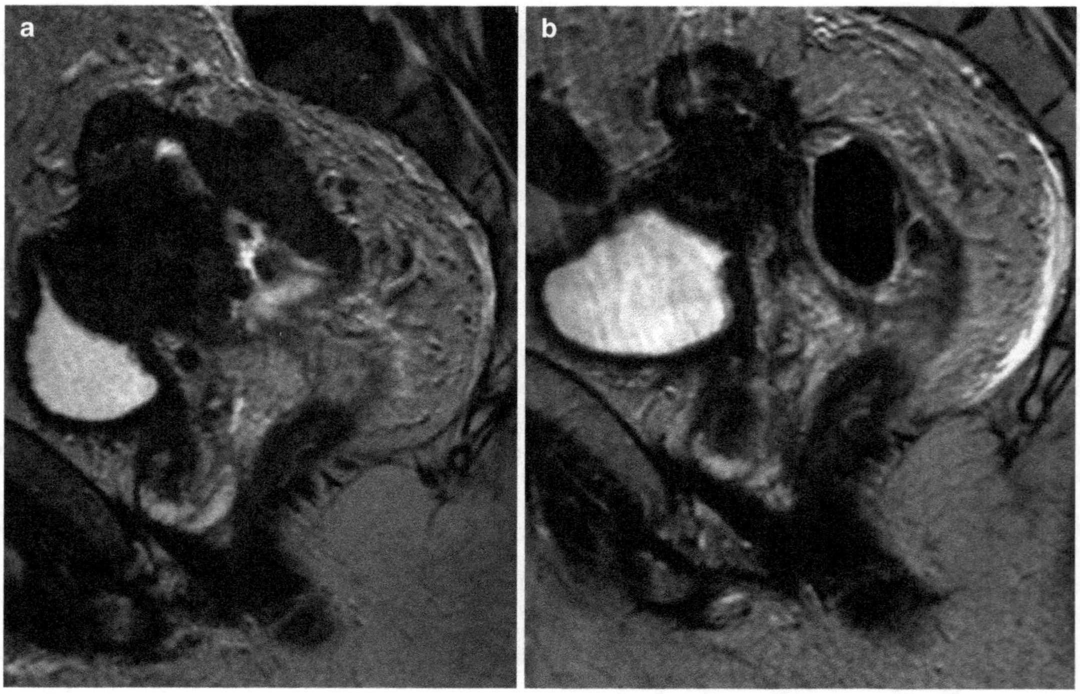

Fig. T2-weighted MRI of a locally advanced rectal tumor before (**a**) and after (**b**) neoadjuvant chemoradiotherapy. The tumor located in the mid-high rectum anteriorly invades the peritoneal reflection and shows a mass effect. It can often be difficult to know whether the tumor is invading in or only pushing the bladder wall and dome. After chemoradiotherapy the tumor has significantly shrunk and for a large proportion becomes fibrotic. Anteriorly it has retracted from the bladder dome but not from the peritoneal reflection, and there is a fibrotically thickened peritoneal reflection. The surgeon should be notified of this finding so that he can perform a wider excision including the peritoneal reflection

Nevertheless, for assessment of the ypT stage of rectal tumors after neoadjuvant treatment, MRI does not outperform ERUS. A meta-analysis of over 1500 patients reported a disappointingly low overall performance with a pooled overall sensitivity of 50% and specificity of 91% [11]. Subgroup analyses showed a pooled sensitivity of only 19% and specificity of 94% for the MRI assessment of pathological complete response (ypT0). Although the performance of MRI for assessment of small tumor remnants limited to the bowel wall (ypT0–2) is higher, the sensitivity of 55% remains insufficient for clinical decision-making. The findings above suggest that both ERUS and MRI are limited in the detection of small tumor remnants within fibrotic tissue after neoadjuvant chemoradiotherapy of rectal cancer. Some authors have shown that the combination of visual assessment of morphological features on post-chemoradiotherapy MRI with objective assessment of tumor shrinkage by magnetic resonance volumetric measurements can yield accuracies as high as 87% [12, 13]. Curvo-Semedo et al. and Ha et al. found AUCs (areas under the ROC curve) of 0.70–0.84 for the assessment of pathological complete response with magnetic resonance volumetric measurements by manual delineation of tumors [14]. This is very time-consuming and thus not a standard practice. Many studies have reported the benefit of diffusion-weighted MRI (DW-MRI) for the detection of residual disease within the fibrotic scar. A meta-analysis has shown that DW-MRI can improve the diagnostic performance of restaging MRI for the assessment of a pathological complete response with an increase in sensitivity from 19% to 84% [11]. A multicenter retrospective study in 120 patients with rectal cancer reported a high NPV of 90% for DW-MRI for the assessment of a pathological complete response, indicating that the visual analysis of DW-MRI is especially valuable for the detection of residual tumor and for ruling out a complete response [15]. Visual analysis of DW-MRI (at b800 or b1000) is now recommended in international clinical guidelines as a valuable adjunct to digital rectal exam and endoscopy. Patients assessed as (near) complete response with these tools can be safely considered for a watch and wait treatment [5]. Figure shows the typical DW-MR and endoscopic image of a clinical complete response.

Overall, there is little evidence concerning restaging with ERUS after neoadjuvant treatment. In a study by Mezzi et al. and Napoleon et al., ERUS after neoadjuvant treatment was only accurate in 47% and 46% of patients, respectively. Fibrotic, necrotic, and inflammatory changes after preoperative radiotherapy can lead to misinterpretation of ERUS images [16, 17]. Radovanovic et al. found a good accuracy rate for restaging rectal cancer after neoadjuvant chemoradiation (75%) [18]. However, ERUS was insufficient in discriminating a complete pathological response, in fact the only key factor of importance in clinical decision-making, as described by the groups of Habr-Gama and Beets [8, 9]. The largest study, by Pastor et al., reported an accuracy of only 47% for the ERUS assessment of complete response. 53% of tumors identified as yT0 by ERUS were understaged [19].

Assessment of Response for Nodal Disease

Node-positive disease is one of the most important risk factors for both local and distant recurrence and is generally considered an indication for neoadjuvant therapy. Identifying mesorectal nodal disease with any imaging technique remains difficult because size criteria used on its own result in only a moderate accuracy. The majority of mesorectal-involved nodes are smaller than 5 mm resulting in inaccuracies when size is used as a cutoff for nodal disease. Meta-analyses showed no significant differences between the three modalities, EUS, CT, or MRI, which were all associated with sensitivities for primary staging around 60–70% [20]. Because the majority of mesorectal nodes disappear or shrink after chemoradiotherapy, restaging nodes after CRT can be more accurate with known improved sensitivities around 70–75%. Nevertheless, assessment of nodal involvement in rectal cancer in general remains a challenging task for any imaging method, and at the moment of writing, this problem has not been solved.

Assessment of Response for Systemic Disease

The World Health Organization (WHO) recognized the need for standardized criteria across clinical trials very early, publishing the initial *WHO handbook for reporting results of cancer treatment* in 1979 [21]. Since then a number of guidelines and updates have been published.

Response Based on Morphology for Chemotherapy

The most commonly applied response criteria for systemic disease are Response Evaluation Criteria in Solid Tumors (RECIST) that have been updated to RECIST 1.1 [22]. Based on the changes of target and nontarget lesions, patients are categorized into four groups: complete response (CR), partial response (PR), stable disease (SD), and progressive disease (PD). To simplify readouts only five target lesions (TL), maximum of two in the same organ, shall be assessed by the maximum diameter. Lymph nodes are measured by the short axis and need to be larger than 1.5 cm to be considered as target lesions. Sclerotic bone lesions are considered nontarget lesions (NTL), as well as cystic lesions, if they do not have large solid components. The sum of all diameters from

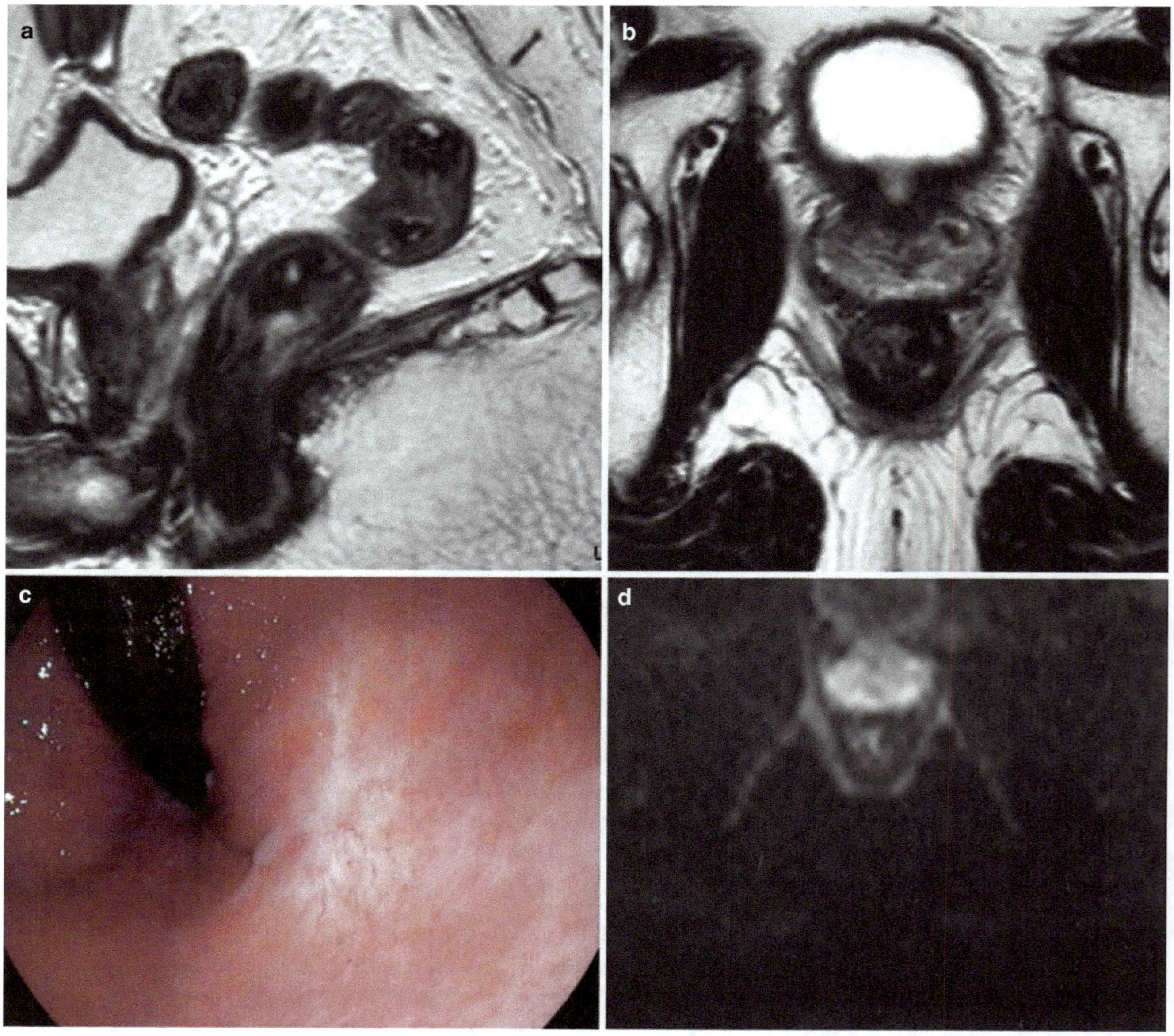

Fig. . DW-MRI and endoscopy of a clinical complete response after neoadjuvant chemoradiotherapy. Endoscopy shows complete regression of the in Fig. visualized tumor with only a white scar tissue with telangiectasia at the irradiated tumor bed (**a**–**d**). T2-weighted MRI shows a minimal fibrotic wall anteriorly without any distortion of the wall anatomy. DWI (b1000) image shows no restricted diffusion in the tumor bed. On the sagittal T2-weighted MR image, the initially suspicious node has decreased in size and shows no suspicious features of malignancy. The patient was successfully treated and closely monitored within a watch and wait regimen. Ten years in follow-up still alive without recurrent disease

TLs needs to decrease more than 30% to be considered as a partial response or increase by 20% (more than 5 mm) to indicate progressive disease.

Response	RECIST 1.1
PD	Increase of TL diameters by ≥20% (with at least an increase of 5 mm), progressive NTL, new lesions
SD	No PR or PD
PR	Decrease of TL diameters by ≥30%, no new lesions
CR	Disappearance of all extranodal TLs, all LN < 1 cm, no progressive NTL, normalization of tumor marker

Response Based on Morphology for Immunotherapy

Classical chemotherapies directly kill tumor cells leading to shrinkage of tumor volume based on the efficacy of the therapy. Immunotherapies activate the immune system of the patient with different response patterns depending on the mechanism of drug action [23]. Summarized morphologic response based on immunotherapy will often need more time compared to conventional therapies, and response patterns can be grouped into four categories:

(1) immediate response, (2) durable stable disease, (3) response after initial increase (flare), and (4) response with new lesions.

For accurate interpretation of the response pattern, understanding of the drug mechanism is crucial. Therapeutics leading to an increasing migration of T cells into the tumor (CTLA-4 blocking, e.g., ipilimumab) will be more likely to have an initial increase in tumor size [24]. iRECIST is based on RECIST 1.1 to select TL and NTL; if however PD is seen on first follow-up, this is interpreted as iUPD (unconfirmed progressive disease); only if tumor increase of more than 30% is confirmed on the second follow-up (4–8 weeks later), a confirmed progression iCPD will be noted. If the tumor remains stable, iUPD will remain the interpretation, and only if criteria for partial or complete response are met, iPR or iCR will be given [23].

Besides accurate interpretation of early pseudoprogression, the recognition of immune-related response (irR) is crucial as well. Inflammatory changes can result in activation of sarcoidosis with enlarged lymph nodes or adrenalitis with enlarged suprarenal glands. This is not only challenging for morphologic imaging but also for PET/CT since irR can show intensive ^{18}F–fluorodeoxyglucose (FDG) uptake [25]. Immunotherapies are already a clinically established option for patients with melanoma or lung cancer. However, more indications also for abdominal diseases will follow soon, such as prostate cancer (sipuleucel-T), kidney cancer (nivolumab), or bladder cancer (pembrolizumab).

Response Based on FDG PET

Numerous publications showed a good correlation between the decrease in FDG accumulation in tumor lesions and therapy response [26]. Therefore, PET response evaluation was postulated, including EORTC PET response recommendations (1999) and the PET response criteria in solid tumors (PERCIST) pioneered by Wahl et al. in 2009 [27]. Both methods follow the model of RECIST with four adapted response categories: complete metabolic response (CMR), partial metabolic response (PMR), stable metabolic disease (SMD), and progressive metabolic disease (PMD). Numerous studies compared the original EORTC PET criteria with PERCIST in the past 8 years showing similar results. However, the use of PERCIST seems preferable for clinical trials due to a better standardization [28]. Both methods recommend the use of standardized uptake values (SUV) normalized to the lean body mass (SUL). However, if possible PERCIST favors the use of a SUL_{peak} (average value in the hottest 1 cm^3 sphere within the tumor), instead of SUL_{max} (only one maximum voxel) to reduce the intrinsic variability.

Response	PERCIST—Based on SUL_{peak} (SUL_{max})
PMD	SUL increase by at least 30% and at least 0.8 SUL units of the target lesion or increase in target lesion size by 30% or development of at least one new lesion or unequivocal progression of nontarget lesions
SMD	Increase or decrease of SUL by less than 30%
PMR	Decrease of SUL by ≥30% and at least 0.8 SUL unit difference and no new FDG-avid lesions and no increase in size >30% of the target lesion and no increase in SUL or size of nontarget lesion
CMR	FDG uptake indistinguishable from surrounding background and SUL less than the liver

It is important to note that all these recommendations are focusing on FDG PET for the evaluation of metabolic response of solid tumors. Tumor dedifferentiation does not correlate with receptor expression in the same way like FDG. Therefore, PERCIST per se is not necessarily applicable for the increasing use of receptor imaging in oncologic diseases, e.g., somatostatin receptor II (SSTR II) for neuroendocrine tumors or prostate-specific membrane antigen (PSMA) for prostate cancer.

Monitoring GIST Molecular Targeted Systemic Therapy

Monitoring GIST with CT/MRI

With the introduction of tyrosine kinase inhibitors imatinib mesylate (Glivec®) in 2002 for gastrointestinal stromal tumors (GIST), a new area of molecular-targeted systemic therapy began, followed by a variety of targeted agents for various indications [29, 30]. Those new therapeutic approaches result in new patterns regarding response assessment, with the classical reduction in tumor size assessed by RECIST criteria often being detected weeks to months later [31]. Classical response patterns that can be observed in liver metastasis include appearance of new lesions, increase in size with decrease in attenuation, increase in attenuation (internal hemorrhage), and temporal changes. These patterns can be explained by the primary effect on tumor vascularity leading to hypoenhancement and therefore pseudoprogression on contrast-enhanced CT scans in the classical portovenous phase, with combination of intratumoral edema and internal hemorrhages [32]. To integrate these observations into clinical response assessment, Choi et al. suggested that either a decrease in size by 10% (largest diameter) or a decrease in attenuation by 15% on portovenous contrast-enhanced CT should be rated as response [33]. More recent approaches for optimal response assessment for GIST included the use of dual-energy CT, with calculation of iodine-related attenuation as a superior predictor for response compared to simple density used for the Choi criteria [34].

MRI can be used in undetermined cases to detect intratumoral hemorrhage and to assess vascularity of the lesions. Furthermore Tang et al. showed that an increase in ADC values after 1 week of therapy is associated with good treatment response [35]. Both methods dual-energy CT and MRI have not been clinically validated to date.

Monitoring GIST with PET

In the first safety and efficacy report on imatinib (2001) including 40 patients, the use of FDG PET was documented for a subgroup of 17 patients, where the decrease in FDG uptake correlated well with the outcome and preceded CT findings according to RECIST criteria [29] (Fig.). This led to numerous studies integrating FDG for response assessment with variable cutoff values to indicate response. Therefore, the ESMO Clinical Practice Guidelines for GIST suggest the use of FDG PET/CT for early detection of tumor response under targeted therapy [36]. Choi et al. used modified EORTC criteria of a decrease in SUV_{max} of more than 70% or an absolute value of $SUV_{max} < 2.5$ as a cutoff [33]. Holdsworth et al. investigated optimal cutoffs for FDG PET based on 63 patients using ROC analysis and suggested a decrease of SUV_{max} of more than 40% or an absolute value of $SUV_{max} < 3.4$ outperformed EORTC criteria in their cohort [37]. Nevertheless, the most commonly used cutoff for new drug trials is still EORTC criteria with a decrease of >25% of SUV_{max} indicating partial response [38]. Recently published data from the Dutch GIST registry on the impact of FDG PET displayed a changed patient management in 27% of GIST patients, due to a lack of metabolic response. Furthermore, the registry data showed that especially patients without KIT exon 11 mutations had limited response to tyrosine kinase inhibitors, with a change in management based on FDG PET in 52% of these patients [39].

Monitoring Liver Disease After SIRT

Selective internal radiotherapy (SIRT) using yttrium-90 (^{90}Y) resins or glass microspheres is an increasingly used palliative therapy option for patients with non-resectable primary liver tumors or metastatic hepatic disease. Clinical evaluation of patients prior to SIRT includes contrast-enhanced CT of the chest and the abdomen to rule out extensive extrahepatic disease, liver MRI to assess tumor burden, and selective angiography to evaluate vascular anatomy and hepatic shunt with technetium-99m labeled aggregated macroalbumin (^{99m}Tc-MAA) [40].

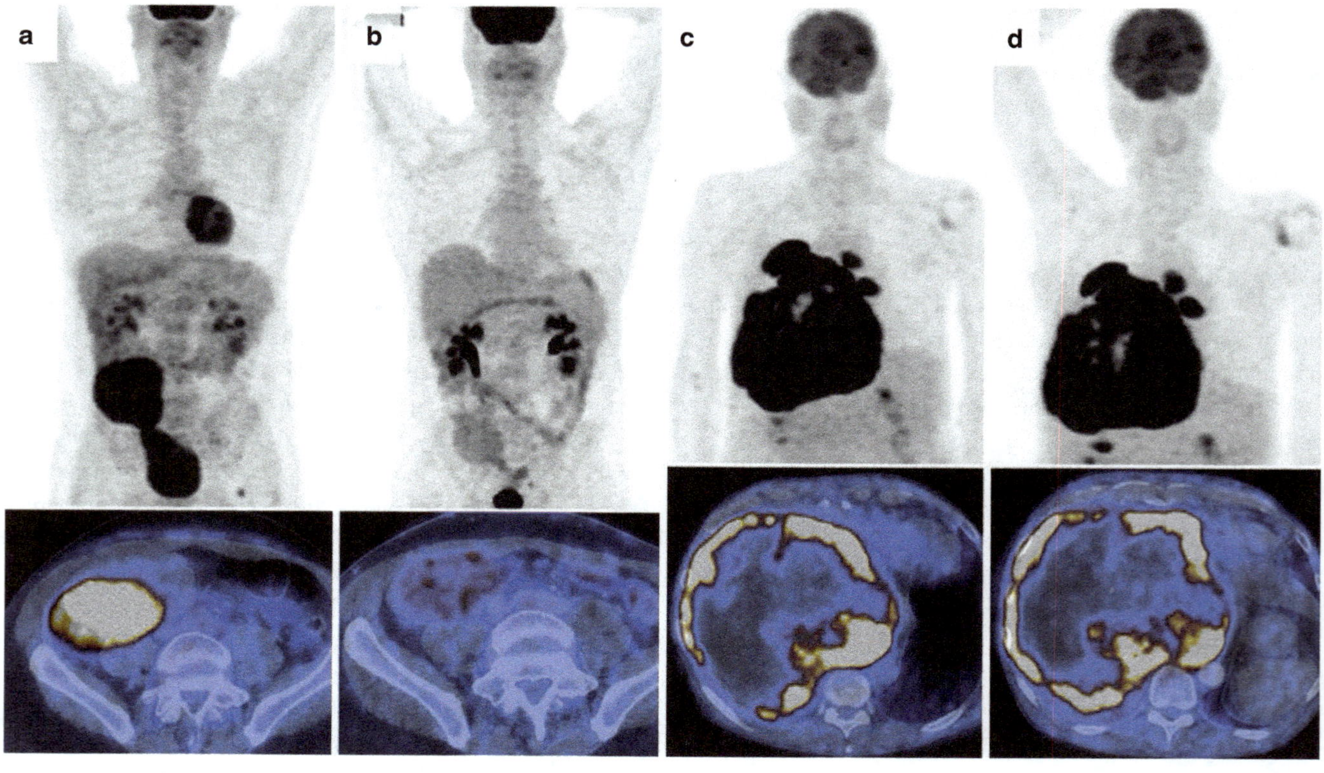

Fig. MIP FDG PET and fused axial FDG PET/CT images of two patients with highly avid GIST tumors. The first patient presented with metastatic small bowel GIST (**a**) and showed subtotal response after 4 weeks of therapy with imatinib (**b**), with only minimal decrease in size. For the second patient with extensive pleural GIST manifestation (**c**), follow-up PET after 4 weeks showed no response to neoadjuvant imatinib (**d**), followed by immediate surgical resection

Monitoring SIRT with CT/MRI

Early response assessment after SIRT using anatomical imaging can be limited due to delayed reduction in tumor size and initial pseudoprogression due to edema and sharper demarcation of tumor boundaries on conventional imaging (Fig.). Early investigations with serial contrast enhanced CT (ceCT) images showed a maximum decrease in tumor size at 3–21 months (median 12 months), concluding that blood tumor markers (e.g., CEA for colorectal metastasis) were superior in therapy response assessment compared to contrast-enhanced CT [41].

The calculation of arterial perfusion (AP) using dynamic contrast-enhanced CT prior to SIRT was the best predictor for good treatment response and overall survival in patients [42]. Furthermore, follow-up perfusion CT showed a significant decrease of AP in hepatic metastasis 4 weeks after SIRT in patients with long-term response, compared to nonresponders [43]. Dual-energy CT is a new technology, allowing the creation of iodine maps as promising tools to evaluate and quantify tumor viability, utilizing iodine maps measuring the amount of iodine per lesion. Although this approach requires validation and standardization, it showed promising first results for hepatic radiofrequency ablation [44] and could also be a promising tool for SIRT therapy response assessment.

Functional MRI was suggested to be used to assess response to SIRT, as well. A post-therapeutic increase in ADC_{min} of more than 22%, 4 weeks after SIRT, was significantly associated with a superior overall survival (18 vs. 5 months, $p < 0.001$), while tumor size did not show any significant decrease after 4 weeks [45].

Monitoring SIRT with PET

Early on FDG PET was used to assess the reduction of hepatic metastatic load after SIRT [46]. Studies comparing response assessment between FDG PET/CT and ceCT gen-

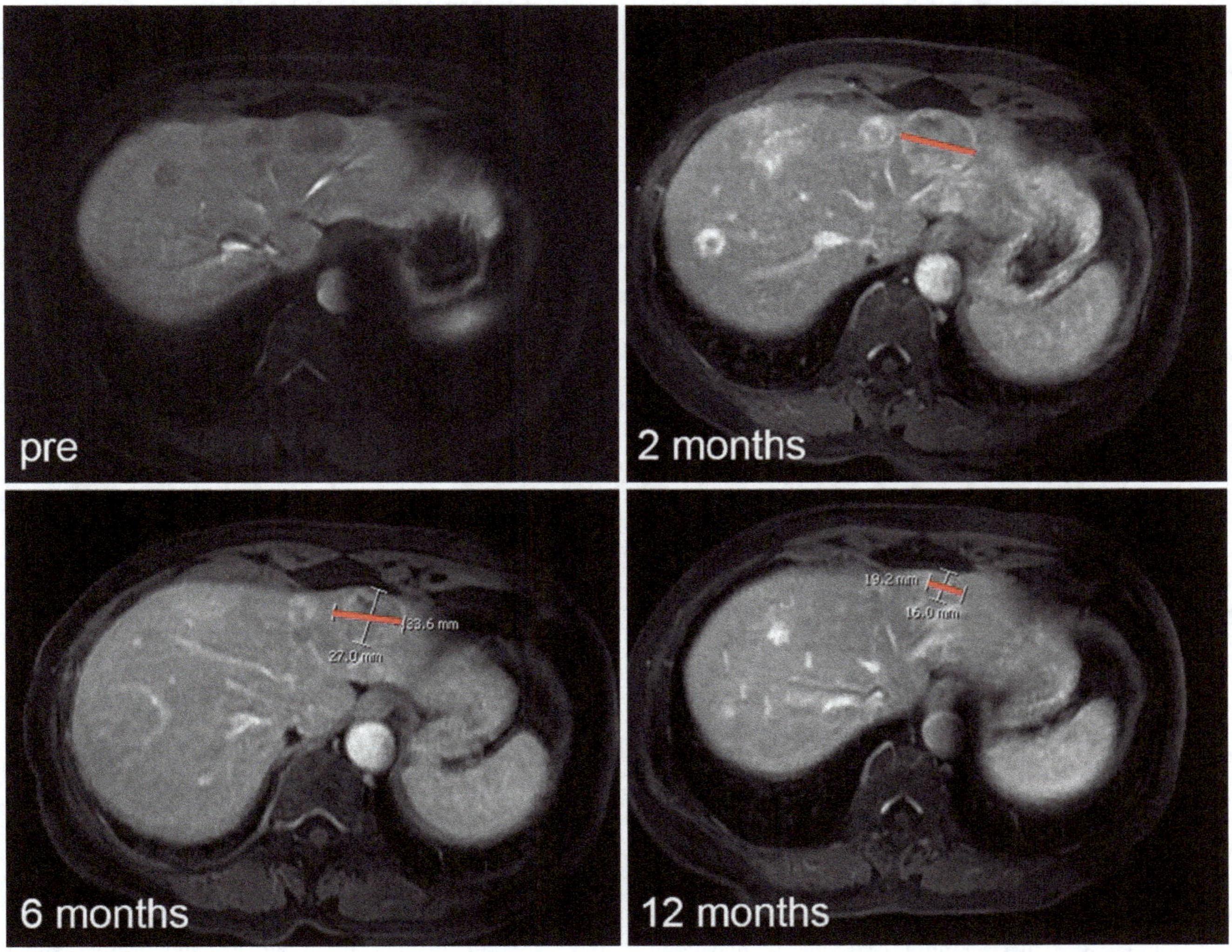

Fig. . Axial post-contrast MRI before and 2, 6, and 12 months after SIRT therapy, showing the long-standing pseudoprogression over 6 months, with improved delineation of metastases on the first scan after SIRT and final partial morphologic response after 12 months erally show a higher predictive value for FDG PET compared to ceCT [47], as published, e.g., in a review article in 2014, where PET/CT revealed superiority over ceCT using RECIST for early response assessment [48]. Other groups investigated the PET-based volume metrics such as the metabolic tumor volume (MTV) or the total lesion glycolysis (TLG) rate and came to the conclusion that those parameters correlate better with outcome compared to plain tumor size or SUV_{max} [49] measured in the PET scan. For accurate response assessment with FDG PET, potential pitfalls have to be considered. The two most prominent limitations are false-negative results caused by partial volume effects in small lesions (<1 cm) or diabetes and false-positive results caused by abscess formation or inflammatory changes [50]. A combination of FDG PET/CT with ceCT can reduce these limita-tions.

Despite the fact that earlier prediction of response to SIRT with FDG PET is possible, there is no established clinical role for FDG PET in assessing tumor response after SIRT. This might be attributable to a lack of additional treatment options. Therefore, early knowledge of a limited response to this palliative therapy will change treatment only in very few cases. Nevertheless, it is crucial to know the potential limitations and possibilities of the various imaging modalities to prevent false interpretation of early morphologic changes for accurate judgment of therapeutic response.

Monitoring Neuroendocrine Tumors

Well-differentiated neuroendocrine tumors (NET) are slow-growing lesions and therefore usually assessed with contrast-enhanced CT scans for staging and detection of progression. New therapeutic approaches such as the combination of everolimus with octreotide long-acting repeatable are systematically assessed based on progression-free survival according to RECIST and chromogranin A blood values [51]. Also the recently published NETTER-1 trial investigated the efficacy of peptide-based systemic radiotherapy (SRT) with ^{177}Lu-Dotatate based on conventional imaging. Tumor progression was defined as a primary endpoint documented with either CT or MRI. The secondary endpoint was overall survival. An increase of progression-free survival from 10.8% in the control group to 65.2% in the ^{177}Lu-Dotatate group was observed after 20 months. On interim analysis of survival, the estimated risk of death was 60% lower in the ^{177}Lu-Dotatate group than in the control group [52].

Similar to SIRT and targeted therapies, the morphologic response lags behind physiologic changes and pseudoprogression due to edema, and improved tumor delineation of liver lesions can be observed. This is crucial, since progression under therapy is a potential reason to stop current treatment according to the European Neuroendocrine Tumor Society (ENETS) consensus guidelines. Therefore, a harmonization and combination of anatomical and molecular imaging as well as biomarkers was suggested for monitoring SRT [53]. No standardized procedures have been established yet on how to interpret molecular imaging (e.g., ^{68}Ga-DOTATATE PET/CT) results after SRT. Only one publication summarizing results of 33 patients undergoing early therapy response assessment with ^{68}Ga-DOTATATE after 1 cycle of SRT was published so far. They came to the conclusion that a decrease of the tumor to spleen ratio ($SUV_{T/S}$) correlated well with progression-free survival ($p = 0.002$), while a decrease in SUV_{max} did not reach significance [54] (Fig.).

Monitoring Metastasized Prostate Cancer (I)

ConventionalMonitoring of Metastasized Prostate Cancer with CT and Bone Scans

Imaging response assessment for prostate cancer is notoriously difficult on anatomical imaging and therefore plays only a secondary role for treatment evaluation in new drug trials that commonly focus on survival and PSA values instead [55, 56]. For the trials investigating efficacy of abiraterone and alpharadin (^{223}Ra), progressive disease was defined as an increase in PSA values or a morphologic progression according to RECIST (lymph nodes (> 2 cm) or visceral metastasis selected as target lesions; progression defined as an increase of >20% of target lesions or two or more new lesions on bone scans not consistent with tumor flare). Bone scans were included since around 68% of prostate cancer patients will develop bone metastasis, and most of these lesions are unmeasurable disease according to RECIST [57]. It is well established that bone scans have a higher sensitivity for bone metastasis compared to CT. However, healing bone metastases will initially react with increasing mineralization and therefore also with an increase in activity on ^{99m}Tc-bone scans or ^{18}F–flouride PET/CT the so-called tumor flare. This typically lasts for 3 months after therapy but can be seen as late as 6 months after treatment [57]. Therefore, ^{99m}Tc-bone scans and ^{18}F–flouride PET/CT alone are both limited for response assessment in prostate cancer patients. To still be able to include bone lesions for response assessment, bone-specific response criteria were suggested by MD Anderson incorporating CT and MRI information indicative for response (e.g., sclerotic fill-in or rim of lytic lesions) together with a decrease of tracer uptake on bone scans to improved evaluation of bone lesions [58] (Fig.).

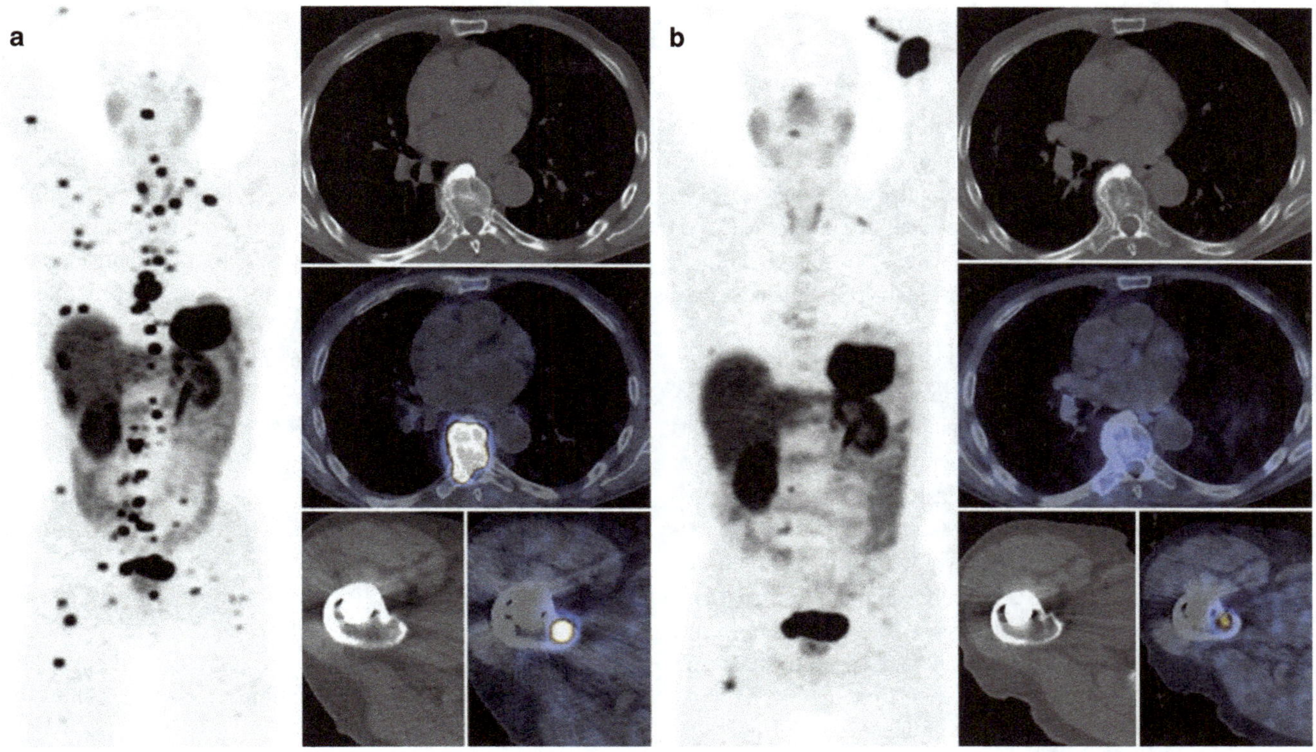

Fig. ^{68}Ga-DOTATATE MIP images of a patient before (**a**) and 12 months after (**b**) SRT with ^{177}Lu-Dotatate. With excellent response of most of the bone metastasis to therapy, without significant changes on CT

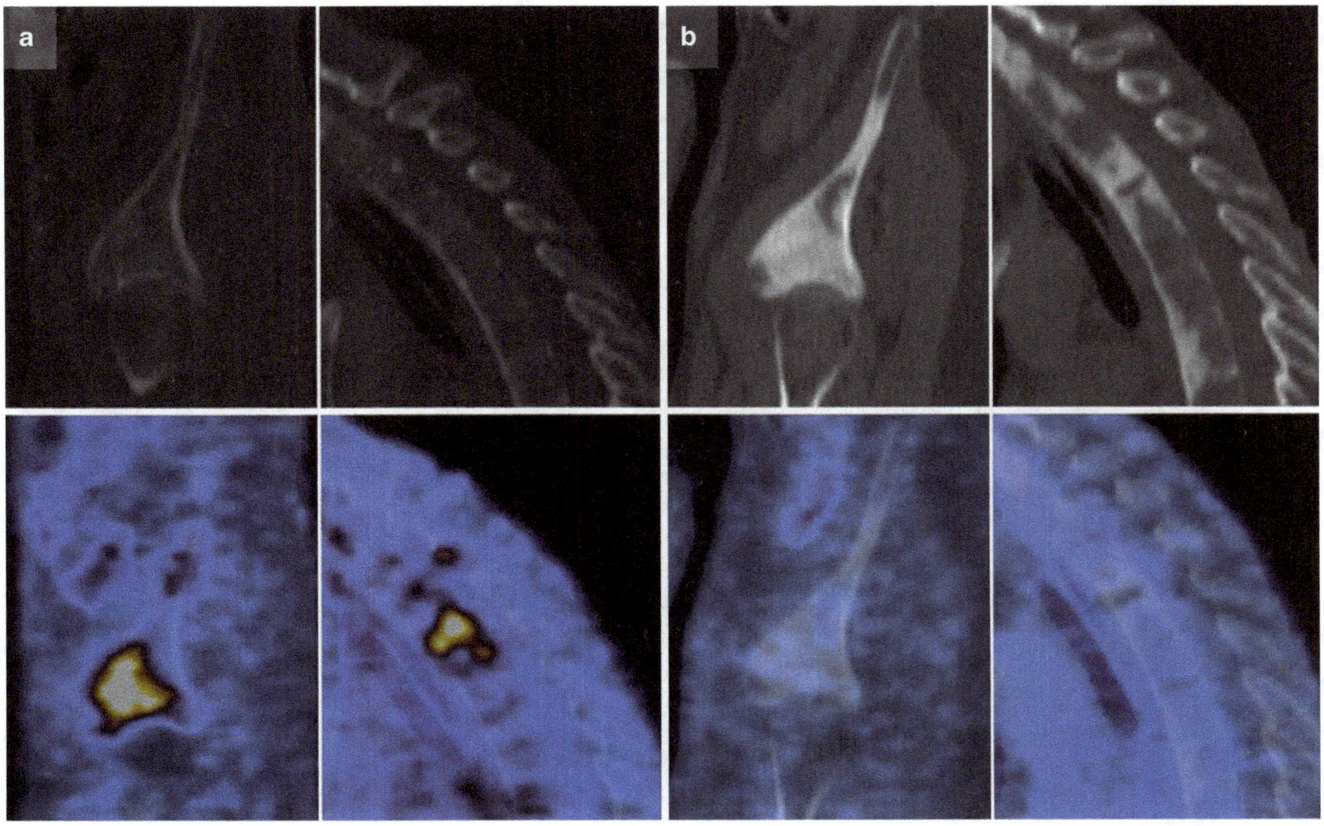

Fig. Sagittal CT and PET/CTs of bone metastasis before (**a**) and after (**b**) chemotherapy showing increasing and new sclerotic lesions with a complete decrease on FDG PET consistent with good metabolic response

Monitoring Metastasized Prostate Cancer with MRI and PET/CT

The use of FDG PET/CT is very limited in prostate cancer patients since only a small subgroup of highly dedifferentiated tumors will have increased glucose uptake. With improvements in technology, the use of diffusion-weighted imaging (DWI) became feasible not only for small areas but for whole-body exams. First preliminary results showed that ADC values could not differentiate between responders and nonresponders in patients undergoing chemotherapy [59]. However, this technology is still in its infancy, and other groups showed a good correlation between decrease in PSA and increase in ADC values for patients under antiandrogen therapy [60]. Assessment of nodal, visceral, and osseous metastasis with one exam is possible with ^{18}F- or ^{11}C–choline or ^{68}Ga-prostate-specific membrane antigen (PSMA) PET/CT. A good correlation between apoptosis and decrease in SUV on ^{11}C–choline PET/CT scans was shown after neoadjuvant docetaxel chemotherapy and complete androgen blockade in locally advanced prostate cancer patients [61]. The prospective use of choline PET/CT for response assessment of standardized docetaxel first-line chemotherapy on the other hand showed no correlation between changes in choline uptake and clinical assessments of progression based on RECIST 1.1 and PSA values [62].

There is a fast-increasing use of ^{68}Ga-PSMA PET/CT for early biochemical recurrence detection in prostate cancer patients. The clinical utility of ^{68}Ga-PSMA PET for treatment response is not established (Fig.). First investigations showed promising results using ^{68}Ga-PSMA PET to evaluate ^{223}Ra therapy response [63]. The use of ^{68}Ga-PSMA PET for response assessment to androgen deprivation therapy (ADT) will need careful prospective evaluation, since preliminary in vitro results showed that ADT is increasing the cellular expression of PSMA; therefore, a novel "tumor flare" might be observed in these patients [64].

Take-Home Messages

- After neoadjuvant therapy, rectal cancer resectability is essential for treatment planning. Restaging MRI shows tumor regression and clearance of the mesorectal fascia. If nonoperative management is considered in very good responders, diffusion-weighted MRI combined with digital rectal examination and endoscopy accurately assesses clinical complete response.
- Systemic therapy response assessment with imaging is generally based on morphology. However,

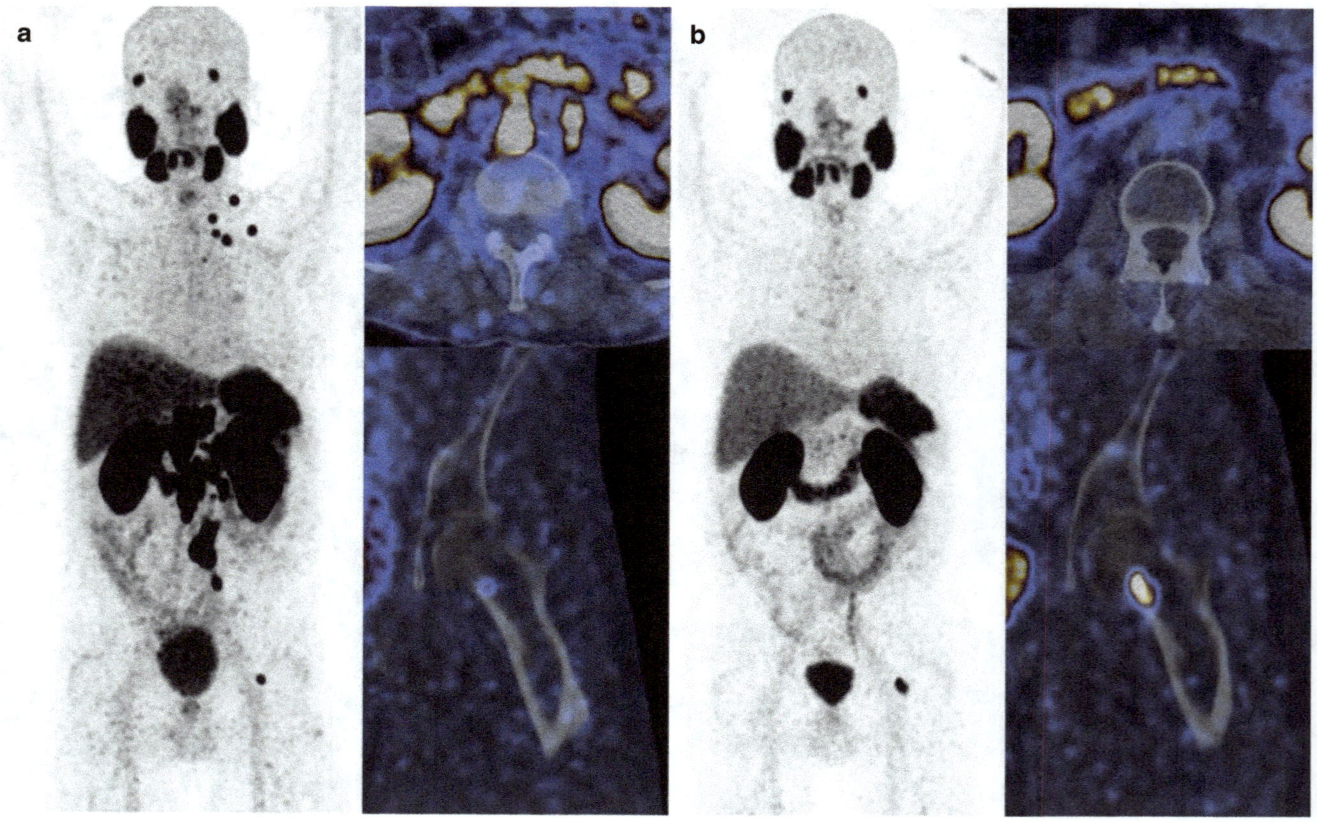

Fig. ^{68}Ga-PSMA PET before (**a**) and after (**b**) two cycles of ^{177}Lu-PSMA therapy with heterogeneous response: significant reduction in PSMA expression and size in all lymph node metastasis; however increase in PSMA expression and size of the bone metastasis

with the introduction of noncytotoxic therapies, response patterns became very heterogeneous. Especially immunotherapy or local therapy of liver metastasis such as SIRT can lead to an initial pseudoprogression as a part of the response pattern with delayed morphologic response.
- PET can be used to identify response before morphologic changes are present in selected cases (GIST).
- Morphologic assessment of bone metastasis is only possible for lytic lesions with a soft tissue component. New sclerotic lesions on CT are not necessarily a sign of tumor progression but might be a sign of response of previously occult lesions.

References

1. Nagtegaal ID, Quirke P. What is the role for the circumferential margin in the modern treatment of rectal cancer? J Clin Oncol. 2008;26:303–12.
2. Beets-Tan RG, Beets GL, Vliegen RF, et al. Accuracy of magnetic resonance imaging in prediction of tumour-free resection margin in rectal cancer surgery. Lancet. 2001;357:497–504.
3. Brown G, Radcliffe AG, Newcombe RG, Dallimore NS, Bourne MW, Williams GT. Preoperative assessment of prognostic factors in rectal cancer using high-resolution magnetic resonance imaging. Br J Surg. 2003;90:355–64.
4. Extramural depth of tumor invasion at thin-section MR in patients with rectal cancer: results of the MERCURY study. Radiology. 2007;243:132–9.
5. Beets-Tan RGH, Lambregts DMJ, Maas M, et al. Magnetic resonance imaging for clinical management of rectal cancer: updated recommendations from the 2016 European Society of Gastrointestinal and Abdominal Radiology (ESGAR) consensus meeting. Eur Radiol. 2017. https://doi.org/10.1007/s00330-017-5026-2.
6. Vliegen RF, Beets GL, Lammering G, et al. Mesorectal fascia invasion after neoadjuvant chemotherapy and radiation therapy for locally advanced rectal cancer: accuracy of MR imaging for prediction. Radiology. 2008;246:454–62.
7. Kulkarni T, Gollins S, Maw A, Hobson P, Byrne R, Widdowson D. Magnetic resonance imaging in rectal cancer downstaged using neoadjuvant chemoradiation: accuracy of prediction of tumour stage and circumferential resection margin status. Color Dis. 2008;10:479–89.
8. Habr-Gama A, Perez RO, Nadalin W, et al. Operative versus nonoperative treatment for stage 0 distal rectal cancer following chemoradiation therapy: long-term results. Ann Surg. 2004;240:711–7. discussion 717–718
9. Maas M, Beets-Tan RG, Lambregts DM, et al. Wait-and-see policy for clinical complete responders after chemoradiation for rectal cancer. J Clin Oncol. 2011;29:4633–40.
10. Beets-Tan RG, Beets GL. Rectal cancer: review with emphasis on MR imaging. Radiology. 2004;232:335–46.
11. van der Paardt MP, Zagers MB, Beets-Tan RG, Stoker J, Bipat S. Patients who undergo preoperative chemoradiotherapy for locally advanced rectal cancer restaged by using diagnostic MR imaging: a systematic review and meta-analysis. Radiology. 2013;269:101–12.
12. Dresen RC, Beets GL, Rutten HJ, et al. Locally advanced rectal cancer: MR imaging for restaging after neoadjuvant radiation therapy with concomitant chemotherapy. Part I. Are we able to predict tumor confined to the rectal wall? Radiology. 2009;252:71–80.
13. Barbaro B, Fiorucci C, Tebala C, et al. Locally advanced rectal cancer: MR imaging in prediction of response after preoperative chemotherapy and radiation therapy. Radiology. 2009;250:730–9.
14. Curvo-Semedo L, Lambregts DM, Maas M, et al. Rectal cancer: assessment of complete response to preoperative combined radiation therapy with chemotherapy--conventional MR volumetry versus diffusion-weighted MR imaging. Radiology. 2011;260:734–43.
15. Lambregts DM, Vandecaveye V, Barbaro B, et al. Diffusion-weighted MRI for selection of complete responders after chemoradiation for locally advanced rectal cancer: a multicenter study. Ann Surg Oncol. 2011;18(8):2224–31.
16. Napoleon B, Pujol B, Berger F, Valette PJ, Gerard JP, Souquet JC. Accuracy of endosonography in the staging of rectal cancer treated by radiotherapy. Br J Surg. 1991;78:785–8.
17. Mezzi G, Arcidiacono PG, Carrara S, et al. Endoscopic ultrasound and magnetic resonance imaging for re-staging rectal cancer after radiotherapy. World J Gastroenterol. 2009;15:5563–7.
18. Radovanovic Z, Breberina M, Petrovic T, Golubovic A, Radovanovic D. Accuracy of endorectal ultrasonography in staging locally advanced rectal cancer after preoperative chemoradiation. Surg Endosc. 2008;22:2412–5.
19. Pastor C, Subtil JC, Sola J, et al. Accuracy of endoscopic ultrasound to assess tumor response after neoadjuvant treatment in rectal cancer: can we trust the findings? Dis Colon Rectum. 2011;54:1141–6.
20. Bipat S, Glas AS, Slors FJ, Zwinderman AH, Bossuyt PM, Stoker J. Rectal cancer: local staging and assessment of lymph node involvement with endoluminal US, CT, and MR imaging—a meta-analysis. Radiology. 2004;232:773–83.
21. Organization WH. WHO handbook for reporting results of cancer treatment; 1979.
22. Eisenhauer EA, Therasse P, Bogaerts J, et al. New response evaluation criteria in solid tumours: revised RECIST guideline (version 1.1). Eur J Cancer. 2009;45:228–47.
23. Seymour L, Bogaerts J, Perrone A, et al. iRECIST: guidelines for response criteria for use in trials testing immunotherapeutics. Lancet Oncol. 2017;18:e143–52.
24. Chiou VL, Burotto M. Pseudoprogression and immune-related response in solid tumors. J Clin Oncol. 2015;33:3541–3.
25. Wong ANM, McArthur GA, Hofman MS, Hicks RJ. The advantages and challenges of using FDG PET/CT for response assessment in melanoma in the era of targeted agents and immunotherapy. Eur J Nucl Med Mol Imaging. 2017;44:67–77.
26. Rymer B, Curtis NJ, Siddiqui MR, Chand M. FDG PET/CT can assess the response of locally advanced rectal cancer to neoadjuvant chemoradiotherapy: evidence from meta-analysis and systematic review. Clin Nucl Med. 2016;41:371–5.
27. Wahl RL, Jacene H, Kasamon Y, Lodge MA. From RECIST to PERCIST: evolving considerations for PET response criteria in solid tumors. J Nucl Med. 2009;50(Suppl 1):122S–50S.
28. Pinker K, Riedl C, Weber WA. Evaluating tumor response with FDG PET: updates on PERCIST, comparison with EORTC criteria and clues to future developments. Eur J Nucl Med Mol Imaging. 2017;44:55–66.
29. van Oosterom AT, Judson I, Verweij J, et al. Safety and efficacy of imatinib (STI571) in metastatic gastrointestinal stromal tumours: a phase I study. Lancet. 2001;358:1421–3.
30. Joensuu H. Treatment of inoperable gastrointestinal stromal tumor (GIST) with Imatinib (Glivec, Gleevec). Med Klin (Munich). 2002;97(Suppl 1):28–30.
31. Van den Abbeele AD. The lessons of GIST--PET and PET/CT: a new paradigm for imaging. Oncologist. 2008;13(Suppl 2):8–13.
32. Shinagare AB, Jagannathan JP, Krajewski KM, Ramaiya NH. Liver metastases in the era of molecular targeted therapy: new faces of treatment response. AJR Am J Roentgenol. 2013;201:W15–28.
33. Choi H, Charnsangavej C, Faria SC, et al. Correlation of computed tomography and positron emission tomography in patients with metastatic gastrointestinal stromal tumor treated at a single institution with imatinib mesylate: proposal of new computed tomography response criteria. J Clin Oncol. 2007;25:1753–9.

34. Apfaltrer P, Meyer M, Meier C, et al. Contrast-enhanced dual-energy CT of gastrointestinal stromal tumors: is iodine-related attenuation a potential indicator of tumor response? Investig Radiol. 2012;47:65–70.
35. Tang L, Zhang XP, Sun YS, et al. Gastrointestinal stromal tumors treated with imatinib mesylate: apparent diffusion coefficient in the evaluation of therapy response in patients. Radiology. 2011;258:729–38.
36. Casali PG, Blay JY, Bertuzzi A, et al. Gastrointestinal stromal tumours: ESMO clinical practice guidelines for diagnosis, treatment and follow-up. Ann Oncol. 2014;25:21–6.
37. Holdsworth CH, Badawi RD, Manola JB, et al. CT and PET: early prognostic indicators of response to imatinib mesylate in patients with gastrointestinal stromal tumor. AJR Am J Roentgenol. 2007;189:W324–30.
38. Benjamin RS, Schoffski P, Hartmann JT, et al. Efficacy and safety of motesanib, an oral inhibitor of VEGF, PDGF, and kit receptors, in patients with imatinib-resistant gastrointestinal stromal tumors. Cancer Chemother Pharmacol. 2011;68:69–77.
39. Farag S, de Geus-Oei LF, Van der Graaf WT, et al. Early response evaluation by 18F-FDG-PET influences management in gastrointestinal stromal tumor (GIST) patients treated with imatinib with neo-adjuvant intent. J Nucl Med. 2017. https://doi.org/10.2967/jnumed.117.196642.
40. Stubbs RS, Cannan RJ, Mitchell AW. Selective internal radiation therapy with 90yttrium microspheres for extensive colorectal liver metastases. J Gastrointest Surg. 2001;5:294–302.
41. Boppudi S, Wickremesekera SK, Nowitz M, Stubbs R. Evaluation of the role of CT in the assessment of response to selective internal radiation therapy in patients with colorectal liver metastases. Australas Radiol. 2006;50:570–7.
42. Morsbach F, Pfammatter T, Reiner CS, et al. Computed tomographic perfusion imaging for the prediction of response and survival to transarterial radioembolization of liver metastases. Investig Radiol. 2013;48:787–94.
43. Reiner CS, Morsbach F, Sah BR, et al. Early treatment response evaluation after yttrium-90 radioembolization of liver malignancy with CT perfusion. J Vasc Interv Radiol. 2014;25:747–59.
44. Lee SH, Lee JM, Kim KW, et al. Dual-energy computed tomography to assess tumor response to hepatic radiofrequency ablation: potential diagnostic value of virtual noncontrast images and iodine maps. Investig Radiol. 2011;46:77–84.
45. Schmeel FC, Simon B, Sabet A, et al. Diffusion-weighted magnetic resonance imaging predicts survival in patients with liver-predominant metastatic colorectal cancer shortly after selective internal radiation therapy. Eur Radiol. 2017;27:966–75.
46. Wong CY, Qing F, Savin M, et al. Reduction of metastatic load to liver after intraarterial hepatic yttrium-90 radioembolization as evaluated by [^{18}F]fluorodeoxyglucose positron emission tomographic imaging. J Vasc Interv Radiol. 2005;16:1101–6.
47. Szyszko T, Al-Nahhas A, Canelo R, et al. Assessment of response to treatment of unresectable liver tumours with 90Y microspheres: value of FDG PET versus computed tomography. Nucl Med Commun. 2007;28:15–20.
48. Annunziata S, Treglia G, Caldarella C, Galiandro F. The role of 18F-FDG-PET and PET/CT in patients with colorectal liver metastases undergoing selective internal radiation therapy with yttrium-90: a first evidence-based review. ScientificWorldJournal. 2014;2014:879469.
49. Fendler WP, Philippe Tiega DB, Ilhan H, et al. Validation of several SUV-based parameters derived from 18F-FDG PET for prediction of survival after SIRT of hepatic metastases from colorectal cancer. J Nucl Med. 2013;54:1202–8.
50. Dierckx R, Maes A, Peeters M, Van De Wiele C. FDG PET for monitoring response to local and locoregional therapy in HCC and liver metastases. Q J Nucl Med Mol Imaging. 2009;53:336–42.
51. Pavel ME, Hainsworth JD, Baudin E, et al. Everolimus plus octreotide long-acting repeatable for the treatment of advanced neuroendocrine tumours associated with carcinoid syndrome (RADIANT-2): a randomised, placebo-controlled, phase 3 study. Lancet. 2011;378:2005–12.
52. Strosberg J, El-Haddad G, Wolin E, et al. Phase 3 trial of 177Lu-Dotatate for Midgut neuroendocrine tumors. N Engl J Med. 2017;376:125–35.
53. Hicks RJ, Kwekkeboom DJ, Krenning E, et al. ENETS Consensus Guidelines for the Standards of Care in Neuroendocrine Neoplasia: peptide receptor radionuclide therapy with radiolabeled somatostatin analogues. Neuroendocrinology. 2017;105(3):295–309.
54. Haug AR, Auernhammer CJ, Wangler B, et al. 68Ga-DOTATATE PET/CT for the early prediction of response to somatostatin receptor-mediated radionuclide therapy in patients with well-differentiated neuroendocrine tumors. J Nucl Med. 2010;51:1349–56.
55. de Bono JS, Logothetis CJ, Molina A, et al. Abiraterone and increased survival in metastatic prostate cancer. N Engl J Med. 2011;364:1995–2005.
56. Parker C, Nilsson S, Heinrich D, et al. Alpha emitter radium-223 and survival in metastatic prostate cancer. N Engl J Med. 2013;369:213–23.
57. Costelloe CM, Chuang HH, Madewell JE, Ueno NT. Cancer response criteria and bone metastases: RECIST 1.1, MDA and PERCIST. J Cancer. 2010;1:80–92.
58. Hamaoka T, Madewell JE, Podoloff DA, Hortobagyi GN, Ueno NT. Bone imaging in metastatic breast cancer. J Clin Oncol. 2004;22:2942–53.
59. Messiou C, Collins DJ, Giles S, de Bono JS, Bianchini D, de Souza NM. Assessing response in bone metastases in prostate cancer with diffusion weighted MRI. Eur Radiol. 2011;21:2169–77.
60. Reischauer C, Froehlich JM, Koh DM, et al. Bone metastases from prostate cancer: assessing treatment response by using diffusion-weighted imaging and functional diffusion maps--initial observations. Radiology. 2010;257:523–31.
61. Schwarzenbock SM, Knieling A, Souvatzoglou M, et al. [^{11}C]choline PET/CT in therapy response assessment of a neoadjuvant therapy in locally advanced and high risk prostate cancer before radical prostatectomy. Oncotarget. 2016;7:63747–57.
62. Schwarzenbock SM, Eiber M, Kundt G, et al. Prospective evaluation of [^{11}C]choline PET/CT in therapy response assessment of standardized docetaxel first-line chemotherapy in patients with advanced castration refractory prostate cancer. Eur J Nucl Med Mol Imaging. 2016;43:2105–13.
63. Bieth M, Kronke M, Tauber R, et al. Exploring new multimodal quantitative imaging indices for the assessment of osseous tumour burden in prostate cancer using 68Ga-PSMA-PET/CT. J Nucl Med. 2017;58(10):1632–7.
64. Meller B, Bremmer F, Sahlmann CO, et al. Alterations in androgen deprivation enhanced prostate-specific membrane antigen (PSMA) expression in prostate cancer cells as a target for diagnostics and therapy. EJNMMI Res. 2015;5:66.

18

Imaging of Testicular and Scrotal Masses: The Essentials

Andreas G. Wibmer and Hebert Alberto Vargas

Learning Objectives

- To identify the clinical scenarios where imaging of the testes and scrotum is indicated
- To learn the association between imaging features and the management of patients with testicular and scrotal masses

Clinical Scenarios Where Imaging Is Indicated

The first key to a meaningful radiology report is to be aware of the clinical indication for which the imaging study was requested.

Scrotal Pain With or Without a Palpable Mass

Infection (i.e., epididymitis/orchitis), torsion of the testis or testicular appendage, vascular pathologies (e.g., varicocele), hydrocele, and trauma are the most common causes of scrotal pain. Ultrasound (US) allows differentiation from testicular neoplasms and helps narrow the differential diagnosis in clinically equivocal cases. From an oncologic perspective, a few factors should be considered before contemplating these diagnoses:

- Their age distribution overlaps with most scrotal and testicular malignancies, and asymptomatic neoplasms can be incidentally identified on imaging.
- About one third of scrotal/testicular malignancies can present with scrotal pain.
- Testicular infection, hematomas, and testicular infarcts can be focal and mimic testicular neoplasms, although the latter are commonly more vascularized on Doppler US. In the right clinical setting and absence of internal vascularity, focal infarct, hematoma, or infection might be an appropriate differential diagnosis and avoid futile surgery. However, these cases need to be followed up closely to document involution and exclude malignancy.

Palpable Painless or Incidental Scrotal Mass

In this scenario, the first and most important task of imaging is localizing the mass to differentiate testicular from extra-testicular origin. In equivocal cases on US, magnetic resonance imaging (MRI) may be used as a problem-solving tool. As a second step, US (and in some selected cases MRI) may narrow the differential diagnosis, most importantly by identifying cysts, cyst-like lesions, and other benign entities with typical appearance (described below). In the absence of unequivocally benign imaging findings, it is important to clearly convey the suspicion for a malignant neoplasm to the referring physician. In case of a testicular mass, this often triggers an intervention (orchiectomy), as further management hinges on adequate histopathologic characterization, which is not always possible through biopsies due to the microscopic heterogeneity of many testicular cancers.

A. G. Wibmer · H. A. Vargas (✉)
Radiology- Memorial Sloan Kettering Cancer Center, New York, NY, USA
e-mail: wibmera@mskcc.org; vargasah@mskcc.org

Isolated Retroperitoneal Lymphadenopathy

Lymphoma, extragonadal germ cell tumors, and testicular cancer metastases are the most common etiology for isolated retroperitoneal lymphadenopathy. Screening testicular US is routinely performed in this scenario. In case of testicular cancer, for which retroperitoneal nodes are the first lymphatic draining points and considered regional spread (i.e., "N") in the TNM staging system, the spatial distribution of the retroperitoneal disease allows for some suggestions on the side of the testicular primary. Left-sided tumors typically metastasize to left periaortic and preaortic nodes, while right-sided cancers metastasize to nodes around the inferior vena cava, including inter-aortocaval nodes. These considerations may seem somewhat academic for the reporting radiologist, who will diligently screen both testes anyway, not least due to the possibility of synchronous bilateral testicular cancers, seen in about 0.6% of all cases [1]. When confronted with equivocal testicular imaging findings, however, this information might help to reach a sound conclusion. If a testicular mass is identified, the objectives of imaging are similar to those described in the previous paragraph. Beyond specific imaging characteristics of some entities, which will be described below, the following facts might be helpful while interpreting these scans:

- Some types of primary testicular cancers, although widely metastatic, might be very small or involuted. On imaging, these primary tumors can be undetectable, or appear as small masses or focal calcifications, a phenomenon that has been referred to as "burned-out" primary tumor (Fig.).
- Some testicular cancers produce high levels of serum tumor markers, most notably alpha-fetoprotein (AFP), human chorionic gonadotropin (hCG), and lactate dehydrogenase (LDH). Although of limited sensitivity and specificity, high levels of these markers indicate a testicular origin of retroperitoneal lymphadenopathy and might help the radiologist to interpret equivocal imaging findings.

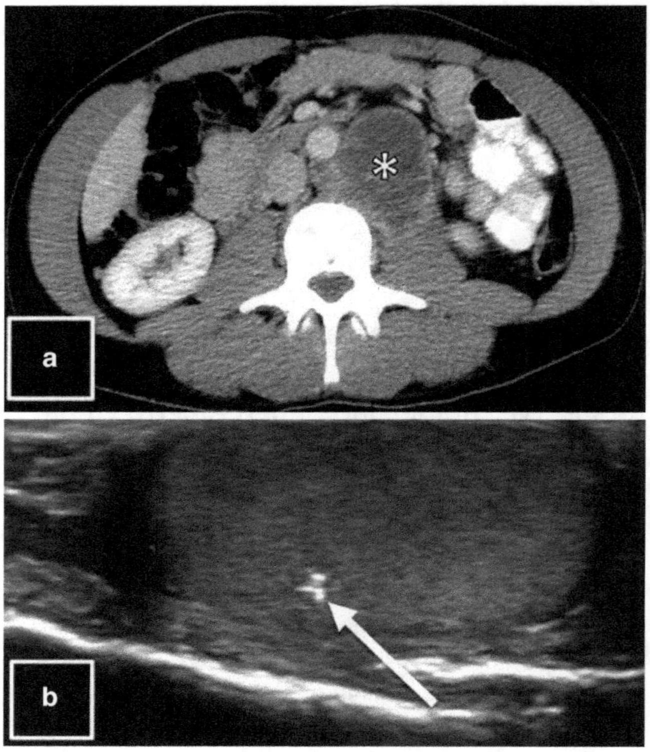

Fig. A 38-year-old with hip pain. (**a**) CT of the abdomen and pelvis shows left para-aortic and preaortic lymphadenopathy (asterisk), raising the suspicion for metastatic left-sided testicular cancer. (**b**) US of the left scrotum shows an intratesticular focal calcification (arrow); the right testis was unremarkable (not shown). Histopathology of the left orchiectomy specimen confirmed a "burned-out" germ cell tumor

Follow-Up After Curative Treatment of Testicular Cancer

Patients with treated testicular cancer are at ≥10-fold increased risk for developing contralateral metachronous cancer with a 15-year cumulative incidence of 1.9% [1]. This elevated pretest probability should be considered when performing surveillance studies. Patients having undergone treatment, particularly those who had metastatic disease, will also need follow-up imaging exams of other parts of the body. In this scenario, the following points deserve consideration:

- Most recurrences occur within the first 2 years after treatment. Late relapses, although less common, have been reported more than 5 years after treatment.
- The most common sites of recurrence are the retroperitoneal lymph nodes. Follow-up studies, especially computed tomography (CT), often spare the pelvis to minimize radiation dose.
  - CAVEAT: In patients with any kind of surgery involving the scrotum or inguinal canal (e.g., hernia repair, orchiopexy, or others), lymphatic drainage is altered, and recurrences can occur in variable anatomic patterns, including inguinal lymph node involvement.
  - In patients initially treated with adequate retroperitoneal lymph node dissection, retroperitoneal recurrence is rare. These patients are more likely to develop lung metastases.

- The most common site of organ metastases is the lung, and CT of the chest is more sensitive and specific for their detection than radiographs.
- After chemo- and/or radiotherapy, there is an increased long-term risk for secondary malignancies, most commonly cancers of the stomach, pancreas, urinary bladder, colon, lung, and esophagus and malignant mesothelioma of the pleura [2].

Imaging Characterization of Testicular and Scrotal Masses

Ultrasound is the initial imaging examination of choice for testicular and scrotal abnormalities; MRI may serve as a diagnostic adjuvant in selected cases. The main task of imaging – and also key to characterization – is to localize the mass. Masses arising within the testis have a higher likelihood of malignancy than those occurring in extra-testicular sites, including the epididymis (although there are some exceptions, as outlined below).

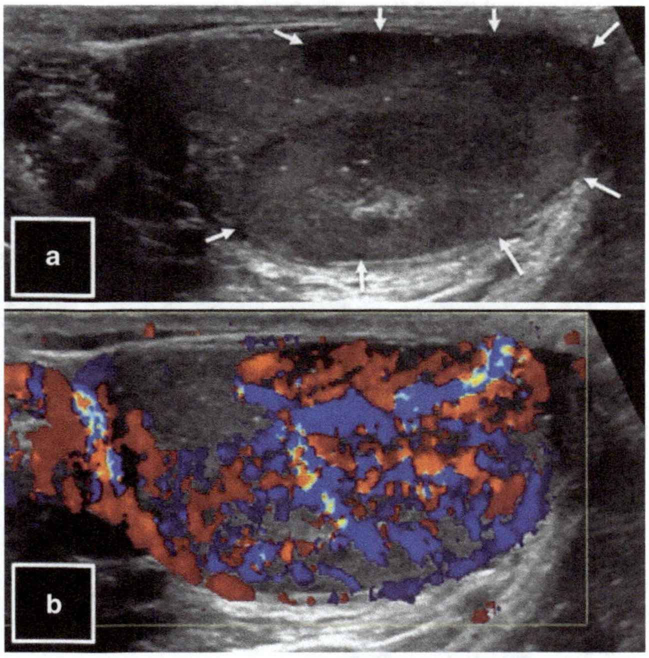

Fig. A 38-year-old with a painless palpable right scrotal mass. (**a**) Gray-scale US of the scrotum shows microlithiasis and an intratesticular, well-circumscribed, lobulated, heterogeneously hypoechoic mass (arrows) with (**b**) internal vascularity on Doppler US. These features are the hallmarks of a malignant testicular neoplasm; the final diagnosis of seminoma was established after orchiectomy

TesticularMasses

Testicular Malignancies

Are typically heterogeneously hypoechoic compared to normal testicular tissue on US. They are well-defined, often lobulated lesions with internal blood flow detectable on Doppler US (Figs.). The likelihood of malig-nancy is high if all these features are present; and this high level of suspicion must be expressed in the radiology report. Characterization of histologic subtypes based on imaging is currently not possible; thus orchiectomy is typically the next step for most of these patients. These imaging features are not specific for testicular cancer and might also be encoun-tered in benign or nonneoplastic tumor mimics (Fig.). The following paragraphs describe typical imaging features of more common benign and nonneoplastic testicular masses that may allow for confident exclusion of malignancy based on imaging.

Testicular Microlithiasis

This frequently encountered entity is defined as the presence of five or more echogenic, non-shadowing foci <3 mm per testis (Fig.). Although it can be associated with testicular cancer, the European Society of Urogenital Radiology recommends against follow-up of isolated microlithiasis in the absence of risk factors (i.e., personal or family history of germ cell tumor, testicular atrophy <12 mL, history of maldescent or orchiopexy) [3].

Cystic TesticularLesions

Similar to other organ systems, cysts in the testes are well-defined, homogeneously hypoechoic lesions with posterior acoustic enhancement on US (Fig.). Complex cysts have some degree of internal echogenicity. However, all cysts lack internal vascularity on Doppler US. The differentiation of tunica albuginea cysts which are found in a peripheral or paratesticular location vs. central cysts has no clinical significance. Ectasia of the rete testis is typically encountered in older men and appears as a cluster of multiple small cysts and tubules along the testicular mediastinum (Fig.). Testicular hematomas and abscesses can have large cystic components and, if considered as a differential diagnosis in the appropriate clinical setting, always need close follow-up. Cystic changes can be seen in testicular malignancies; however, purely cystic cancers are exceedingly rare.

Epidermoid Cysts

This benign lesion can have typical features on US allowing for confident diagnosis in most cases. Multiple concentric

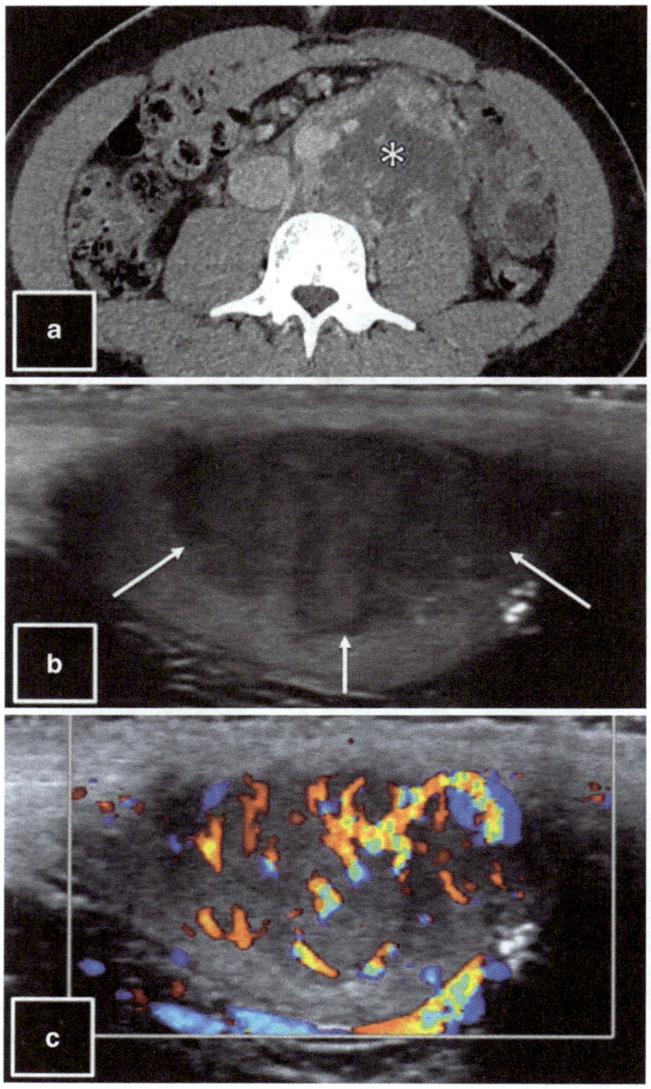

Fig. A 24-year-old with back pain. (**a**) CT of the abdomen and pelvis shows left para-aortic and preaortic lymphadenopathy (arrow), suspicious for metastatic left-sided testicular cancer. (**b**) Gray-scale US of the scrotum shows a left-sided intratesticular, well-circumscribed, lobulated, heterogeneously hypoechoic mass (arrows) with (**c**) internal flow on Doppler US. These features are the hallmarks of a malignant testicular neoplasm; the final diagnosis of mature teratoma was established after orchiectomy

layers of keratinous debris give it a more solid appearance of a round hypoechoic lesion with multiple concentric hyperintense internal layers resembling an "onion skin" and lacking internal blood flow (Fig.. Although these findings are specific for the entity, some epidermoid cysts can also mimic testicular cancers on imaging (Fig.).

Focal Infections, Hematomas, and Infarcts

In the adequate clinical context, these entities might be considered in the differential diagnoses: local or systemic signs of infection (Fig.) and recent history of inguinal or scro-

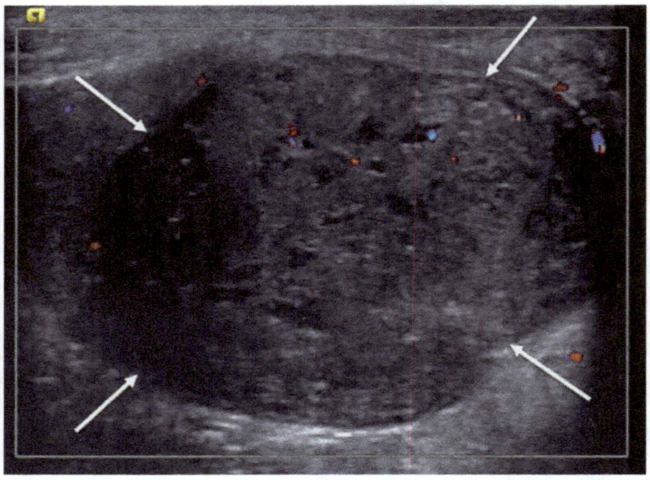

Fig. A 54-year-old with a painless palpable right scrotal mass. (**a**) US of the scrotum shows an intratesticular, well-circumscribed, lobulated, heterogeneously hypoechoic mass (arrows) with low-level internal vascularity on Doppler US. These features are the hallmarks of a malignant testicular neoplasm, justifying orchiectomy; the final histopathologic diagnosis was epidermoid cyst

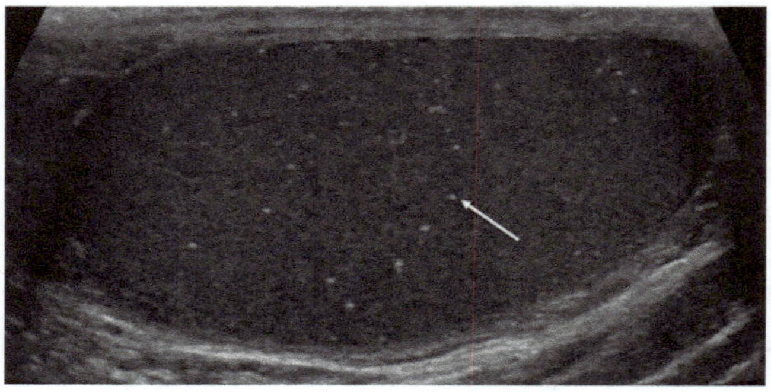

Fig. Imaging features of microlithiasis. Multiple (i.e., ≥5 per tes-tis) microcalcifications (i.e., <3 mm) within the testicular parenchyma; one microcalcification is marked with an arrow

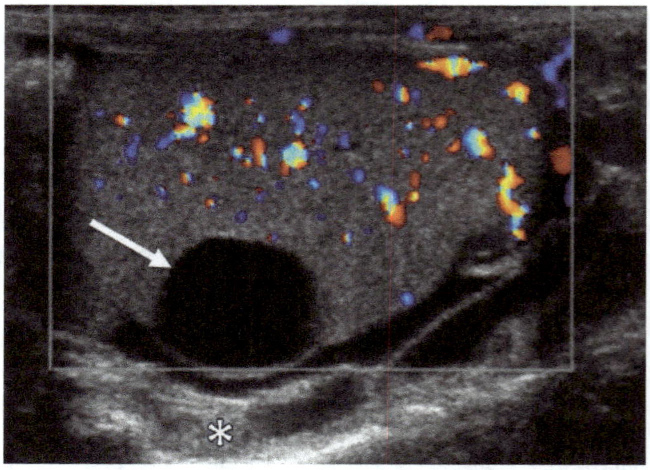

Fig. Imaging features of a simple testicular cyst. A round, well-defined, homogeneously hypoechoic lesion (arrow) with posterior acoustic enhancement (asterisk) and lack of internal flow

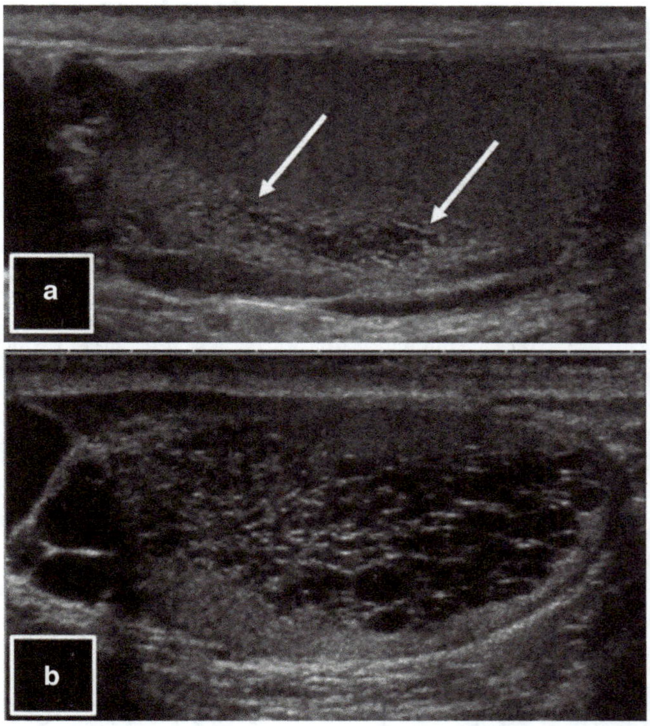

Fig. Two cases of ectasia of the rete testis. (**a**) 67-year-old patient with prostate cancer and an incidentally discovered testicular lesion. US of the scrotum shows a cluster of multiple small cysts and tubules along the testicular mediastinum (arrows), consistent with rete testis ectasia. (**b**) In this example of a 70-year-old patient with prostate cancer and a remote history of scrotal surgery, rete ectasia is more extensive, occupying large parts of the testis

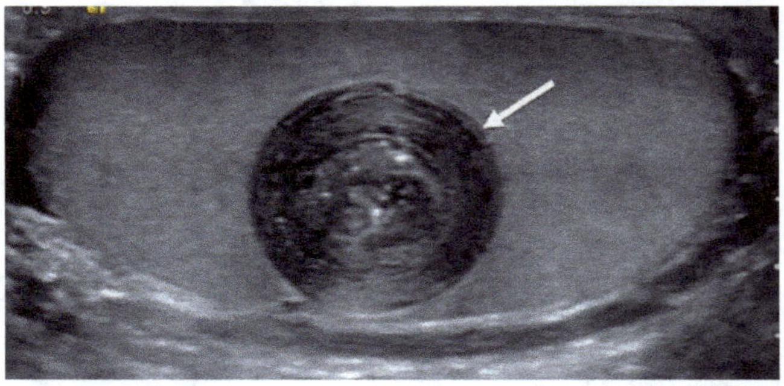

Fig. A 23-year-old with a painless palpable scrotal mass. US of the scrotum shows a round, well-delineated lesion with multiple concentric hyperintense internal layers, resembling an "onion skin," consistent with epidermoid cyst, justifying a nonsurgical, observational approach. The appearance of the mass did not change over the course of 3 years

tal surgery/trauma, torsion, or abnormal states of coagulation for hematoma and infarction (Fig.). All these entities share the lack of internal vascular flow on Doppler US. As previously mentioned, all cases must be monitored to docu-ment involution and exclude malignancy.

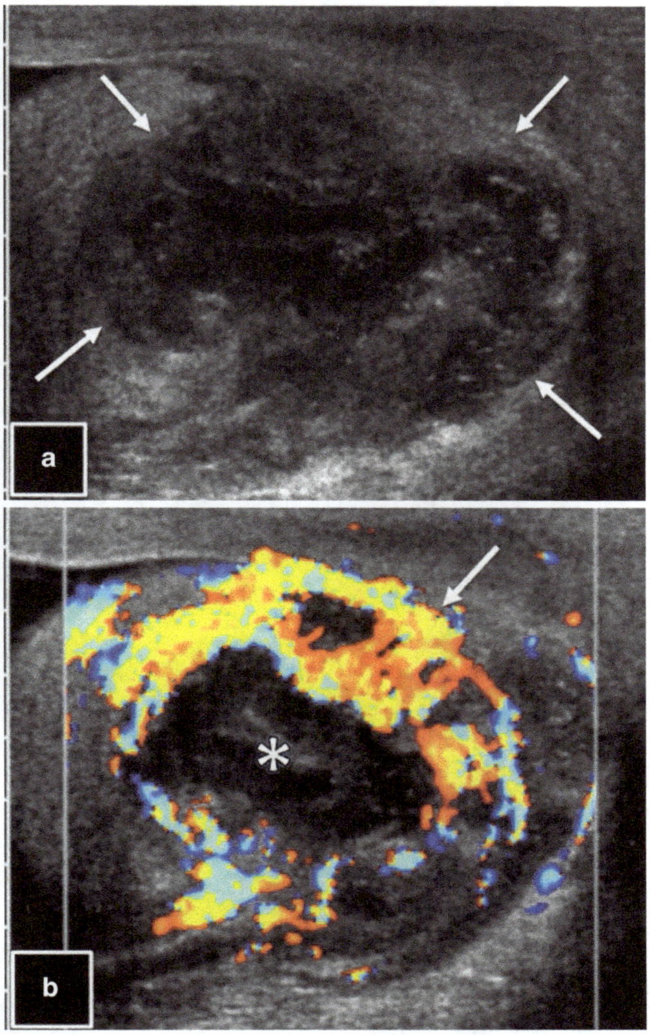

Fig. An 88-year-old with anastomotic leakage after rectal sur-gery, pelvic abscesses, sepsis, and painful scrotal swelling. (**a**) US of the scrotum shows a well-circumscribed, lobulated, heterogeneously hypoechoic mass (arrows) with (**b**) intense peripheral (arrow) but no central (asterisk) flow on Doppler US. The patient underwent orchiectomy, which confirmed the infectious etiology

Testicular Adrenal Rest

These benign masses occur in patients with congenital adrenal hyperplasia. In addition to clinical history, bilaterality is the key to the diagnosis [4], although unilateral appearance has been reported [5]. Their imaging features are otherwise similar to testicular cancer.

Epididymal Masses

Epididymal masses or mass-like lesions are frequently encountered as incidental findings on scrotal ultrasound. They are almost always benign and do not require specific treatment. Cysts are well-defined, homogeneously

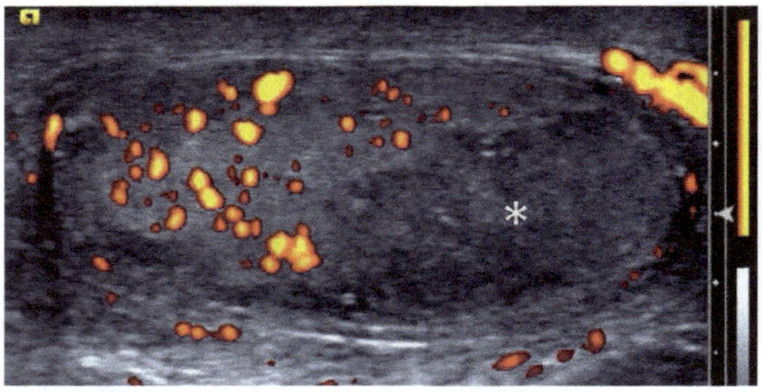

Fig. A 56-year-old with painless right scrotal swelling after recent right nephrectomy with reported gonadal vein tie off/thrombosis. US of the scrotum shows an intratesticular, well-circumscribed, lobulated, heterogeneously hypoechoic mass without internal flow on Power Doppler ultrasound (asterisk). The clinical history and imaging appearance suggest partial/focal testicular infarction, and involution was documented on follow-up US (not shown)

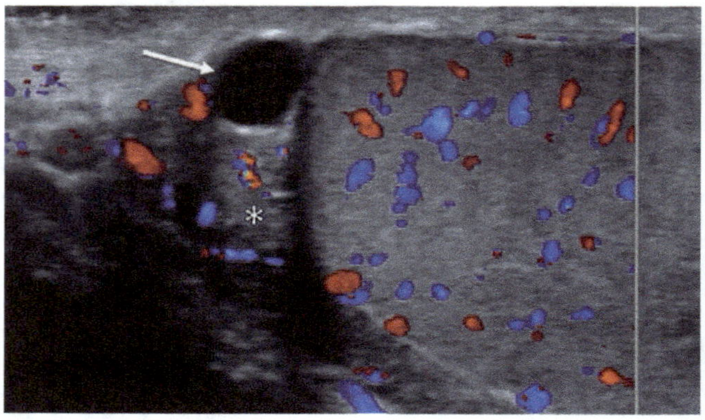

Fig. Imaging features of a simple epididymal cyst. A round, well-defined, homogeneously hypoechoic lesion within the epididymis (arrow) with posterior acoustic enhancement (asterisk) and lack of internal flow.

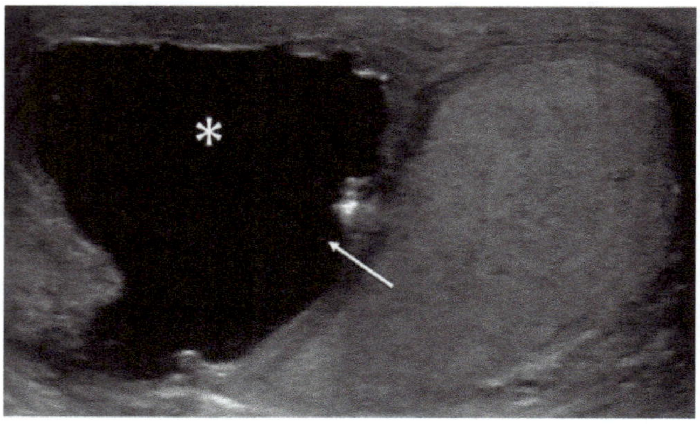

Fig.A 61-year-old with resolved scrotal pain but persistent swelling after antibiotic therapy for epididymitis. US of the scrotum shows a cystic epididymal lesion (asterisk) with multiple small internal low-level echoes (the arrow is pointing at one), consistent with spermatocele

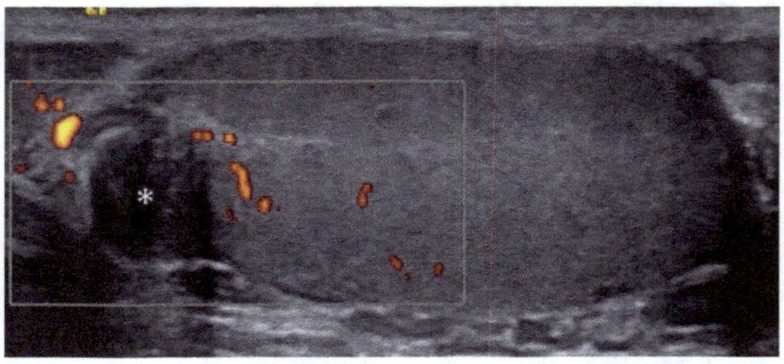

Fig. A 35-year-old with scrotal pain without a palpable mass. US of the scrotum shows a round, well-delineated, heterogeneously hypoechoic mass within the epididymis without detectable flow on Doppler US (asterisk). These imaging findings are non-specific; however, the epididymal location suggests a benign entity; excisional biopsy showed adenomatoid tumor

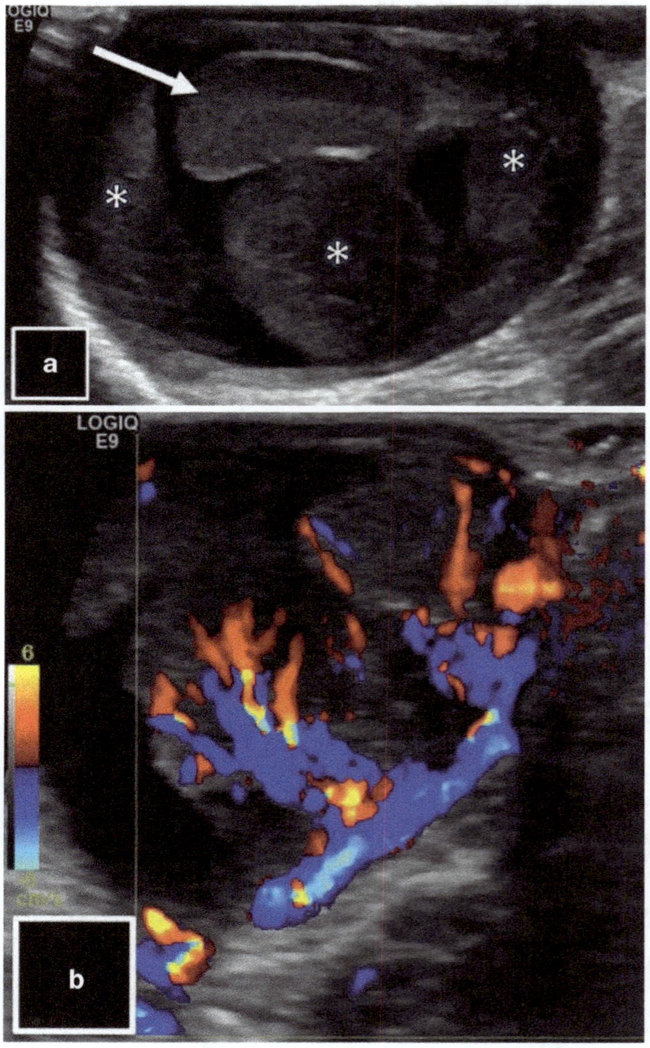

Fig. A 2-year-old with scrotal swelling and mild scrotal pain. (**a**) Gray-scale US of the scrotum shows a large extra-testicular, hypoechoic mass (asterisk); the normal testis is marked with an arrow. (**b**) Doppler US demonstrates intense intralesional blood flow. In this age group, the suspicion for extra-testicular rhabdomyosarcoma, which was confirmed on histopathology, has to be unequivocally conveyed to the referring physician

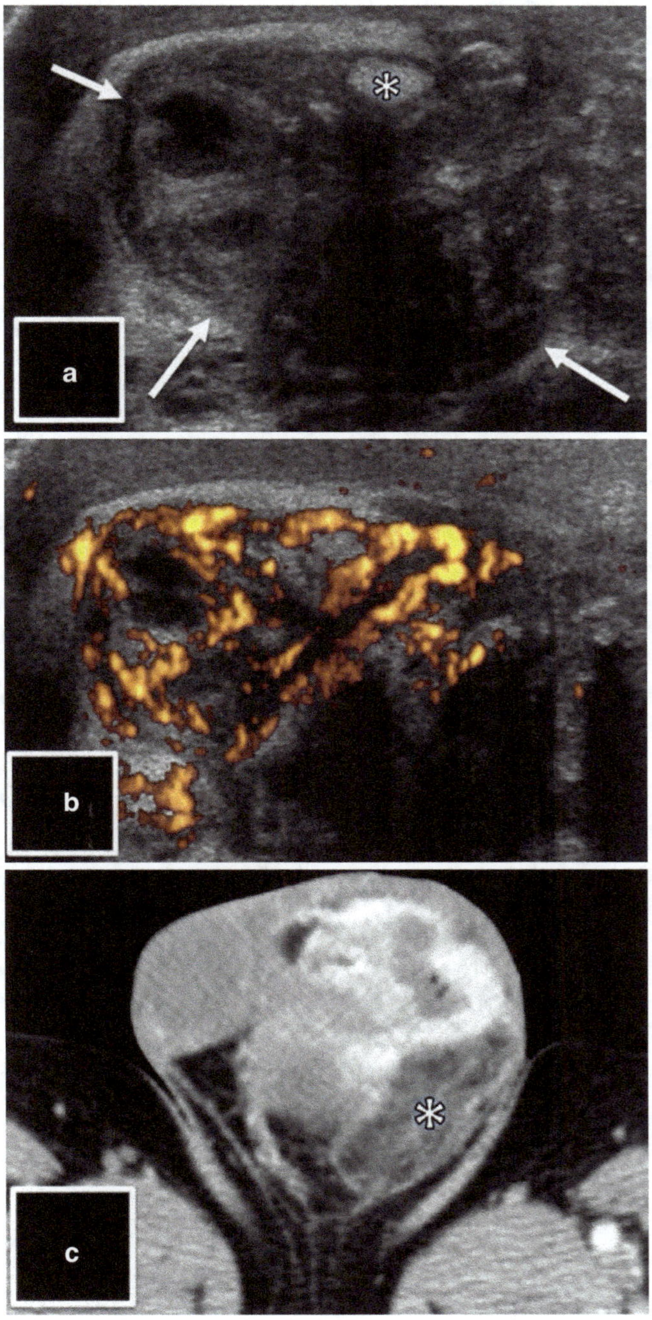

Fig. A 61-year-old with a long-standing history of hydrocele and a recent increase of scrotal swelling. (**a**) Gray-scale US shows an extra-testicular, heterogeneously hypointense mass (arrows) with (**b**) intense internal flow on Doppler US; the normal epididymis is marked within (asterisk) (**a**). These findings are suspicious for malignancy; (**c**) the presence of intralesional fat (asterisk) on staging CT suggests liposarcoma, which was confirmed on histopathology

hypoechoic lesions of varying size, most frequently located in the epididymal head (Fig.). Multiple small low-level echoes within a cystic lesion in a patient with prior vasec-tomy or other inguinal/scrotal surgery are suggestive of a spermatocele (Fig.). The most common solid neo-plasms of the epididymis are adenomatoid tumors and leio-myomas. Both entities are well defined and show variable size, echogenicity, and vascular flow (Fig.). The dif-ferentiation of these benign neoplasms from sperm (cell) granulomas is rarely possible and not necessary from a clini-cal perspective.

Extra-TesticularMasses

As with epididymal tumors, most scrotal neoplasms outside the testes are benign, most commonly lipomas and fibrous pseudotumors. Scrotoliths are calcified tumor-like masses that can be encountered in any part of the scrotum. The rare exceptions are paratesticular rhabdomyosarcomas in children and adolescents, as well as sarcomas, metastases, and locally advanced scrotal skin cancer in adults.

Malignant Paratesticular Tumors

Key to the diagnosis of a rhabdomyosarcoma is patient age in conjunction with a hypoechoic extra-testicular mass that is highly vascular on Doppler US (Fig.). Paratesticular sarcomas are heterogeneous, markedly hypervascular tumors of adult men; liposarcomas can contain macroscopic fat (Fig.). The diagnosis of metastases and locally advanced skin cancer can be made in the adequate clinical context.

Fat-Containing Paratesticular Lesions

The presence of fat in an extra-testicular mass, most accurately assessed on MRI, can guide the radiologist toward the correct diagnosis. The most common fat-containing paratesticular neoplasm is lipoma of the spermatic cord. Large, markedly hypervascular fat-containing masses in an adult are suspicious for liposarcoma (Fig.). Fat-containing tumor mimics are inguinal-scrotal hernias and fat necrosis after trauma or surgery.

Key Points

- The role of imaging testicular and scrotal masses will vary according to the clinical scenario.
- Imaging is helpful to establish or narrow the differential diagnoses.

ConcludingRemarks

Understanding the clinical scenario in which a scrotal imaging exam is performed is pivotal for meaningful radiology reports. Solid testicular masses with internal vascular flow must prompt a high level of suspicion for testicular malignancy, unless unequivocal imaging findings suggest a benign diagnosis. Most epididymal and paratesticular masses are benign; however, irregularly shaped, ill-defined, hypervascular masses may represent malignant tumors.

References

1. Fossa SD, Chen J, Schonfeld SJ, McGlynn KA, McMaster ML, Gail MH, et al. Risk of contralateral testicular cancer: a population-based study of 29,515 U.S. men. J Natl Cancer Inst. 2005;97(14):1056–66.
2. Travis LB, Fossa SD, Schonfeld SJ, McMaster ML, Lynch CF, Storm H, et al. Second cancers among 40,576 testicular cancer patients: focus on long-term survivors. J Natl Cancer Inst. 2005;97(18):1354–65.
3. Richenberg J, Belfield J, Ramchandani P, Rocher L, Freeman S, Tsili AC, et al. Testicular microlithiasis imaging and follow-up: guidelines of the ESUR scrotal imaging subcommittee. Eur Radiol. 2015;25(2):323–30.
4. Wang Z, Yang Z, Wang W, Chen LD, Huang Y, Li W, et al. Diagnosis of testicular adrenal rest tumors on ultrasound: a retrospective study of 15 cases report. Medicine. 2015;94(36):e1471.
5. Stikkelbroeck NM, Suliman HM, Otten BJ, Hermus AR, Blickman JG, Jager GJ. Testicular adrenal rest tumours in postpubertal males with congenital adrenal hyperplasia: sonographic and MR features. Eur Radiol. 2003;13(7):1597–603.

19

Benign Diseases of the Colon and Rectum (Incl. CT Colonography)

Thomas Mang and Philippe Lefere

> **Learning Objectives**
> - To illustrate the spectrum of benign conditions of the colon and rectum, seen at CT colonography and conventional cross-sectional imaging
> - To learn how to characterize and differentiate benign polypoid and stenotic filling defects with 3D and 2D CT colonography imaging criteria
> - To discuss both specific and unspecific cross-sectional imaging criteria of various infectious and noninfectious inflammatory conditions of the colon

Introduction

Diagnostic imaging of the colon and the rectum has undergone a remarkable evolution over the last few decades. Routine cross-sectional imaging techniques, such as standard abdominal CT scans, provide the possibility to evaluate the course of the colon for mural and extracolonic changes. With the introduction of CT colonography (CTC) to the clinical routine, a noninvasive and safe diagnostic test for imaging the endoluminal aspect of the entire colon became available. CTC has been shown to be as accurate as optical colonoscopy (OC) for the detection of advanced colonic neoplasia, including advanced adenomas and cancers [1]. Since its performance is clearly superior to that of the barium enema, it is now recommended as the radiological method of choice for the detection of colorectal neoplasia [2, 3]. The barium enema is no longer recommended for this indication. Indeed, the role of the barium enema in daily radiological imaging has been fading over the last several years due to the emerging use of endoscopic techniques. Today, OC represents the diagnostic and therapeutic gold standard in colonic imaging. CTC has become a valuable complementary diagnostic tool to OC, serving as an alternative colonic screening test, and it represents the method of choice in patients with incomplete colonoscopy or with contraindications to colonoscopy [3].

The purpose of this contribution is to focus on benign conditions of the colon and rectum that can be detected during CTC and routine cross-sectional imaging techniques.

T. Mang
Department of Biomedical Imaging and Image-guided Therapy, Medical University of Vienna, Vienna, Austria

P. Lefere (✉)
Department of Radiology, AZ Delta, Roeselare, Belgium

Benign Colonic Findings Seen at CTC

Benign Mucosal Colonic Polyps

Polyps are the most common benign lesions of the colon. In addition to malignant tumors, polyps are the main targets of CTC. According to the Paris classification, they are categorized by their morphologic appearance as sessile, pedunculated, or flat [4]. On CTC, polypoid findings of the colon are characterized by their outer morphology, their internal structure and attenuation characteristics, and their mobility between the supine and prone patient positions [5].

A sessile polyp (0-Is) presents as a round, oval, or lobulated intraluminal filling defect, with a base that is equal to or larger than its vertical height (Fig. .

A pedunculated polyp (0-Ip) presents with a round, oval, or lobulated polyp head that is connected to the mucosa by a stalk. On 2D planar images, colorectal polyps typically show a homogeneous internal structure with a soft tissue attenuation. Polyps arise from the colonic wall. Therefore, they maintain their intraluminal position when the prone and supine scanning positions are compared. This criterion may help to differentiate true polyps from untagged residual stool that is not attached to the colonic wall and that shows a positional movement. Pedunculated polyps, however, may show a

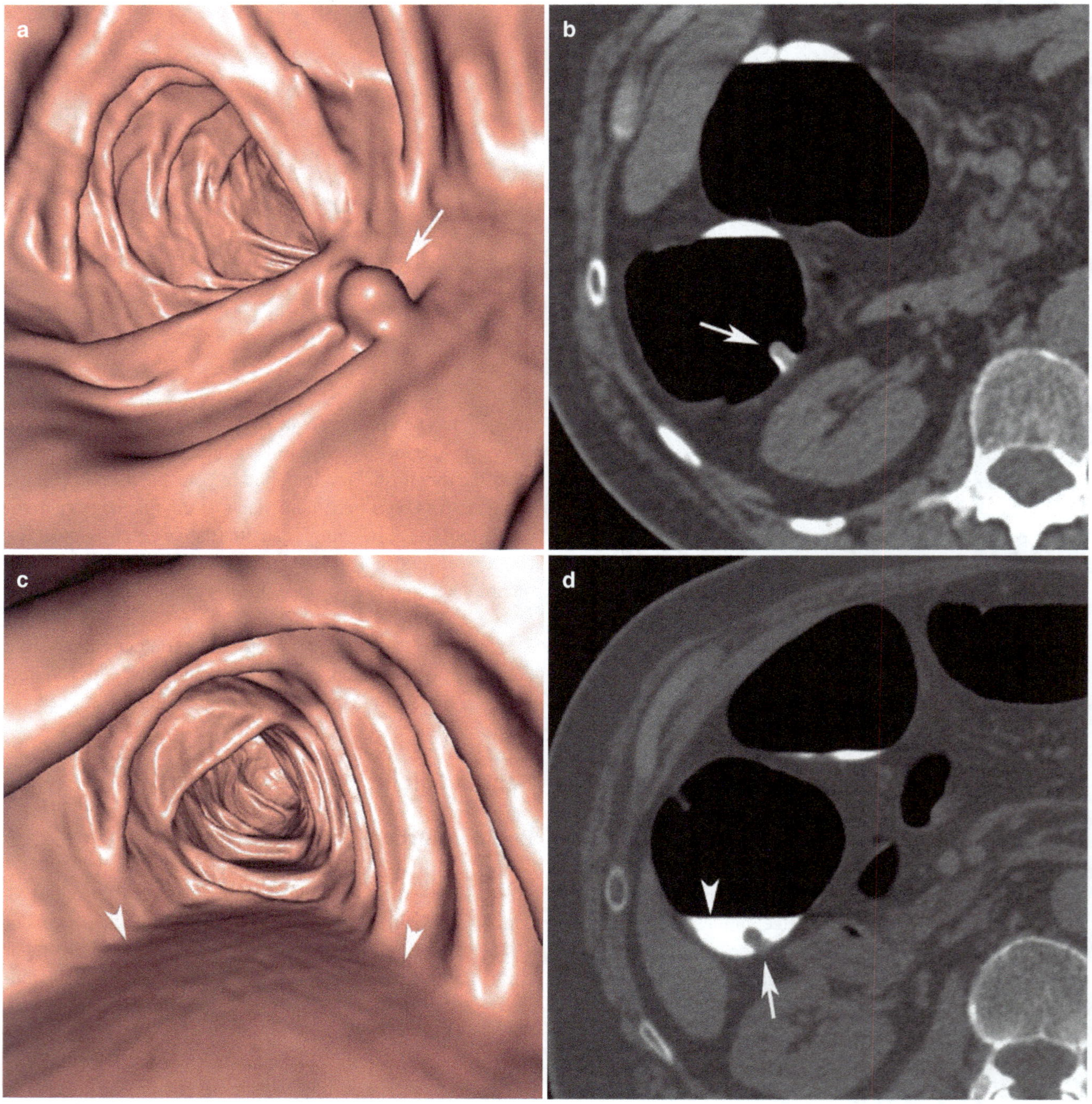

Fig. (**a–d**) Sessile oval polyp located in the ascending colon. (**a**)The endoluminal 3D view shows a round polypoid lesion (arrow) (**b**) The corresponding prone axial 2D image shows the homogeneous soft-tissue density (arrow) of the lesion. (**c**) The corresponding supine endoluminal 3D view shows a horizontal fluid layer (arrowheads). No polyp is seen. (**d**) The supine axial 2D image shows that the lesion (arrow) is submerged unter tagged residual fluid (arrowhead)

considerable positional shift between the supine and prone acquisitions because of their stalk (Fig.). This so-called pseudo mobility may cause confusion with the untagged stool, showing true mobility, i.e., a pseudo-stool appearance. Flat or non-polypoid lesions are morphologically character-ized by their low elevation compared to their width (Fig.). On CTC, non-polypoid lesions are defined as lesions that mea-sure 6 mm or larger above the surrounding mucosa, with a height of 3 mm or less [6]. Endoscopically, they are categorized according to their predominant direction of growth, which defines their morphology: flat elevated (0-IIa), truly flat (0-IIb), and depressed flat (0-IIc). Non-polypoid lesions are generally less common than their polypoid counterparts.

On CTC, they are less conspicuous than polypoid lesions. On endoluminal 3D views, flat lesions present as a plaque-like elevation of the colonic wall, with a smooth or nodular surface. A flat lesion, located on a semilunar fold, typically leads to a circumscribed thickening of the fold. On 2D pla-

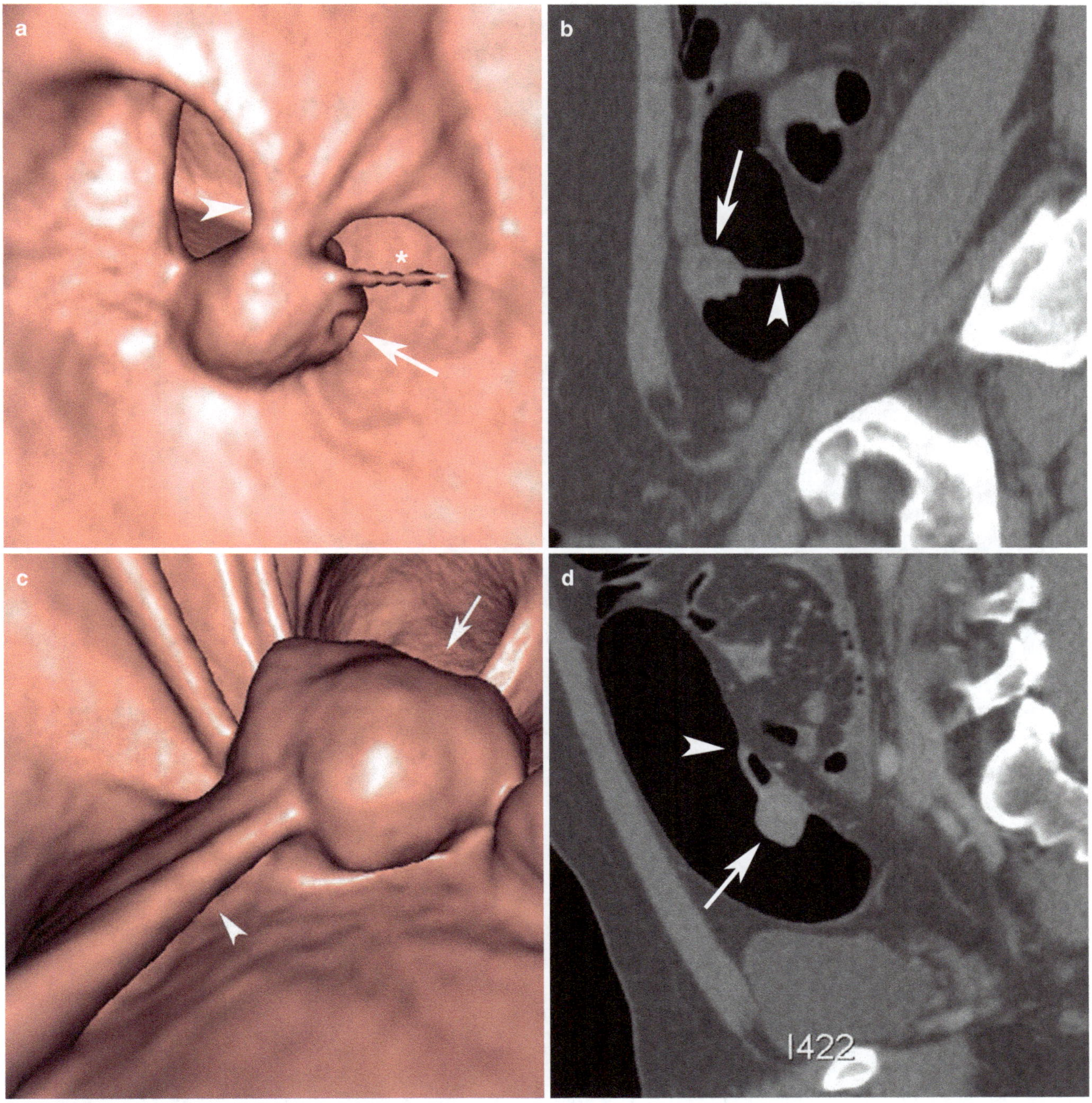

Fig. Large pedunculated polyp located in the sigmoid colon. (**a**) The prone endoluminal 3D view shows the polyp head (arrow), connected to the mucosa by its stalk (arrowhead). A small mucus tear is attached to the polyp head (asterisk). (**b**) The corresponding prone sagittal 2D image shows the soft tissue dense polyp head (arrow) located on the anterior sigmoid wall. It is connected by the stalk (arrowhead) to the dorsal sigmoid wall. (**c**) The corresponding supine endoluminal 3D view and (**d**) sagittal 2D image show that the polyp head (arrow) moves on its stalk (arrowhead) to the dorsal sigmoid wall

nar views, flat lesions typically appear as circumscribed, plaque-like wall thickening with a homogeneous soft-tissue attenuation [5]. Flat lesions with a central depression have been shown to have a higher risk for malignancy. Flat lesions are frequently covered by tagged residue, which may aid detection. This is called "contrast coating" [7].

Larger non-polypoid tumors, spreading over ≥1 cm (on CTC ≥ 3 cm), are laterally spreading tumors (LSTs). An older, commonly used term is a "carpet lesion." They are an important subset of flat lesions, with a predilection for the cecum and the rectum. They typically present with advanced histological features. Based on their surface appearance, they are endoscopically categorized as granular or non-granular types [8].

On CTC, they typically present with a broad-based flat morphology, with a size ≥3 cm. They may exceed 3 mm in

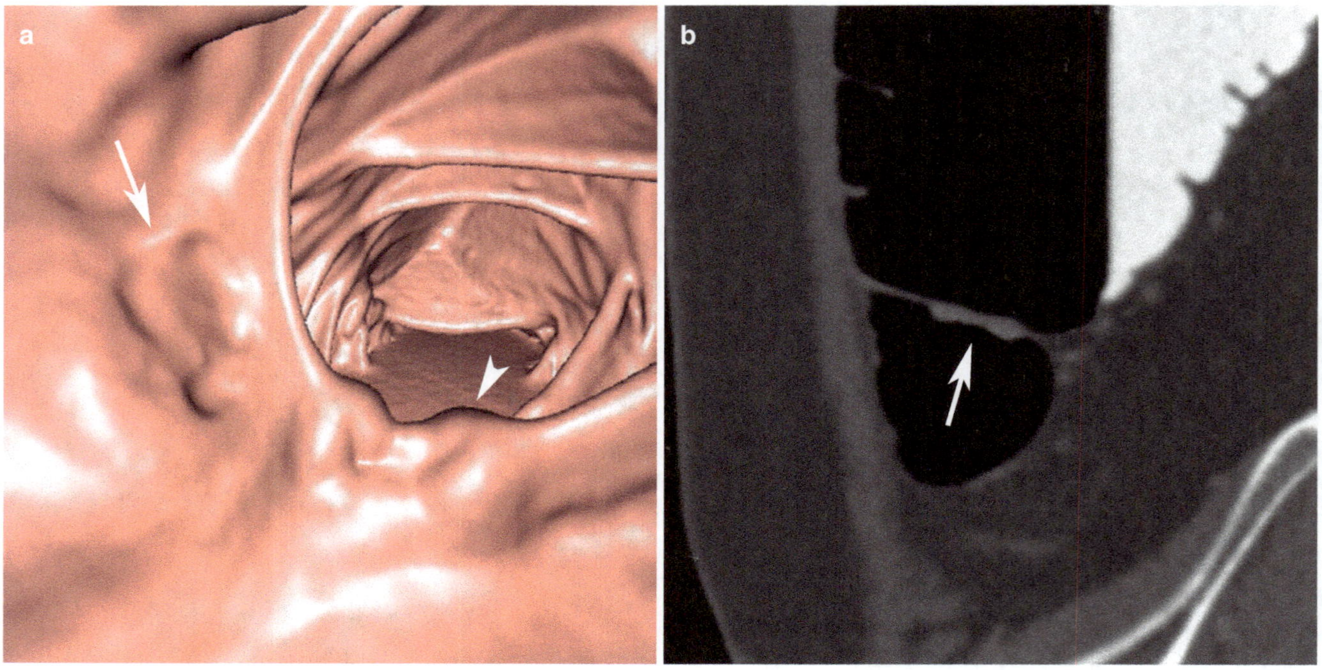

Fig. (**a**, **b**) A 12 mm slightly elevated flat lesion with a central depression. (**a**) The endoluminal 3D image shows a flat slightly elevated filling defect with a central depression (arrow), located on a haustral fold adjacent to the ileocecal valve (arrowhead). (**b**) The corresponding sagittal 2D view shows a flat elevation of the bowel wall leading to a plaque-like soft tissue thickening of the haustral fold. Note the slight central depression at the center of the lesion (arrow)

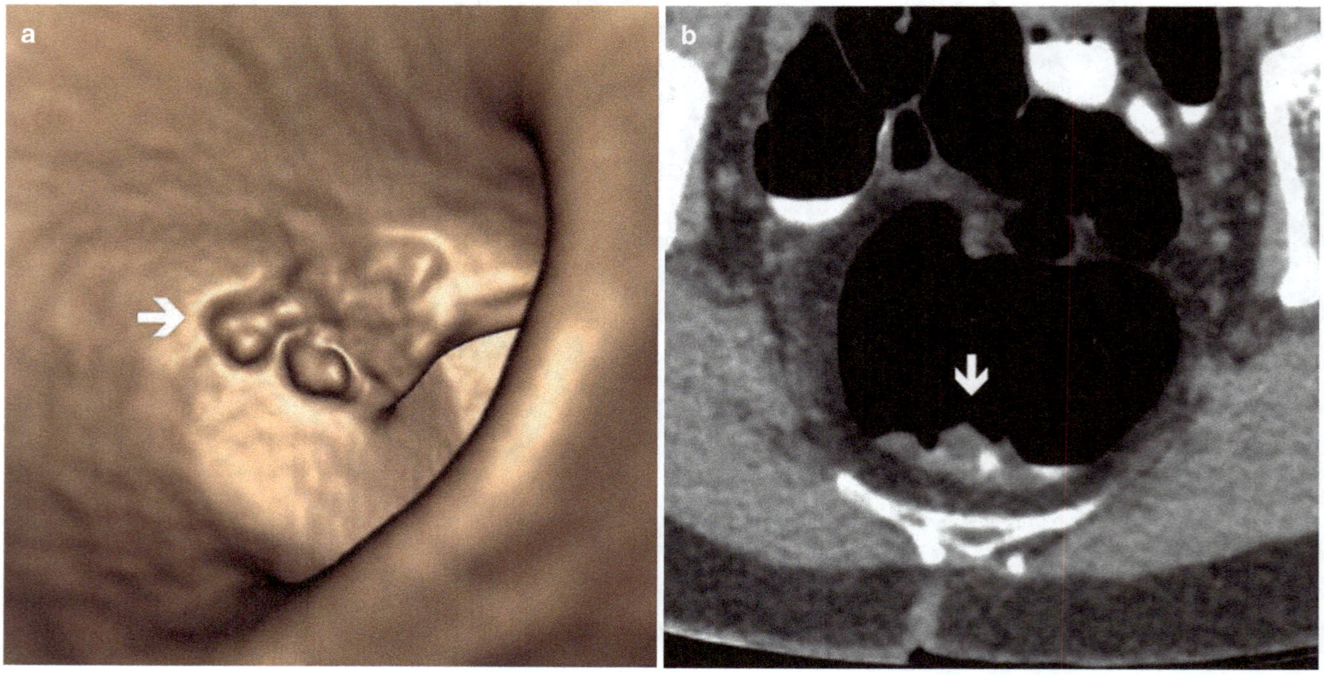

Fig. (**a**, **b**) Laterally spreading tumor of the mixed granular type in the rectum. (**a**) The endoluminal 3D view shows a flat irregular filling defect with a nodular surface (arrow). (**b**) The corresponding axial 2D image shows a nodular wall thickening with soft tissue attenuation (arrow). The lesion is covered by a small amount of tagged fluid

height but are still flat and may have superficially raised edges. Surface coating with oral contrast material is fre-quently seen 9] (Fig.).

Correct CTC size measurement is important because the size of a polyp, as measured by the radiologist, has a direct influence on the selection of the appropriate therapeutic procedures. There is general consensus that all polyps measuring 6 mm or larger need to be reported, and endoscopic polypectomy should be recommended [3, 6]. Polyps smaller than 6 mm are frequently ignored. For sessile and flat polyps, the greatest diameter is measured, which is most often at the base of the lesion. For pedunculated lesions, only the largest diameter for the polyp head should be measured, excluding the stalk [6].

Benign Submucosal Tumors

Lipomas

Lipomas are the most common submucosal tumors in the colon. They are typically between 1 and 3 cm in size. A lipoma can have a sessile, pedunculated, or even flat morphology. On endoluminal 3D views, they present as filling defects, typically with a smooth surface. A correct diagnosis is obtained with 2D views: lipomas typically have a homogeneous fatty attenuation. Often, a thin mucosal stripe covering the fatty tissue is seen. Since lipomas are relatively soft lesions, they may change their shape when the position of the patient is changed (Fig.). Lipomas are benign. No diagnostic or therapeutic investigation is needed. Large lipomas, however, can be symp-tomatic and lead to intussusceptions [10].

RareSubmucosal Tumors

Lymphangiomas are rare benign lesions which may be simple, cavernous, or cystic. In case of the cystic type, the lesion appears with a cystic morphology on 2D views. However, whenever the finding is ≥6 mm on OC, it is necessary to exclude a true neoplastic lesion. There is a wide range of other submucosal tumors that are typically very rare, including leiomyoma, hemangioma, and ganglioneuroma. These cannot be differentiated from adenomatous polyps or tumors based on CT imaging criteria [10].

Pneumatosis Cystoides Coli

Pneumatosis coli is a rare entity with intramural collections of gas. The primary type is benign and self-limiting. The secondary type is related to bowel wall necrosis. It usually requires immediate treatment according to the clinical presentation. On CTC, the primary type has been reported as a rare finding. Primary pneumatosis coli presents with pseudopolypoid filling defects on endoluminal 3D views, corresponding to submucosal cystic or linear pockets of air. Two-dimensional views reveal the pathognomonic air attenuation on these findings. Primary pneumatosis coli is a totally innocuous, asymptomatic, and self-limiting "complication," which requires no further medical action [11].

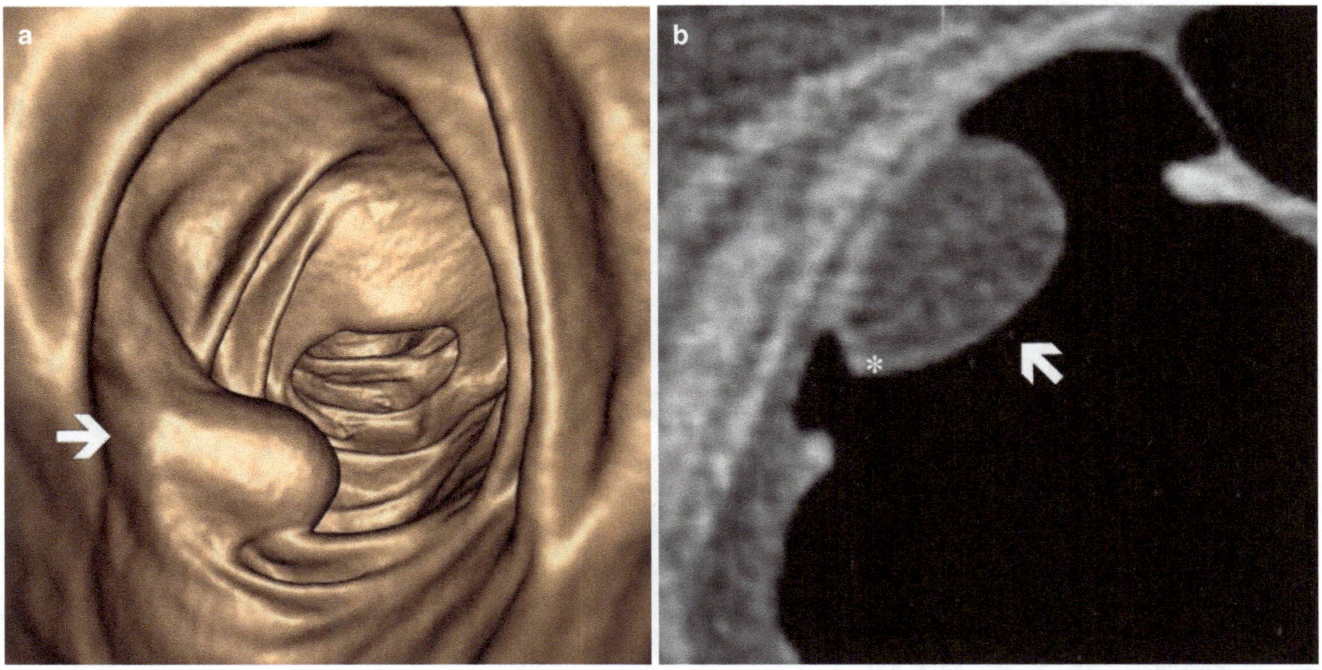

Fig. (**a**, **b**) Lipoma in the ascending colon. (**a**) The endoluminal 3D view shows a large polypoid lesion with smooth appearance (arrow). (**b**) The corresponding axial 2D image shows the homogeneous fat tissue density (arrow) of the lesion, covered by a thin mucosal stripe confirming its submucosal origin (asterisk)

Endometriosis

Endometriosis is a condition related to the growth of the endometrium outside the uterus. Colonic involvement occurs mostly in the rectosigmoid and rarely in the cecum. This occurs via peritoneal implants of endometrial tissue. These implants may develop trans-serosal growth with submucosal extension. From there, intraluminal extension may occur in a small number of patients. According to the grade of invasion, CTC shows different aspects. With serosal/submucosal infiltration, there is mural thickening, which leads to a marginal luminal filling defect, showing a smooth delin-eation (Fig.). In case of extension to the mucosa, the wall becomes irregular and ends in a polypoid lesion or mass [12].

Anatomy-RelatedFindings

Segmental Colonic Spasm

Colonic spasm is a physiological narrowing of the intestinal lumen due to muscular contraction of the colonic wall that can simulate circular stenotic tumors. The degree of colonic distension and the intraluminal aspect of the colon also depend on the muscular contraction of the taenia coli. Optimal colonic distension prevents spasms and possible false-positive findings. In the sigmoid, the taenia is more or less subtle. When contracted, they cause the narrowed lumen to be round, with smoothly thickened folds without overhanging edges. In the descending colon, the taenia becomes slightly more prominent with, in contraction, a slightly more triangular aspect of the colonic lumen. In the transverse and ascending colon, the triangular shape of the lumen is obvious. However, the folds are not distorted, and there is usually no shoulder formation, which is typical of malignancy. Due to redistribution of intracolonic gas, the spasm will frequently either change in morphology or even disappear between the supine and prone acquisitions [5].

Flexural Pseudotumor

The colon presents with many loops and flexures. At each flexure, the structure at the inner side is more compressed than that on the outer side. This can cause complex structures that consist of crowded and thickened colonic folds. This thickening is accentuated by the pericolic fat and its vascular structures. On 2D planar views, this may lead to an apparent wall thickening that may be mistaken for a colonic mass. Therefore, such thickening is referred to as a flexural pseudotumor. Such pseudolesions can become real tumor mimics in case of a flexure over an acute angle with the convergence of many folds. A comparison of both acquisitions will help to detect any change in appearance. A thorough analysis of the appearance on 3D and 2D images is helpful to exclude a tumoral process. The pseudolesion most frequently consists of a convergence of many folds that show regular smooth contours on endoluminal 3D views. On 2D views, pericolic fat is sometimes demonstrated in the thickened fold [13].

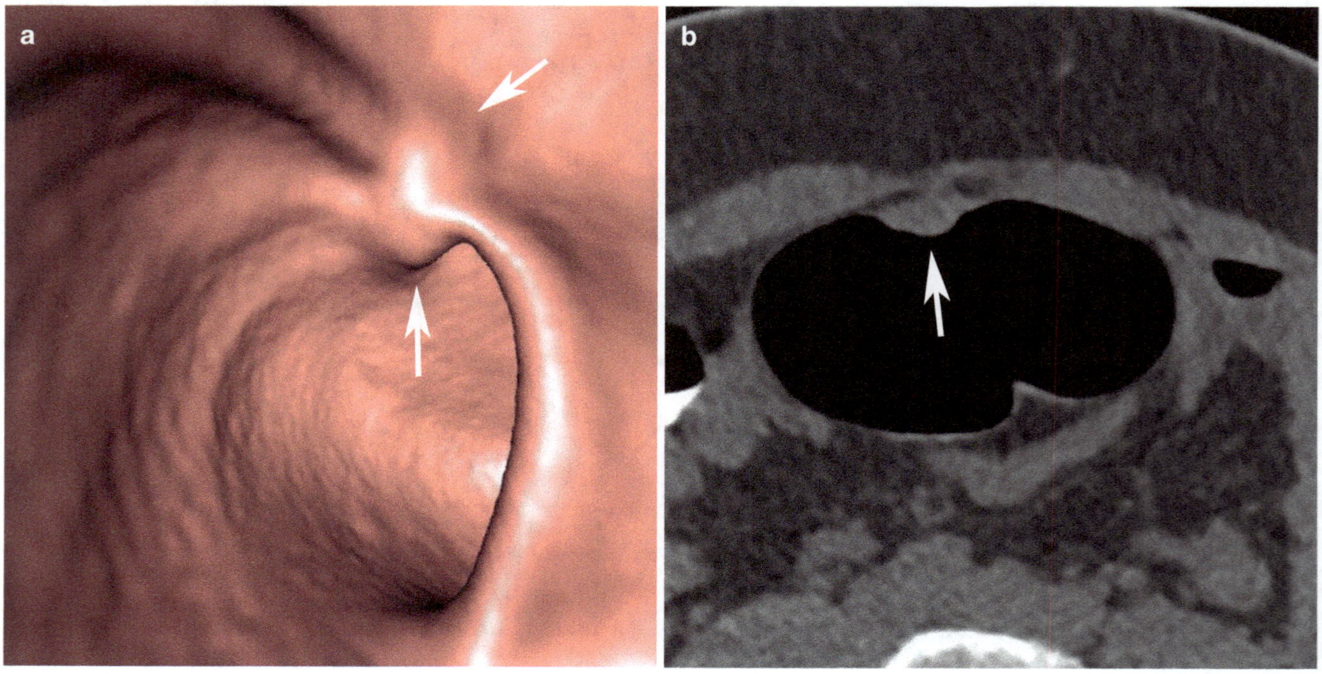

Fig. (**a**, **b**) Endometriosis implant in the sigmoid colon. (**a**) The endoluminal 3D view shows a flat intraluminal filling defect with a smooth delineation (arrows). (**b**) The corresponding axial 2D image shows a homogeneous soft tissue dense lesion (arrow) infiltrating the colonic wall

The Anorectal Region

For the evaluation of the rectum, it is important to inspect the anal margin. This is done by turning the virtual camera to the anus. In this part of the rectum, several benign and/or tumor-like conditions are possible [5, 13, 14].

The Hypertrophied Anal Papilla

The hypertrophied anal papilla is a frequent finding. It is a papillary projection of a rectal column (Morgagni) and appears as a fibrous white polyp of any size at OC. On CTC, it is impossible to differentiate from a true polyp, necessitating rectoscopy in case of a polypoid structure ≥6 mm.

Internal Hemorrhoids

Internal hemorrhoids are varicosities of the superior hemorrhoidal plexus. They arise at the anal margin and are a very frequent finding (±50% of patients). They typically appear as smooth filling defects surrounding the rectal catheter with thin folds converging toward the catheter. On rare occasions, they may have a polypoid appearance.

Other Findings

The rectal varix is a dilated submucosal vein that causes a long, serpiginous filling defect. It is important to be aware of its existence, as, on rare occasions, polyps may also have a serpiginous aspect. A venous bleb is a small venous malformation that may present with a polypoid morphology and mimic true polypoid lesions. However, usually they are <5 mm.

The Cecum

The cecum has a complex topography including the ileocecal valve and the appendix. As with the rectum, its CTC examination requires specific attention [15–17].

The Ileocecal Valve

The normal ileocecal (IC) valve consists of twofolds (upper and lower lip), converging at both sides in a prominent fold, the frenulum. When examining the cecum, it is always essential to identify the IC valve and check its anatomic appearance, excluding polyps and cancers located on the valve. The normal IC valve, however, may show some pseudotumoral aspects that should not be confused with colonic pathology.

Lipomatous Transformation

Lipomatous transformation refers to fatty infiltration of both lips of the IC. The IC valve is typically enlarged and may have a dome-like appearance. Correct characterization of this benign anatomical variant is obtained by assessing the typical fat attenuation (0/−100 H.U.) in an abdominal window setting.

Papillary Transformation

Papillary transformation is less frequently observed than the normal labial appearance. The papillary IC valve is caused by protrusion of the terminal ileum into the IC valve. This is considered a normal functional status, with the IC valve preventing fluid reflux from the colon into the ileum. A papillary IC valve is recognized by a bulbous or polypoid morphology and a smooth surface. It may also appear slightly distorted and presents as a bulky, mass-like lesion. In such cases, the diagnosis is not always straightforward. Most often, this condition is characterized by a smooth delineation of the IC valve with some fatty infiltration on 2D images. The appearance frequently changes with dual acquisition (i.e., supine-prone). However, any accumulation of soft tissue should raise the suspicion for neoplasia.

The Appendix

As the appendix is part of the colon, it is necessary to inspect it. On endoluminal 3D views, the orifice of appendix is identified as a small orifice or depression frequently located in the vicinity of small fold. On 2D planar views the appendix presents as a thin-walled tubular structure, which may be filled with air or tagged fluid. Any global or focal wall thickening should prompt further investigation to rule out malignancy (appendectomy). Tumoral conditions of the appendix are rare and are frequently asymptomatic [18].

Mucocele of the Appendix

An appendiceal mucocele corresponds to a mucus-dilated appendix. It typically appears as a tubular cystic lesion in the course of the appendix and may present with a mural calcification. This may correspond to a simple mucocele (retention cyst) or a hyperplastic mucocele (hyperplastic polyp) in 5–20% of cases, to mucinous cystadenoma in 63–84%, and to mucinous cystadenocarcinoma in 11–20%. Rarely, it corresponds to endometriosis. A mucocele can protrude into the cecal lumen and presents as a polypoid lesion on endoluminal 3D views (Fig.) [19]. A malignant cause has to be excluded by surgery.

Inverted Appendiceal Stump

Following inversion-ligation appendectomy, which is an older appendectomy technique, an appendiceal stump may be seen as a polypoid lesion in the region of the expected appendiceal orifice. It presents as a round smooth polypoid filling defect at the site of the appendiceal orifice with a homogeneous soft-tissue attenuation. This postsurgical polypoid finding cannot be differentiated from a true colonic polyp based on CT imaging criteria. If there is uncertainty concerning previous appendectomy, OC should be recommended, the same as for any polypoid lesion ≥6 mm. Furthermore, on rare occasions, a polyp or malignancy may develop in the stump [20].

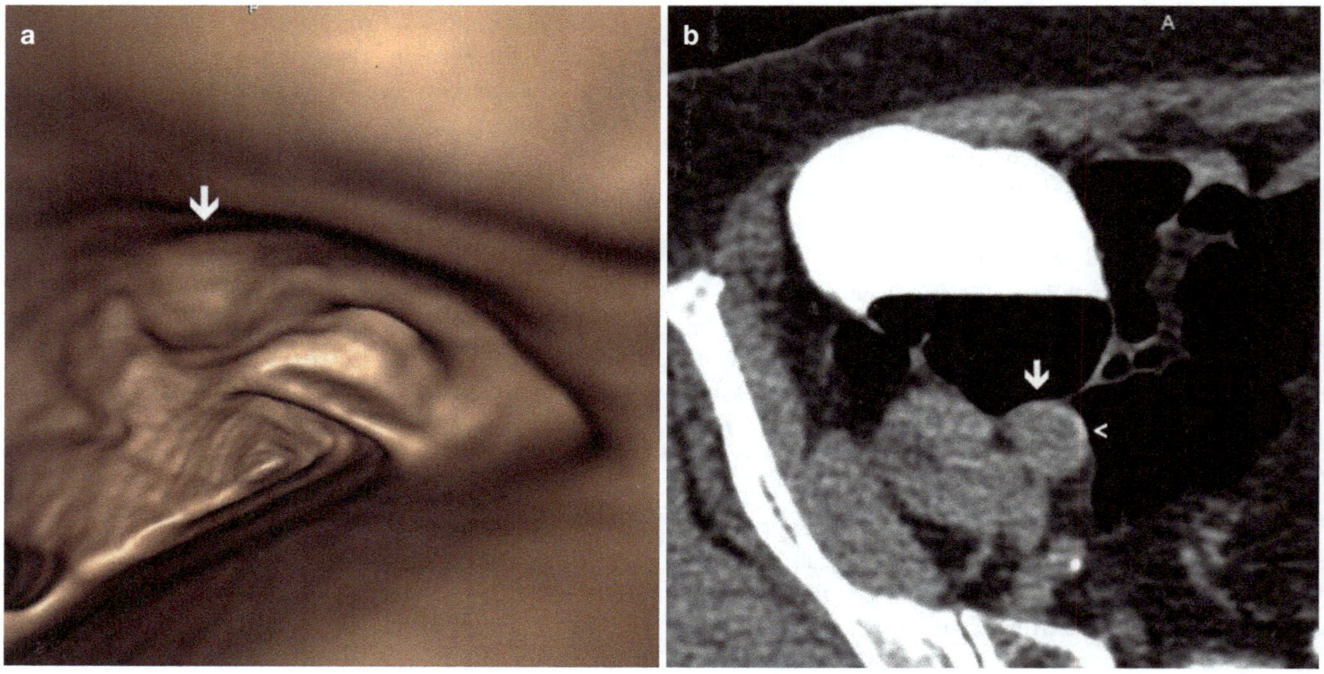

Fig. (**a**, **b**) Mucocele of the appendix. (**a**) The endoluminal 3D view of the partially fluid-filled cecum showing a broad-based polypoid intraluminal filling with a smooth surface (arrow). (**b**) The corresponding axial 2D image shows a cystic structure, causing a subtle extrinsic impression on the colonic lumen (arrow). The lesion had a thin mural calcification (open arrowhead) and was contiguous with the appendix

Diverticular Disease

Diverticular disease is the most common disease of the colon in the Western population, with a frequency of about 30% at age 50 and more than 50% at age 60. It is mostly located in the sigmoid colon. In its early stage, diverticular disease is characterized by myochosis: a triad of muscular wall thickening, shortening of the taenia, and luminal narrowing. This results in restricted colonic distensibility with prominent and narrow stranding semilunar folds and deep haustrations, with shortening of the interhaustral segments (concertina appearance). On endoluminal 3D views, there is restricted mucosal visualization behind and between the prominent semilunar folds (blind spots). Dedicated 3D inspections are required, which involve turning the virtual camera around to visualize the backside of the folds and the interhaustral segment. To improve colonic distension, the use of hyoscine-*N*-butylbromide is justified [6]. Distension can also be improved by repositioning the patient to the right or left lateral decubitus position, with an additional low-dose CT scan of the affected segment.

With progression of myochosis, the diverticula appear and the semilunar folds become more prominent. On 2D images, the diverticula are characterized by gas-filled outpouchings on the colonic wall. On endoluminal 3D views, they appear as a well-defined complete dark ring that may simulate a small sessile polyp lesion. Polyps, in contrast, often present with an incomplete or vague ring shadow when viewed en face. Two-dimensional views make differentiation of diverticula and polyps straightforward. Diverticular disease gives rise to pseudopolypoid lesions [21].

The Diverticular Fecalith

Diverticula are often impacted with fecal residue that can protrude through the neck of the diverticulum into the colonic lumen. This causes a polypoid filling defect on endoluminal 3D views, with a pathognomonic aspect on 2D views: the diverticular fecalith almost invariably presents as a round structure with a hyperdense ring and a hypodense center corresponding to an air occlusion [22]. It can protrude from the diverticulum into the colonic lumen. Diverticular fecaliths can be the source of inflammation that leads to focal diverticulitis.

The Inverted Diverticulum

A diverticulum may invert into the colonic lumen. Although infrequent, radiologists need to be aware of this possibility. On endoluminal 3D views, the inverted diverticulum mimics a true polyp with, on 2D planar views, mostly an air or fat inclusion. Sometimes, a central umbilication can be distinguished.

Chronic Diverticular Disease or Stenosing Cancer

Patients with repetitive episodes of acute diverticulitis may develop chronic diverticular disease, a common reason for

Table CT colonography imaging characteristics suggestive of chronic diverticular disease in the left column, and a stenosing colonic cancer in the right column

Findings suggesting chronic diverticular disease	Findings suggesting a stenosing colonic cancer
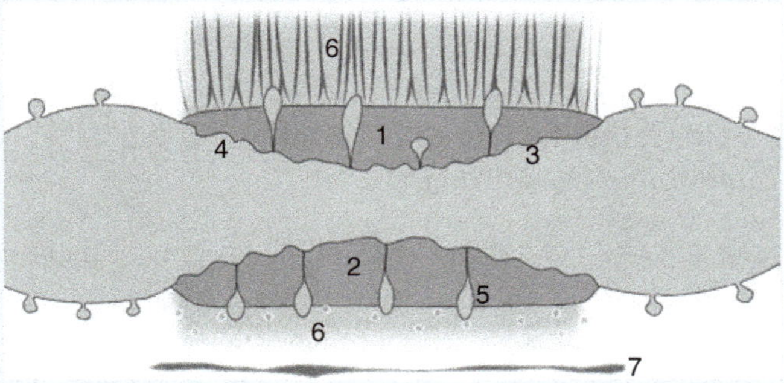	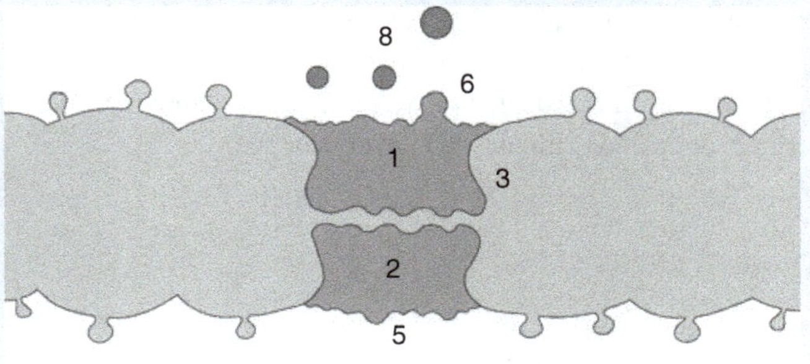
1. Long segment ≥10 cm	1. Shorter segment
2. Milder wall thickening (<2 cm)	2. Wall thickening ++ (≥2 cm)
3. Cone-shaped aspect, tapered margins	3. Shoulder formation, overhanging edges
4. Preserved folds	4. Completely distorted fold pattern
5. Diverticula in the thickened segment	5. No diverticula in the thickened segment
6. Pericolic fat infiltration	6. Pericolic tumor infiltration
7. Thickened local facia	7. No thickened local facia
8. No pericolic lymphadenopathy	8. Pericolic lymphadenopathy

Note that these signs overlap each other, making an exact diagnosis difficult and sometimes impossible. However, the absence of diverticula within the affected segment and the presence of shoulder formation are strong indicators for cancer

incomplete OC. CTC is the method of choice to complete the colonic evaluation. However, differential diagnosis between chronic diverticular disease and a stenosing cancer can be challenging. Each entity presents with imaging characteristics which, unfortunately, are not entirely specific. Interference of signs is quite frequent. Features, characteristic of chronic diverticular disease and malignant tumor, are presented in Table . Studies comparing both entities concluded that it seems reasonable that the presence of divertic-ula in the affected segment, together with wall thickening over a rather long segment, thickening of the local fascia (fascia sign) without lymphadenopathy, cone-shaped or tapered margins, and the preserved more or less thickened colonic folds, is likely indicative of chronic diverticular dis-ease. Conversely, the absence of diverticula in the thickened segment and thickening of the local fascia, a more prominent wall thickening with a short extension, shoulder formation or overhanging edges, and a completely distorted or fold pat-tern are more likely indicative of a stenosing colonic cancer [23, 24].

Postoperative Colon

According to the surgical technique used (end-to-end or side-to-end), the anastomosis will have a different morphology. The anastomosis should show a smooth transition, with, occasionally, a subtle, smooth, circumferential ridge, or a web-like appearance. On 2D views, the surgical staples, if used, are easily identified. Sometimes, the staples protrude into the colonic lumen, causing a tiny luminal filling defect on 3D views that can be easily identified on 2D views by its high internal density. Polypoid granulation tissue as well as inflammatory and hyperplastic polyps may develop at the anastomosis. These findings will present with the same imaging features as adenomatous polyps. In the postoperative period, fibrosis may develop, causing a pseudotumoral narrowing at the anastomosis [25]. Therefore, any increase of soft tissue at the site of, or adjacent to, the anastomosis should raise the suspicion for tumor recurrence, indicating OC.

Inflammatory Diseases of the Colon

In addition to benign polypoid and stenotic findings and their pitfalls, several other benign colonic conditions may be encountered with diagnostic imaging techniques. They include a wide range of inflammatory diseases, including diverticulitis, chronic inflammatory bowel diseases (CIBDs), infectious and noninfectious colitis, as well as mechanical colonic obstruction and perforation. In almost all of these acute conditions, CTC is contraindicated since the distension of the colon with gas may lead to colonic wall perforation. For these indications, standard cross-sectional imaging is the method of choice. Furthermore, some of these entities require histologic workup to achieve a correct diagnosis or identification of dysplasia.

In the large bowel, inflammation typically leads to bowel wall thickening, with or without mural stratification, which is the ability to distinguish the different layers of the colonic wall on cross-sectional imaging [26, 27]. Various inflammatory bowel diseases differ in their primary location within the GI tract, length of segmental involvement, degree of wall thickening, mural enhancement pattern, and extraintestinal involvement.

Diverticulitis

Inflammation of diverticula leads to symptomatic diverticulitis, which occurs, in two-thirds of cases, in the sigmoid colon. This can affect a single or a few adjacent diverticula, called focal diverticulitis, or the entire colonic segment. If a single diverticulum is inflamed, t here i s f ocal, e dematous m ural thickening, typically surrounding a stool-impacted diverticulum, with increased mural enhancement and focal pericolonic fat stranding [28]. Imaging findings of acute colonic diverticulitis are cone-shaped inflammatory wall thickening, involving a long segment (>10 cm), and increased mural contrast enhancement, as well as submucosal edema. Acute inflammation is typically accompanied by pericolic fat stranding and fluid at the root of the mesentery (Fig.). The presence of diverticula is pathognomonic. Their absence makes diverticu-litis unlikely [29]. Complications that may develop are perico-lic abscess, contained or free perforation, hemorrhage, fistula formation, and post-inflammatory stenosis. The most important differential diagnosis for diverticulitis is colon cancer. In contrast, extensive wall thickening with short extension (<5 cm), especially with shoulder formation and pericolonic lymph nodes, is suspicious for neoplasms [30].

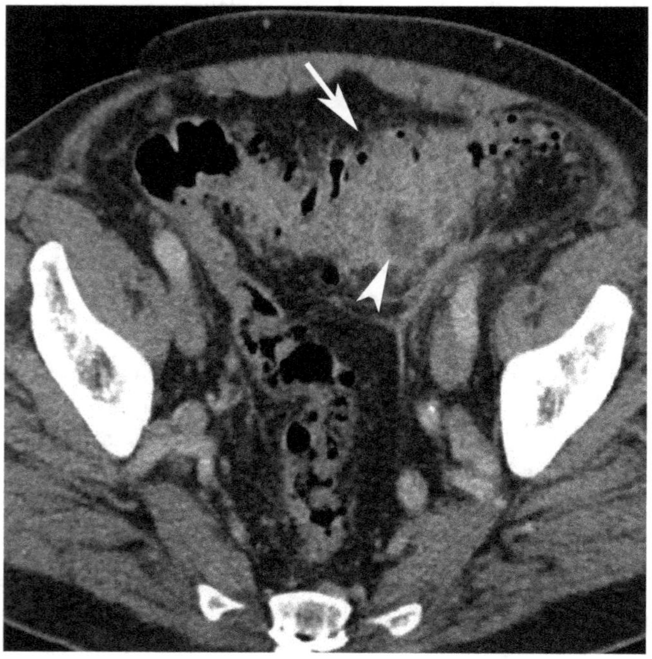

Fig. Acute diverticulitis. The contrast-enhanced axial CT image shows wall thickening of the sigmoid colon (arrow) with adjacent inflammatory stranding of the pericolic fat tissue. Note the fluid collection representing abscess formation (arrowhead)

Colonic Involvement in Chronic Inflammatory Bowel Disease

Within the group of CIBD, Crohn's disease (CD) and ulcerative colitis (UC) represent the most important conditions. OC with biopsy is the examination of choice to evaluate colonic involvement in CIBD, specifically for the detection of colonic dysplasia, and to differentiate between an inflammatory stenosis and cancer. Standard abdominal CT is indicated for the detection of acute complications. CTC is not indicated and may be an option only in patients with incomplete OC in chronic inactive disease.

Ulcerative Colitis

Ulcerative colitis is an inflammatory bowel disease limited to the mucosa and submucosa of the colon. The disease typically begins in the rectum and continuously extends proximally to involve parts of the colon or the entire colon. In 10–40% of cases, the distal ileum is also inflamed, which is referred to as backwash ileitis.

Early, subtle, and inflammatory mucosal changes, such as the granular pattern of the mucosa or tiny punctuate ulcers, may be beyond the current spatial resolution of modern cross-sectional imaging.

Progression of the disease leads to mucosal hyperemia and submucosal edema, which then result in thickening and stratification of the wall, accompanied by increased pericolic vascularity. Increased ulceration and pseudopolyps appear, and the mucosa becomes friable. Typically, the outer contour of the affected colonic wall is regular and smooth (Fig.). Lymph node enlargement is only slight. The appearance of abscess or fistula formation is uncommon.

Subacute and chronic forms lead to thickening and rigidity of the wall. Narrowing of the colonic lumen and foreshortening of the colon may occur. The bowel loses its haustral pattern, which can result in a tubular "lead pipe" appearance. Post-inflammatory polyps may be present. The deposition of submucosal fat in the large bowel is found in up to 61% of cases and may result in additional wall thickening and, consequently, in luminal narrowing. As a result of inflammation, there may be proliferation of the pericolic/rectal fat, resulting in widening of the presacral space.

The most severe complication is the toxic megacolon, which appears in up to 5% of cases and carries the risk of perforation and peritonitis. The risk development of colorectal cancer increases with the extent and the duration of the disease [28, 29, 31].

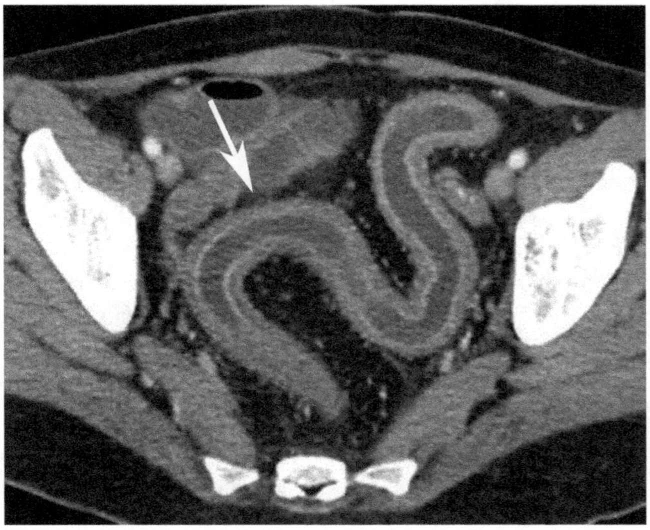

Fig. Ulcerative colitis. The contrast-enhanced axial CT image shows continuous wall thickening of the sigmoid colon with mural stratification (arrow). Note that the outer contour of the colon is regular and smooth

Crohn's Disease

Crohn's disease may involve segments of the whole GI tract. However, Crohn's disease most often affects the terminal ileum and the proximal colon. Unlike ulcerative colitis, Crohn's disease typically affects the GI tract in a discontinuous way (so-called skip lesions), and the inflammatory process is transmural in nature.

CT usually misses the early stages of Crohn's disease. With progression of the disease, distinct mural thickening and luminal narrowing occur. In the acute stage of the disease, wall thickening presents with mural stratification mostly related to submucosal edema. The degree of contrast enhancement of the bowel wall correlates with the severity of the disease. Compared to ulcerative colitis, the outer contour of the colonic wall is irregular. As a result of the hyperemia from the inflammatory process, the local mesenteric vessels are dilated and widely spaced. This has been described as the "comb sign," indicating disease activity (Fig.). A progressive increase in higher-density pericolic fat is called fibrofatty proliferation, resulting in separation of the bowel loops. Usually, multiple mesenteric lymph nodes, measuring <10 mm in the short-axis diameter, are present. Extensive, intersecting linear transverse and longi-tudinal ulcerations can result in the so-called cobblestone pat-tern. With progression of the disease, the transmural inflammation is accompanied by irreversible fibrosis. On cross-sectional imaging, this presents with a loss of mural stratifica-tion, with mural thickening and homogeneous attenuation [28, 29, 31].

Frequent complications are fistula, abscesses, adhesions, and stenosis, leading to bowel obstruction. Fistula can appear as ill-defined soft tissue bands extending either to another part of the gastrointestinal tract or to the skin. Abscesses are most

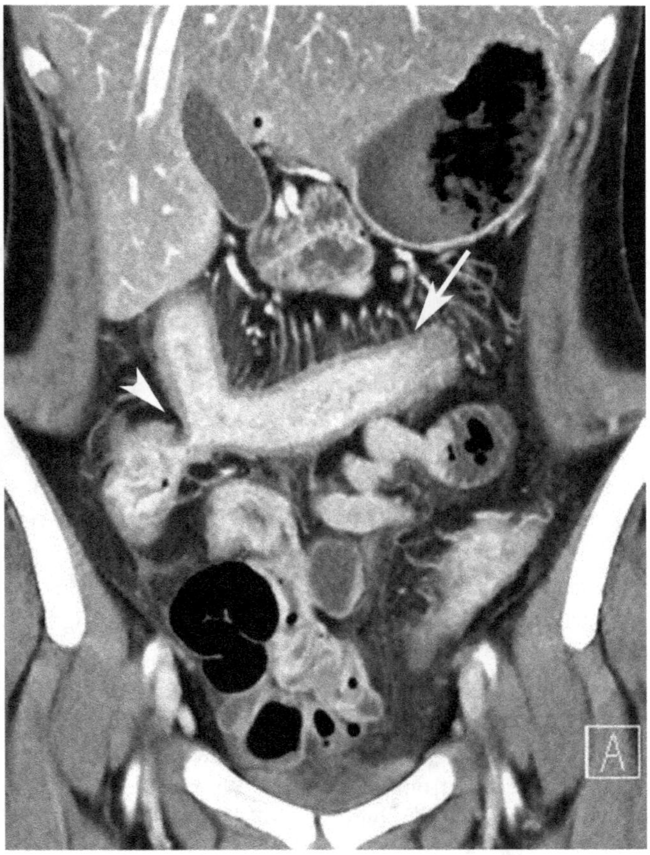

Fig. Crohn's disease. The contrast-enhanced coronal CT image shows mural thickening of the transverse colon with dilated mesenteric vessels (comb sign) and fistula formation to the ascending colon (arrowhead). Note the inflammatory mural enhancement of small bowel loops

frequently associated with the penetrating type of Crohn's disease, affecting the small bowel with or without the colon. Stenosis in Crohn's disease shows, in many cases, circular, cone-shaped wall thickening with increased contrast enhancement and involvement of a longer segment. In other cases, short stenosis with wall thickening and abrupt shoulders at the proximal and distal end occur, which renders differentiation from malignant stenosis impossible. Perforations are uncommon and usually contained. Conglomerate masses are present if there is involvement of multiple bowel segments or a large bowel segment with fistulization and abscess formation. There is a slightly increased risk of developing colorectal cancer and lymphoma as a complication of the disease. These neoplasms mostly affect the small bowel. The presence of lymph node enlargement >10 mm in the short-axis diameter should raise the suspicion of malignancy.

Infectious Colitis

Inflammation of the colon can be caused by bacterial, viral, fungal, or parasitic infection. The diagnosis of infectious colitis is readily achieved, based on the typical presentation of GI symptoms. Stool culture may be required to identify specific organisms. In general, most of these diseases are self-limiting, and dedicated imaging is not required for diagnosis. However, cross-sectional imaging may be required to assess the extent, the severity, and the potential complications of the disease.

Radiologic imaging features are not specific for a particular microorganism. Infectious colitis presents with diffuse colonic wall thickening, frequently with a so-called target appearance caused by mural stratification. This phenomenon is caused by mucosal CM enhancement and submucosal edema. Colonic air-fluid levels may be present. Extracolonic changes may include pericolonic fat stranding as well as ascites.

The affected colonic segment may suggest a specific organism. For instance, colonic infection with shigella or salmonella is limited to the right colon, while diffuse involvement may be seen with CMV and *E. coli*. Gonorrhea, herpes virus, and *C. trachomatis* typically involve the rectosigmoid area (Fig.) [32, 33].

Pseudomembranous Colitis

Pseudomembranous colitis (PMC) is an acute infectious colitis that results from an unopposed bacterial overgrowth of Clostridium difficile, typically following broad-spectrum antibiotic therapy or chemotherapy. Bacterial enterotoxins lead to superficial ulceration and subsequent formation of pseudomembranes. Often, the whole colon is involved; however, both the rectosigmoid colon and the right colon may be affected in isolation.

Typical imaging findings include marked circumferential diffuse colonic wall thickening, caused by distinct mucosal and submucosal edema. The edema leads to a typical low attenuation aspect of the colonic wall. Wall thickening is more pronounced than in other types of colitis. After IV CM administration, mucosal and serosal enhancement reveals a target enhancement pattern, consisting of three concentric rings of different attenuation. Edematous thickening of the haustral outpouchings, as well as semilunar folds, leads to the appearance of an accordion on longitudinal cross-sectional (accordion sign). Pericolonic changes include fat stranding and, often, ascites (Fig.). Potential complica-tions include toxic megacolon and colonic perforation [34].

Noninfectious Colitis

This summarizes a colonic inflammatory involvement related to either a heterogeneous range of disorders or secondary to medical treatment.

Ischemic Colitis

Ischemic colitis is a disease of elderly patients with atherosclerotic disease, hypotension, or heart failure. Vascular insufficiency and ischemia can lead to a secondary inflammation of the colon. Low-flow states and nonocclusive vessel disease are

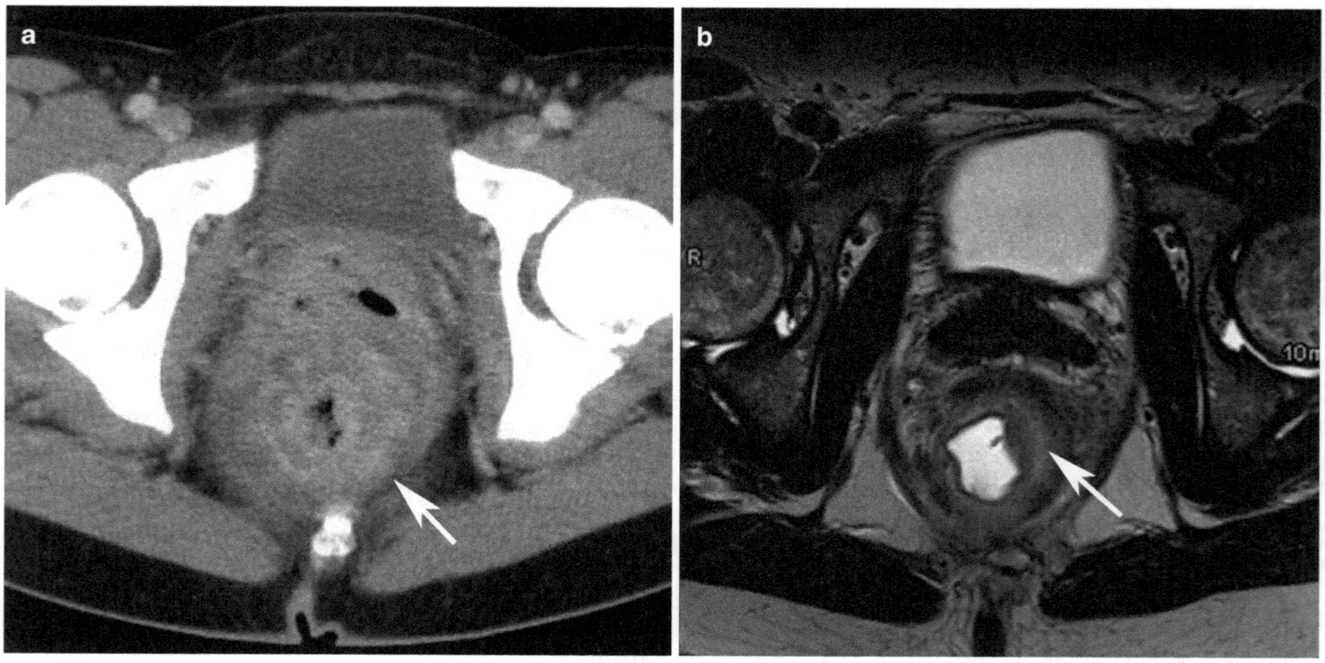

Fig. (**a**, **b**) Rectal syphilis mimicking rectal cancer. (**a**) The contrast-enhanced axial CT image shows a large circumferential mass-like rectal structure of with soft tissue density suggestive for a rectal carcinoma (arrow). (**b**) Axial T2-weighted image of the rectum reveals a mural stratification caused by hyperintense, oedematous thickening of the submucosal layer, indicating an inflammatory process

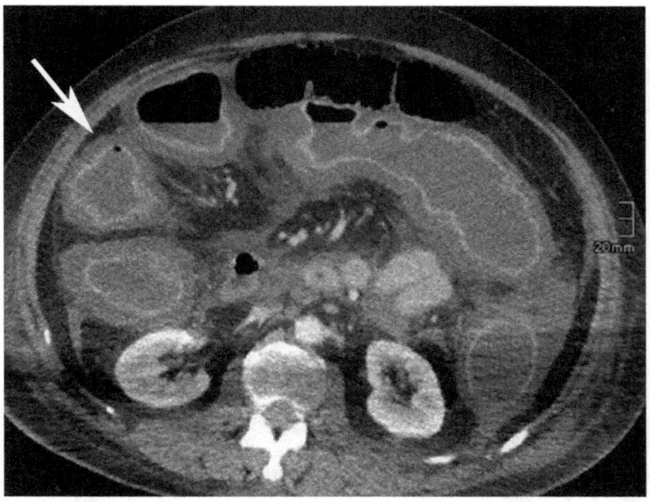

Fig. Pseudomembranous colitis. The contrast-enhanced axial CT image shows marked mural thickening with intense enhancement of the mucosa and distinct submucosal edema of the entire colon (target sign) (arrow). Note the ascites

most common and typically lead to ischemic colitis in watershed areas at the splenic flexure and the rectosigmoid junction. The left colon is more frequently affected than the right colon. Imaging findings are nonspecific and may include mural thickening associated with submucosal edema. A target sign may be present. Following the acute event, fibrosis may lead to chronic strictures of the colonic lumen (Fig.) [29].

Neutropenic Colitis

Neutropenic colitis, also referred to as typhlitis, is a necrotizing inflammation of the cecum, ascending colon, and sometimes the terminal ileum seen in immunocompromised patients with severe neutropenia. It is caused by the transmural invasion of various microorganisms, including bacteria, virus, or fungi, without an inflammatory reaction. Imaging findings include a marked circumferential mural thickening of the right colon, typically the cecum, with distinct submucosal edema. Pneumatosis indicates the severity of the disease. Pericolonic fat stranding is a common finding. Complications include wall necrosis and perforation [29].

Graft-Versus-Host Disease

In graft-versus-host disease (GvHD), after allogenic bone marrow transplantation, donor lymphocytes attack the host tissues. GvHD is more frequently present in the small bowel but may also affect the colon. Imaging findings are nonspecific and include mural thickening associated with submucosal edema, which also affects mucosal enhancement (target sign). Typically, longer bowel segments are affected. Engorged mesenteric vascularization, fat stranding, and ascites may be present. In chronic stages, submucosal edema is replaced by fat tissue [35]. Clinical history leads to the specific diagnosis.

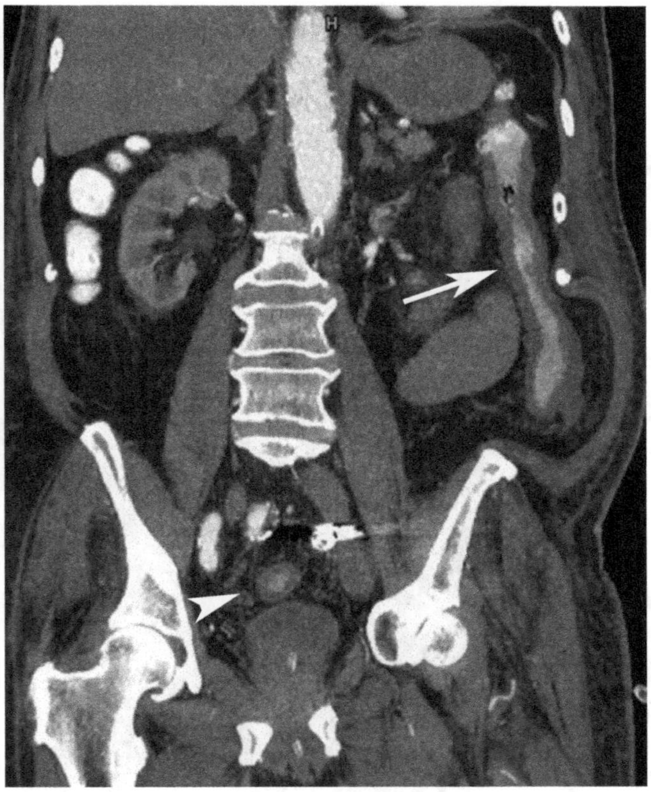

Fig. Ischemic colitis. The contrast-enhanced axial CT image shows mural thickening of the descending (arrow) and sigmoid colon (arrowhead)

Drug-Induced Colitis

Drug-induced injury to the colon most frequently presents as colitis [36]. Cancer treatment with chemotherapeutics may lead neutropenic enterocolitis, pseudomembranous colitis, or pneumatosis intestinalis [37, 38]. With the introduction of new anticancer drugs, such as checkpoint inhibitors, a new range of potential side effects from these therapies has been encountered. Checkpoint inhibitor-induced (e.g., ipilimumab- associated) colitis may occur in melanoma patients under immunotherapy (Fig.). On cross- sectional imaging, it may present as mild, diffuse, bowel- wall thickening, with fluid-filled colonic distention, and mesenteric vessel engorgement. It can also present as seg-mental colitis in the sigmoid colon in an area of pre-existing diffuse diverticulosis [39].

Long-term abuse of nonsteroidal anti-inflammatory drugs (NSAIDs) can induce colitis [40]. NSAID-induced colitis typically affects the right colon, with diffuse or segmental inflammation and ulcerations, as well as diaphragm-like fibrotic strictures. CT imaging findings are nonspecific, and wall thickening may simulate malignancy. Diaphragm-like strictures in the right colon on CTC may raise the suspicion for an inflammatory cause. A clinical history of NSAID abuse and an ischemic appearance at pathohistology leads to the diagnosis.

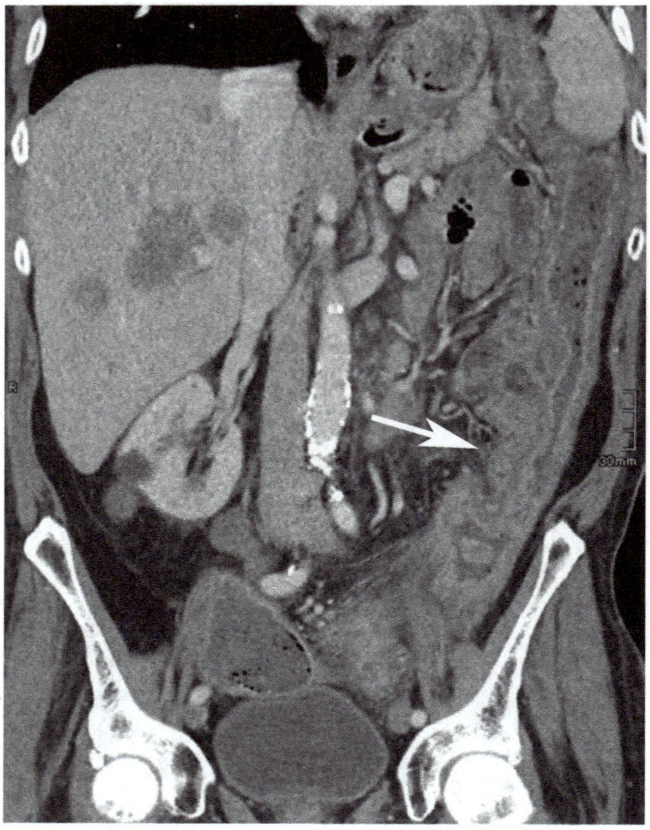

Fig. Severe ipilimumab-associated colitis in a patient with met-astatic melanoma. The contrast-enhanced coronal CT image shows marked thickening of the left colon with pericolic fat stranding and mesenteric vessel engorgement (arrow). Note the liver metastasis

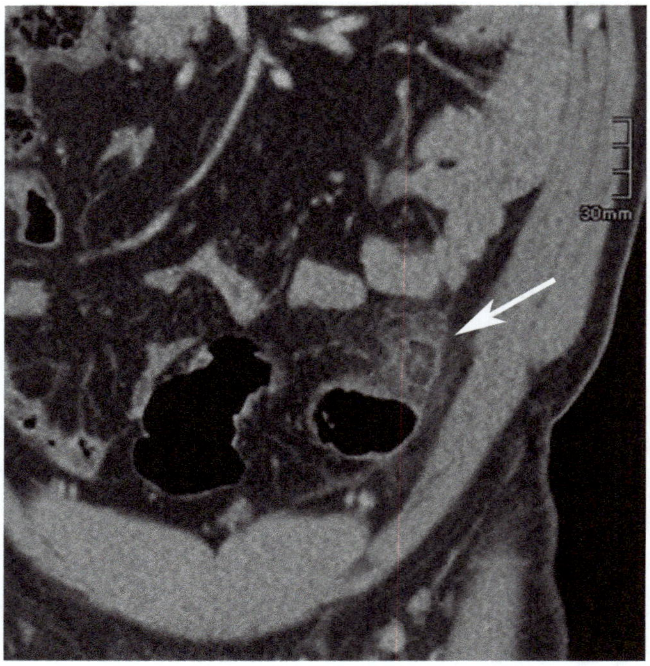

Fig. Epiploic appendagitis. The contrast-enhanced coronal CT image shows a round fat containing pericolic lesion with stranding of the surrounding fat tissue (arrow). A central hyperdense "dot" within the lesion corresponds to the thrombosed vein

Radiation Colitis

Since radiation therapy is often given for pelvic disease, the sigmoid colon and rectum are most commonly affected. Acute radiation injury, within 8 weeks after treatment, is typically self-limited and treated symptomatically. It is diagnosed clinically and does not require imaging. Imaging findings include nonspecific wall thickening and inflammatory stranding in the affected segments. In chronic radiation injury, 6–12 months after treatment, which results from radiation-induced endarteritis, smooth wall thickening and fibrosis may narrow the colonic lumen. Strictures and fistulas are possible complications. Increased pelvic fat may be present [29, 37].

Epiploic Appendagitis

Epiploic appendagitis is an uncommon inflammatory/ischemic process that results from torsion with infarction or spontaneous venous thrombosis of the appendices epiploicae. Patients may present clinically with sudden, focal abdominal pain, indistinguishable from diverticulitis or appendicitis. CT is diagnostic, typically showing an ovoid 1.5–3.5 cm fat-containing pericolic lesion with stranding of the surrounding fat tissue (Fig.). A central hyperdense "dot" can be identified within the lesion that corresponds to the thrombosed vein. Chronically, an infarcted epiploic appendix may calcify. Epiploic appendagitis is a self- limiting condition and does not require invasive intervention [41].

Take Home Messages

- Cross-sectional imaging techniques have become the most important radiologic tool for the evaluation of diseases of the colon and rectum.
- CTC is a reliable technique for the detection and classification of polypoid and stenotic lesions of the colon.
- At CTC, the most important imaging features to characterize a finding are morphology, internal structure and attenuation characteristics, and mobility. Inflammatory conditions of the colon represent a heterogeneous spectrum of diseases, showing, however, a considerable overlap of their imaging criteria.
- Radiologic differentiating features at standard cross-sectional imaging include the primary location within the GI tract, length of segmental involvement, degree of wall thickening, mural enhancement pattern, pericolonic and extraintestinal findings.

References

1. Kim DH, et al. CT colonography versus colonoscopy for the detection of advanced neoplasia. N Engl J Med. 2007;357(14):1403–12.
2. Halligan S, et al. Computed tomographic colonography versus barium enema for diagnosis of colorectal cancer or large polyps in symptomatic patients (SIGGAR): a multicentre randomised trial. Lancet. 2013;381(9873):1185–93.
3. Spada C, et al. Clinical indications for computed tomographic colonography: European Society of Gastrointestinal Endoscopy (ESGE) and European Society of Gastrointestinal and Abdominal Radiology (ESGAR) guideline. Eur Radiol. 2015;25(2):331–45.
4. Endoscopic Classification Review, G. Update on the paris classification of superficial neoplastic lesions in the digestive tract. Endoscopy. 2005;37(6):570–8.
5. Mang T, et al. Evaluation of colonic lesions and pitfalls in CT colonography: a systematic approach based on morphology, attenuation and mobility. Eur J Radiol. 2013;82(8):1177–86.
6. Neri E, et al. The second ESGAR consensus statement on CT colonography. Eur Radiol. 2013;23(3):720–9.
7. Kim DH, et al. Contrast coating for the surface of flat polyps at CT colonography: a marker for detection. Eur Radiol. 2014;24(4):940–6.
8. Kudo S, et al. Nonpolypoid neoplastic lesions of the colorectal mucosa. Gastrointest Endosc. 2008;68(4 Suppl):S3–47.
9. Pickhardt PJ, et al. Carpet lesions detected at CT colonography: clinical, imaging, and pathologic features. Radiology. 2014;270(2):435–43.
10. Pickhardt PJ, et al. Evaluation of submucosal lesions of the large intestine: part 1. Neoplasms. Radiographics. 2007;27(6):1681–92.
11. Pickhardt PJ, et al. Evaluation of submucosal lesions of the large intestine: part 2. Non neoplastic causes. Radiographics. 2007;27(6):1693–703.
12. Jeong SY, et al. The usefulness of computed tomographic colonography for evaluation of deep infiltrating endometriosis: comparison with magnetic resonance imaging. J Comput Assist Tomogr. 2013;37(5):809–14.
13. Lefere P, Gryspeerdt S. CT colonography: avoiding traps and pitfalls. Insights Imaging. 2011;2(1):57–68.
14. Dachman AH, et al. CT colonography: visualization methods, interpretation, and pitfalls. Radiol Clin N Am. 2007;45(2):347–59.
15. Silva AC, et al. Spectrum of normal and abnormal CT appearances of the ileocecal valve and cecum with endoscopic and surgical correlation. Radiographics. 2007;27(4):1039–54.
16. Mang T, Schima W. CT colonography: a guide for clinical practice. 1st ed. Stuttgart: Georg Thieme Verlag KG; 2013.
17. Regge D, et al. Ileocecal valve imaging on computed tomographic colonography. Abdom Imaging. 2005;30(1):20–5.
18. Pickhardt PJ, et al. Primary neoplasms of the appendix: radiologic spectrum of disease with pathologic correlation. Radiographics. 2003;23(3):645–62.
19. Lange N, Barlow D, Long J. Mucocele of the appendix on screening CT colonography: a case report. Abdom Imaging. 2008;33(3):267–9.
20. Johnson EK, Arcila ME, Steele SR. Appendiceal inversion: a diagnostic and therapeutic dilemma. JSLS. 2009;13(1):92–5.
21. Lefere P, et al. Diverticular disease in CT colonography. Eur Radiol. 2003;13(Suppl 4):L62–74.
22. Mang T, et al. Pitfalls in multi-detector row CT colonography: a systematic approach. Radiographics. 2007;27(2):431–54.
23. Gryspeerdt S, Lefere P. Chronic diverticulitis vs. colorectal cancer: findings on CT colonography. Abdom Imaging. 2012;37(6):1101–9.
24. Lips LM, et al. Sigmoid cancer versus chronic diverticular disease: differentiating features at CT colonography. Radiology. 2015;275(1):127–35.
25. Choi YJ, et al. CT colonography for follow-up after surgery for colorectal cancer. AJR Am J Roentgenol. 2007;189(2):283–9.
26. Macari M, Balthazar EJ. CT of bowel wall thickening: significance and pitfalls of interpretation. AJR Am J Roentgenol. 2001;176(5):1105–16.
27. Wittenberg J, et al. Algorithmic approach to CT diagnosis of the abnormal bowel wall. Radiographics. 2002;22(5):1093–107; discussion 1107–9.
28. Mang T, et al. Virtual colonoscopy: beyond polyp detection, in virtual colonoscopy: a practical guide. Berlin: Springer; 2009. p. 199–217.
29. Horton KM, Corl FM, Fishman EK. CT evaluation of the colon: inflammatory disease. Radiographics. 2000;20(2):399–418.
30. Chintapalli KN, et al. Diverticulitis versus colon cancer: differentiation with helical CT findings. Radiology. 1999;210(2):429–35.
31. Gore RM, et al. CT features of ulcerative colitis and Crohn's disease. AJR Am J Roentgenol. 1996;167(1):3–15.
32. Thoeni RF, Cello JP. CT imaging of colitis. Radiology. 2006;240(3):623–38.
33. Cha JM, Choi SI, Lee JI. Rectal syphilis mimicking rectal cancer. Yonsei Med J. 2010;51(2):276–8.
34. Kawamoto S, Horton KM, Fishman EK. Pseudomembranous colitis: spectrum of imaging findings with clinical and pathologic correlation. Radiographics. 1999;19(4):887–97.
35. del Campo L, et al. Abdominal complications following hematopoietic stem cell transplantation. Radiographics. 2014;34(2):396–412.
36. McGettigan MJ, et al. Imaging of drug-induced complications in the gastrointestinal system. Radiographics. 2016;36(1):71–87.
37. Viswanathan C, et al. Imaging of complications of oncological therapy in the gastrointestinal system. Cancer Imaging. 2012;12:163–72.
38. Torrisi JM, et al. CT findings of chemotherapy-induced toxicity: what radiologists need to know about the clinical and radiologic manifestations of chemotherapy toxicity. Radiology. 2011;258(1):41–56.
39. Kim KW, et al. Ipilimumab-associated colitis: CT findings. AJR Am J Roentgenol. 2013;200(5):W468–74.
40. Klein M, Linnemann D, Rosenberg J. Non-steroidal anti-inflammatory drug-induced colopathy. BMJ Case Rep. 2011;2011:bcr1020103436.
41. Singh AK, et al. Acute epiploic appendagitis and its mimics. Radiographics. 2005;25(6):1521–34.

20

Emergency Radiology of the Abdomen and Pelvis: Imaging of the Non-traumatic and Traumatic Acute Abdomen

Jay P. Heiken, Douglas S. Katz, and Yves Menu

Learning Objectives

- To distinguish the roles of ultrasound, computed tomography, and magnetic resonance imaging in evaluating traumatic and non-traumatic emergencies of the abdomen and pelvis.
- To discuss the differential diagnosis of acute abdominal and pelvic disorders that present with diffuse abdominal pain and with pain in each abdominal quadrant.
- To evaluate the imaging findings in acute non-traumatic disorders of the abdomen and pelvis.
- To evaluate the imaging findings after blunt or penetrating abdominal trauma.

Imaging Techniques

General Considerations

Acute abdominal and pelvic pain is often non-specific, and even under the best of circumstances, physical examination findings and laboratory investigations may not reveal a diagnosis, which is why the radiologist has such a major role in the evaluation of these patients. Because of their substantial limitations compared with cross-sectional imaging examinations, abdominal radiographs have a limited role but are still obtained selectively, primarily to evaluate suspected bowel obstruction and/or perforation. Multiple studies have demonstrated the superiority of CT as well as its impact on patient management for imaging the acute abdomen, whether in the trauma or non-trauma setting. Conventional radiographs include supine and upright views, as well as lateral decubitus views. Multi-detector CT, as noted, is the primary imaging examination for evaluation of adult patients with acute abdominal pain, as well as for patients of all ages following acute abdominal and pelvic trauma.

CT

The use of CT in patients with an acute abdomen requires careful attention to protocol. In suspected or known urolithiasis, if rupture of an abdominal aortic aneurysm (AAA) is suspected, or if there is a suspected non-traumatic hemorrhage, then generally no intravenous (IV) contrast is administered for initial CT evaluation. In most other cases of non-traumatic acute abdominal and pelvic pain, IV contrast is generally indicated. Typically, 2–3 mL per second of an appropriate per weight amount of iodinated contrast is administered through a peripheral IV catheter, and portal venous phase images are acquired from the dome of the diaphragm to the inferior aspect of the symphysis pubis, with routine image reconstruction in the transaxial plane using 3 mm slice thickness and 2 mm intervals. Thinner sections can be generated in selected cases, but coronal reformations should be created routinely by the CT technologists, sent to PACS, and reviewed by the radiologist. Sagittal (or other) reformations may be helpful in selected cases, especially in patients with bowel obstruction. The data set should be reviewed using routine abdominal windows, bone windows, and lung windows (e.g., to look for extraluminal gas and for pneumothorax at the lung bases in trauma patients). Protocols

J. P. Heiken (✉)
Mallinckrodt Institute of Radiology, Washington University School of Medicine, St. Louis, MO, USA
e-mail: heikenj@wustl.edu

D. S. Katz · Y. Menu
Hôpital Saint Antoine, Paris, France
e-mail: yves.menu@aphp.fr

can be modified by the radiologist, in conjunction with the referring physician, for specific situations. For example, a CT angiography protocol can be used for evaluation of suspected bowel ischemia, with thin-section arterial and then routine portal venous phase images acquired.

On post-contrast CT images, hyperattenuating areas can correspond to contrast enhancement or hematoma. Similarly, some calcifications can mimic contrast enhancement. To avoid this ambiguity, some centers recommend acquisition of images using dual energy to allow the reconstruction of virtual unenhanced images whenever necessary. However, the need for dual energy CT acquisition would have to be anticipated, as it is not routinely performed.

In the trauma setting, IV contrast should be given to all patients if possible, but oral contrast is not given (although combined water-soluble oral and rectal contrast may be indicated in selected patients with penetrating trauma, to evaluate for colonic injury). Trauma CT protocols vary depending on the practice and the specific situation and are often combined with CT imaging of other portions of the body. In general a single acquisition is obtained in the late arterial/early portal venous phase, which is then immediately checked by the radiologist. If there are any substantial abnormalities on these images, or if initial plain radiography of the pelvis demonstrates fractures, then a delayed (and ideally relatively low dose) CT acquisition through the area(s) of interest can be performed, to sort out the nature of injuries (i.e., whether a pseudoaneurysm versus an area of active vascular hemorrhage is present; or CT cystography can be performed in suspected bladder injury).

Oral contrast is used less frequently or not at all in an increasing number of practices, for a variety of reasons, in patients undergoing CT for non-traumatic abdominal and pelvic pain. The yield of oral contrast has been questioned, administration of such contrast adds time and minor expense, the contrast does not always reach the distal bowel, and subtle bowel wall pathology may be obscured. However, other practices prefer to give oral contrast for CT of suspected appendicitis and/or when the patient has non-specific abdominal pain. For imaging of suspected solid organ abnormalities, and for suspected urinary tract and gynecologic pathology, oral contrast is not indicated. In suspected high-grade small bowel obstruction or in the setting of mesenteric ischemia or gastrointestinal bleeding, positive oral contrast is contraindicated.

Increased attention has recently been paid to the radiation exposure from diagnostic CT examinations. Although CT appropriately remains the workhorse examination for the acute abdomen, radiation dose reduction strategies should be employed routinely, including the use of mAs reduction and, if available, iterative reconstruction in conjunction with radiation dose reduction (such as lowering the kVp in thin patients). Multiple CT phases should be acquired only when needed. For patients requiring repeat cross-sectional imaging examinations, alternative strategies, particularly MRI, should be strongly considered whenever feasible.

Ultrasound

Ultrasound (US) is the initial imaging examination of choice for patients with suspected acute cholecystitis and acute gynecological abnormalities. It is also the primary method for evaluating pregnant women and pediatric patients with acute abdominal or pelvic pain, in most clinical situations. Although somewhat less sensitive and specific than CT for appendicitis in adult patients, US is a very good first imaging examination when employed by experienced radiologists (and technologists). It also can be used to evaluate the bowel wall (in patients with a body habitus permitting such evaluation) and has a role for rapid triage of trauma patients. A variety of probes and techniques are routinely employed, including Doppler imaging and graded compression for right lower quadrant evaluation.

Magnetic Resonance Imaging

Magnetic resonance imaging (MRI) has a growing role in the imaging of pregnant women with abdominal pain who have undergone a nondiagnostic US examination. In a variety of mostly retrospective, small- to medium-sized studies, MRI has been shown to have high accuracy in the evaluation of appendicitis (Fig.) and has utility for identification and evaluation of alternative conditions, including other bowel

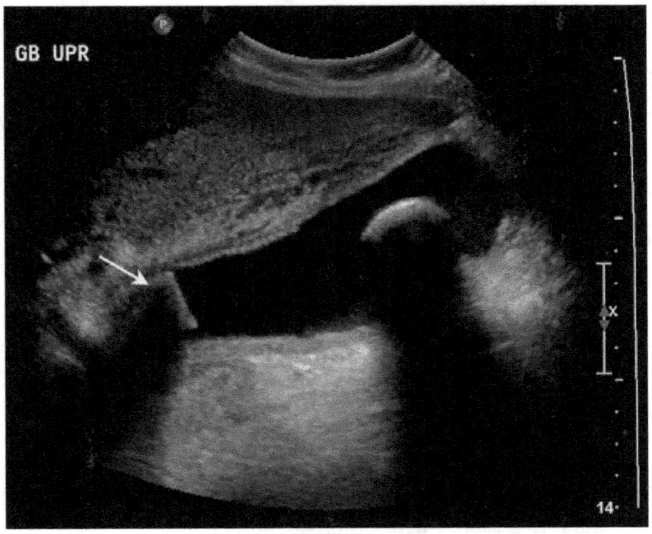

Fig. Acute cholecystitis. Ultrasound image demonstrates moder-ate distention of the gallbladder with wall thickening, sludge, and stones, including one impacted in the gallbladder neck (arrow)

pathology (such as Crohn disease), and for urinary and biliary tract pathology. Non-contrast sequences are obtained at 1.5 Tesla (or lower), with an emphasis on fast, multi-planar gradient echo/T2-weighted sequences.

Acute Pain in an Abdominal Quadrant

The differential diagnosis in a patient with an acute abdomen is greatly influenced by the nature and location of the pain. Therefore, the imaging strategies localized to each of the four abdominal quadrants will be discussed first, followed by pain which is diffuse or localized to the flank or the epigastric region.

Right Upper Quadrant

Pain from gallstones, particularly acute cholecystitis, is by far the most common group of disorders to present with acute right upper quadrant pain. Other differential diagnostic considerations include hepatitis from a variety of etiologies, liver abscess, and rarely a ruptured liver mass (usually hepatocellular adenoma or carcinoma).

US is the imaging examination of choice for evaluation of acute right upper quadrant pain. It is an accurate examination for diagnosing or excluding acute cholecystitis. Sonographic findings include gallstones, a sonographic Murphy's sign, wall thickening of 3 mm or greater, and pericholecystic fluid/inflammatory changes (Fig). The more these findings are present, particularly gallstones combined with a sono-graphic Murphy's sign, the more likely acute cholecystitis is present. Isolated gallbladder wall thickening may be due to a variety of etiologies in addition to acute cholecystitis. Recent publications have shown that CT and MRI also are relatively accurate imaging examinations for cholecystitis, although the findings may be more subtle compared with sonography, especially early on. In our experience, patients with non-specific abdominal pain and the eventual diagnosis of cholecystitis may be sent for CT on a relatively frequent basis rather than for sonography, and radiologists need to be aware of the potential for establishing or suggesting this diagnosis based on the initial CT findings, which are very similar to those on sonography, although pericholecystic inflammatory changes may be more obvious on CT and MRI. If the CT findings suggest cholecystitis but are not definitive, US can then be performed. CT also is an excellent examination for demonstrating complications and severe forms of cholecystitis, including perforation/abscess formation, hemorrhage, gas (in diabetic patients with emphysematous cholecystitis), and wall gangrene. The CT findings of a stone lodged in the gallbladder neck or cystic duct and areas of absent wall enhancement have been shown to correlate with the need for an open rather than a laparoscopic cholecystectomy. CT is also accurate in differentiating cholecystitis from gallbladder cancer, which sometimes is challenging.

US, CT, and MRI are all accurate examinations for the diagnosis (and follow-up) of liver abscesses (Fig. 13.2), which usually are pyogenic but which also may be amebic. US usually demonstrates a round or oval hypoechoic mass or masses, which may contain low-level echoes. Occasionally a hepatic abscess may simulate a solid (or partially solid)

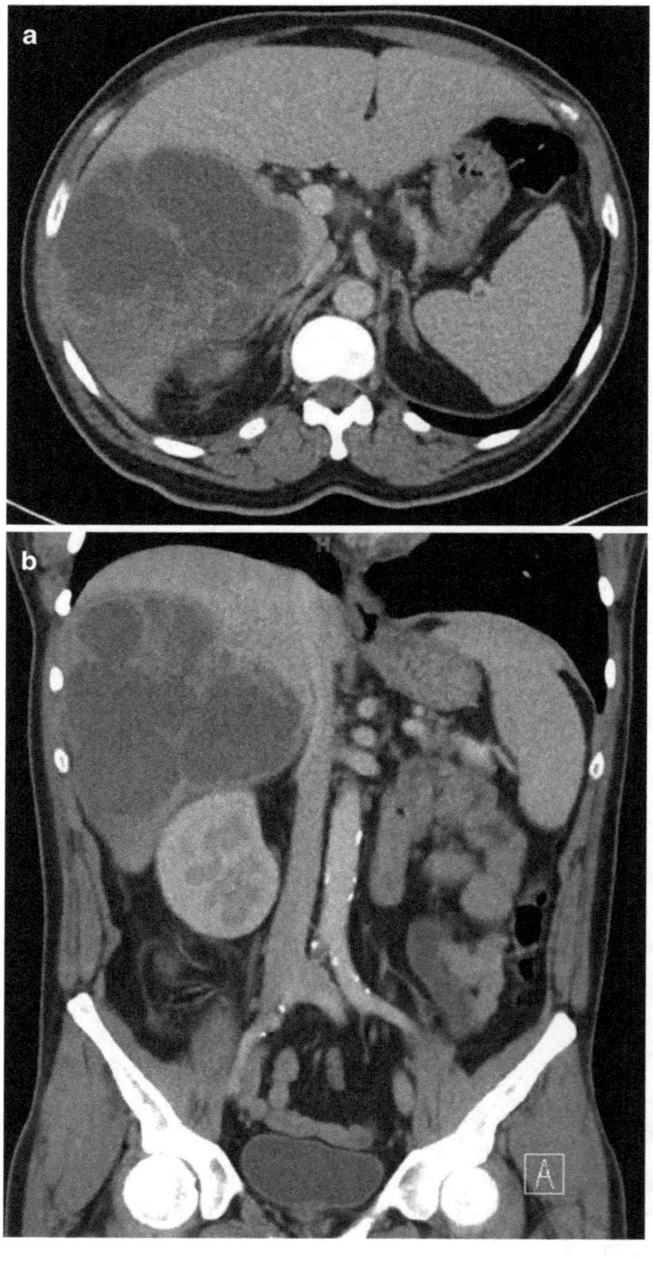

Fig. Hepatic abscess. 48-year-old man with right upper quadrant abdominal pain, fever, and leukocytosis. Transaxial (**a**) and coronal (**b**) contrast-enhanced CT images demonstrate a large fluid attenuation mass in the right hemiliver with a thick enhancing wall and septations. A drainage catheter was placed, and cultures grew *Streptococcus anginosus-constellatus-intermedius* group hepatic mass on cross-sectional imaging examinations (especially with certain *Klebsiella* species). Pyogenic liver abscesses may be idiopathic or may result from seeding from infection in the biliary tract, from the luminal gastrointestinal tract or from the portal/mesenteric venous system. An enhancing wall and a peripheral zone of edema are common on CT and MRI, but are not universally present.

Spontaneous rupture of a hepatocellular carcinoma with associated hemoperitoneum is a frequent complication in countries with a high incidence of this tumor, but is very uncommon in Western countries (less than 2% of cases). Hepatocellular carcinoma usually is highly vascular, and tumor necrosis with associated hepatic capsular rupture and rupture of vessels within the tumor is the presumed etiology. The differential diagnosis includes spontaneous hemorrhage within a hepatic adenoma or a hepatic metastasis. Patients present with acute pain and blood loss. Rapid diagnosis and therapy are essential. Transcatheter embolization is the treatment of choice.

Left Upper Quadrant

Although infrequent, acute left upper quadrant pain is most often caused by splenic infarction or splenic abscess (e.g., secondary to bland or septic emboli to the spleen) (Fig.), but may also occur in the setting of acute gas-tric disorders including gastritis and ulcer. Generally CT is performed first, although US may occasionally be the first imaging examination in such patients. The diagnosis of gastric pathology is best established by endoscopy, although patients may present with left or right upper abdominal pain, and with other non-specific s igns a nd

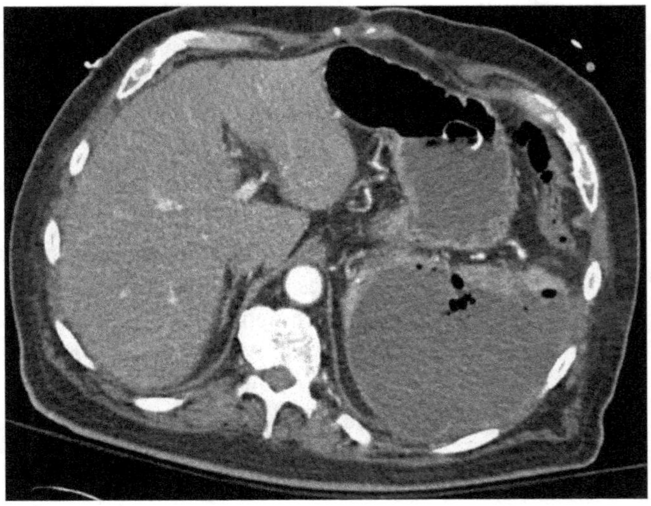

Fig. Splenic abscess. 73-year-old man with left upper quadrant pain, fever, and leukocytosis. Transaxial contrast-enhanced CT image shows a gas-containing fluid collection in the spleen. A drainage catheter was placed percutaneously, and cultures grew *Escherichia coli*

symptoms, and CT may reveal the diagnosis when it is not clinically suspected. CT findings include focal or diffuse gastric wall thickening, increased mucosal enhancement, submucosal edema, and perigastric inflammatory changes. Focal ulceration with or without perforation also may be identified, which is generally of benign but occasionally of malignant etiology.

Splenic infarction may be focal and less commonly global. Other etiologies of splenic infarction include marked splenomegaly with outgrowth of the splenic blood supply and pancreatitis. Typical infarcts are wedge-shaped and hypoattenuating on CT. Most splenic abscesses are secondary to hematogenous dissemination of infection and are seen primarily in immunocompromised individuals and IV drug abusers. On CT, splenic abscesses demonstrate low attenuation centrally with an enhancing rim and occasionally have central gas. Spontaneous splenic rupture can occur in patients with splenomegaly caused by hematologic malignancy or viral infection (e.g., mononucleosis).

Right Lower Quadrant

Appendicitis is the most frequent cause of acute right lower quadrant pain and the most commonly encountered diagnosis leading to surgery. Other disorders that can present with acute right lower quadrant pain include Crohn disease, right-sided colitis or diverticulitis, and, in women, pelvic inflammatory disease, ovarian cysts (and their complications, including rupture, hemorrhage, and torsion), and other obstetric and gynecologic conditions. Less common causes include omental infarction (which also can present with upper or mid right abdominal pain), epiploic appendagitis, and small bowel diverticulitis (ileal or Meckel's).

Preoperative cross-sectional imaging continues to play an important role in the diagnosis or exclusion of appendicitis, as well as in the identification of complications or alternative diagnoses. At most centers, even when the clinical presentation is typical (in up to one-third of patients, it is not), CT usually is obtained to confirm the diagnosis and to serve as a surgical road map (Fig.). The most specific CT finding is a thick-walled, dilated, fluid-filled appendix (occasionally containing gas), which may have one or more liths. Contrast-enhanced CT often demonstrates "stratification," in which the individual layers of the appendiceal wall can be identified, with mucosal hyperenhancement and submucosal edema. As the disorder progresses, there is increasing inflammation of the adjacent fat, especially in the retroperitoneal planes. Findings indicative of perforation include periappendiceal abscess, extraluminal gas or lith(s), a defect in the appendiceal wall, and associated small bowel obstruction. Determination of the severity of appendicitis is increasingly important as treatment strategies continually evolve. Surgery

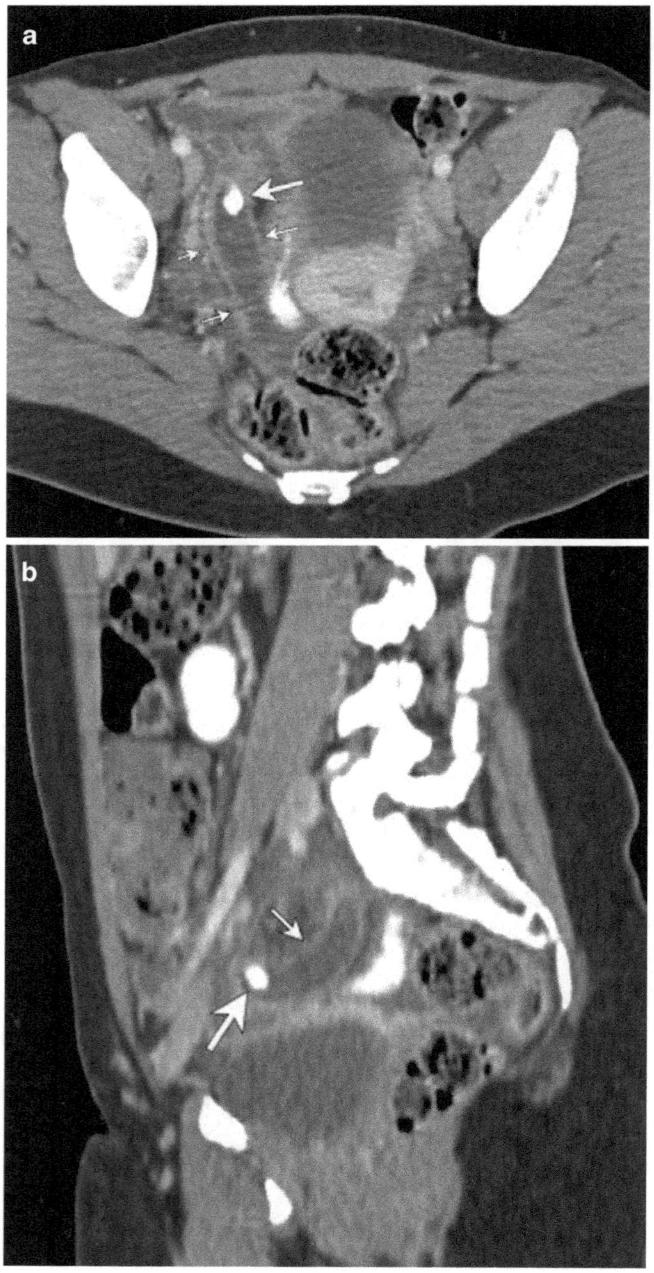

Fig. Acute appendicitis. Transaxial (**a**) and sagittal (**b**) contrast-enhanced CT images demonstrate a dilated, thick-walled, fluid-filled appendix (small arrows) with an appendicolith (large arrow) at the appendiceal orifice

should be performed emergently for severe forms of appendicitis, but alternative options that are increasingly used at some centers include delayed surgery, either the next day or on an outpatient basis, and medical treatment with imaging follow-up.

Opacification of the entire appendiceal lumen is a helpful finding to exclude appendicitis, if oral contrast is administered; however, as noted, some institutions/practices have eliminated the routine use oral contrast for CT of the acute abdomen. Regardless of the specific CT protocol used, interpretation depends in part on the experience of the interpreting radiologist. In a minority of cases, particularly in early and subacute/chronic appendicitis, the imaging findings can be subtle. It should be noted that the appendix can be larger than 6 mm in transverse diameter and can still be normal on CT, if other findings o f a ppendicitis a re absent. In the evaluation of suspected appendicitis in chil-dren (Fig.) (and in selected nonpregnant women of childbearing age), US is considered the initial examination of choice, if available, although CT has a higher accuracy. Demonstration of a swollen, noncompressible appendix >7 mm in diameter, with a target configuration (and with pain corresponding to the site of the appendix), is the primary US criteria. An appendicolith or multiple appendicoliths may be identified.

In pregnant women, appendicitis has a more variable presentation, and diagnosis is more challenging with all cross-sectional imaging modalities. US remains the initial imaging examination, despite its poor sensitivity and specificity in this clinical setting. Non-contrast MRI (Fig.) is being used increasingly in such patients after nondiagnostic US and has demonstrated high accuracy for diagnosis and exclu-sion of appendicitis and for identification of alternative diagnoses. CT should be reserved as a third-line examination, used only if needed.

A potential pitfall of image interpretation in patients with suspected acute appendicitis is the occurrence of "secondary appendicitis." In patients with adjacent inflammatory processes such as enteritis or pelvic inflammatory disease, the appendix may be inflamed secondarily as an extension of the regional process. Differentiation between secondary and primary appendicitis may be difficult as some thickening of adjacent bowel loops, including the terminal ileum, may occur in cases of "primary appendicitis."

The CT findings of right-sided diverticulitis are similar to those of the more common left-sided diverticulitis, including an inflamed diverticulum, adjacent diverticula, colonic wall thickening, and pericolonic inflammatory changes. Localized inflammation may be substantial. When considering a diagnosis of cecal diverticulitis, it is important to identify a normal appendix. Microperforation may occur, but more substantial complications, which are common in left-sided diverticulitis, including abscess formation, fistula, and obstruction, are highly unusual in right-sided diverticulitis.

Crohn disease often is first evaluated with CT; however, because patients with known Crohn disease usually are young and require serial imaging, follow-up imaging with MR enterography has become increasingly important to reduce radiation exposure (Fig.). Cross-sectional imaging permits evaluation of wall thickening and enhancement; changes of the adjacent fat, vessels, and lymph nodes; and assessment of complications, including formation of abscesses, strictures, and fistulas.

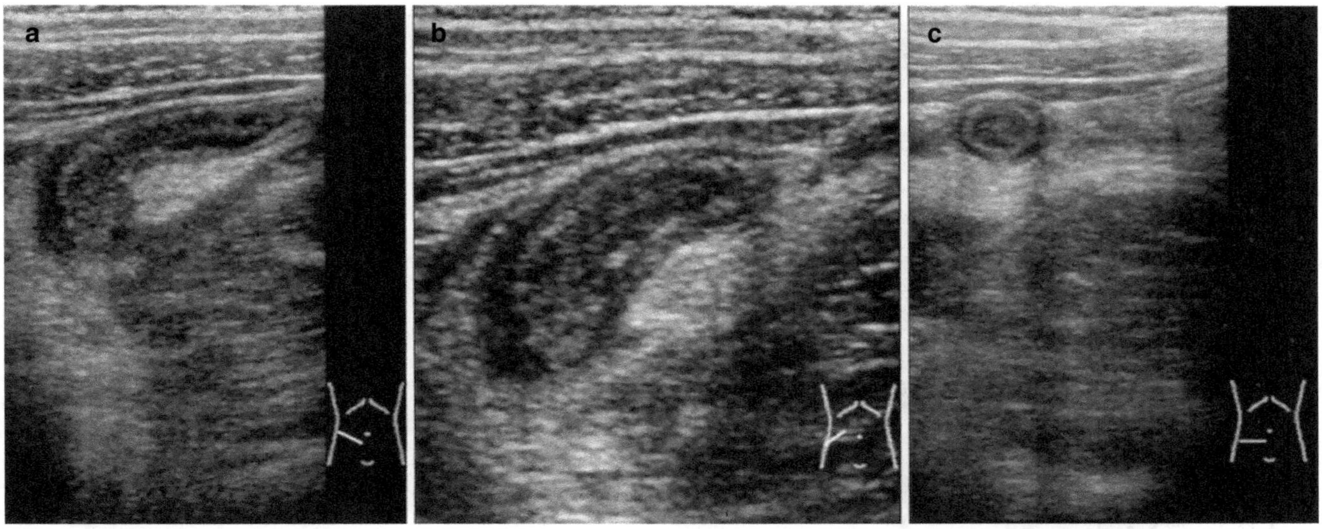

Fig. (**a**–**c**) Ultrasonography of acute appendicitis in a 12-year-old girl. Oblique and transverse views show a swollen appendix (diameter 10 mm), with a target configuration

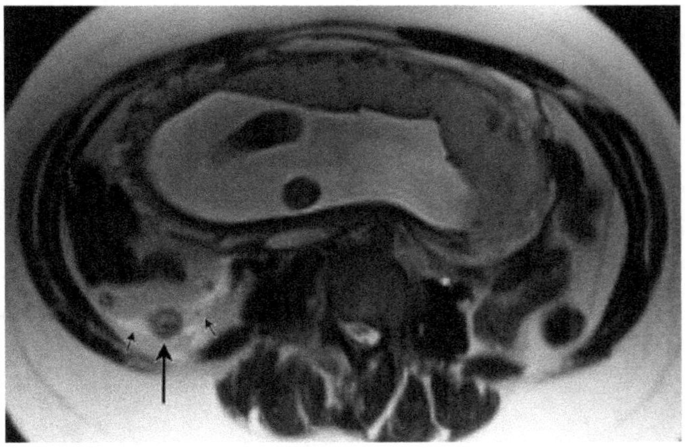

Fig. Acute appendicitis. 30-year-old woman who is 21 weeks pregnant with right lower quadrant pain. Transaxial T2-weighted unenhanced MR image shows a thick-walled retrocecal appendix (large arrow) with surrounding inflammation (small arrows)

Left Lower Quadrant

Diverticulitis of the sigmoid or descending colon is a very common disorder in middle-aged and older patients, but also can affect young individuals. CT is the examination of choice, which is typically performed with IV contrast, with or without oral or rectal contrast. Other protocols include non-contrast CT. In uncomplicated disease, the CT (or MR) findings a re t he s ame a s w ith r ight c olonic d iverticulitis. Patients with redundancy of the sigmoid colon may present with midline or right lower quadrant pain. CT also demonstrates complications, including microperforation/ extralu-minal gas (Fig.), fistula/abscess formation, and unusual complications such as venous thrombosis, liver abscess, urinary tract obstruction, and adnexal involvement. Recent data suggest that only selected patients identified with what is believed to be left colonic diverticulitis on CT require follow-up optical colonoscopy to exclude underlying carcinoma (i.e., those with CT findings that are atypical and/or complicated).

Other diagnostic considerations in patients presenting with left lower quadrant pain include colitis of a variety of etiologies, including infection (especially from *C. difficile*, in the correct clinical setting) and ischemia; functional colonic disorders (especially constipation and also obstruction from a variety of other etiologies); urinary tract infection; and gynecologic disease.

Epiploic appendagitis is a relatively common, self-limiting condition, in which an appendage of fat along the external aspect of the colon, left side much more common than right, undergoes torsion, with subsequent venous thrombosis. CT findings include a swollen, ovoid, 1.5–3.5 cm fat-containing focus with peripheral thickening and associated inflammation. The adjacent colon is usually normal or nearly normal.

GynecologicDisorders

US is the primary imaging examination in females with suspected gynecologic pathology. A human chorionic gonadotropin (HCG) level should be checked emergently in all women of childbearing age with acute non-traumatic abdominal and pelvic pain to exclude ectopic or incidental pregnancy. MRI is being used increasingly as a problem-solving examination after pelvic US and

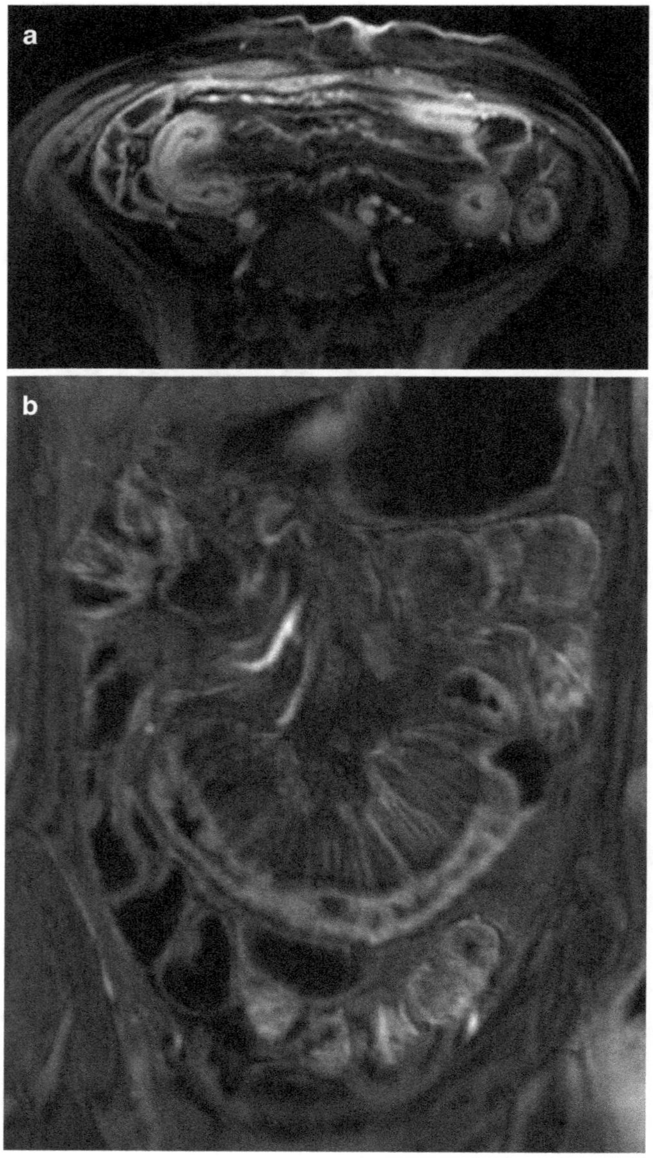

Fig. Crohn disease. 55-year-old woman with abdominal pain, diarrhea, and gastrointestinal bleeding. Transaxial (**a**) and coronal (**b**) contrast-enhanced T1-weighted images with fat suppression demonstrate ileal wall thickening, mucosal hyperenhancement, submucosal edema, and mesenteric vascular engorgement indicative of disease flair

for follow-up. However, because women with acute gynecologic disorders often present with non-specific signs and symptoms, CT is frequently ordered to evaluate their abdominal pain. Therefore radiologists interpreting CT of the acute abdomen and pelvis must be familiar with the findings of a wide variety of gynecologic disorders that may present emergently. CT also can be used selectively as a problem-solving tool in patients with known or suspected gynecologic disorders.

If ovarian torsion is suspected prospectively, pelvic US is performed emergently. However, CT and MR findings also are characteristic, are similar to US findings, and may complement

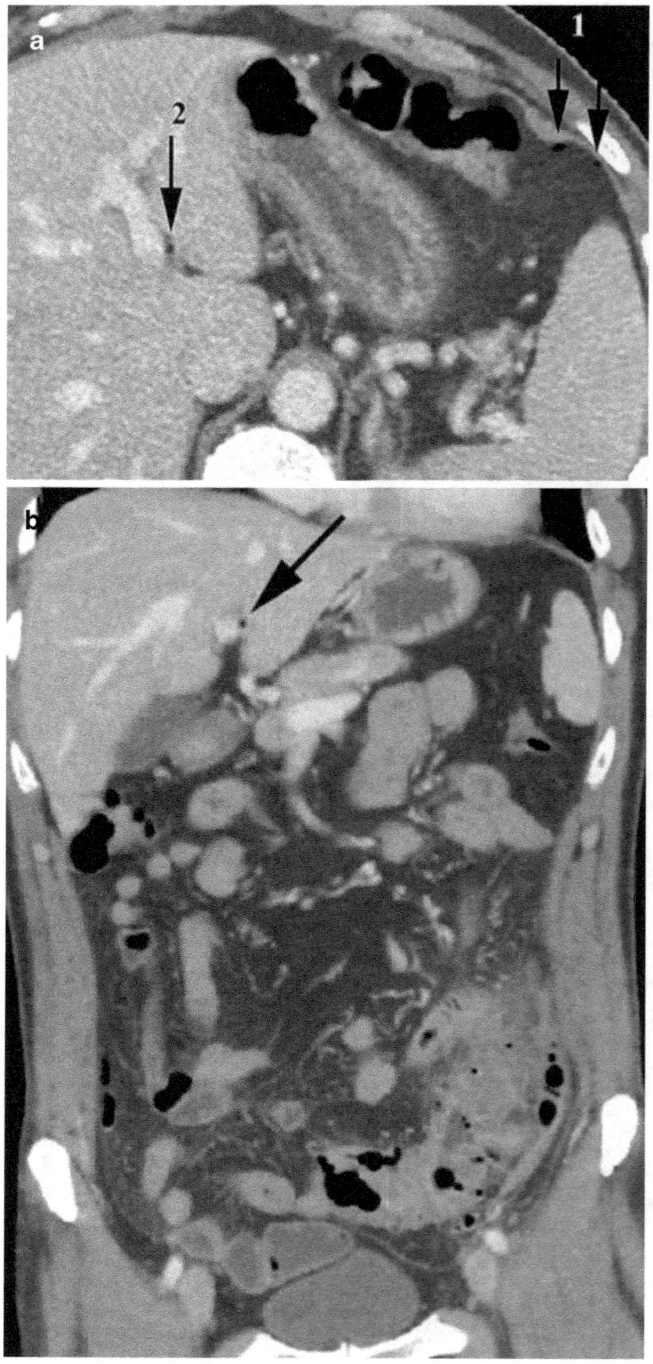

Fig. (**a**, **b**) Perforated sigmoid diverticulitis. (**a**) Axial CT image demonstrates tiny bubbles of extraluminal gas within the left subphrenic space (arrows, *1*) and hepatic pedicle (arrow, *2*). (**b**) Coronal CT reformation shows thickened sigmoid colon, with associated diverticular disease, inflammation of the adjacent fat, and thickening of the root of the sigmoid mesocolon. Note the tiny bubble of extraluminal gas (arrow) within the hepatic pedicle

US if the sonographic examination is initially equivocal. Radiologists must maintain a high index of suspicion for ovarian torsion as the clinical presentation is variable; the possibility of torsion should be raised if the imaging findings suggest or strongly point to this diagnosis. Cross-sectional imaging findings include an enlarged, edematous ovary, with or without an associated cyst or mass (most commonly a teratoma), deviation of the adnexal structures to the contralateral side, deviation of the uterus to the side of torsion, twisting of the adnexal/vascular structures, decreased ovarian vascularity, multiple peripheral ovarian follicles, inflammation of the adjacent fat, and ascites which may be high attenuation due to blood.

Ovarian cysts are very common and may be complicated by hemorrhage. Associated hemoperitoneum, if present, usually is self-limited. The differential diagnosis of a hemorrhagic ovarian cyst is endometrioma. It is particularly critical to check the HCG level in a woman with otherwise unexplained hemoperitoneum, to ensure that a ruptured ectopic pregnancy is not present.

Pelvic inflammatory d isease (PID) i s c ommon a nd h as a broad spectrum of findings and presentations. If PID is known or suspected, US is done first. H owever, C T m ay b e i nitially performed if the diagnosis is not known and the clinical presen-tation is non-specific (Fig.). The most common causative organisms are gonococcus and chlamydia. Because PID most commonly results from ascending infection, it usually involves both adnexa. In the earlier stages of PID, there may be no find-ings or subtle findings on cross-sectional imaging. There may be swelling of the ovaries and/or fallopian tubes, abnormal enhancement of the adnexal structures, and mild adjacent edema. In later stages, tubo-ovarian abscesses and/or hydrosal-pinx/ pyosalpinx may be identified, and adjacent organs also may be involved in complicated cases. Imaging findings include thickening and increased enhancement of the dilated, tortuous fallopian tube(s), a septated mass in the ovary or ovaries, and adjacent edema. Other presentations of PID include endometri-tis, cervicitis, and Fitz-Hugh-Curtis syndrome in which peri-hepatitis leads to increased on cross-sectional imaging examinations include less common forms of PID (e.g., actinomycosis), endometritis, ovarian vein thrombosis (typically following cesarean section), uterine rupture following delivery, gynecologic tumors, and complicated uterine leiomyomas (e.g., hemorrhage/degeneration, torsion, and acute prolapse).

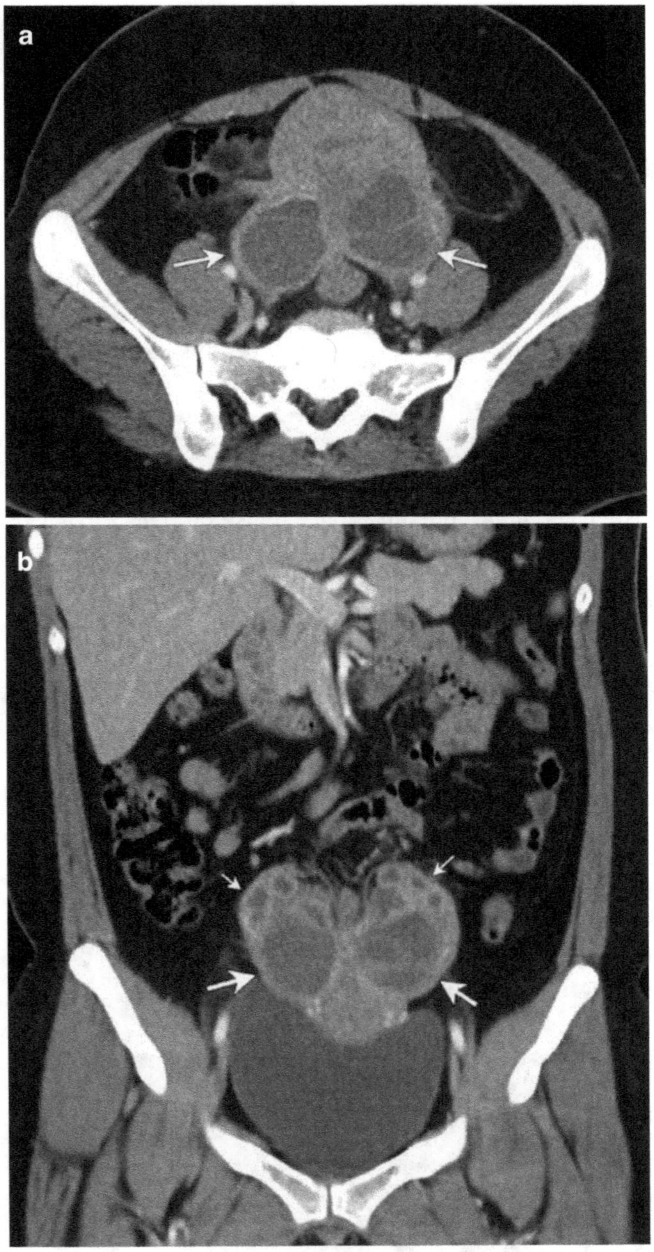

Fig. Pelvic inflammatory disease. 27-year-old woman with lower abdominal pain, fever, and leukocytosis. Transaxial (**a**) and coronal (**b**) contrast-enhanced CT images show hydrosalpinx (small arrows) and a thick-walled fluid collection (large arrows) in both adnexa

Acute Abdomen with Diffuse Pain

Any disorder that involves a large portion of the gastrointestinal tract or irritates the peritoneum can cause diffuse abdominal pain. The most common disorder is gastroenteritis, in which the CT findings often are normal or may show mild bowel wall thickening and increased intraluminal fluid. Patients with colitis have varying degrees of colonic wall thickening/edema, with inflammation of the adjacent fat. Other important disorders that present with diffuse abdominal pain include bowel obstruction and ischemia.

Bowel Obstruction

Bowel obstruction is a very frequent cause of abdominal pain in the emergency setting. Small bowel obstruction (SBO) usually is due to adhesions (more commonly in patients with previous surgery, but occasionally in patients without prior surgery) and less commonly due to a hernia (external or internal), obstructing tumor, perforated appendicitis, inflammatory bowel disease, or complicated diverticulitis. Less common etiologies include gallstone ileus, intussusception, intramural small bowel hematoma, and radiation enteritis.

Large bowel obstruction (LBO) is most commonly due to colorectal carcinoma, but diverticulitis and sigmoid or cecal volvulus also are important etiologies.

Bowel obstruction usually is diagnosed on clinical grounds and then confirmed and further evaluated as needed by imaging, typically with CT, with or without initial plain radiographs. However, not infrequently the diagnosis of bowel obstruction is not clear or known clinically, and obstruction is established on the basis of imaging. CT reveals the presence or absence of obstruction, as well as the site, level, and cause of obstruction, and permits identification of associated ischemia (Fig.). In SBO, the radiologist should search for the transition zone between the dilated proximal small bowel and the collapsed distal small bowel. There often is a segment of small bowel containing feces-like material, just proximal to the transition zone. Review of multi-planar CT reformations is important to help identify the site of transition, which may be difficult to find conclusively on review of transaxial images alone. In a minority of cases, CT reveals a closed-loop SBO (Fig.), which usually requires emergency surgery. In this situation, two points along the course of the small bowel are obstructed at a single site, usually associated with an adhesive band or hernia. Less commonly, closed-loop SBO may be due to volvulus of the small bowel.

SBO needs to be differentiated from LBO and from ileus and motility disorders involving the small and/or large bowel. Ileus of the small and/or large bowel is common after abdominal surgery and has multiple etiologies. In LBO, CT demonstrates distension of the colon to the point of obstruction, with collapse of the colon. The small bowel may demonstrate varying degrees of associated dilation. Colonic volvulus should be readily identified (Fig.), particu-larly on review of multi-planar reformations. A variety of CT signs have been reported, and volvulus may be complicated by ischemia and subsequent perforation. Marked dilation of most or all of the colon may be seen in toxic megacolon from a variety of etiologies, as well as in "pseudo-obstruction," the latter of which also can lead to subsequent volvulus. A very common cause of abdominal pain in emergency department patients is constipation, which may be of varying degrees of severity, usually without an associated focal obstructing lesion. Other motility disorders, such as scleroderma and

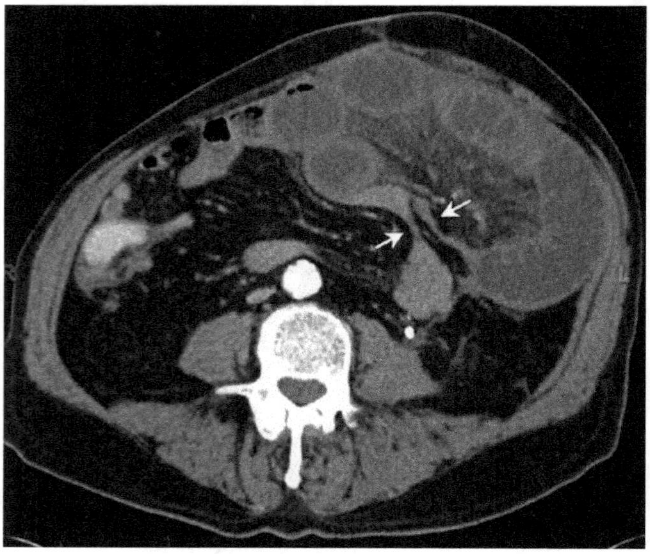

Fig. Closed-loop small bowel obstruction. 62-year-old man with metastatic colon cancer who presented with severe abdominal pain, nausea, and vomiting. Transaxial contrast-enhanced CT image shows a fluid-filled, distended loop of small bowel in the left mid-abdomen. Mesenteric edema and mild wall thickening indicate bowel ischemia. Note the two adjacent collapsed segments of small bowel (arrows), where the loop of small bowel had entered an internal hernia

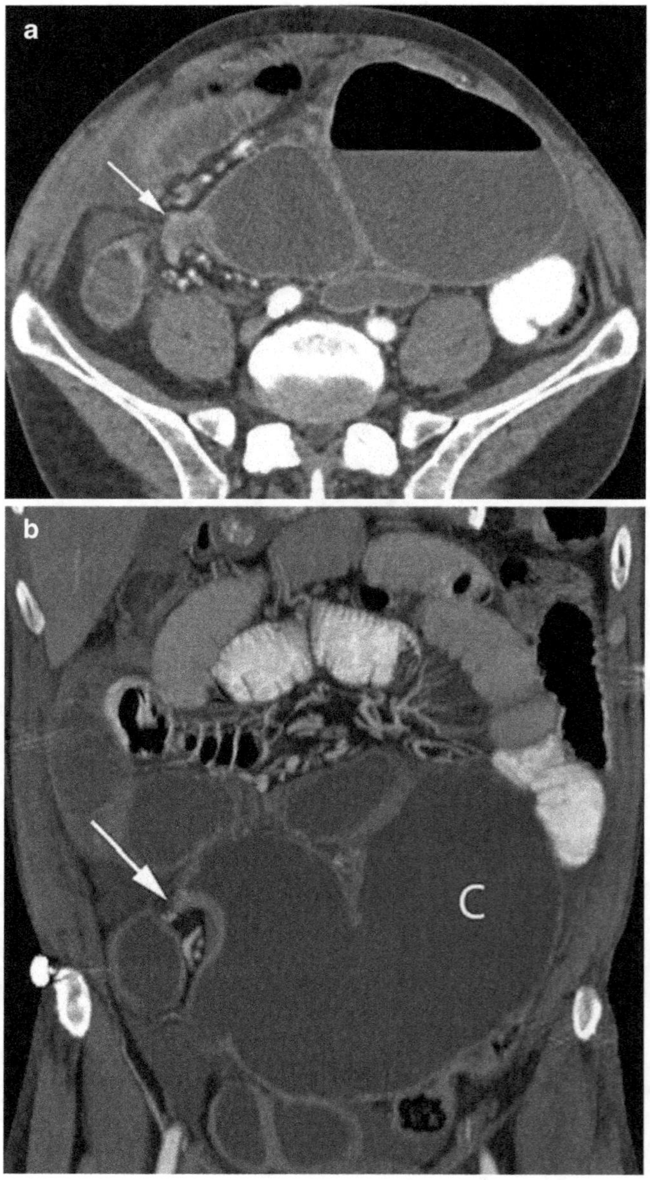

Fig. (**a**, **b**) Cecal volvulus. Transverse CT image (**a**) and coronal CT reformation (**b**) demonstrate a markedly dilated cecum (*C*) located in the midline and left lower abdomen and upper pelvis. The arrow points to the area of colonic twisting. Note the dilated small bowel loops, due to the proximal colonic obstruction

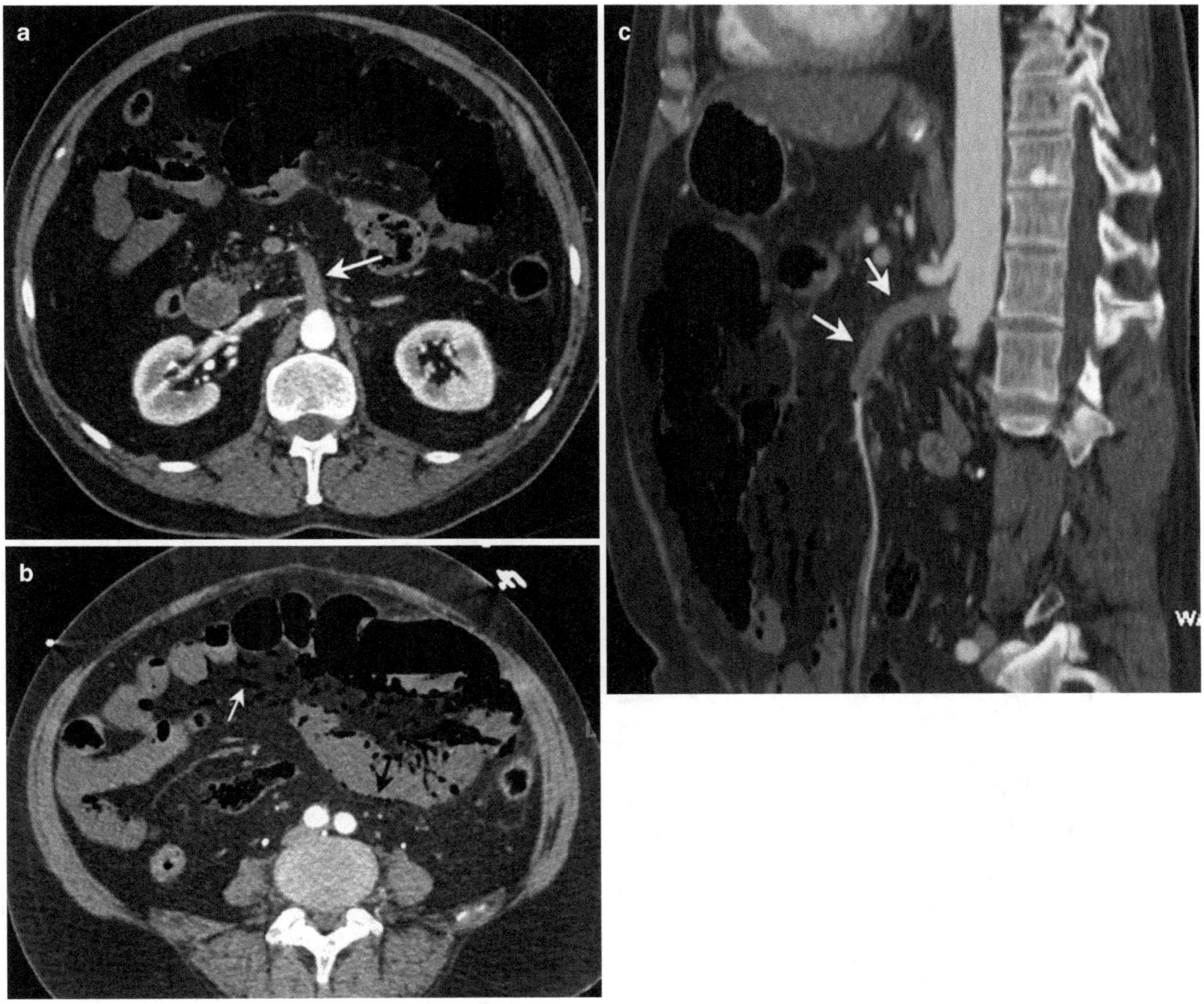

Fig. Acute bowel ischemia secondary to superior mesenteric artery thrombosis. 52-year-old man with 4-day history of severe diffuse abdominal pain. Transaxial (**a**, **b**) and sagittal curved planar reformatted (**c**) contrast-enhanced CT images demonstrate thrombosis of the superior mesenteric artery (large white arrow). Note the bowel pneumatosis (small black arrow) and gas within the mesenteric veins (small white arrow) indicative of bowel ischemia

administration of anticholinergic or opioid medications, also may lead to the performance of CT, in patients presenting with acute abdominal pain.

One of the most important responsibilities of the radiologist in the case of acute bowel obstruction is to help determine if the patient should undergo surgery or conservative management. Today, more than 50% of patients with bowel obstruction do not undergo surgery. Imaging criteria for surgical intervention include findings indicative of bowel ischemia (see Sect. 13.4.2) or a closed-loop obstruction.

Bowel Ischemia

Bowel ischemia has a variety of etiologies, including arterial thrombosis or embolism, venous thrombosis, hypoperfusion, and vasculitis. Occlusive disease involves the mesenteric arteries, most commonly the superior mesenteric artery (Fig.), whereas bowel ischemia secondary to venous thrombosis is much less common. The only direct CT (or MRI) sign of vascular impairment of the bowel is diminished wall enhancement, whereas increased bowel wall enhancement is seen in a wide variety of disorders, including in a subset of patients with bowel ischemia due to reactive hyperemia, loss of autoregulation, or compromised venous outflow. Other cross-sectional imaging findings include direct visualization of embolus or thrombus in the mesenteric arterial circulation or thrombus in the mesenteric venous circulation. Bowel distension and wall edema are non-specific findings that may be identified in ischemia, but also may be present in various infectious, inflammatory, or immunologic conditions and in primary bowel obstruction. Nonocclusive acute mesenteric ischemia usually is due to hypoperfusion secondary to severe cardiac disease; generalized decreased caliber of the arterial circulation is present.

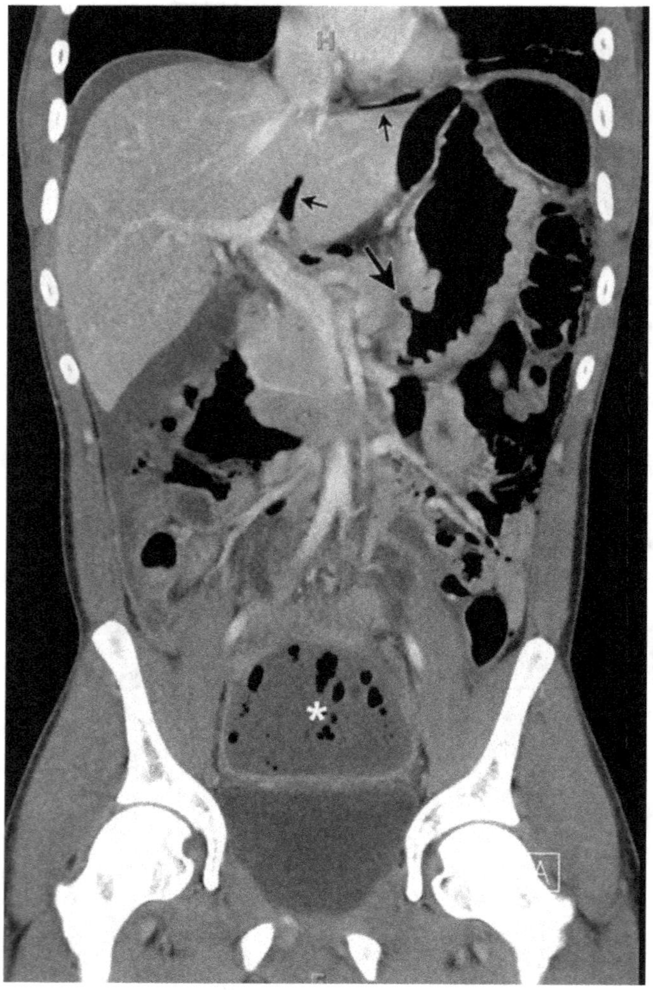

Fig. Perforated gastric ulcer. 26-year-old man with left upper quadrant pain, fever, and leukocytosis. Coronal CT image shows an ulcer (large arrow) along the lesser curvature of the stomach with surrounding wall thickening. Note free intraperitoneal gas (small arrows) and large pelvic abscess (asterisk)

Bowel ischemia also may be secondary to bowel obstruction, particularly a closed-loop SBO, but may also be identified secondary to large bowel obstruction or volvulus. Focal or regional bowel wall thickening due to edema and hemorrhage may be seen on CT, with decreased bowel wall enhancement and edema adjacent to the affected bowel. With frank infarction, pneumatosis, portal/mesenteric venous gas, peritonitis/ascites, and free gas can be found.

Gastrointestinal Perforation

Gastrointestinal perforation usually causes localized pain initially, which becomes more diffuse if peritonitis devel-ops. Perforation due to peptic ulcer disease (Fig.) or a necrotic neoplasm has become less frequent, due to earlier diagnosis and improved therapy (Fig). However, perforation resulting from endoscopic procedures has increased in incidence. Perforation of the small bowel is relatively uncommon, but may be secondary to a foreign body, diverticulitis, or trauma, among other possibilities. Perforation of the colon is more frequent and can occur when the colon becomes markedly distended proximal to an obstructing lesion (e.g., tumor, volvulus) or when the colonic wall is friable (e.g., diverticulitis, ischemia, ulcerative colitis, tumor).

Pneumoperitoneum can be recognized by gas under the diaphragm on an upright chest radiograph or an upright or lateral decubitus abdominal radiograph. Detection of subtle pneumoperitoneum often is difficult. CT is the examination of choice in suspected bowel perforation as is much more sensitive for the identification of such perforations compared with plain radiographs and can be used to identify the source of perforation in the vast majority of such cases. Viewing the CT images using lung window settings improves demonstration of small amounts of extraluminal gas. Examining all three orthogonal planes (axial, sagittal, and coronal) improves the sensitivity for detection of small volume pneumoperitoneum. The sagittal plane is especially helpful as a minimal amount of gas in the umbilical area may be very difficult to see under the transverse mesocolon on axial images.

Identifying the cause of perforation may be difficult. The first step is to determine if the perforation is in the upper or lower abdomen. Some simple rules are helpful. If the pneumoperitoneum is localized only under the transverse mesocolon, the perforation likely is of colonic origin. If gas accumulates in the lesser omentum and along the left portal vein in the liver hilum, gastroduodenal perforation is likely. If gas is found in the lesser sac, gastroduodenal perforation is almost certain. In cases of abundant pneumoperitoneum, localizing the site of perforation may be difficult.

Gas from retroperitoneal bowel perforation typically has a more mottled appearance and initially may be contained locally. As with intraperitoneal perforation, it is more readily identified and its etiology more clearly defined on CT. Diagnostic considerations include a perforated duodenal ulcer, complicated diverticulitis, perforated colon cancer, and iatrogenic perforation.

Acute Abdomen with Flank or Epigastric Pain

Acute flank pain or upper abdominal pain that radiates to the back most commonly is a manifestation of retroperitoneal pathology, particularly ureteral colic, acute pancreatitis, and ruptured abdominal aortic aneurysm (AAA). If AAA rupture is suspected, or if retroperitoneal (or other site of hemorrhage) is suspected, then an emergency non-contrast CT is performed. An additional CT acquisition with IV contrast to evaluate the vascular anatomy in more detail and to determine if there is ongoing active hemorrhage usually is obtained as part of the same examination.

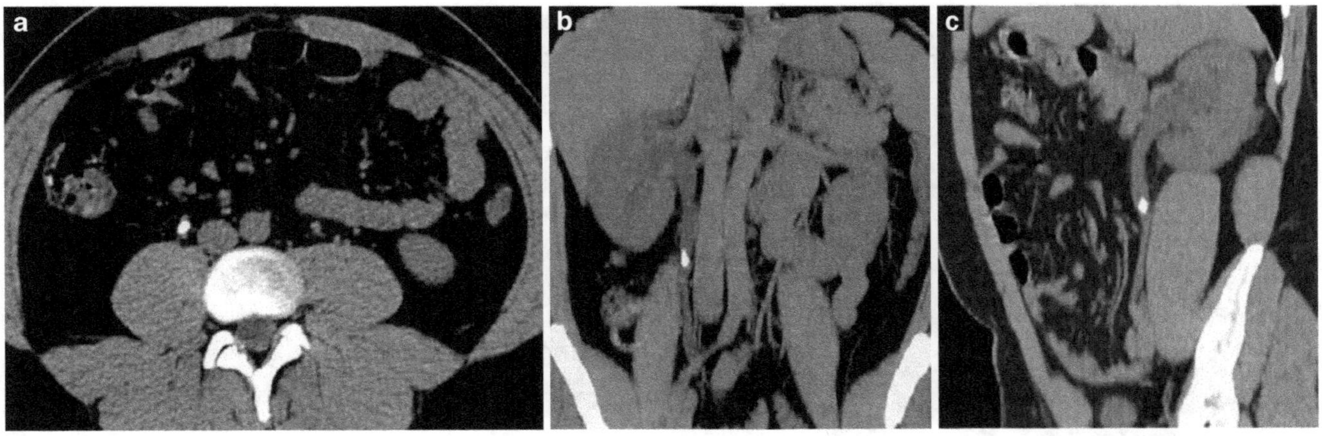

Fig. (**a–c**) Right-sided urinary colic. Axial CT image (**a**) and coronal (**b**) and oblique sagittal (**c**) CT reformations show dilatation of the proximal right urinary tract, due to a ureteral calculus

Urinary Colic

The lifetime incidence of an obstructing ureteral calculus is estimated at upward of 12%. The clinical diagnosis often is not initially clear (and CT with IV contrast may therefore be obtained). For evaluation of known or suspected urolithiasis, non-contrast CT is the imaging examination of choice. It is extremely accurate for the identification of urinary tract calculi, as well as for stone sizing, determination of overall stone burden, identification of complications, and demonstration of alternative or additional significant diagnoses (in upward of 10–15% of cases).

Virtually all urinary tract stones are radiopaque, regardless of their specific chemical composition. The non-symptomatic side acts as an intrinsic control, as bilateral ureteral calculi are rare. Secondary signs of obstruction, including hydronephrosis, hydroureter, renal swelling, and perinephric and periureteric edema, are present in 95% of patients with a ureteral stone (Fig.). Coronal reformations are routinely used and may help the radiologist distinguish between a ureteral calculus and an adjacent phlebolith. Phleboliths, which are calcifications in veins, increase in incidence with age, usually are located lateral and posterior to the ureter, and typically have a "tail" or "comet" sign, whereas most ureteral calculi are surrounded by a rim of soft tissue. In patients who present with symptoms of renal colic but do not have a ureteral calculus, CT demonstrates a wide variety of alternative diagnoses in a substantial minority of such patients.

CT is used to determine management of patients with urolithiasis, as almost all ureteral calculi <5 mm, especially if distally located, will pass spontaneously with conservative treatment (unless there is concurrent infection, in which case more aggressive management usually is indicated). Renal calculi frequently are found concurrently with ureteral calculi and occasionally may be the source of pain. Repeat CT, for short-term follow-up and for additional episodes of colic, should be used selectively, especially in younger patients, and attention should be paid to reducing radiation dose. In very selected situations, repeat CT with IV contrast is indicated, for evaluation of suspected superinfection or to clarify an equivocal alternative diagnosis.

Acute Pancreatitis

Pancreatitis is common and has a broad spectrum of presentations and outcomes. On initial clinical evaluation, pancreatitis frequently is confused with other disorders, and amylase and lipase levels may either be pending or not obtained. Therefore it is important for the radiologist to identify pancreatitis, usually on CT but occasionally on sonography, when the diagnosis is not suspected clinically. The vast majority of cases are due to gallstones or alcohol abuse. Less common etiologies include trauma, interventional pancreatobiliary procedures, medications, elevated triglycerides, congenital anomalies (i.e., pancreas divisum, annular pancreas, absent dorsal pancreas), and underlying tumor. Less common presentations include chronic pancreatitis, autoimmune pancreatitis, and paraduodenal (groove) pancreatitis.

A routine CT protocol is used when pancreatitis is not specifically suspected, but a tailored protocol can be used when it is suspected or for follow-up of known pancreatitis. Specifically, no oral contrast is given, or water is used as a neutral oral contrast agent. IV contrast is administered, if not contraindicated, to assess for necrosis, to characterize fluid collections, and to identify vascular complications including venous thrombosis and pseudoaneurysm formation. Imaging is performed in a late arterial ("pancreatic") phase. CT findings range from a normal or nearly normal pancreas with mild focal or diffuse peripancreatic inflammation to marked pancreatic edema and associated necrosis (Fig.). In the initial few days, CT findings do not necessarily correlate with patient outcome, but later in the patient's course, the CT findings have greater prognostic significance.

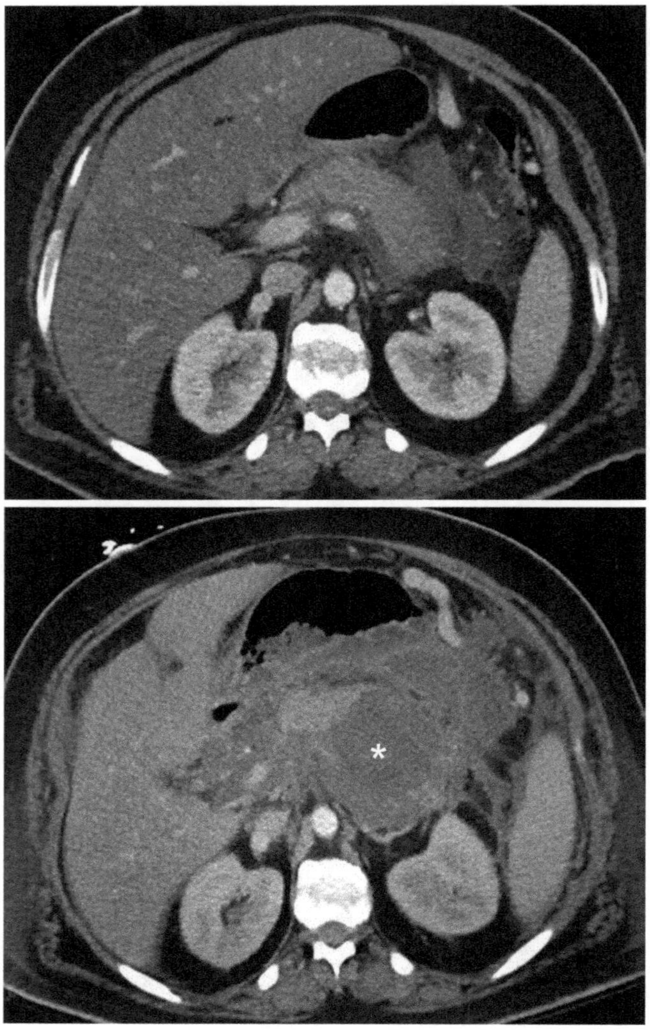

Fig. Evolution of acute interstitial edematous pancreatitis (**a**) to acute necrotizing pancreatitis (**b**). 34-year-old man with abdominal pain. (**a**) Transaxial contrast-enhanced CT image shows diffuse edema of the pancreas and peripancreatic fluid. (**b**) Transaxial contrast-enhanced CT image obtained 2 weeks later shows necrosis of the pancreatic tail which is now replaced by an acute necrotic collection (asterisk)

There are two main types of acute pancreatitis: interstitial edematous versus necrotizing. The revised Atlanta classification system attempts to better characterize the disease process, to standardize terminology—including the description of cross-sectional imaging findings—and to provide better correlation with prognosis. Other CT scoring systems also are in use to characterize the findings of pancreatitis and provide prognostic information. In the revised Atlanta classification system, in the first 4 weeks, there may be acute peripancreatic fluid collections (APFCs) associated with interstitial edematous pancreatitis versus acute necrotic collections (ANCs) associated with necrotizing pancreatitis, the latter of which can be pancreatic and/or peripancreatic and which may be sterile or infected. After 4 weeks, APFCs usually resolve, but can become pseudocysts (which may be sterile or infected), whereas ANCs may evolve into areas of walled-off necrosis (WON), which may be pancreatic and/or peripancreatic and which may be sterile or infected.

CT-guided aspiration is very useful when indicated, to distinguish sterile from infected necrosis/fluid collections. Additionally, MRI should be strongly considered when follow-up imaging is needed, to reduce radiation exposure, as these patients often require multiple repeat examinations in the short term and may also have repetitive episodes of pancreatitis.

Imaging of Abdominal and Pelvic Trauma

Blunt Abdominal Trauma

MDCT has become the primary imaging examination for evaluating blunt abdominal trauma and has replaced diagnostic peritoneal lavage (DPL) in almost all circumstances. US plays an important role in the detection of hemoperitoneum in hemodynamically unstable patients. The intra-abdominal injuries expected after blunt abdominal trauma depend upon the mechanism of injury, whether or not a restraint device was used, and patient body habitus. Knowledge of the common patterns of injury resulting from different types of motor vehicle collisions (frontal, lateral, and rear impact; sideswipe, rollover, etc.) and other traumatic events aids identification of specific types of injuries, but a discussion of these factors is beyond the scope of this chapter.

Imaging Techniques

Intravenous contrast enhancement for MDCT is critical to enable detection of abdominal and pelvic injuries. As noted above, mages generally are obtained in the portal venous phase of enhancement (approximately 65–80 s after administration of 100–150 mL injected at 3–5 mL per second). Arterial phase images may be helpful in some severely injured patients to demonstrate vascular injuries of the solid organs that may not be apparent on the portal venous phase images and to characterize areas of active extravasation as arterial versus venous. When injuries are suspected on the portal venous phase images, 5–10-min delayed images are helpful to detect injuries of the urinary tract and to further characterize solid visceral organ injuries that involve the vasculature. Patients with suspected bladder injury should undergo CT cystography. Oral contrast material is no longer administered at almost all trauma centers for patients with blunt abdominal trauma.

Focused assessment with sonography for trauma (FAST) is a limited abdominal ultrasound examination designed primarily to identify peritoneal fluid. A six-point examination generally is performed using a 3.5 MHz sector transducer. Images of the right subphrenic space (above the liver), left subphrenic space (above the spleen), hepatorenal fossa, perisplenic space (at the inferior margin of the spleen), peritoneal recess of the pelvis, and pericardium are recorded. Although FAST has been shown to be 86% sensitive for detection of abdominal injuries requiring surgery, liver and spleen injuries are not always associated with hemoperitoneum, and a negative FAST does not exclude an intra-abdominal injury. On the other hand, patients with a positive FAST do not always require surgery. Therefore, hemodynamically stable patients with a positive FAST should undergo MDCT for staging of their injuries. In addition, FAST is not reliable for assessment of the retroperitoneum.

Pneumoperitoneum

On MDCT, pneumoperitoneum may consist of free gas beneath the anterior abdominal wall or small bubbles of gas trapped between leaves of the mesentery or within peritoneal recesses. Review of images using lung window settings can be helpful in identifying small amounts of intraperitoneal gas. In the setting of trauma, pneumoperitoneum is highly suggestive of bowel perforation. A localized collection of gas may be identified adjacent to the site of bowel perforation. It is important to keep in mind that pneumoperitoneum is not always present on CT scans of patients with documented bowel perforation. In addition, pneumoperitoneum occasionally may be present in patients without bowel injury, secondary to multiple other potential causes including barotrauma, intraperitoneal spread of air from a large pneumothorax, or DLP.

Peritoneal Fluid

In trauma patients, peritoneal fluid m ost c ommonly r epresents blood resulting from injury to the liver, spleen, bowel, or mesentery. In most patients hemoperitoneum has an atten-uation value ranging from 20 to 45 HU or greater (Fig.); however, in up to one-quarter of patients, hemoperitoneum has an attenuation value less than 20 HU. Blood located adja-cent to the source of hemorrhage often is partially clotted and higher in attenuation (the "sentinel clot" sign), which can be helpful in identifying the site of bleeding. Free peritoneal fluid in the absence of direct signs of solid or hollow visceral injury may be problematic, especially in men. However, recent studies have shown that small amounts of simple peri-toneal fluid are found in up to 5% of male blunt trauma patients in the absence of hollow or solid organ injury. Therefore, immediate surgical intervention is not mandated in such patients, but careful review of the CT images for subtle injuries and hospital admission with close clinical follow-up and repeat CT if necessary are recommended.

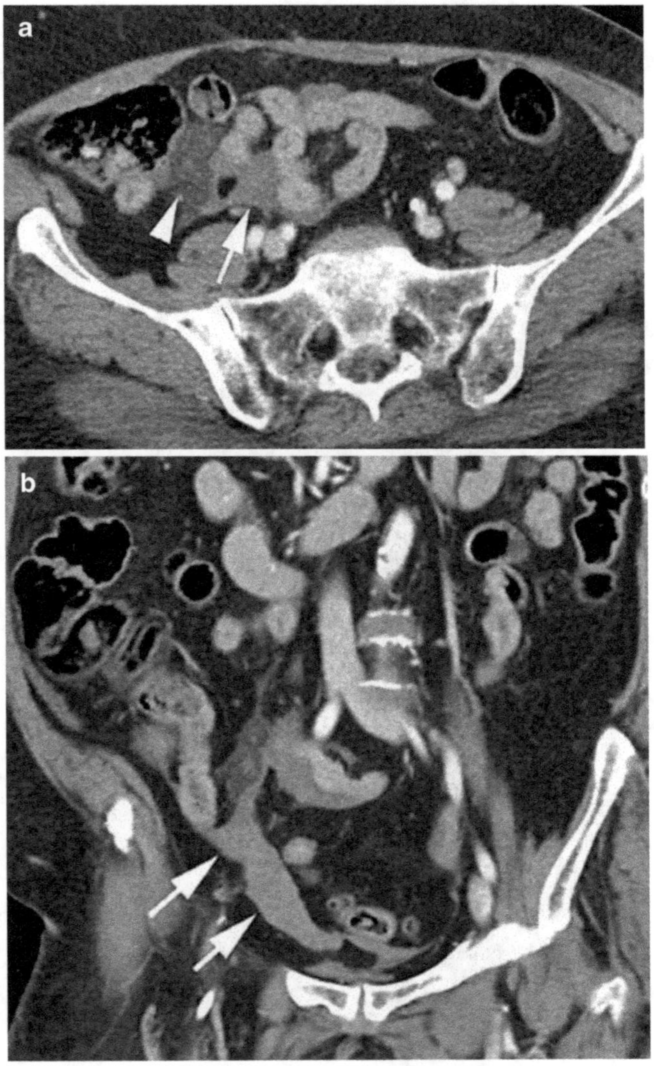

Fig.(**a**, **b**). Hemoperitoneum due to mesenteric injury from motor vehicle collision. Transaxial CT image (**a**) demonstrates high-attenuation fluid (arrow) adjacent to small bowel loops. Increased attenuation within the mesenteric fat (arrowhead) is due to a mesenteric contusion. Coronal image (**b**) shows blood layering dependently within the peritoneal cavity

Splenic Injuries

The spleen is the most commonly injured abdominal organ in blunt trauma. In the large majority of cases, splenic injuries can be managed nonsurgically. The need for surgical intervention is based on patient factors, clinical findings, and the CT-based splenic injury scale developed by the American Association for the Surgery of Trauma (AAST) (Table). The AAST splenic injury scale takes into account the size and location of splenic lacerations and hematomas. Higher- grade injuries (generally AAST grade III and higher) more often require surgical therapy; how-ever, this grading scale has been shown to be a relatively poor predictor of the success of nonsurgical management. More recently an MDCT- based splenic injury grading sys-

Table American Association for the Surgery of Trauma (AAST) Splenic Injury Scale

Injury grade and type	Description
I	
Hematoma	Subcapsular, <10% surface area
Laceration	Capsular tear, <1-cm parenchymal depth
II	
Hematoma	Subcapsular, 10–50% of surface area or intraparenchymal hematoma <5-cm diameter
Laceration	1–3 cm parenchymal depth; does not involve trabecular vessels
III	
Hematoma	Subcapsular hematoma, >50% surface area or expanding; ruptured subcapsular or intraparenchymal hematoma; intraparenchymal hematoma >5 cm or expanding
Laceration	>3-cm parenchymal depth or involves trabecular vessels
IV	
Laceration	Laceration, involves segmental or hilar vessels, producing major devascularization (>25% of spleen)
V	
Laceration	Completely shattered spleen
Vascular	Hilar vascular injury that devascularizes spleen

Note: Increase by one grade (up to grade III) for multiple injuries. Adapted from Moore et al. (1995), with permission

Table Multidetector computed-tomography-based splenic injury grading system

Injury grade	Description
I	Subcapsular hematoma <1-cm thick; laceration <1-cm parenchymal depth; parenchymal hematoma <1-cm diameter
II	Subcapsular hematoma 1- to 3-cm thick; laceration 1- to 3-cm parenchymal depth; parenchymal hematoma 1- to 3-cm diameter
III	Splenic capsular disruption; subcapsular hematoma <3-cm thick; laceration <3-cm parenchymal depth; parenchymal hematoma <3-cm thick
IVA	Active intraparenchymal or subcapsular splenic bleeding; splenic vascular injury (pseudoaneurysm or arteriovenous fistula); shattered spleen
IVB	Active intraperitoneal bleeding

Adapted from Marmery et al. (2007), with permission

tem (Table) has been proposed, which takes into account additional CT features of splenic trauma including the presence of active hemorrhage (Fig.), a pseudoaneurysm, or an arteriovenous (AV) fistula. Active hemorrhage appears as a localized area of hyperattenuation within the injured splenic parenchyma, which persists and grows larger on delayed images. In contradistinction, a pseudoan-

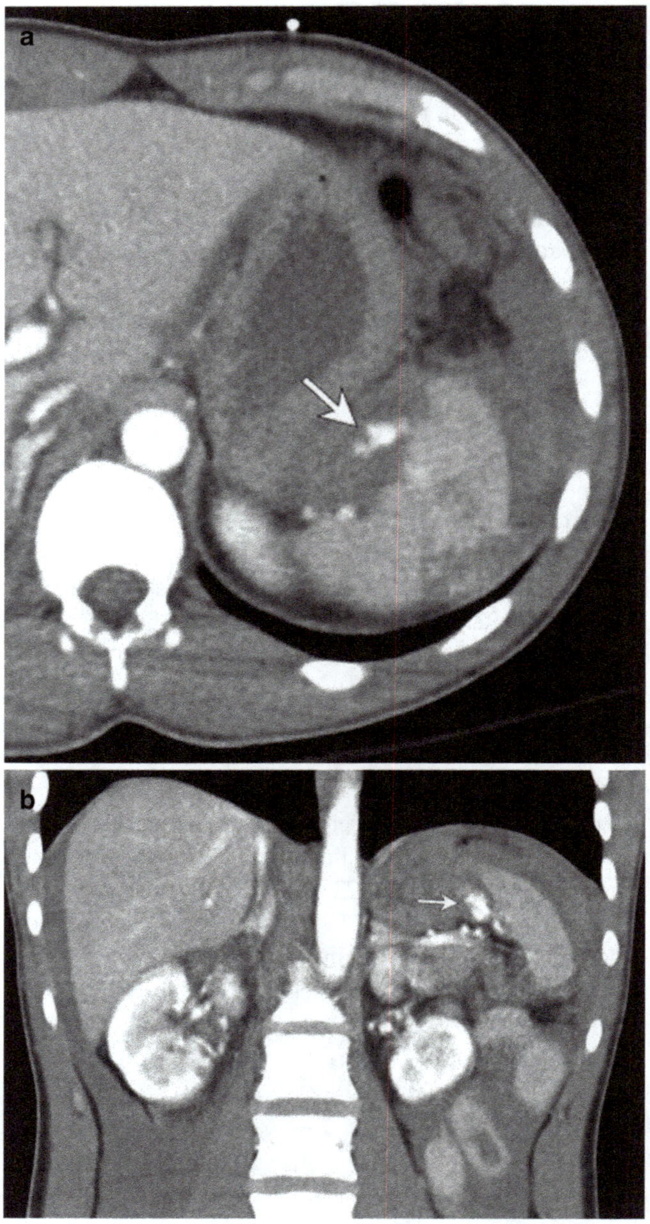

Fig. Splenic laceration. Transaxial (**a**) and coronal (**b**) contrast-enhanced CT images show a splenic laceration with contrast extravasation (arrow) and intraperitoneal bleeding (grade IVB)

eurysm or AV fistula washes out on delayed phase images. Some trauma specialists now advocate the acquisition of arterial phase CT images of the abdomen, in addition to the portal venous and delayed phase images after blunt trauma, because not all vascular injuries of the spleen are identified on portal venous and delayed phase images. Further study is required to validate this proposal.

Hepatic Injuries

Hepatic injuries are only slightly less common than splenic injuries and more frequently involve the right lobe. As with

Table American Association for the Surgery of Trauma (AAST) Liver Injury Scale

Injury grade and type	Description
1	
Hematoma	Subcapsular, <10% surface area
Laceration	<1 cm in depth
2	
Hematoma	Subcapsular, 10–50% of surface area; intraparenchymal hematoma <10 cm in diameter
Laceration	1–3 cm in depth or <10 cm in length
3	
Hematoma	Subcapsular, >50% surface area or expanding; ruptured subcapsular or parenchymal hematoma; intraparenchymal hematoma >10 cm or expanding
Laceration	>3-cm parenchymal depth
4	
Laceration	Parenchymal disruption involving 25–75% of hepatic lobe or one to three Couinaud segments in a single lobe
5	
Laceration	Parenchymal disruption involving >75% of hepatic lobe, or more than three Couinaud segments in a single lobe
Vascular	Juxtahepatic venous injuries (i.e., retrohepatic vena cava and/or central major hepatic veins)
6	
Vascular	Hepatic avulsion

Adapted from Moore et al. (1995), with permission

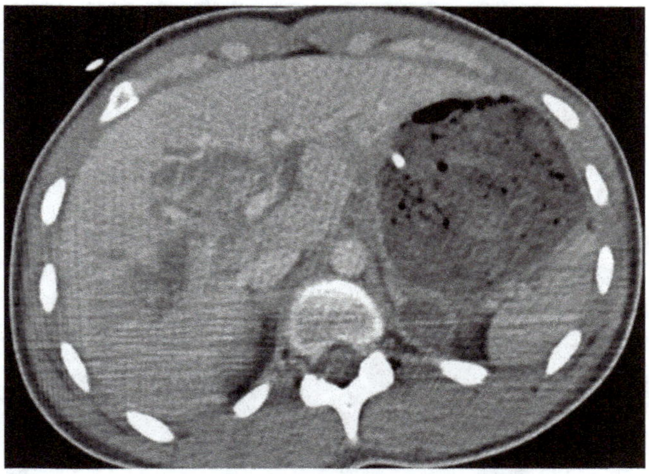

Fig. Grade V liver laceration. Transaxial CT image shows a large ill-defined area of hypoattenuation surrounding the central hepatic blood vessels

splenic injuries, the majority of blunt liver injuries are successfully managed nonoperatively. The AAST liver injury scale (Table) is commonly used to assess the severity of hepatic injuries. Lacerations appear as linear or branching areas of hypoattenuation that frequently travel along vascu-lar planes. Perihilar lacerations may be associated with bili-ary tract injuries. As with the AAST splenic injury scale, the AAST liver injury scale has limitations in guiding clinical management. Additional useful CT findings include exten-sion of the injury to the major hepatic veins (Fig.), the presence of active bleeding into the peritoneal cavity, and the presence of large volume hemoperitoneum. Extension to the major hepatic veins usually requires surgery to control hem-orrhage, and active bleeding into the peritoneum often can be treated with endovascular interventions.

Bowel and Mesenteric Injuries

Injuries to the hollow viscera and mesentery occur in only approximately 5% of patients with blunt abdominal trauma, and the CT findings may be subtle; however, identification of bowel and mesenteric injuries is critical, as delay in diagnosis increases the morbidity and mortality from peritonitis and sepsis. The bowel segments affected most commonly are the proximal jejunum and the distal ileum. The most specific signs of bowel injury are focal discontinuity of the bowel wall (transection), extraluminal oral contrast (when administered), pneumoperitoneum, and retropneumoperitoneum. Less specific (but m ore frequently encountered) signs of bowel trauma include focal wall thickening, abnormal bowel wall enhancement, mesenteric stranding, and free intraperitoneal fluid. The a ssociation o f a focal bowel abnormality with adjacent or free fluid increases the likelihood that bowel injury is present. The most specific signs of mesenteric injury are active extravasation from a mesenteric vessel (Fig.), mesenteric hematoma, and abrupt termina-tion or beading of mesenteric vessels. Small isolated mesenteric hematomas do not always require immediate surgery and can be managed with observation. Larger hematomas and mesenteric vascular injuries have a higher risk of subsequent bowel isch-emia and usually require

In the setting of trauma, the combination of diffuse thickening and hyperenhancement of the bowel generally is not an indication of direct bowel injury but is a component of the hypoperfusion complex (Fig.), which is seen in trauma patients who have persistent hypovolemia after initial intrave-nous fluid resuscitation. Other CT features of the hypoperfusion complex include collapse of the inferior vena cava, flattening of the renal veins, decreased caliber of the aorta, delayed nephro-grams, increased enhancement of the adrenal glands, decreased enhancement of the spleen, and pancreatic enlargement with peripancreatic and retroperitoneal edema. These findings usu-ally are reversible with additional fluid resuscitation.

Pancreatic Injuries

Pancreatic injuries typically occur after blunt trauma to the upper abdomen. Pancreatic contusions appear as focal areas of hypoattenuation or enlargement, whereas lacerations are linear low attenuation defects that may be superficial or

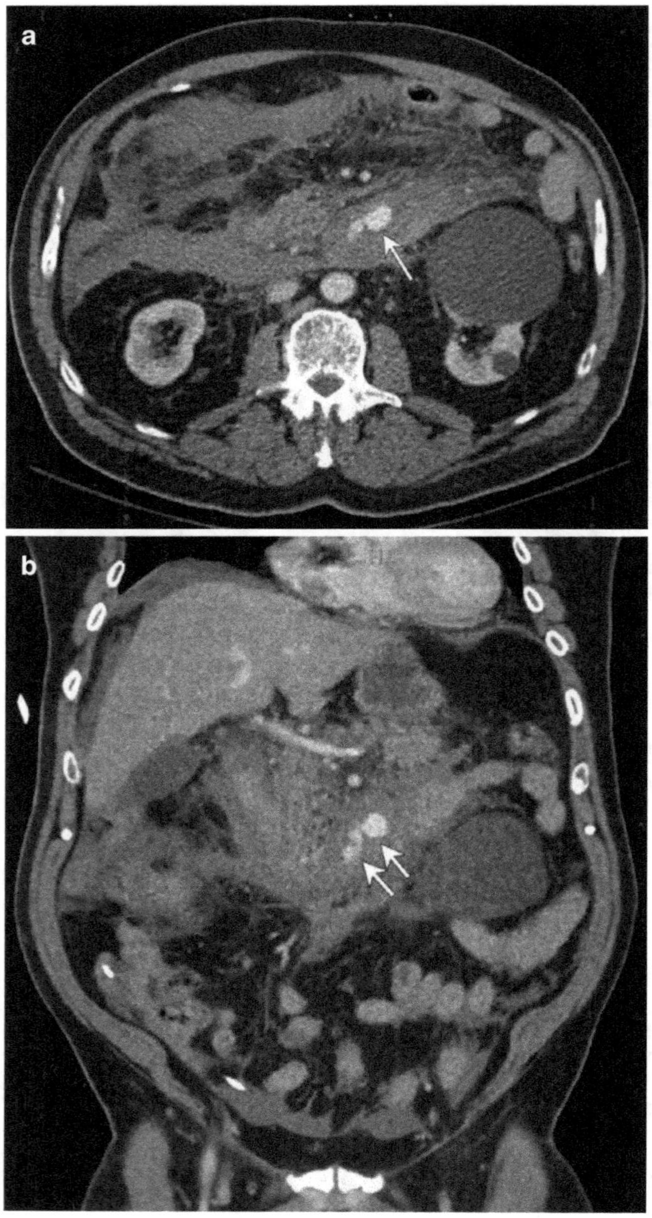

Fig. Severe mesenteric injury. 81-year-old man who suffered blunt abdominal trauma from a fall. Transaxial (**a**) and coronal (**b**) contrast-enhanced CT images demonstrate a large mesenteric hematoma with extravasation from a mesenteric artery (arrows)

extend completely through the pancreas, resulting in transec-tion (Fig.). Lacerations that involve more than 50% of the pancreatic thickness usually cause pancreatic ductal injury. Indirect signs of pancreatic injury include fluid in the peripancreatic fat or transverse mesocolon and thickening of the left anterior renal fascia. The injured pancreas may appear normal at CT in the first 12 hours after trauma. Therefore a 24–48-h repeat CT is warranted in patients who subsequently develop abdominal

Magnetic resonance cholangiopancreatography (MRCP) may be useful to document noninvasively injury of the main pancreatic duct; however, endoscopic retrograde cholangiopancreatography (ERCP) may be necessary for diagnosis. Although some patients with pancreatic ductal injury may be successfully treated with endoscopic pancreatic duct stenting, most require surgical repair.

Urinary Tract Injuries

As with the liver and spleen, an AAST grading system classifies the severity of renal trauma based on the size and location of renal lacerations and hematomas (Table). Most renal injuries are treated conservatively, with surgical intervention reserved for collecting system disruptions and vascular injuries (Fig.). Delayed CT images are necessary to assess the integrity of the collecting system. Avulsion of the renal pedicle, characterized on CT as very poor or absent enhancement of the kidney, carries a high risk of renal devascularization. Rupture of the urinary bladder is a complication of pelvic trauma. Patients with gross hematuria or pelvic fractures should undergo CT cys-tography. Intraperitoneal rupture requires surgical repair, whereas extraperitoneal rupture can be treated conservatively. However, there may be combined intraperitoneal and extraperi-toneal bladder rupture in some trauma patients.

Diaphragmatic Injuries

Diaphragmatic injuries are caused by sudden increase in intra-abdominal pressure from blunt abdominal trauma. CT findings include diaphragmatic discontinuity, herniation of abdominal viscera into the thorax, constriction of herniated abdominal contents through a diaphragmatic defect, and dependent position of the herniated viscera along the posterior chest wall (dependent viscera sign). Multiplanar CT imaging can be helpful in identifying diaphragmatic injuries.

Vascular Injuries

Abdominal aortic injuries in high-speed motor vehicle collisions can be life-threatening. Obvious findings include large retroperitoneal hematoma and active extravasation. More subtle injuries include pseudoaneurysm, intimal flap, and thrombosis. Thoracic aortic transection usually requires emergency surgical repair, preferably utilizing endovascular techniques, but selected less severe aortic injuries can be watched closely initially without repair. Abdominal aortic injuries most commonly result from high-speed motor vehicle collisions in which the aorta is compressed between a lap belt and the lumbar spine. It is important to note that a substantial amount of blood loss in the retroperitoneum may be clinically occult and will not be detected with FAST. Extraperitoneal hemorrhage in the pelvis often is

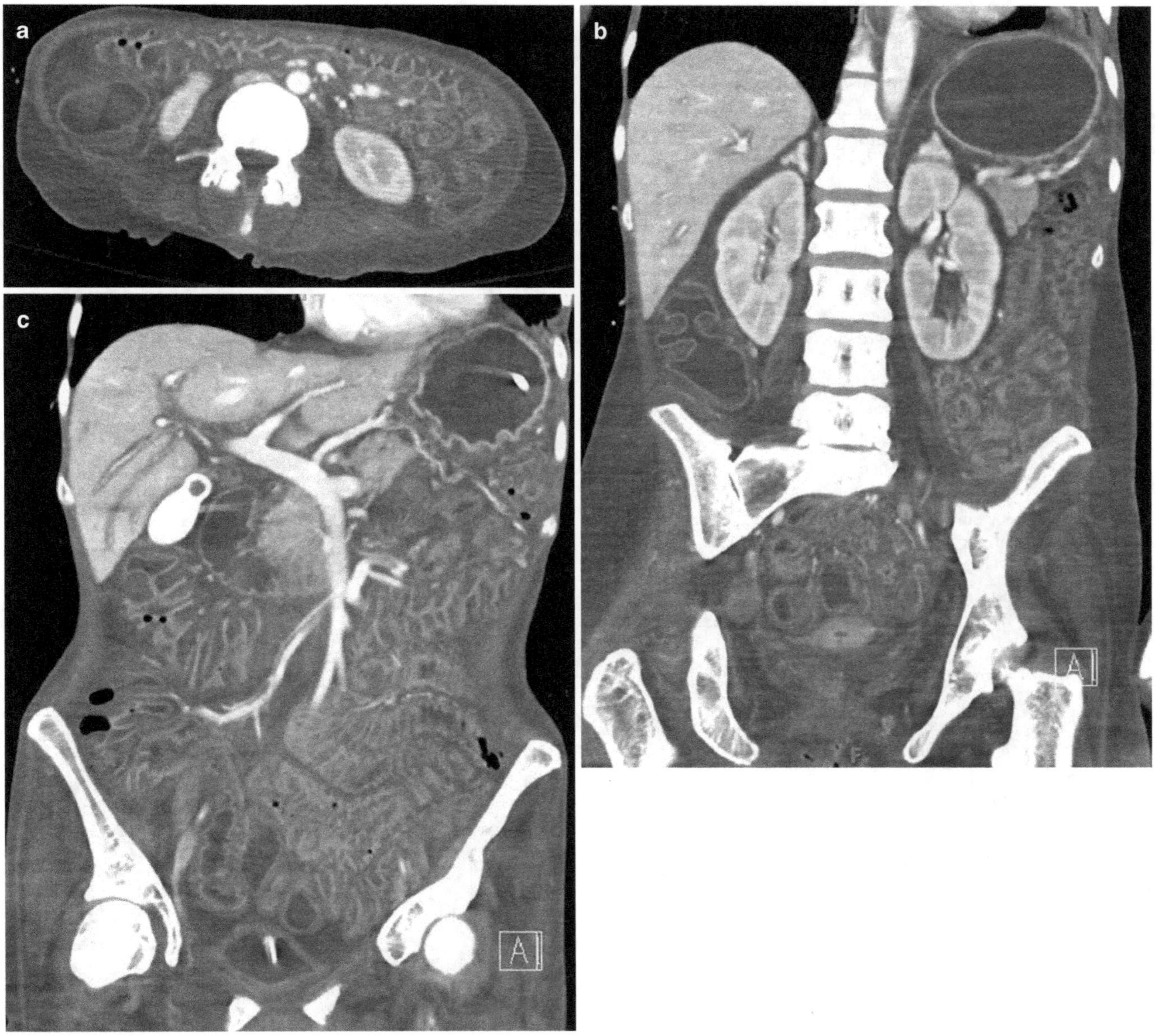

Fig. Hypoperfusion complex. 42-year-old woman with acute blood loss. Transaxial (**a**) and coronal (**b, c**) contrast-enhanced CT images show diffuse edema, bowel wall thickening, collapse of the inferior vena cava, and hyperenhancement of the adrenal glands

associated with pelvic fractures. CT angiography is useful in this setting to evaluate for active extravasation, which can be treated in most cases with endovascular embolization.

Penetrating Abdominal Trauma

The need for surgery after a stab wound depends upon the location and depth of penetration. Wounds in any location that penetrate the peritoneum require surgical exploration because of the likelihood of bowel injury. Anterior wounds that penetrate the deep fascia usually require laparoscopy or laparotomy because of the possibility of bowel injury. In contradistinction, posterior stab wounds that penetrate the deep muscular fascia may be confined to the paraspinal muscles and may not be deep enough to penetrate the peritoneum, thus not necessitating surgical exploration. CT with intravenous, oral, and rectal contrast is useful in determining the depth of wound penetration and in identifying organ injury, retroperitoneal hematoma, and hemoperitoneum.

Gunshot wounds are much more complex injuries that often are difficult to evaluate clinically. If clinical examination or radiographs indicate that the bullet might have crossed bowel, laparoscopy or exploratory laparotomy is indicated, and CT is not necessary. Similarly, patients who are hemodynamically unstable require surgical exploration. In the remainder of patients who are hemodynamically stable, CT is effective in delineating the path of the bullet and identifying solid and hollow organ injuries. Solid organ injuries are staged using the AAST criteria. Findings of bowel perforation including pneumoperitoneum and extraluminal leakage of orally or rectally administered contrast material require surgical exploration; however, small perforations of bowel may be very difficult to diagnose with CT. If CT demonstrates peritoneal fluid or the bullet path crossing bowel in the absence of pneumoperitoneum or contrast leakage, surgical exploration is indicated.

Table American Association for the Surgery of Trauma (AAST) Kidney Injury Scale

Injury grade and type	Description
I	
Contusion	Microscopic or gross hematuria, with normal urologic studies
Hematoma	Subcapsular nonexpanding, without parenchymal laceration
II	
Hematoma	Nonexpanding perirenal hematoma confined to renal retroperitoneum
Laceration	<1-cm parenchymal depth of renal cortex, without urinary extravasation
III	
Laceration	>1-cm parenchymal depth of renal cortex, without collecting system rupture or urinary extravasation
IV	
Laceration	Parenchymal laceration extending through renal cortex, medulla, and collecting system
Vascular	Main renal artery or vein injury, with contained hemorrhage
V	
Laceration	Completely shattered kidney
Vascular	Avulsion of renal hilum, which devascularizes the kidney

Adapted from Moore et al. (1989), with permission

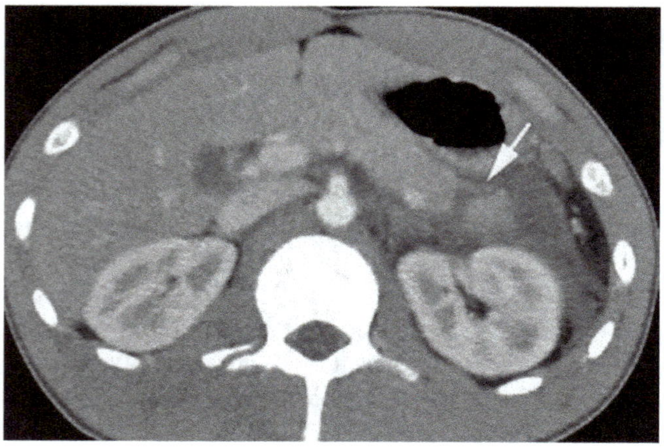

Fig. Pancreatic laceration. Transaxial CT image demonstrates a linear hypoattenuating defect (arrow) extending through the tail of the pancreas. The pancreatic tail is surrounded by fluid

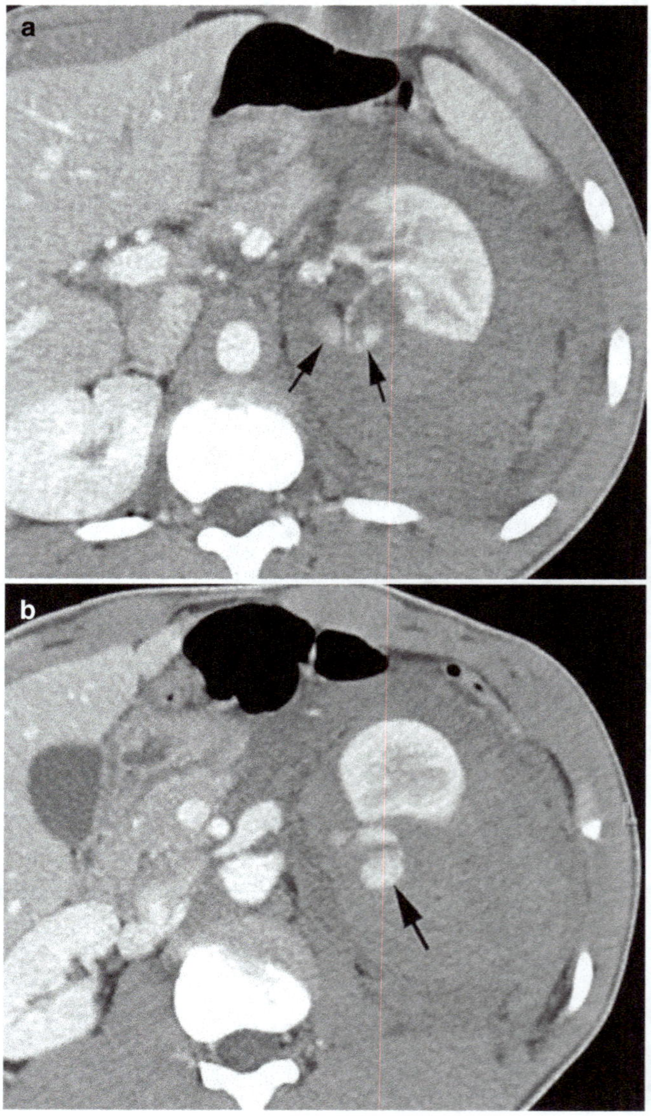

Fig.(**a**, **b**) Deep (grade III) renal laceration with active extrava-sation. Transaxial CT images (**a**, **b**) show a deep laceration of the left kidney that extends to the renal hilum. Arrows indicate active extravasa-tion. A large hematoma surrounds the kidney and displaces it anteriorl

Take-Home Messages

- Imaging of non-traumatic abdominal and pelvic pain, as well as imaging of acute abdominal and pelvic trauma, continues to evolve.
- CT, using a variety of protocols, remains the mainstay for imaging acute traumatic as well as non-traumatic conditions, especially in adults, although US frequently is used as the first examination in children and in the non-trauma setting, with subsequent CT utilized in children when necessary.
- MRI has a growing role, especially for follow-up examinations in the non-trauma setting and for initial imaging or following US in pregnant patients and in pediatric patients, to reduce radiation exposure.
- Close cooperation with the referring physician immediately prior to imaging remains essential for rapid and accurate diagnosis, as the character and location of the patient's pain, and other considerations, strongly influence the specific imaging examination(s) performed and the protocol(s) utilized, as well as the resulting imaging differential diagnosis.

References

Ahn SH, Mayo-Smith WW, Murphy BL, Reinert SE, Cronan JJ. Acute nontraumatic abdominal pain in adult patients: abdominal radiography compared with CT evaluation. Radiology. 2002;225:159–64.

Anderson SW, Soto JA, Lucey BC, et al. Abdominal 64-MDCT for suspected appendicitis: the use of oral and IV contrast material versus IV contrast material only. AJR. 2009;193:1282–8.

Atri M, Hanson JM, Grinblat L, et al. Surgically important bowel and/or mesenteric injury in blunt trauma: accuracy of multidetector CT evaluation. Radiology. 2008;249:524–33.

Balthazar EJ, Robinson DL, Megibow AJ, Ranson JH. Acute pancreatitis: value of CT in establishing prognosis. Radiology. 1990;174:331–6.

Boscak AR, Shanmuganathan K, Mirvis SE, et al. Optimizing trauma multidetector CT protocol for blunt splenic injury: need for arterial and portal venous phase scans. Radiology. 2013;268:79–88.

Desir A, Ghaye B. CT of blunt diaphragmatic rupture. Radiographics. 2012;32:477–98.

Dewhurst C, Beddy P, Pedrosa I. MRI evaluation of acute appendicitis in pregnancy. J Magn Reson Imaging. 2013;37:566–75.

Drasin TE, Anderson SW, Asandra A, et al. MDCT evaluation of blunt abdominal trauma: clinical significance of free intraperitoneal fluid in males with absence of identifiable injury. AJR. 2001;191:1821–6.

Duke E, Kalb B, Arif-Tiwari H, et al. A systematic review and meta-analysis of diagnostic performance of MRI for evaluation of acute appendicitis. AJR. 2016;206:508–17.

Fuks D, Mouly C, Robert B, Hajji H, Yzet T, Regimbeau JM. Acute cholecystitis: preoperative CT can help the surgeon consider conversion from laparoscopic to open cholecystectomy. Radiology. 2012;263:128–38.

Gans B, Sodickson A. Imaging of blunt bowel, mesenteric, and body wall trauma. Semin Roentgenol. 2016;51:230–8.

Gordon RW, Anderson SW, Ozonoff A, et al. Blunt pancreatic trauma: evaluation with MDCT technology. Emerg Radiol. 2013;20:259–66.

Gore RM, Miller FH, Pereles FS, Yaghmai V, Berlin JW. Helical CT in the evaluation of the acute abdomen. AJR. 2000;174:901–13.

Hines J, Rosenfeld J, Duncan DR, Friedman B, Katz DS. Perforation of the mesenteric small bowel: etiologies and CT findings. Emerg Radiol. 2013;20:155–61.

Katz DS, Klein MA, Ganson G, Hines JJ. Imaging of abdominal pain in pregnancy. Radiol Clin North Am. 2012;50:149–71.

Katz DS, Khalid M, Coronel EE, Mazzie JP. Computed tomography imaging of the acute pelvis in females. Can Assoc Radiol J. 2013a;64:108–18.

Katz DS, Scheirey CD, Bordia R, Hines JJ, Javors BR, Scholz FJ. Computed tomography of miscellaneous regional and diffuse small bowel disorders. Radiol Clin North Am. 2013b;51:45–68.

Kereshi B, Lee KS, Siewert B, Mortele KJ. Clinical utility of magnetic resonance imaging in the evaluation of pregnant females with suspected acute appendicitis. Abdom Radiol. 2017 (published online: 28 August 2017).

Keyzer C, Cullus P, Tack D, De Maertelaer V, Bohy P, Gevenois PA. MDCT for suspected acute appendicitis in adults: impact of oral and IV contrast media at standard-dose and simulated low-dose techniques. AJR. 2009;193:1272–81.

LeBedis CA, Anderson SW, Soto JA. CT imaging of blunt traumatic bowel and mesenteric injuries. Radiol Clin North Am. 2012;50:123–36.

Lee SS, Park SH. Computed tomography evaluation of gastrointestinal bleeding and acute mesenteric ischemia. Radiol Clin North Am. 2013;51:29–43.

Levenson RB, Camacho MA, Horn E, Saghir A, McGillicuddy D, Sanchez LD. Eliminating routine oral contrast use for CT in the emergency department: impact on patient throughput and diagnosis. Emerg Radiol. 2012;19:513–7.

Lucey BC, Varghese JC, Anderson SW, Soto JA. Spontaneous hemoperitoneum: a bloody mess. Emerg Radiol. 2006;14:65–75.

MacKersie AB, Lane MJ, Gerhardt RT, et al. Nontraumatic acute abdominal pain: unenhanced helical CT compared with three-view acute abdominal series. Radiology. 2005;237:114–22.

Marmery H, Shanmuganathan K, Alexander MT, Mirvis SE. Optimization of selection of nonoperative management of blunt splenic injury: comparison of MDCT grading systems. AJR. 2007;189:1421–7.

Mellnick VM, McDowell C, Lubner M, et al. CT features of blunt abdominal aortic injury. Emerg Radiol. 2012;19:301–7.

Mirvis SE, Shanmuganagthan K. Imaging hemidiaphragmatic injury. Eur Radiol. 2007;17:1411–21.

Moore EE, Shackford SR, Pachter HL, et al. Organ injury scaling: spleen, liver, and kidney. J Trauma. 1989;29:1664–6.

Moore EE, Cogbill THJ, Jurkovich GJ, et al. J Trauma. 1995;38:323–4, with permission from Lippincott Williams and Wilkins/Wolter Kluwer Health.

Orwig D, Federle MP. Localized clotted blood as evidence of visceral trauma on CT: the sentinel clot sign. AJR. 1989;153:747–9.

Pooler BD, Lawrence EM, Pickhardt PJ. Alternative diagnoses to suspected appendicitis at CT. Radiology. 2012;265:733–42.

Rapp EJ, Naim F, Kadivar K, Davarpanah A, Cornfeld D. Integrating MR imaging into the clinical workup of pregnant patients suspected of having appendicitis is associated with a lower negative laparotomy rate: a single-institution study. Radiology. 2013;267:137–44.

Revzin MV, Mathur M, Dave HB, Macer ML, Spektor M. Pelvic inflammatory disease: multi-modality imaging approach with clinical-pathologic correlation. Radiographics. 2016;36:1579–96.

Robinson JD, Sandstrom CK, Lehnert BE, Gross JA. Imaging of blunt abdominal solid organ trauma. Semin Roentgenol. 2016;51:215–29.

Rosen MP, Ding A, Blake MA, et al. ACR Appropriateness Criteria right lower quadrant pain - suspected appendicitis. JACR. 2011;8:749–55.

Santillan CS. Computed tomography of small bowel obstruction. Radiol Clin North Am. 2013;51:17–27.

Shakespear JS, Shaaban AM, Rezvani M. CT findings of acute cholecystitis and its complications. AJR. 2010;194:1523–9.

Singh AK, Gervais DA, Hahn PF, Sagar P, Muller PR, Novelline R. Acute epiploic appendagitis and its mimics. Radiographics. 2005;25:1521–34.

Smith RC, Varanelli M. Diagnosis and management of acute ureterolithiasis. AJR. 2000;175:3–6.

Soto JA, Anterson SW. Multidetector CT of blunt abdominal trauma. Radiology. 2012;265:678–93.

Stojer J, van Randen A, Lameris W, Boermeester MA. Imaging patients with acute abdominal pain. Radiology. 2009;253:31–46.

Stuhlfaut JW, Lucey BC, Varghese JC, Soto JA. Blunt abdominal trauma: utility of 5-minute delayed CT with a reduced radiation dose. Radiology. 2006;238:473–9.

Thoeni RF. The revised Atlanta classification of acute pancreatitis: its importance for the radiologist and its effect on treatment. Radiology. 2012;262:751–64.

Werner A, Diehl SJ, Farag-Soliman M, Duber C. Multi-slice spiral CT in routine diagnosis of suspected acute left-sided colonic diverticulitis: a prospective study of 120 patients. Eur Radiol. 2003;13:2596–603.

Wieseler KM, Bhargava P, Kanal KM, Vaidya S, Stewart BK, Dighe MK. Imaging in pregnant patients: examination appropriateness. Radiographics. 2010;30:1215–29.

Yu J, Fulcher AS, Wang DB, et al. Frequency and importance of small amount of isolated pelvic free fluid detected with multidetector CT in male patients with blunt trauma. Radiology. 2010;256:799–805.

21

Magnetic Resonance Imaging of the Prostate in the PI-RADS Era

Bernd Hamm and Patrick Asbach

Learning Objectives

- To understand the current role of prostate MRI for imaging-based targeted prostate biopsy, staging, and active surveillance
- To learn how to optimize the multiparametric prostate MR imaging protocol
- To illustrate how to use the PI-RADS classification for prostatic lesion assessment
- To understand the need of structured reporting in communicating with the urologists
- To discuss the most common pitfalls in multiparametric MRI of the prostate

Introduction

Over the past years, continuing technical innovation in combination with a broad research activity has resulted in a high diagnostic accuracy of magnetic resonance imaging (MRI) of the prostate. At the same time, the Prostate Imaging Reporting and Data System (PI-RADS) has standardized image acquisition and reporting and facilitated the communication of imaging findings to the urologist and can therefore be considered an obligatory key element in prostate MRI. This has had a tremendous impact on the diagnostic workup of patients with suspected prostate cancer, with MRI being incorporated in multiple prostate cancer guidelines (e.g., NICE, AUA, German S3-Guideline) by now. As a direct result, imaging-based targeted prostate biopsy has increased almost at the same speed, and urologists not only heavily rely on accurate interpretation of MRI of the prostate but actively claim high-quality MRI scans for their daily practice because prostate MRI has direct impact on their cancer detection rate. Furthermore, a paradigm shift is taking place in the urological community regarding the care of low-grade prostate cancer patients, where therapy is more and more replaced by active surveillance (AS). Prostate MRI plays an important role in AS not only during the initial assessment whether the patient is a candidate for AS but also during the surveillance of the disease.

Therefore, any abdominal and genitourinary radiologist if not already performing prostate MRI will subsequently be involved, and we forecast prostate MRI to be an indispensable diagnostic step for *any* patient with a clinical suspicion for prostate cancer or during surveillance of low-grade prostate cancer in the near future.

PI-RADS

The European Society of Uroradiology (ESUR) has introduced PI-RADS (**P**rostate **I**maging **R**eporting and **D**ata **S**ystem) in 2012. An updated version (PI-RADS v2) was published in 2015 in collaboration with the American College of Radiology (ACR) and the AdMeTech Foundation. PI-RADS is not based on evidence from clinical research trials rather than on expert knowledge; however, several studies have confirmed that the PI-RADS system improves the diagnostic accuracy of mpMRI. The overall rationale for implementation of PI-RADS was to "improve detection, localization, characterization, and risk stratification in patients with suspected cancer in treatment naïve prostate glands." PI-RADS is currently not applicable to assess treatment response in prostate cancer patients. The following specific definitions and aims regarding MR imaging and reporting are targeted by PI-RADS:

B. Hamm (✉) · P. Asbach
Department of Radiology, Charité—Universitätsmedizin Berlin, Berlin, Germany
e-mail: bernd.hamm@charite.de

Clinical Considerations

Timing of mpMRI after prostate biopsy does not necessarily need to be postponed since clinically significant cancer is likely in a location not altered by post biopsy hemorrhage when the biopsy was negative. For local staging of prostate cancer, a delay of a minimum of 6 weeks might be advantageous. No specific patient preparation is necessary; however, the administration of a spasmolytic drug may be beneficial. Bowel cleaning is not recommended; however, the patient should evacuate the rectum if possible.

Technical Considerations

The field strengths of 1.5 and 3 T can both be adequate (even without an endorectal coil at 1.5 T) when the scan parameters are tailored to small field-of-view imaging of the prostate and contemporary scanner technology is used (specifically multichannel phased-array surface coils and high-performance gradients); however, 3 T is the preferred field strength (higher signal-to-noise ratio, shorter scan time).

Multiparametric MRI of the prostate should include the following sequences:

T2-weighted imaging: 2D turbo spin-echo sequence, slice thickness ≤3 mm (no interslice gap), and in-plane spatial resolution ≤0.7 mm (phase-encoding direction) x ≤ 0.4 mm (frequency-encoding direction).

Diffusion-weighted imaging (DWI): spin-echo EPI (echo planar imaging) sequence with fat saturation, slice thickness ≤4 mm (no interslice gap), in-plane spatial resolution ≤2.5 mm (phase- and frequency-encoding direction), and at least two *b*-values (low *b*-value of 50–100 s/mm^2 and a high *b*-value of 800–1000 s/mm^2) with consecutive calculation of an ADC map. If SNR allows, a very high *b*-value of 1400–2000 s/mm^2 should be measured. An alternative is to calculate a high *b*-value, which is less SNR critical.

Dynamic contrast-enhanced (DCE) imaging: 2D or 3D gradient-echo sequence with a temporal resolution below 10 s (preferably below 7 s) per acquisition, slice thickness ≤ 3 mm (no interslice gap), and in-plane spatial resolution ≤2 mm (phase- and frequency-encoding direction).

Slice orientation and slice thickness should match for all mpMRI sequences to allow side-by-side comparison. Also, a large field-of-view sequence covering the pelvic lymph nodes and the skeleton should be acquired.

Assessment of Prostatic Lesions

One major key element of PI-RADS is scoring the likelihood of a prostatic lesion to be *clinically significant* prostate cancer on a 5-point Likert-type scale (Table).

Since several different definitions of clinically significant prostate cancer exist, PI-RADS defines it as "Gleason score ≥7 (including 3+4 with prominent but not predominant Gleason 4 component), and/or volume ≥0.5 cc, and/or extra prostatic extension (EPE)." The scoring system is based on typical imaging findings on the respective multiparametric MR sequence (exact definitions according to PI-RADS, see Tables ; for examples, see Figs.). For this purpose, typical examples for each score and sequence are included in the

Table PI-RADS classification (5-point Likert-type scale)

PI-RADS 1	Very low (clinically significant cancer is highly unlikely to be present)
PI-RADS 2	Low (clinically significant cancer is unlikely to be present)
PI-RADS 3	Intermediate (the presence of clinically significant cancer is equivocal)
PI-RADS 4	High (clinically significant cancer is likely to be present)
PI-RADS 5	Very high (clinically significant cancer is highly likely to be present)

Table T2-weighted imaging

Score	Peripheral zone (PZ)	Transition zone (TZ)
1	Uniform hyperintense signal intensity (normal)	Homogeneous intermediate signal intensity (normal)
2	Linear or wedge-shaped hypointensity or diffuse mild hypointensity, usually indistinct margin	Circumscribed hypointense or heterogeneous encapsulated nodule(s) (BPH)
3	Heterogeneous signal intensity or non-circumscribed, rounded, moderate hypointensity, includes others that do not qualify as 2, 4, or 5	Heterogeneous signal intensity with obscured margins, includes others that do not qualify as 2, 4, or 5
4	Circumscribed, homogenous moderate hypointense focus/mass confined to prostate and <1.5 cm in greatest dimension	Lenticular or non-circumscribed, homogeneous, moderately hypointense, and <1.5 cm in greatest dimension
5	Same as 4 but ≥1.5 cm in greatest dimension or definite extraprostatic extension/invasive behavior	Same as 4, but ≥1.5 cm in greatest dimension or definite extraprostatic extension/invasive behavior

Table Diffusion-weighted imaging (DWI)

Score	Peripheral zone (PZ) or transition zone (TZ)
1	No abnormality (i.e., normal) on ADC and high *b*-value DWI
2	Indistinct hypointense on ADC
3	Focal mildly/moderately hypointense on ADC and isointense/mildly hyperintense on high *b*-value DWI
4	Focal markedly hypointense on ADC and markedly hyperintense on high *b*-value DWI; <1.5 cm in greatest dimension
5	Same as 4 but ≥1.5 cm in greatest dimension or definite extraprostatic extension/invasive behavior

Table Dynamic contrast-enhanced (DCE) imagin

Score	Peripheral zone (PZ) or transition zone (TZ)
Negative	No early enhancement or diffuse enhancement not corresponding to a focal finding on T2-weighted and/or DWI or focal enhancement corresponding to a lesion demonstrating features of BPH on T2-weighted imaging
Positive	Focal and earlier than or contemporaneously with enhancement of adjacent normal prostatic tissues and corresponds to suspicious finding on T2-weighted and/or DWI

PI-RADS publication. The goal is to increase the diagnostic accuracy for detection of prostate cancer and to reduce the variability in image interpretation. Most preliminary studies report a good reader agreement which is higher for peripheral zone (PZ) lesions as compared to transition zone (TZ) lesions. Also, agreement is higher for PI-RADS score 4 and 5 compared to lower scores.

In the PI-RADS version 2, the diagnostic weighting of the multiparametric sequences has been changed compared to the first version. Now, a concept of a dominant sequence has

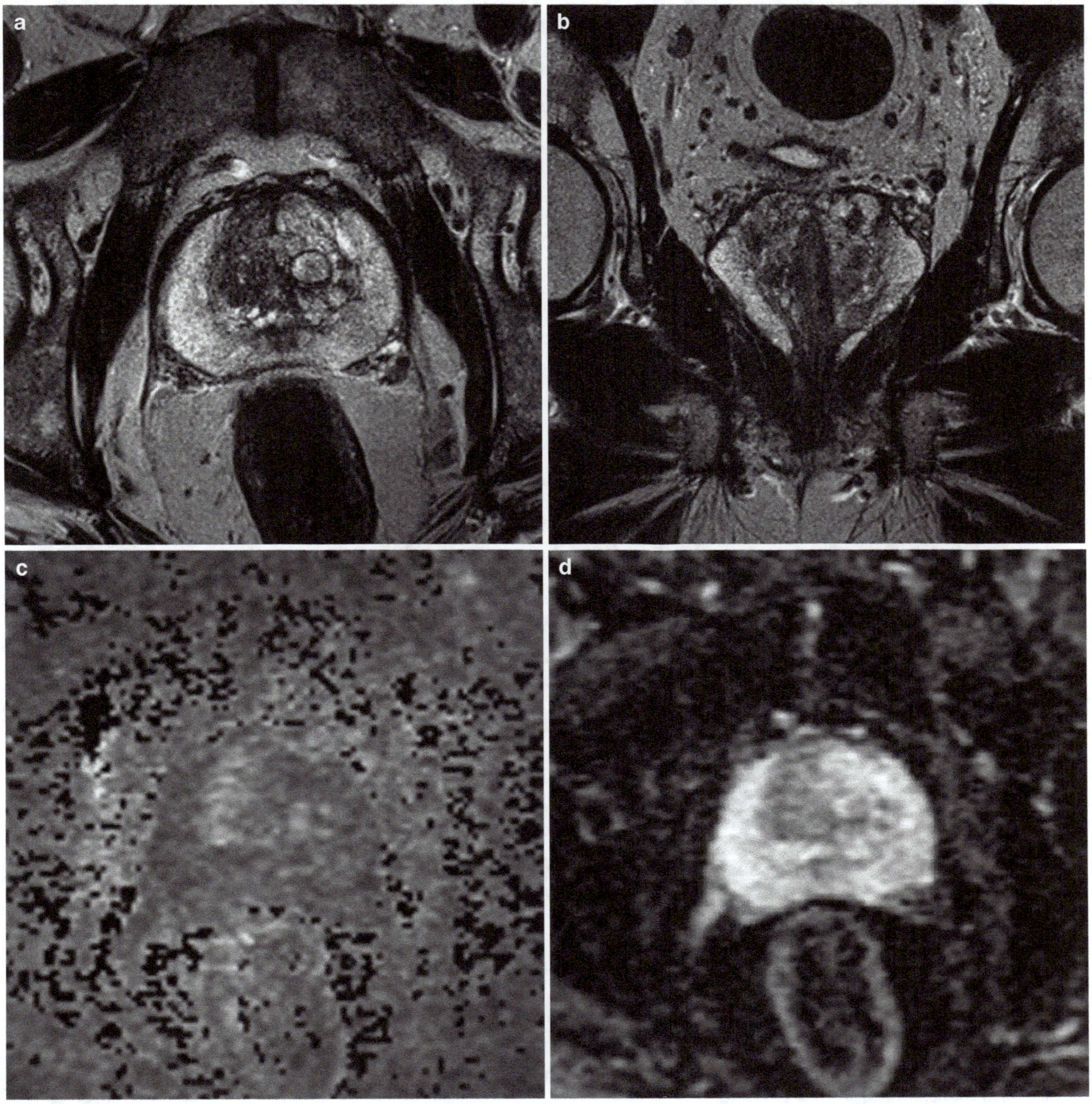

Fig.(**a**–**d**) Normal peripheral zone. (**a**) Axial and (**b**) coronal T2-weighted sequence showing uniform hyperintense signal intensity of the peripheral zone (PI-RADS score 1). (**c**) Diffusion-weighted high *b*-value (calculated b = 1400 s/mm^2) image and (**d**) ADC map (dominant sequence for the peripheral zone) with no abnormality consistent with an overall PI-RADS score of 1

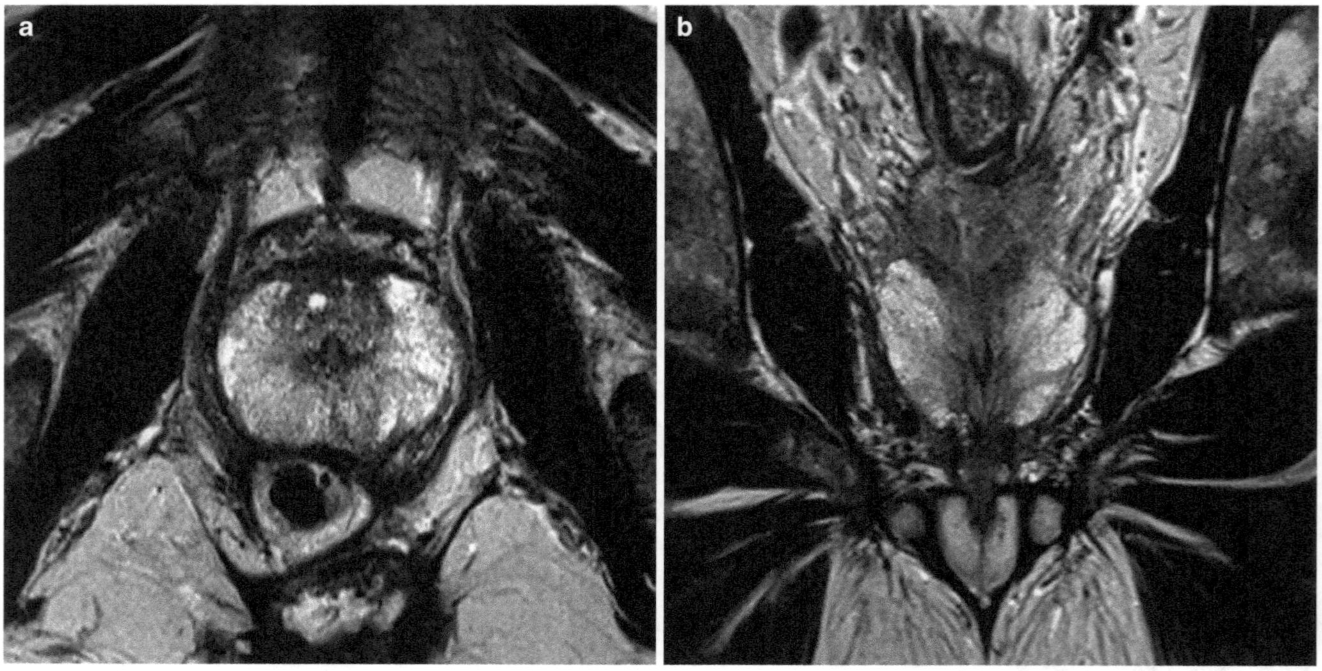

Fig. (**a**, **b**) Normal transition zone. (**a**) Axial and (**b**) coronal T2-weighted sequence (dominant sequence for the transition zone) showing homogeneous intermediate signal intensity of the non-enlarged transition zone (PI-RADS score 1)

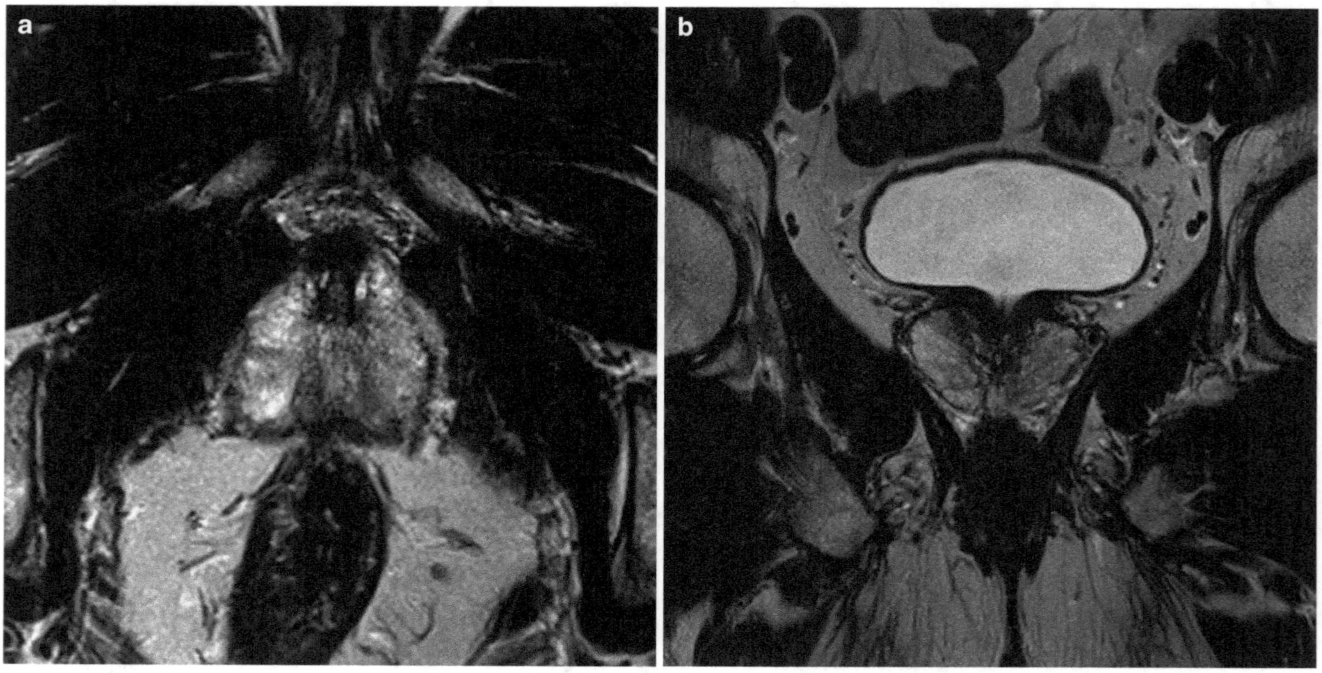

Fig. (**a–e**) PI-RADS 2 changes of the peripheral zone. (**a**) Axial and (**b**) coronal T2-weighted sequence showing linear hypointensities in the bilateral peripheral zone (PI-RADS score 2). (**c**) Diffusion-weighted high *b*-value (calculated $b = 1400$ s/mm^2) image shows no areas of increased signal intensity. (**d**) ADC map shows no focal hypointense areas (dominant sequence for the peripheral zone) in the peripheral zone (PI-RADS score 2). (**e**) DCE sequence shows no focal or early enhancement (DCE negative) consistent with an overall PI-RADS score of 2. Linear T2 hypointensities in the peripheral zone are a frequent finding and may represent changes related to chronic prostatitis or post biopsy scarring

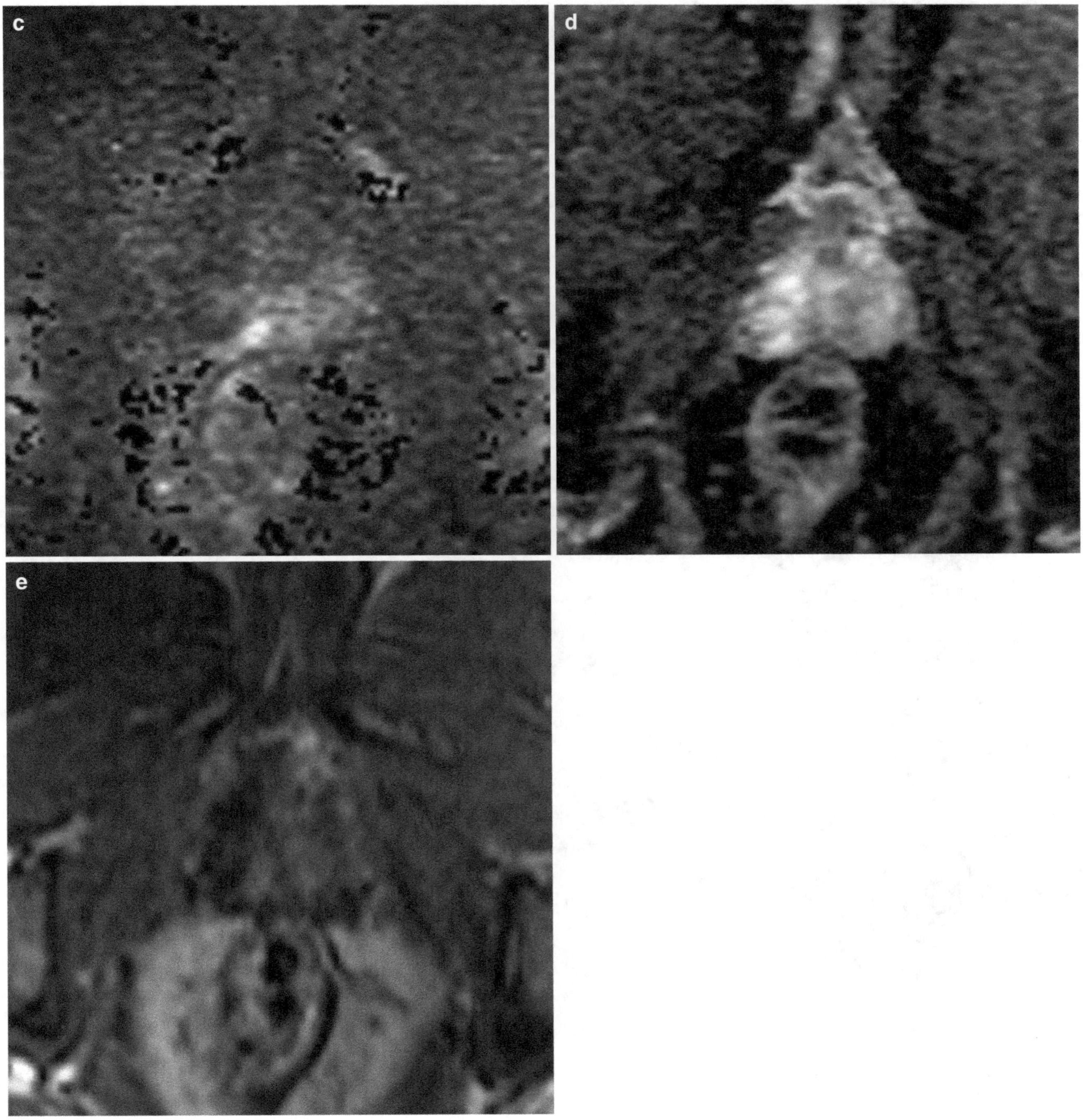

Fig. (continued)

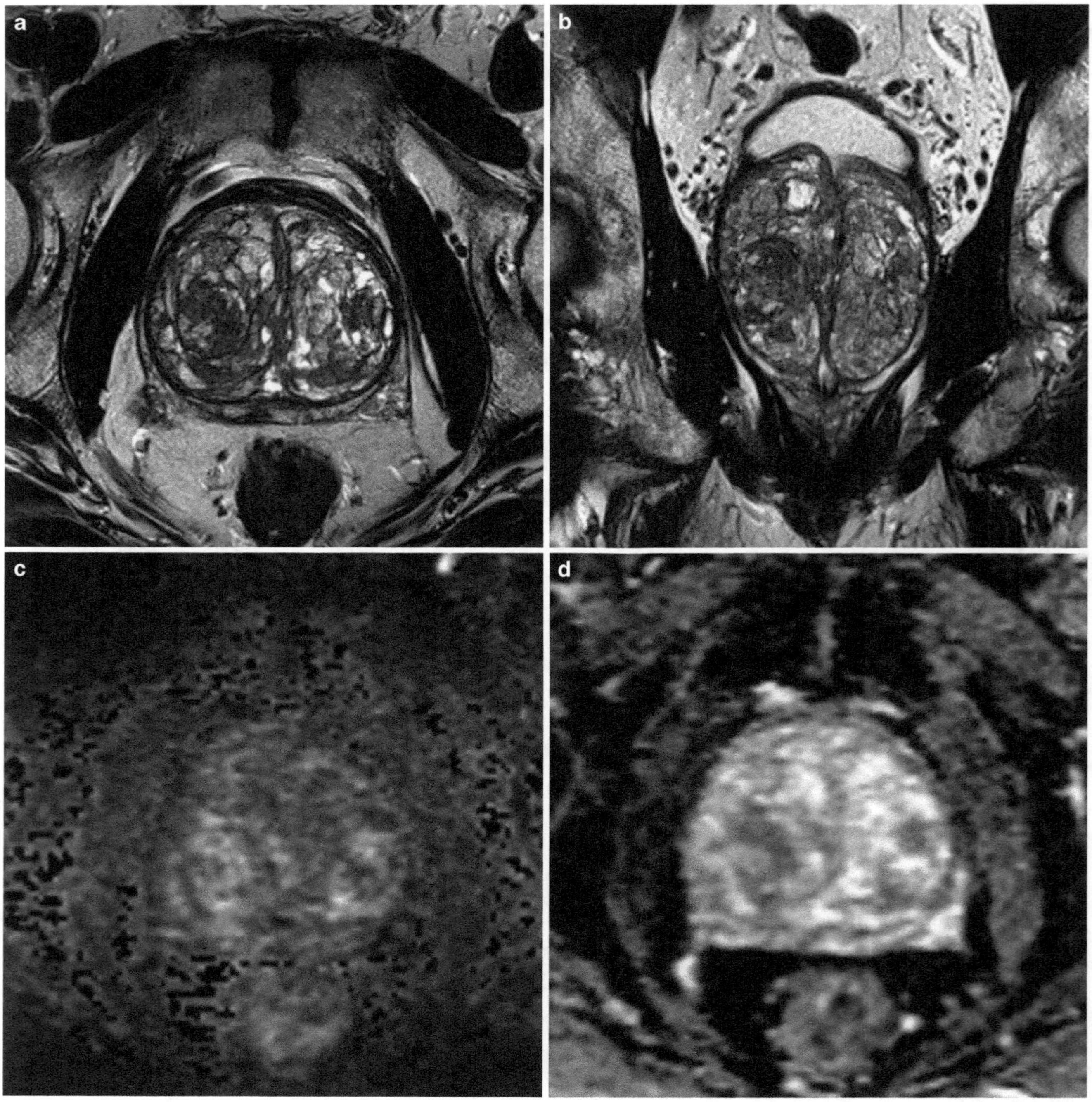

Fig. (**a**–**d**) PI-RADS 2 findings of the transition zone in a patient with benign prostatic hyperplasia (BPH). (**a**) Axial and (**b**) coronal T2-weighted sequence (dominant sequence for the transition zone) showing multiple circumscribed heterogeneous encapsulated nodules (dark T2-rim) within the enlarged transition zone (overall PI-RADS score 2). (**c**) Diffusion-weighted high *b*-value (calculated b = 1400 s/mm^2) image shows no focal areas of moderately increased signal intensity. (**d**) ADC map shows no focal hypointense areas (PI-RADS score 2)

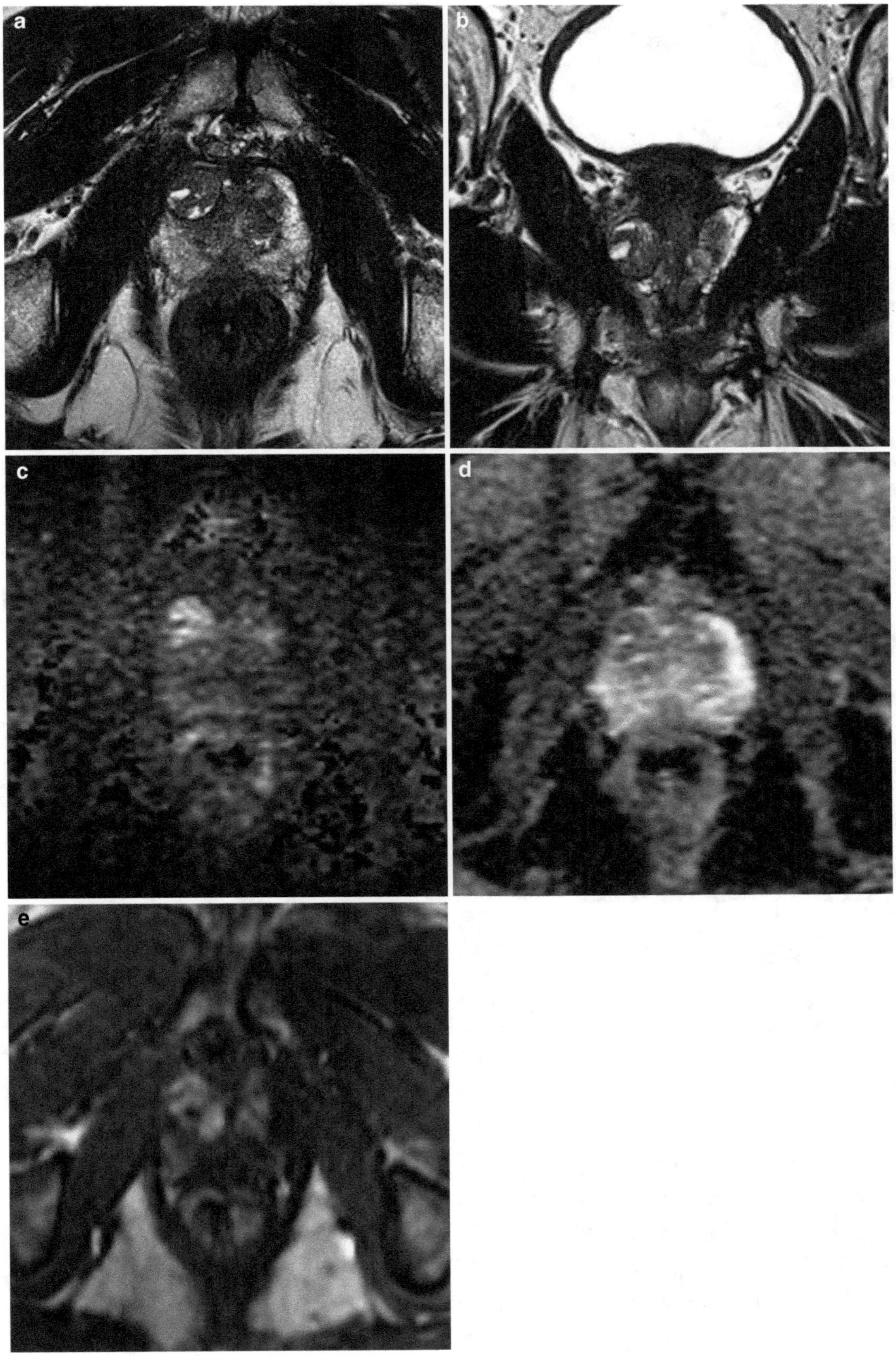

Fig. (**a**–**e**) Protruded BPH node in the right anterior gland. (**a**) Axial and (**b**) coronal T2-weighted sequence (dominant sequence for the transition zone) showing a circumscribed heterogeneous encapsulated nodule (overall PI-RADS score 2). (**c**) Diffusion-weighted high *b*-value (calculated $b = 1400$ s/mm^2) image shows increased signal intensity. (**d**) ADC map shows a focal hypointensity which is related to stromal BPH components which corresponds to the BPH nodule (therefore PI-RADS score of 2). (**e**) DCE sequence showing focal enhancement which corresponds to the lesion that demonstrates clear features of a BPH node (therefore DCE negative) consistent with an overall PI-RADS score of 2

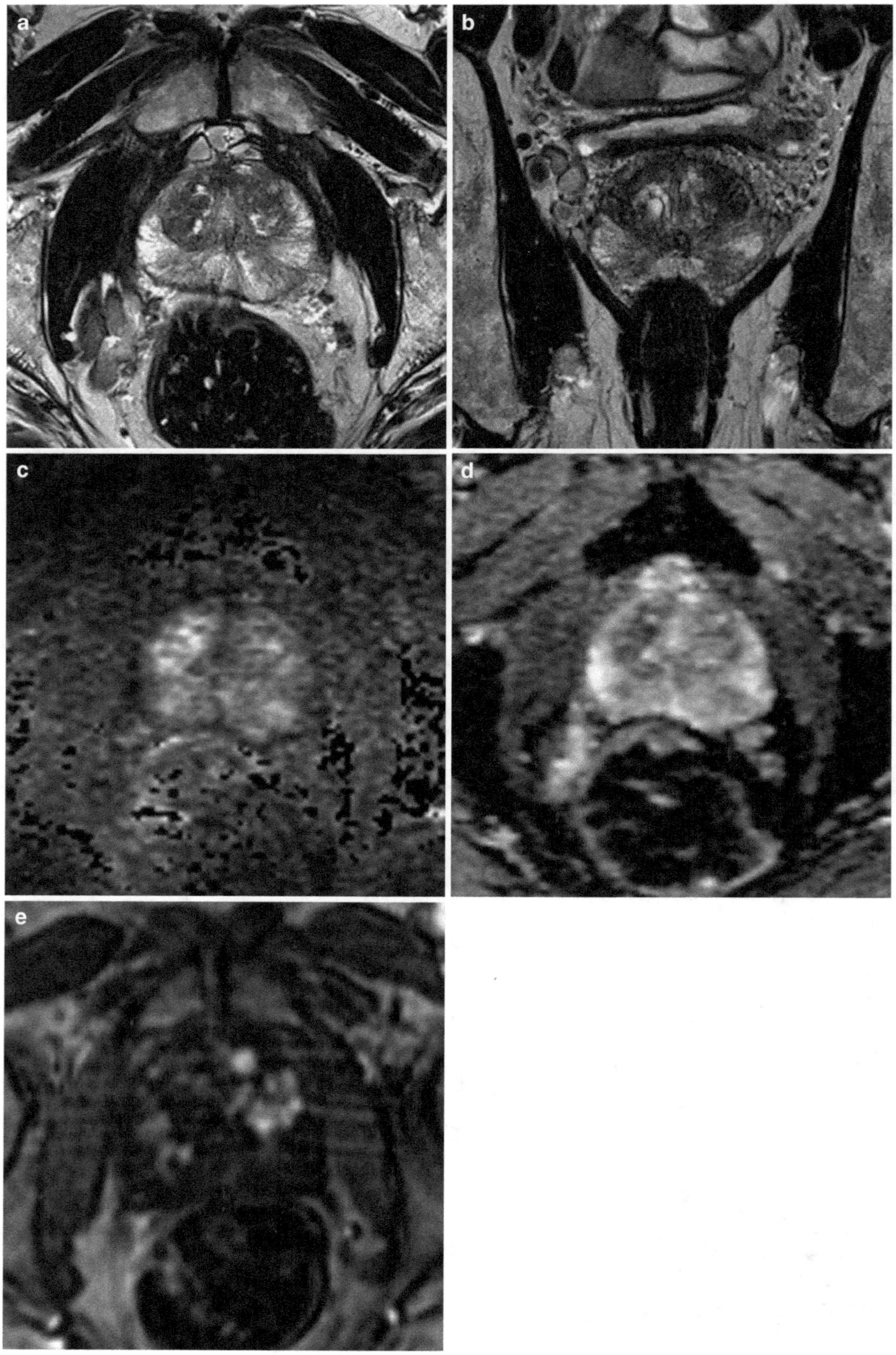

Fig. (**a**–**e**) PI-RADS 3 changes of the peripheral zone. (**a**) Axial and (**b**) coronal T2-weighted sequence showing heterogeneous non-circumscribed changes of the bilateral peripheral zone (PI-RADS score 3). (**c**) Diffusion-weighted high *b*-value (calculated $b = 1400$ s/mm^2) image shows a mildly hyperintense signal intensity. (**d**) ADC map (dominant sequence for the peripheral zone) shows moderately hypointense changes in the bilateral peripheral zone (PI-RADS score 3). (**e**) DCE sequence shows no focal early enhancement (DCE negative) consistent with an overall PI-RADS score of 3. Randomized TRUS-guided prostate biopsy revealed mild chronic prostatitis with no evidence for prostate cancer

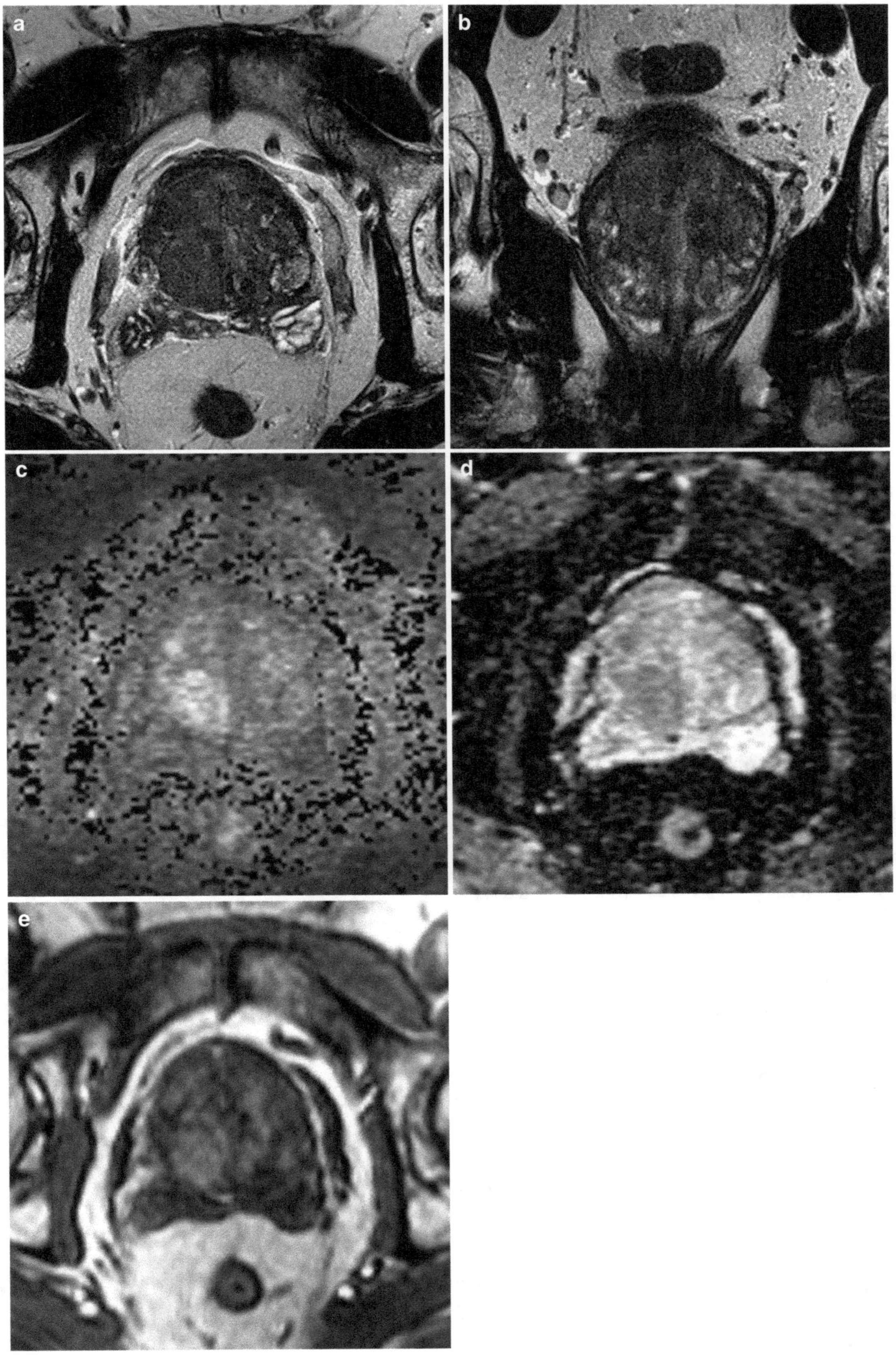

Fig. (**a**–**e**) PI-RADS 3 changes of the transition zone in a patient with benign prostatic hyperplasia (BPH). (**a**) Axial and (**b**) coronal T2-weighted sequence (dominant sequence for the transition zone) showing heterogeneous signal intensity with obscured margins within the enlarged transition zone (overall PI-RADS score 3). (**c**) Diffusion-weighted high *b*-value (calculated $b = 1400$ s/mm^2) image shows mildly hyperintense signal intensity. (**d**) ADC map shows moderately hypointense areas (PI-RADS score 3). (**e**) DCE sequence shows diffuse enhancement not corresponding to a focal finding on any other sequence (DCE negative). Randomized TRUS-guided biopsy revealed no malignancy; therefore, the findings can be attributed to BPH with predominantly stromal (T2 hypointense) components

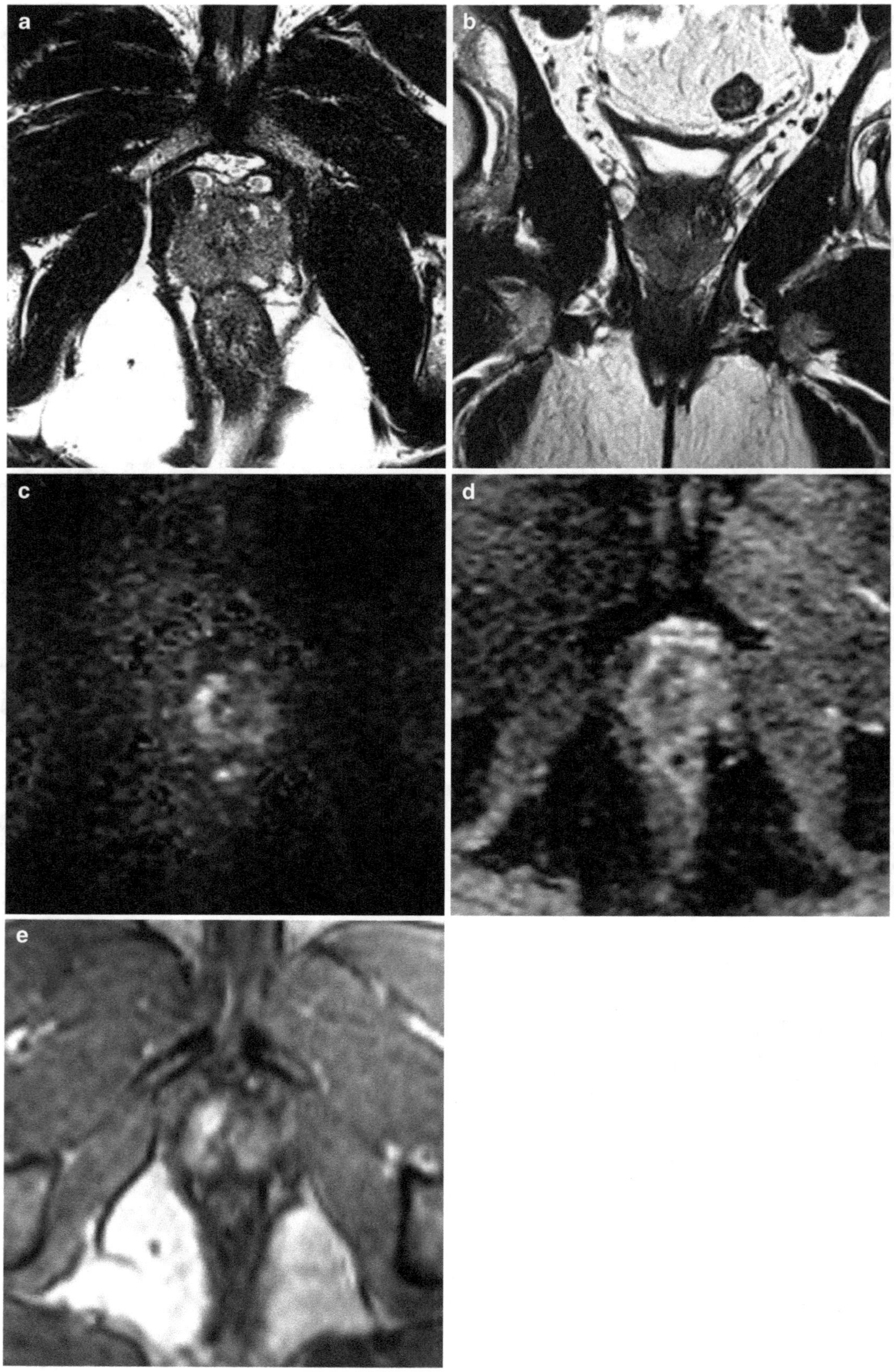

Fig. (**a**–**e**) PI-RADS 4 lesion in the peripheral zone. (**a**) Axial and (**b**) coronal T2-weighted sequence showing moderate diffuse (non-circumscribed) hypointensity of the bilateral peripheral zone (PI-RADS score 3). (**c**) Diffusion-weighted high *b*-value (calculated b = 1400 s/mm^2) image shows mildly hyperintense signal intensity in the right anterior and lateral peripheral zone (PI-RADS score 3). (**d**) ADC map correspondingly shows moderate hypointense signal intensity (dominant sequence for the peripheral zone) in the right anterior and lateral peripheral zone (PI-RADS score 3). (**e**) DCE sequence shows focal and contemporary enhancement (DCE positive) consistent with an upgrading to an overall PI-RADS score of 4. MRI/US fusion-guided biopsy revealed a Gleason 3 + 4 = 7 adenocarcinoma (PSA level was 6.9 ng/mL)

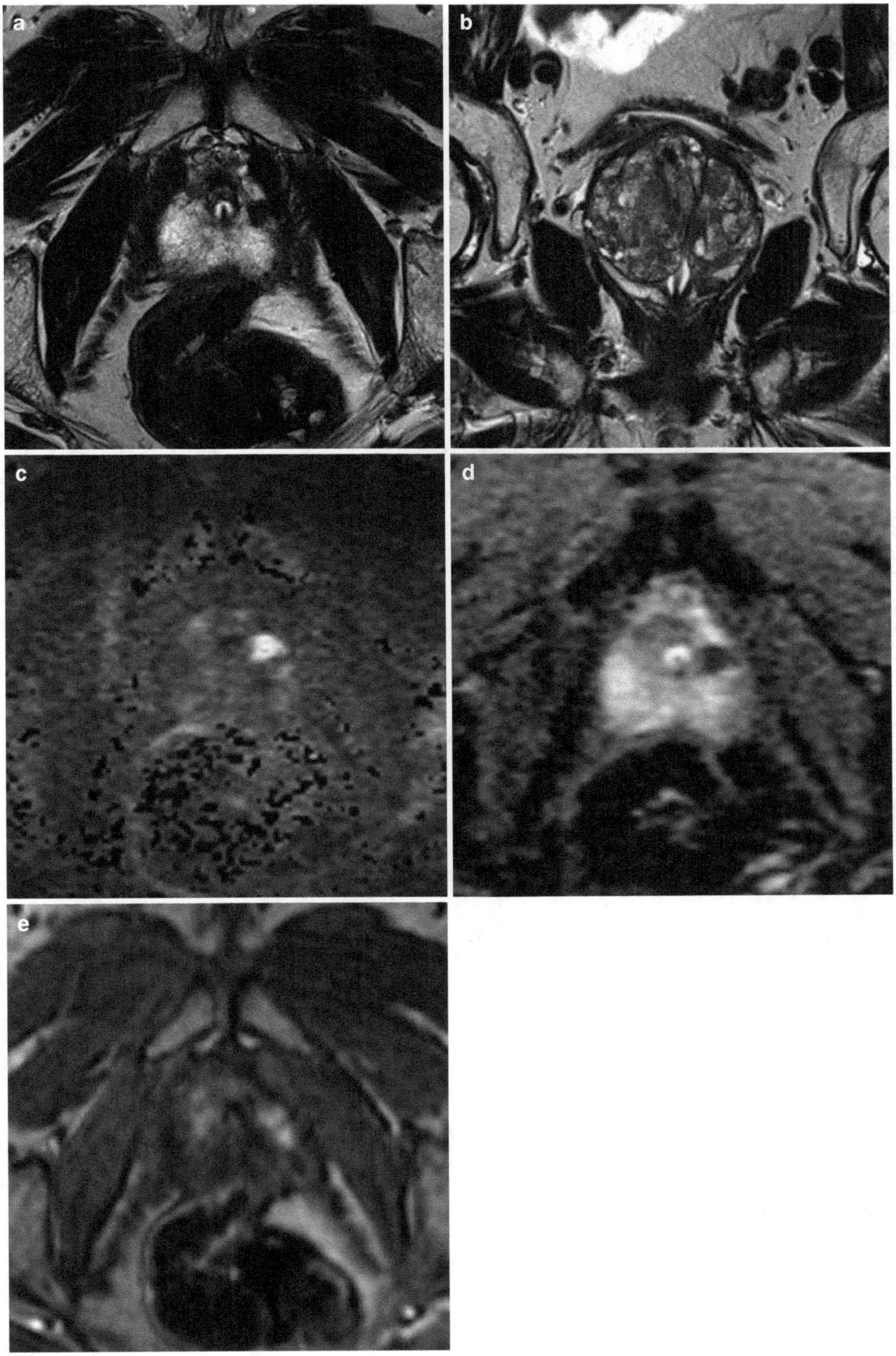

Fig.(**a**–**e**) PI-RADS 4 lesion in the peripheral zone. (**a**) Axial and (**b**) coronal T2-weighted sequence showing a circumscribed 11 mm hypointense mass in the left lateral peripheral zone (PI-RADS score 4). (**c**) Diffusion-weighted high *b*-value (calculated $b = 1400$ s/mm^2) image shows focal markedly hyperintense signal intensity of the mass. (**d**) ADC map (dominant sequence for the peripheral zone) correspondingly shows focal markedly hypointense signal intensity of the mass (PI-RADS score 4). (**e**) DCE sequence shows focal and early enhancement (DCE positive) corresponding to the focal mass seen on T2-weighted and DWI consistent with an overall PI-RADS score of 4. MRI/US fusion-guided biopsy revealed a Gleason 4 + 3 = 7 adenocarcinoma (PSA level was 8.1 ng/mL)

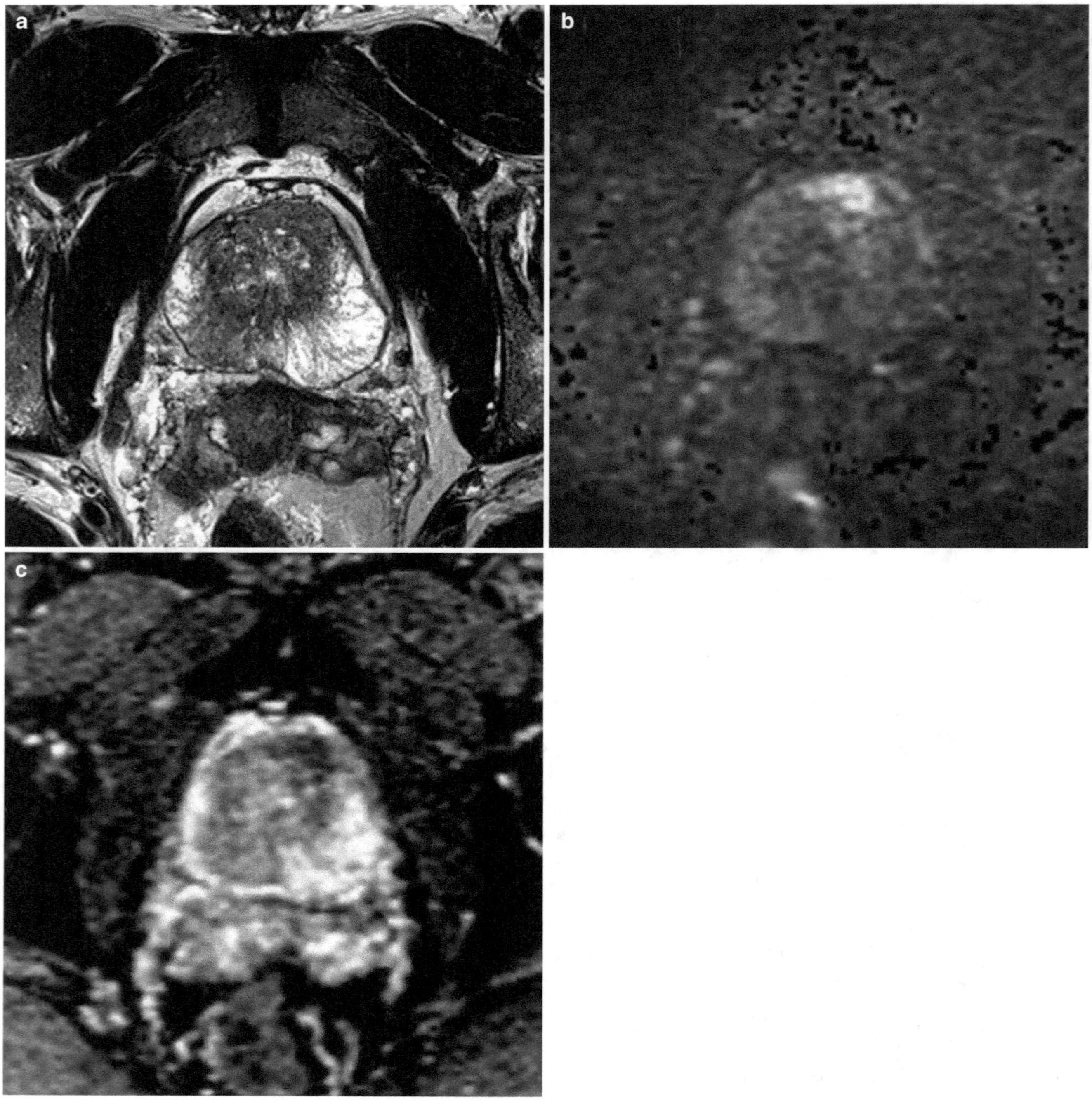

Fig. (**a–c**) PI-RADS 4 lesion in the transition zone. (**a**) Axial T2-weighted sequence (dominant sequence for the transition zone) showing a circumscribed lenticular 14 mm hypointense mass in the left anterior transition zone with bulging of the prostatic capsule (PI-RADS score 4). (**b**) Diffusion-weighted high *b*-value (calculated b = 1400 s/mm^2) image shows focal markedly hyperintense signal intensity of the mass. (**c**) ADC map correspondingly shows focal markedly hypointense signal intensity of the mass (PI-RADS score 4). MRI/US fusion-guided biopsy revealed a Gleason 4 + 4 = 8 adenocarcinoma (PSA level was 9.8 ng/mL). The patient had undergone a randomized TRUS-guided biopsy 3 months earlier with no evidence for malignancy. The anterior location is typical for adenocarcinoma missed by randomized biopsy; therefore, MRI is particularly useful in patients with negative randomized biopsy and persisting clinical suspicion for prostate cancer

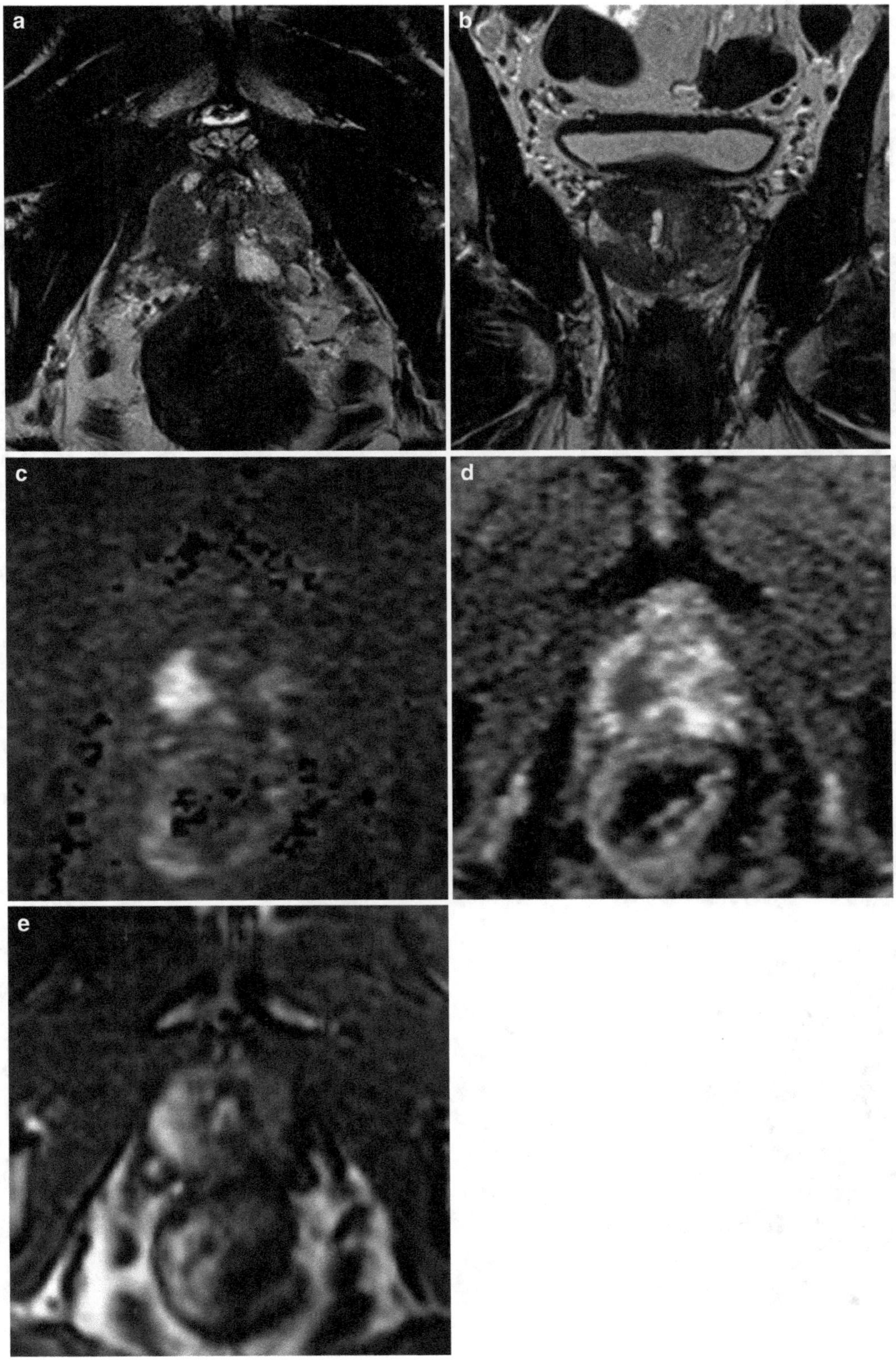

Fig. (**a**–**e**) PI-RADS 5 lesion in the peripheral zone. (**a**) Axial and (**b**) coronal T2-weighted sequence showing a circumscribed 18 mm hypointense mass in the right lateral peripheral zone (PI-RADS score 5). (**c**) Diffusion-weighted high *b*-value (calculated $b = 1400$ s/mm^2) image shows focal markedly hyperintense signal intensity of the mass. (**d**) ADC map (dominant sequence for the peripheral zone) correspondingly shows focal markedly hypointense signal intensity of the mass (PI-RADS score 5). (**e**) DCE sequence shows focal and early enhancement (DCE positive) corresponding to the focal mass seen on T2-weighted and DWI consistent with an overall PI-RADS score of 5. MRI/US fusion-guided biopsy revealed a Gleason 4 + 3 = 7 adenocarcinoma (PSA level was 11.2 ng/mL). Also note the wedge-shaped T2 hypointensities in the left lateral peripheral zone which demonstrate moderately hypointense signal on the ADC map and no focal enhancement (PI-RADS 3). On biopsy multifocal prostate cancer was diagnosed with Gleason 3 + 3 = 6 pattern in the left prostatic lobe

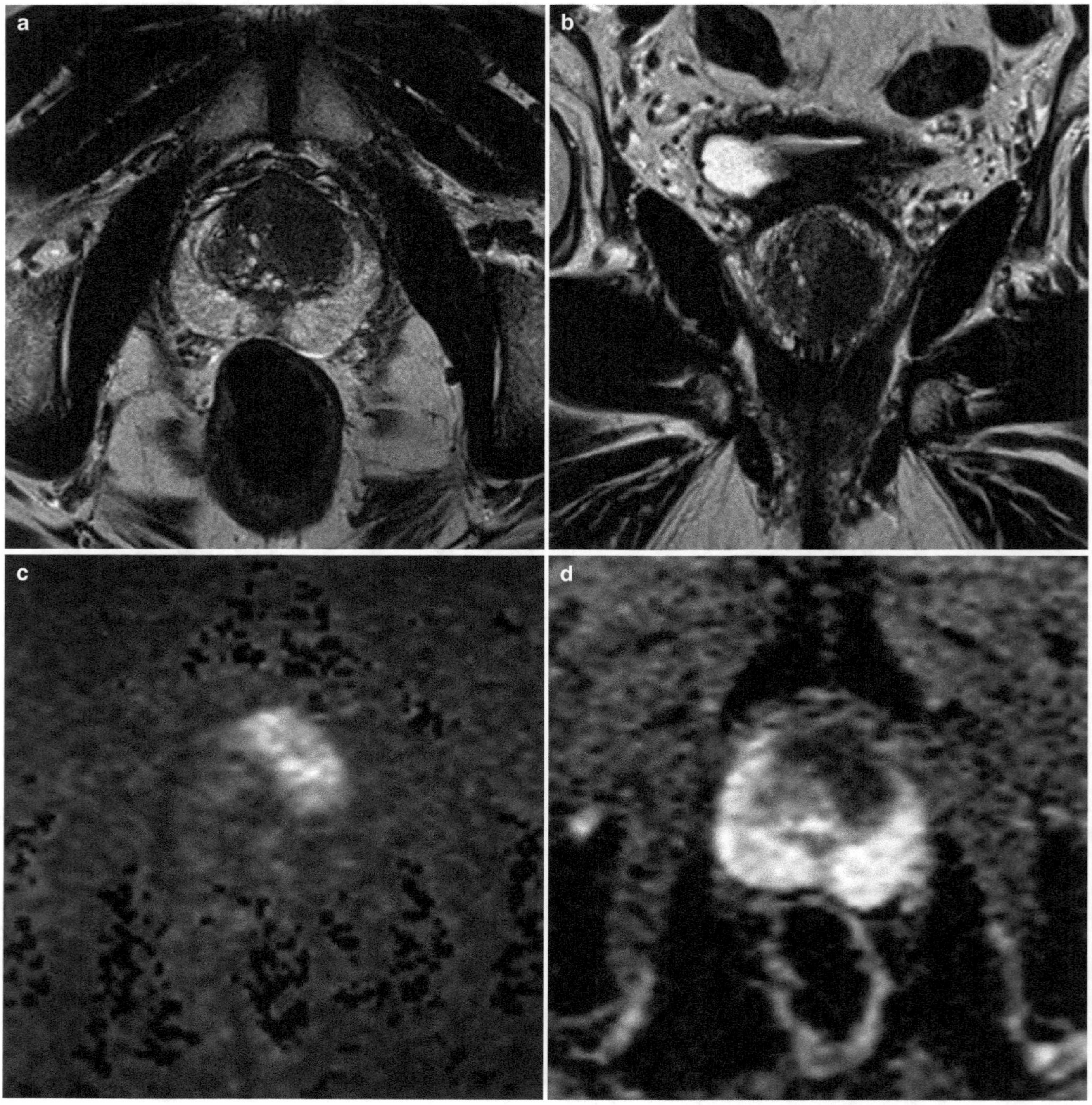

Fig. (**a**–**d**) PI-RADS 5 lesion in the transition zone. (**a**) Axial and (**b**) coronal T2-weighted sequence (dominant sequence for the transition zone) showing a circumscribed lenticular 20 mm hypointense mass in the anterior transition zone with minimal bulging of the prostatic capsule (PI-RADS score 5). (**c**) Diffusion-weighted high b-value (calculated $b = 1400$ s/mm^2) image shows focal markedly hyperintense signal intensity of the mass. (**d**) ADC map correspondingly shows focal markedly hypointense signal intensity of the mass (PI-RADS score 4). MRI/US fusion-guided biopsy revealed a Gleason 4 + 3 = 7 adenocarcinoma (PSA level was 14.7 ng/mL)

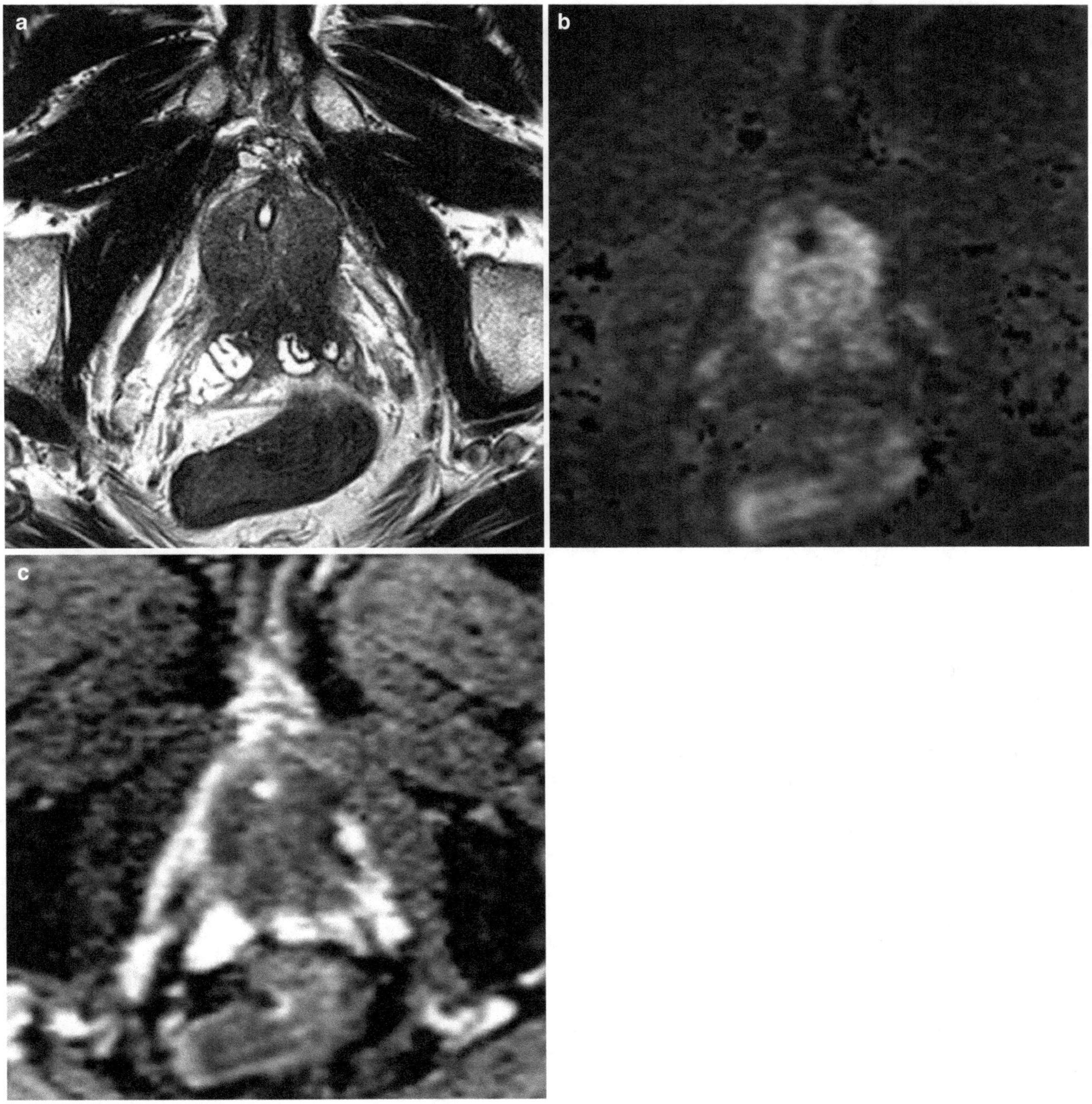

Fig.(**a–c**) Locally advanced prostate cancer with seminal vesi-cle infiltration. (**a**) Axial T2-weighted sequence showing diffuse hypointensity of the entire prostate (zonal anatomy not visible) with extension into the bilateral seminal vesicles (PI-RADS score 5). (**b**) Diffusion-weighted high *b*-value (calculated $b = 1400$ s/mm^2) image shows markedly hyperintense signal intensity of the entire prostate. (**c**) ADC map correspondingly shows markedly hypointense signal intensity of the prostate (PI-RADS score 5). Randomized TRUS-guided biopsy revealed a Gleason 4 + 5 = 9 adenocarcinoma (PSA level was 26.5 ng/mL)

Table Peripheral zone (PZ)

DWI	T2	DCE	PI-RADS score
1	Any	Any	1
2	Any	Any	2
3	Any	Negative	3
		Positive	4
4	Any	Any	4
5	Any	Any	5

Table Transition zone (TZ)

T2	DWI	DCE	PI-RADS score
1	Any	Any	1
2	Any	Any	2
3	≤ 4	Any	3
	5		4
4	Any	Any	4
5	Any	Any	5

been introduced. The dominant sequence depends on the prostatic zone the lesion is located; therefore identification of the zonal anatomy is crucial. The area at the base of the prostate where the central zone borders the peripheral zone and the anterior gland where the anterior horn of the peripheral zone borders the transition zone and the anterior fibromuscular stroma might be challenging in this respect. The DWI sequence is the dominant sequence for the peripheral zone where most prostate cancers are located. The T2-weighted sequence is the dominant sequence for the transition zone. The dominant sequence defines the fi nal PI-RADS score with the exception of PI-RADS 3 lesions, where for the peripheral zone the DCE sequence and for the transition zone the DWI sequence defines the final PI-RADS score (see Tables).

If a particular sequence cannot be acquired or is nondiagnostic due to artifacts (e.g., DWI when certain hip implants are present), it should be marked with "x." In this situation, the following rules apply:

Assessment without DWI (applies to PZ and TZ): the T2-weighted sequences define the final PI-RADS score with the exception of PI-RADS 3—if the lesion is DCE negative, the final score remains 3; if the lesion is DCE positive, the final score is 4.

Assessment without DCE (only applies to the peripheral zone since DCE is not needed for transition zone scoring): the DWI score represents the final PI-RADS score.

Structured Reporting

A very important task of PI-RADS is to "simplify and standardize the terminology and content of radiology reports" and to "enhance interdisciplinary communications with referring clinicians." A comprehensive mpMRI report should therefore include the following contents:

The volume of prostate should be reported according to the ellipsoid formula: maximum AP diameter x maximum transverse diameter x maximum longitudinal diameter × 0.52.

The aforementioned PI-RADS score is assigned to up to four intraprostatic lesions with a score ≥3. In case of multiple lesions, an index lesion should be defined. The index lesion is the one with the highest PI-RADS score. In case multiple lesions qualify for the highest PI-RADS score, extraprostatic extension (EPE) outclasses lesion size. For each lesion a PI-RADS score is assigned to *the series* and *the image number* where the lesion is best visualized should be reported to assist the urologist in selecting optimal images for MRI/US fusion-guided prostate biopsy. The lesion size also needs to be reported. Measurement of each lesion is preferred on the axial images; the DWI sequence should be used for peripheral zone lesions and the T2-weighted images for transition zone lesions. If a lesion is not well delineated on the axial sequences, then another plain should be used.

Another crucial element of a full PI-RADS report is a sector map in which the lesions should be indicated, since this particularly enhances the communication with the urologist. For this matter, the prostate is subdivided into three axial heights, the base, the midgland, and the prostatic apex, respectively. The seminal vesicles should also be included for cases of extraprostatic extension. The zonal anatomy (peripheral zone, transition zone, central zone, and anterior fibromuscular stroma) and the urethra should also be incorporated into the sector map.

Concluding Remarks

Comprehensive multiparametric MRI of the prostate should include lesion scoring and reporting according to the PI-RADS system. This will assist to achieve a high level of diagnostic accuracy and assure a thriving communication with the urologist.

Key Points

- Continuing technical innovation and broad research activity have resulted in a high diagnostic accuracy of MRI of prostate.
- Prostate MRI plays an important role for imaging-based targeted prostate biopsy.
- In patients undergoing active surveillance of prostate carcinoma, MRI has become indispensable for initial assessment as well as during the surveillance of the disease.
- PI-RADS standardizes image acquisition and facilitates communication with the urologists. It is considered an obligatory key element in prostate MRI.
- Comprehensive multiparametric MRI of the prostate should include lesion scoring and reporting according to the PI-RADS system.

Suggested Reading

Ahmed HU, El-Shater Bosaily A, Brown LC, PROMIS Study Group, et al. Diagnostic accuracy of multi-parametric MRI and TRUS biopsy in prostate cancer (PROMIS): a paired validating confirmatory study. Lancet. 2017;389:815–22.

Barentsz JO, Richenberg J, Clements R, European Society of Urogenital Radiology, et al. ESUR prostate MR guidelines 2012. Eur Radiol. 2012;22:746–57.

Cash H, Günzel K, Maxeiner A, et al. Men with a negative real-time MRI/ultrasound-fusion guided targeted biopsy but prostate cancer detection on TRUS-guided random biopsy – what are the reasons for targeted biopsy failure? BJU Int. 2016;118:35–43.

Cash H, Maxeiner A, Stephan C, et al. The detection of significant prostate cancer is correlated with the prostate imaging reporting and data system (PI-RADS) in MRI/transrectal ultrasound fusion biopsy. Word J Urol. 2016;34:525–32.

Greer MD, Shih JH, Lay N, et al. Validation of the dominant sequence paradigm and role of dynamic contrast-enhanced imaging in PI-RADS version 2. Radiology. 2017;285(3):859–69.

Haas M, Günzel K, Penzkofer T, et al. Implications of PI-RADS version 1 and updated version 2 on the scoring of prostatic lesions on multiparametric MRI. Aktuelle Urol. 2016;47:383–7.

http://www.esur.org/esur-guidelines/prostate-mri/. Accessed 4 Aug 2017.

Polanec S, Helbich TH, Bickel H, et al. Head-to-head comparison of PI-RADS v2 and PI-RADS v1. Eur J Radiol. 2016;85:1125–31.

Purysko AS, Bittencourt LK, Bullen JA, et al. Accuracy and interobserver agreement for Prostate Imaging Reporting and Data System, Version 2, for the characterization of lesions identified on multiparametric MRI of the prostate. AJR Am J Roentgenol. 2017;209:339–49.

Rosenkrantz AB, Ginocchio LA, Cornfeld D, et al. Interobserver reproducibility of the PI-RADS version 2 lexicon: a multicenter study of six experienced prostate radiologists. Radiology. 2016;280:793–804.

Ullrich T, Quentin M, Oelers C, et al. Magnetic resonance imaging of the prostate at 1.5 versus 3.0 T: a prospective comparison study of image quality. Eur J Radiol. 2017;90:192–7.

Weinreb JC, Barentsz JO, Choyke PL, et al. PI-RADS prostate imaging - reporting and data system: 2015, version 2. Eur Urol. 2015;69:16–40.

22

Focal Liver Lesions

Wolfgang Schima, Dow-Mu Koh, and Richard Baron†

Learning Objectives

- To learn the optimal imaging techniques and the relevance of differential diagnosis for liver diseases
- To discuss current indications for liver-specific contrast agents
- To review the imaging features of benign and malignant focal liver lesions
- To discuss the differential diagnosis of primary and secondary hepatic tumors

Introduction

Multidetector computed tomography (MDCT) and magnetic resonance (MR) imaging provide noninvasive insights into liver anatomy and the pathophysiology of liver diseases, which allows for better disease diagnosis, monitoring of disease evolution and treatment response, as well as for guiding treatment decisions. Understanding the application of different imaging techniques is critical for the management of focal liver lesions. In the current climate of challenging health economics, the most appropriate and cost effective modality should always be utilized. For liver imaging, ultrasonography (US) is widely available, noninvasive, and often used in the community for disease screening but has unfortunately limited diagnostic sensitivity and specificity. Contrast-enhanced MDCT remains the modality of choice for routine liver imaging. MR imaging is still used largely as a problem-solving tool when MDCT or US is equivocal or if there is concern for malignancy in high-risk populations.

In this chapter, we will highlight imaging of focal liver lesions, focusing on the use of MDCT and MR imaging for disease detection and characterization. The reader should learn how to optimize CT and MR imaging in his/her own practice, understand how to apply and interpret CT and MR imaging for the management of focal liver lesions, and appreciate the expanding role of liver-specific MR contrast agents for lesion characterization.

MDCT Imaging Techniques

MDCT allows imaging to be performed in multiple planes. Using a 64-plus-detector-row system, the entire liver can be scanned within 1–4 s using a submillimeter detector configuration allowing for high-quality multiplanar reconstructions (MPR) [1]. When viewed axially, reconstructed sections of 2.5–3 mm thickness with an overlap of 0.5–1 mm are usually used in clinical practice. Thinner slices do not improve lesion conspicuity because of increased image noise [2] that can decrease diagnostic specificity [3]. The amount of contrast material administered can be calculated by a patient's weight, but 0.5 g iodine/kg b.w. is typical (i.e., 1.7 mL/kg b.w. at 300 mg/mL). The total amount of iodine administered determines the quality of the portal venous imaging phase, with the aim of increasing the liver attenuation by 50 HU after contrast injection [4]. To achieve good arterial phase imaging, a relatively high contrast medium injection rate of 4–5 mL/s is recommended [5]. On the other hand, studies have shown that a fixed injection duration of 30 s (meaning that the injection rate will differ

†Author was deceased

W. Schima, M.D., M.Sc. (✉)
Department of Radiology, Göttlicher Heiland Krankenhaus, Barmherzige Schwestern Krankenhaus, Sankt Josef Krankenhaus, Vinzenzgruppe, Vienna, Austria
e-mail: wolfgang.schima@khgh.at

D.-M. Koh
Department of Radiology, Royal Marsden Hospital, Sutton, UK

according to patient's weight) also provides consistent image quality.

The timing of the image acquisition in relation to contrast media administration depends on whether imaging is required during early arterial phase (for arterial anatomy only), late arterial phase (for hypervascular tumor detection and characterization), or venous phase (for follow-up imaging and hypovascular tumor detection). For the detection and characterization of focal liver lesions, late arterial phase imaging (with a delay of aortic transit time plus 15–18 s) [6, 7] and a venous phase scan (20–30 s interscan delay or with fixed delay of ~60–70 s) are performed. However, the use of combinations of these imaging phases also depends on specific indications [8]. Automated methods of measuring arterial enhancement (aortic transit time) on CT, often termed bolus tracking, have replaced the use of fixed scan-delay times because it provides better coincidence of scanning with peak enhancement of liver tumors (in the late arterial phase) and the liver parenchyma (in the venous phase).

Different techniques for dose reduction and optimization of image quality are now widely in use: automatic exposure control by tube current (mA) modulation, selection of lower tube potential (kVp), and adaptive dose shielding to minimize overscanning in the z-axis, to name a few. Conventional filtered back projection (FBP), the standard CT image reconstruction technique for many years, has given way to iterative reconstruction (IR). IR uses loop-wise raw data correction to reduce image noise, thus allowing imaging to be performed at reduced kVp or mAs, with lower radiation dose but comparable image quality. All major manufacturers now provide iterative reconstruction techniques (SAFIRE, ADMIRE, Siemens; iDose, IMR, Philips; ASIR, MBIR, GE Healthcare; AIDR, AIDR 3D, Toshiba) [9]. Stepwise IR reduces CT noise levels. However, high levels of IR may induce a pixelated (plastic-like) image texture and may render image quality unacceptable [10]. A substantial dose reduction of 38–55% is possible with IR without compromising image quality [11–13] (Fig.). In recent years, dual-energy and spectral CT technique has emerged, where the utilization of dual-source or polychromatic X-ray beams and the differential attenuation of such beams of different energies in tissues are applied to improve the detection of hypervascular hepatocellular carcinomas [14] or for the quantification o f h epatic i ron c ontent [15]. H owever, dual-energy CT technology is still not widely employed in clinical practice despite potential merits, in part because of the post-processing time required to generate the appropriate images.

MR Imaging Technique

MR imaging of the liver can now be performed at both 1.5 and 3.0 T; the latter has significantly improved in image quality due to advancements in both imaging hardware and software. MR examination of the liver should include unenhanced T1-weighted and T2-weighted sequences, as well as contrast-enhanced sequences. Specific acquisition sequences vary by manufacturer, patient compliance, and the clinical question being addressed.

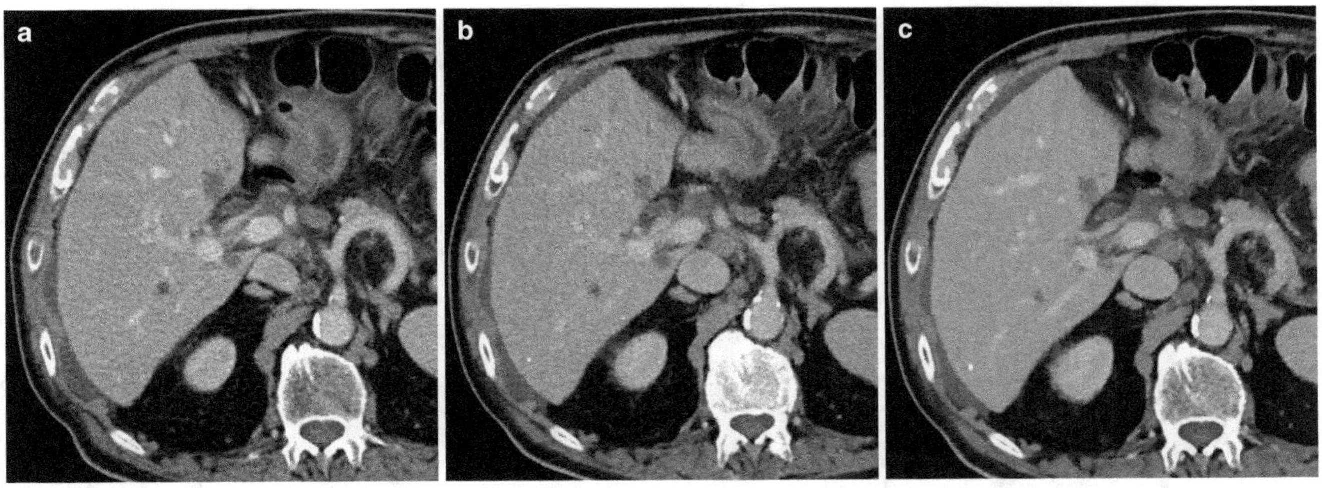

Fig. Dose reduction using iterative reconstruction techniques at MDCT. (**a**) Normal dose MDCT in the venous phase (120 kVp, ref. mAs 230) reconstructed with standard filtered back projection shows colorectal liver metastases. (**b**) Image appearance (120 kVp, ref. mAs 150) using iterative reconstruction (SAFIRE level 3) is slightly different in general, due to reduced image noise. The lesions are shown with the same conspicuity. Patient dose is reduced by 36%. (**c**) At higher iterative reconstruction levels (SAFIRE level 5), the image appearance is pixelated ("plastic-like"), especially seen at the liver parenchyma and the perirenal fat

In- and opposed-phase (or out-of-phase) T1-weighted imaging is recommended for maximal tumor detection and for characterization of fat containing tumors and the presence of steatosis. T1-weighted MRI can be now performed using a 3D DIXON technique, which can generate in-phase, out-of-phase, water-only, and fat-only images of the whole liver volume in a single breath-hold acquisition. The resultant water-only images have been shown to improve the uniformity of fat suppression at 3 T, compared with conventional spectral fat suppression technique [16]. The use of the DIXON images for dynamic contrast-enhanced acquisition has also been shown to improve the detection of hepatocellular carcinoma compared with standard fat-suppressed sequences.

Another useful recent implementation is non-Cartesian radial T1-weighted imaging, which allows 3D volume T1-weighted imaging of the liver to be performed in free breathing. This allows good quality T1-weighted of the liver to be obtained in patients with poor breath holding (e.g., elderly, breathless adults, or young children) (Fig.), especially during dynamic contrast-enhanced acquisitions [17]. T2-weighted pulse sequences with fat suppression provide better lesion contrast than nonfat-suppressed sequences and are also widely used.

Diffusion-weighted imaging (DWI) has become a standard technique in liver imaging, and it is now available on all scanners. In general, DWI depends upon the microscopic mobility of water, called Brownian motion, in tissue. Water-molecule diffusion (and thus the measured signal intensity) depends on tissue cellularity, tissue organization, integrity of cellular membranes, and extracellular space tortuosity. Usually, lower water diffusion is found in most solid tumors, which are attributed to their high cellularity [18]. Thus, DWI is helpful for detecting liver solid focal liver lesions [19–21]. By performing diffusion-weighted imaging using two or more b-values, we can quantify the apparent diffusion coefficient (ADC) of liver tissues. Benign focal liver lesions have been shown to have higher ADC value than malignant liver lesions, although there is significant overlap [22]. Nonetheless, quantitative ADC values may be useful to support lesion characterization and for identifying early tumor response to treatment, which is currently being investigated.

Imaging after the administration of intravenous contrast agents remains the cornerstone for liver MR imaging. Of these, nonspecific extracellular gadolinium contrast medium is still most widely used. Following the intravenous (IV) bolus injection of extracellular gadolinium-based contrast agents, dynamic imaging (using volumetric T1-weigthed imaging) is performed in characterizing lesion, detecting lesion, evaluating tumor response to therapy, and detecting marginal recurrences after tumor ablation.

Liver-specific (or hepatobiliary) MR contrast agents are available and have specific roles in the management of focal liver lesions. These include gadobenate dimeglumine (MultiHance®, Bracco) and gadoxetic acid (Primovist® or Eovist®, Bayer Healthcare). Liver-specific MR contrast agents are also usually administered IV as a bolus, as with nonspecific gadolinium chelates for dynamic imaging. However, imaging is also performed at a delayed liver-specific or hepatobiliary phase, the timing of this differs according to the contrast agent. These liver-specific agents are taken up into hepatocytes to varying extent (gadobenate dimeglumine 4–5%; gadoxetic acid ~50%), resulting in avid T1 enhancement of the liver parenchyma in the hepatobiliary

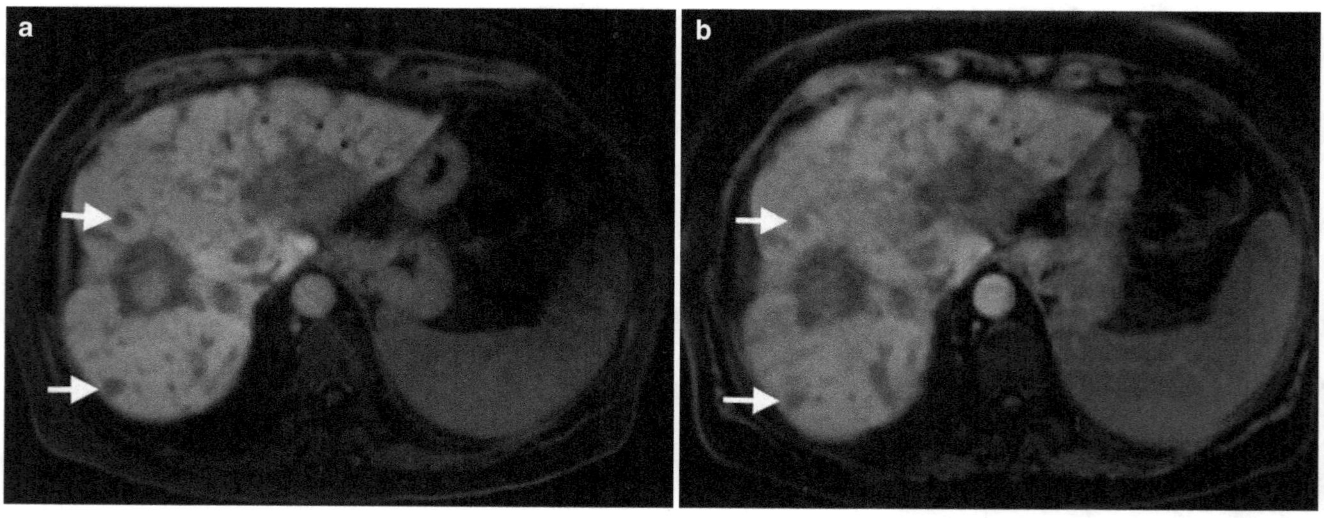

Fig. Radial acquisition technique. Colorectal liver metastases. Hepatobiliary phase imaging performed at 20 min after gadoxetate contrast administration using (**a**) free breathing radial acquisition fat-suppressed gradient echo and (**b**) breath-hold volume interpolated fat-suppressed gradient echo technique. Note that the free-breathing acquisition in this patient resulted in better delineation of the smaller liver metastases as T1 hypointense lesions against the enhancing liver parenchyma (arrows)

phase, which is performed at 20 min for gadoxetic acid and about 1–2 h for gadobenate dimeglumine after contrast administration. Liver-specific contrast agents have been shown to improve the detection of liver metastases [23–26], especially when used in combination with diffusion-weighted MR imaging.

Benign Hepatic Lesions

Cysts

Simple hepatic cysts are common, occurring in 5–14% of the general population. As they are usually asymptomatic, they are detected incidentally on US, CT, or MR imaging. On CT, hepatic cysts are well circumscribed and typically show attenuation values similar to water (0–15 HU), although smaller cysts may show higher attenuation values due to partial volume effects. Cysts should not show mural thickening, nodularity, or contrast enhancement. Small cysts (≤3 mm in size) may pose a diagnostic challenge in the cancer patient on CT as they are too small to fully characterize and stability on follow-up imaging is important to reassure. Nonetheless, the majority of small hypodense liver lesions even in the oncology patient are usually benign.

On MR imaging examinations, cysts are well-defined, homogeneous lesions that appear hypointense on T1-weighted images and markedly hyperintense on T2-weighted images. Their marked hyperintensity on T2-weighted imaging provides greater confidence toward the diagnosis of small cysts on MRI.

Hemangioma

Hemangioma is the most common benign liver tumor. On US, liver hemangioma appears circumscribed, well-defined, hyperechoic, and associated with distal acoustic enhancement. Small hemangiomas usually appear homogeneous, but larger hemangiomas (>4 cm) can show a heterogeneous appearance.

On CT, hemangiomas are well-defined hypodense masses. They are hypointense on T1-weighted and markedly hyperintense on T2-weighted imaging, sometimes with a lobular contour. Hyperintensity on T2-weighted MRI helps to differentiate hemangiomas from other solid neoplasms [27, 28]. At a relatively long T2 echo time (140 ms or longer), a homogeneously bright lesion is characteristic of a benign lesion, such as a cyst or hemangioma. Exceptions include cystic or mucinous metastases, gastrointestinal stromal tumor (GIST), and neuroendocrine tumor metastases.

Hemangiomas show three distinctive patterns of enhancement at CT/MRI (type I to III) [29], where there is characteristically enhancement that closely follows the enhancement of blood pool elsewhere [30]. Small lesions (up to ~2 cm) may show immediate and complete enhancement in the arterial phase, with sustained enhancement in the venous and delayed phases (type I, "flash filling") [31] (Fig.. On delayed imaging, the enhancement usually fades to a similar extent as the blood pool. The most common enhancement pattern is peripheral nodular discontinuous enhancement, which progressively fill-in over time (type II). Larger lesions (>5 cm) or lesions with central thrombosis/fibrosis may lack central fill-in (type III) (Fig.). When evaluated using liver-specific contrast agents, the appearance of hemangiomas in the dynamic arterial and venous phases is similar to that with nonspecific gadolinium chelates. However, in the delayed phase, after 3 min, there may be "pseudowashout" (hypointensity) due to early hepatocellular enhancement of liver parenchyma (Fig.). In the hepatobiliary phase, hemangiomas may appear hypointense to the parenchyma, thus mimicking liver metastases. In this instance, DWI may help to differentiate between hemangioma and other solid lesions, as the apparent diffusion coefficient (ADC) of uncomplicated hemangiomas is significantly higher (typi-cally $>1.70 \times 10^{-3}$ s/mm^2) than in malignant solid lesions [22, 32].

Focal Nodular Hyperplasia

Focal nodular hyperplasia (FNH) is a benign lesion that can cause confusion when incidentally detected during abdominal imaging. On ultrasound, the lesion is usually isoechoic or slightly hypoechoic [33] to liver, but appears hypoechoic in patients with diffuse hepatic steatosis. Typically, FNH demonstrates a lobular contour, which is uncommon in malignant lesions. A central scar is present in about 67% of larger lesions and about 33% of smaller lesions [34]. The central scar in FNH is usually hyperintense on T2-weighted images, with a comma-shaped or spoke-wheel appearance, which can be distinguished from fibrolamellar HCC, where the central scar, when present, is predominately low signal intensity on T2-weighted MR. Color/power Doppler US may show blood flow within the scar [35].

FNH is isodense or minimally hypodense on unenhanced and equilibrium-phase post-contrast CT and may be only suspected because of the presence of mass effect on adjacent vessels. On unenhanced T1- and T2-weighted MR images, FNH returns signal intensity similar to hepatic parenchyma but is usually slightly different on either T1- or T2-weighted

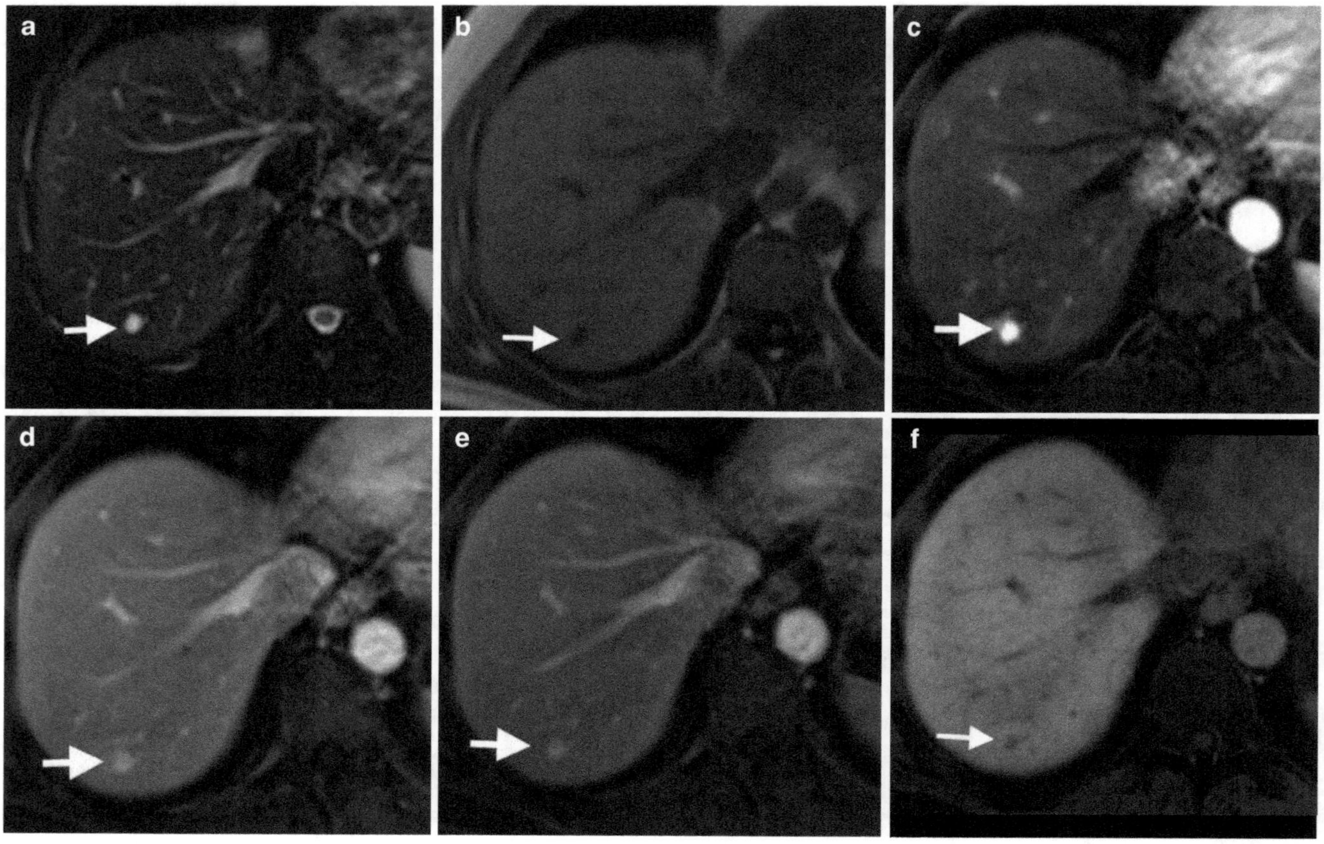

Fig. Hemangioma type 1. Liver-specific MR contrast agent. A 45-year-old woman with incident lesion (arrows) in the right lobe of the liver. This appears as (**a**) high signal intensity on T2-weighted imaging and (**b**) low signal intensity on T1-weighted imaging and (**c–e**) shows uniform enhancement on dynamic T1-weighted contrast-enhanced imaging, isointense to the vascular signal at all phases. The lesion appears (**f**) hypointense in the hepatobiliary phase of gadoxetic acid-enhanced MRI

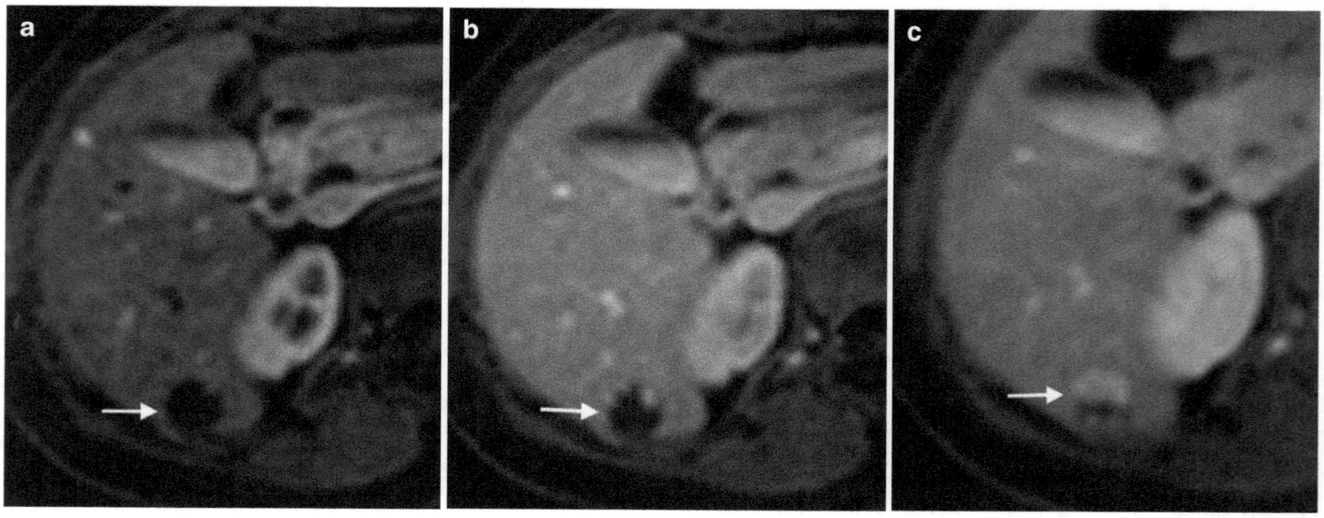

Fig. Hemangioma type 3: nonspecific gadolinium chelate. (**a–c**) T1-weighted dynamic enhanced T1-weighted GRE in the (**a**) arterial and (**b**) portal venous and (**c**) delayed phase shows nodular peripheral enhancement of the lesion with centripetal filling. There is incomplete enhancement of the lesion

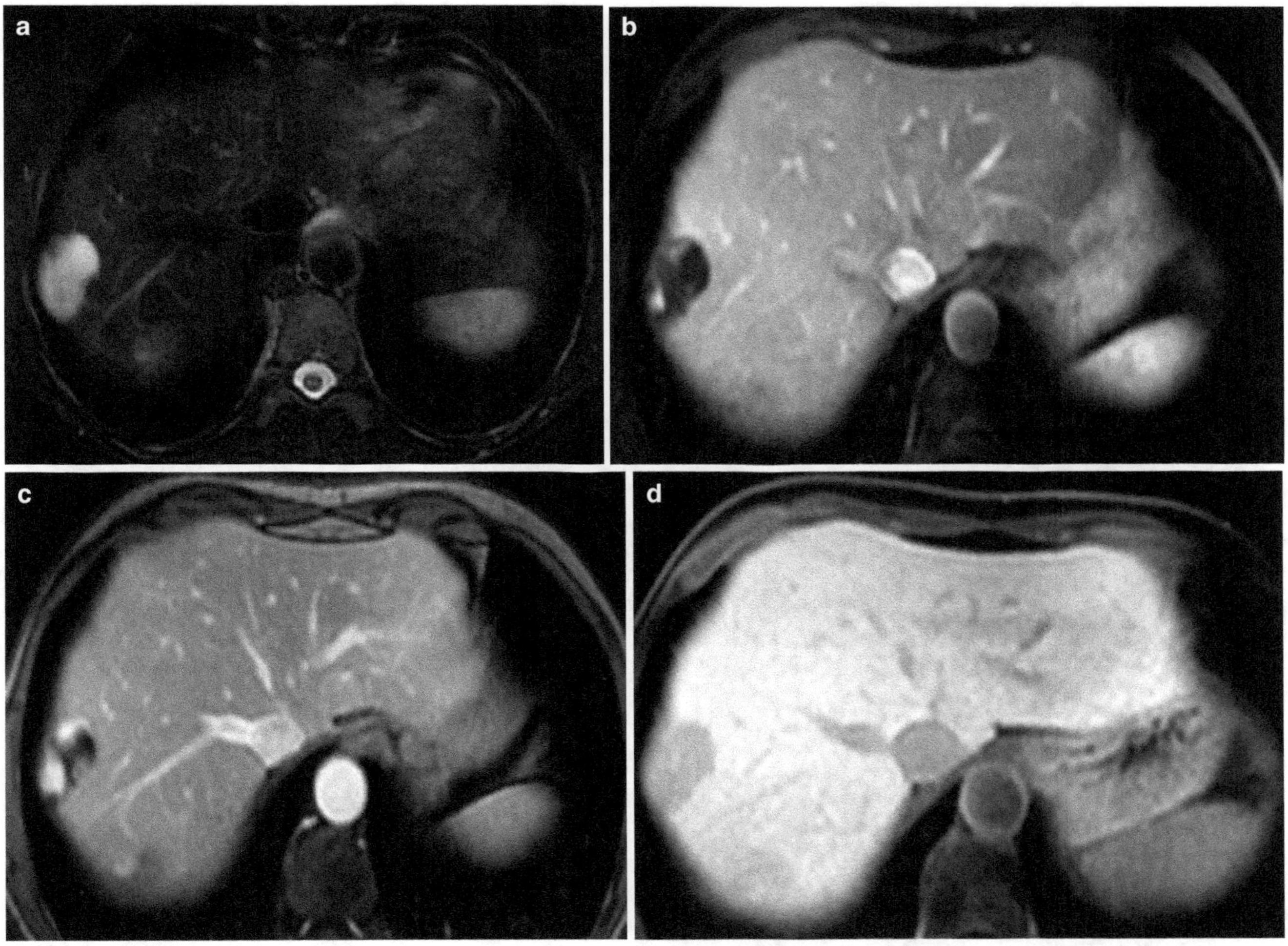

Fig. Hemangioma type 3: liver-specific MR contrast agent. (**a**) T2-weighted TSE shows a large lobulated lesion of very high signal intensity. (**b–d**) Dynamic gadoxetic acid-enhanced imaging shows peripheral nodular enhancement in the arterial (**b**) and venous phases (**c**). In the hepatobiliary phase (**d**) there is marked hypointensity of the lesion due to lack of hepatocellular uptake in the lesion and enhancement of surrounding liver parenchyma

images. Due to the prominent arterial vascular supply, FNH demonstrates marked homogenous enhancement during the arterial phase of contrast-enhanced CT/MR imaging, which becomes rapidly isodense/isointense to liver parenchyma in the portal venous phase [34]. The central scar often showed delayed enhancement (Fig.) [33] because of its vascular component. Another key feature is that other than the scar, FNH are usually homogeneous in appearance compared with the heterogeneous appearance encountered in fibrolamellar HCC.

Using liver-specific M R c ontrast a gents, F NH f requently shows enhancement on delayed images after administration of hepatobiliary contrast agents (such as gadoxetic acid or gadobenate dimeglumine) because of the presence of normal biliary ductules within the lesion and the expression of OATP receptors (Fig.). However, the uptake of hepatobiliary contrast agents within FNH may be rarely heterogeneous or absent [36]. Nonetheless, a recent meta-analysis showed that the lesion T1 isointensity or hyperintensity at delayed hepatobiliary phase MRI has a high sensitivity (91–100%) and specificity (87–100%) for diagnosing FNH [36]. This feature can be helpful for differentiating FNH from hypervascular metastases or hepatic adenomas (HCA) and hepatocellular carcinomas (HCC) (which do not usually take up liver-specific agents) [31, 37]. However, it should be noted that some HCAs (particularly inflammatory HCA and beta-catenin-activated HCA) and HCC can appear isointense or hyperintense at delayed imaging after hepatobiliary contrast media administration. While differentiating FNH from variants of HCA remains challenging, it has been suggested that the presence of contrast washout (i.e., lesion hypointensity compared to liver parenchyma) of HCC in the portal venous or transitional phase of dynamic contrast enhancement can be used to distinguish between HCC (that shows contrast uptake in the hepatobiliary phase) and FHN nodules. The majority of FNH tend to remain static in size, although FNH may increase in size on follow-up (3–11%), although oral contraceptives do not appear to stimulate FNH growth [38, 39].

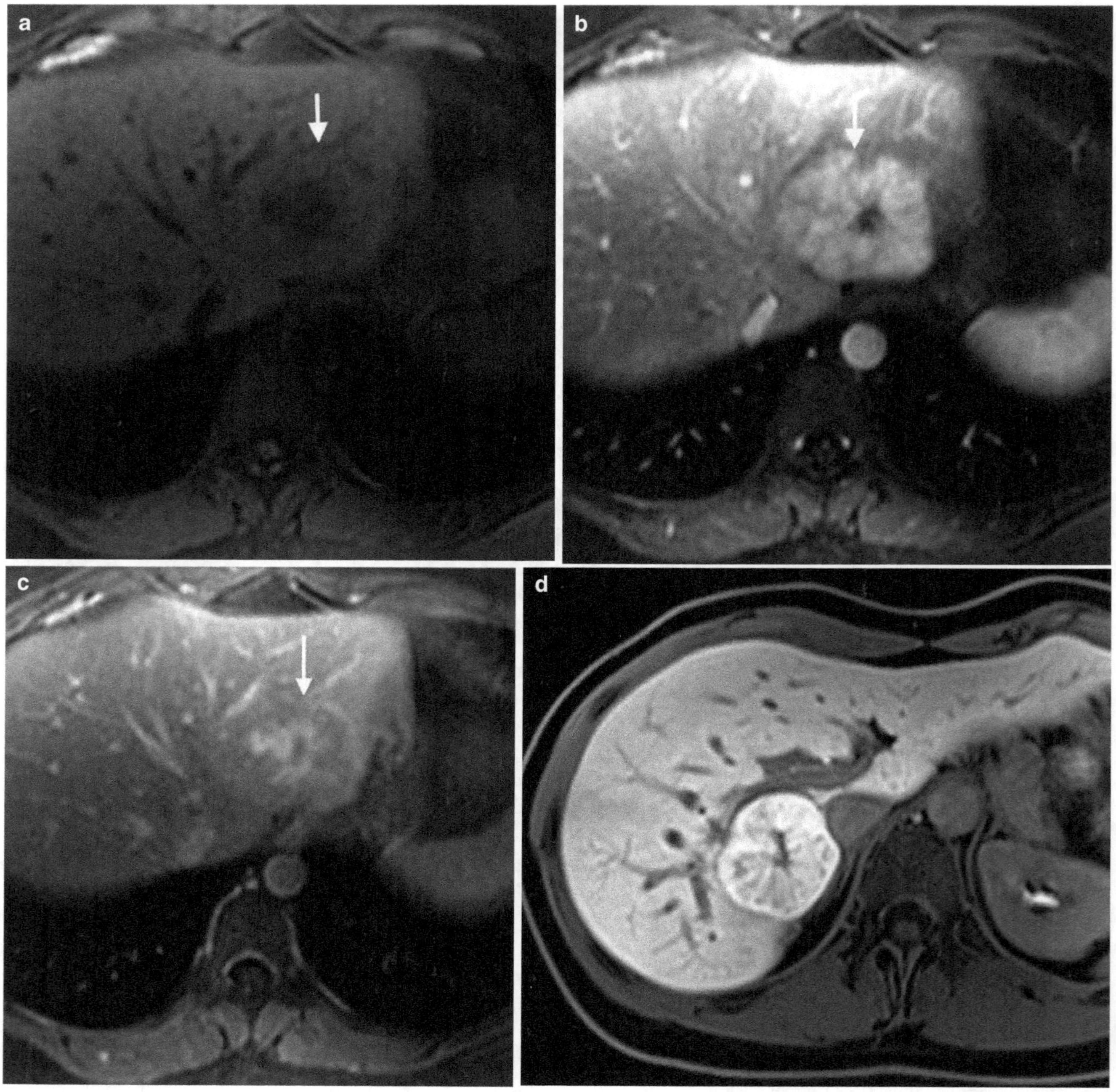

Fig. FNH. Incidental lesion in the left lobe of the liver (arrows). (**a**) Pre-contrast T1-weighted image shows an isointense lesion with a central hypointense scar, which shows minimal mass effect upon adjacent vasculature. (**b**) Arterial phase T1-weighted contrast-enhanced image shows hypervascularity of the lesion. (**c**) T1-weighted delayed phase imaging after contrast shows that the lesion is now predominantly isointense to the liver but with late enhancement of the (vascular) central scar. The enhancement pattern is typical for FNH. (**d**) Hepatobiliary phase imaging of another FNH: homogenous uptake of the liver-specific MR contrast agent, the spoke-wheel central scar is typically not enhanced

Hepatocellular Adenoma

Hepatocellular adenoma (HCA) is uncommon, but has an association with oral contraceptive and anabolic steroid usage. Histologically, HCA is composed of cells resembling normal hepatocytes but lacking bile ducts, which distinguishes them from FNH [39].

The imaging features of HCA are heterogeneous and varied. HCA are often hypervascular and may appear heterogeneous due to the presence of fat, necrosis, or hemorrhage [39, 40]. T1-weighted chemical shift or DIXON imaging is useful for detecting intratumoral fat, while the presence of high T1-signal before contrast administration will raise the suspicion of spontaneous hemorrhage. The reader should be familiar with the differential diagnoses of fat containing focal liver lesions on MRI, which include focal fat infiltration, HCA (particularly the HNF1A inactivating subtype), hepatocellular carcinoma (usually well differentiated), angiomyolipoma, lipoma, teratoma, and liver metastases from fat containing malignancies (e.g., liposarcomas). The presence of intratumoral fat helps to narrow the differential diagnosis of a hypervascular lesion, as hemangioma can be excluded and metastases and FNH rarely contain fat.

On dynamic contrast-enhanced CT or MR, adenomas usually show marked arterial-phase enhancement, with rapid transition to either iso- or hypoattenuating/intense to hepatic parenchyma on portal venous phase imaging. Our understanding of the molecular aberrations associated with HCA has improved our understanding of HCA subtypes, which is linked to risk factors, histological features, clinical presentation, and imaging appearances [41, 42]. The latest molecular classification categorizes HCA into the following six subgroups: HNF1A-inactivated HCA, inflammatory HCA, CTNNB1-mutated HCA in exon 3, CTNNB1 mutated in exon 7 and 8 HCA, sonic hedgehog HCA, and unclassified HCA [43, 44].

What is important for radiologists? Inactivating mutations of hepatocyte nuclear factor 1 alpha (HNF1A) are observed in 40–50% of HCA. HNF1A-inactivated HCA usually contains fat as evidenced by diffuse and homogenous signal loss on chemical shift T1-weighted imaging (Fig.). They return variable T2 signal. At contrast-enhanced T1-weighted MRI, they are hypervascular, often with contrast washout in the portal venous or delayed phase. They are typically hypointense on hepatobiliary-phase MRI using liver-specific contrast medium. HNF1A-inactivated HCAs have a very low risk of malignant transformation.

Inflammatory HCA accounts for 35–45% of HCA cases. Obesity and a history of oral contraceptives intake are risk factors for their development. Inflammatory HCA appear strongly hyperintense on T2-weighted MRI, which may be diffuse or rim-like in the periphery of the lesion (Atoll sign). Intralesional fat is uncommon and, when present, is often patchy or heterogeneous. On contrast-enhanced imaging, there is usually intense arterial enhancement, with persistent enhancement on delayed phase imaging (Figs.). Although the majority of inflammatory HCA are hypointense on hepatobiliary phase using liver-specific con-trast media, about 30% may appear iso- or hyperintense. Inflammatory HCA may also harbor activating mutations of b-catenin in exon 3 and are therefore at risk of malignant transformation.

Mutations of catenin b1 (CTNNB1) in exon 3 (coding for b-catenin) are seen in 10–15% of HCA. These are associated with a higher risk of malignant transformation. By contrast, a subset of HCA (5–10%) is associated with mutations of CTNNB1 in two hot spots in exon 7 and 8, which does not confer an increased risk of malignancy. These variants of HCA do not have typical imaging features and may be difficult to differentiate from HCC or FNH. HCA with mutations of catenin b1 may also show contrast uptake in the hepatobiliary phase of MRI using liver-specific contrast media.

Activation of sonic hedgehog pathway occurs in approximately 5% of HCA. As these are relatively uncommon, the spectrum of imaging features associated with these is yet to be fully described. Nonetheless, these lesions have a higher propensity to undergo spontaneous hemorrhage. About 7% of HCA remains unclassified. These do not have typical clinical or imaging appearances.

Overall, the imaging features at MRI, including their appearances using liver-specific MR contrast agents (gadobenate, gadoxetic acid) are helpful in distinguishing between FNH and HCA. In the hepatobiliary phase of contrast enhancement, FNH typically show contrast uptake, whereas NHF1A-inactivated HCA and the majority of other HCA subtypes do not [44]. Of note is that diffusion-weighted MRI has little value in helping to distinguish between HCA and FNH or HCC because of the substantial overlap in the ADC values.

Biliary Hamartomas (Von Meyenburg Complex)

Bile duct hamartomas are congenital malformations of the ductal plate without connections to the bile ducts. They are usually discovered incidentally at abdominal imaging. Although of no clinical significance, they can mimic disseminated small liver metastases in the patient with cancer. Biliary hamartomas are typically small (5–10 mm in size) and usually widely distributed in both lobes of the liver. On ultrasound, they appear as small hyperechoic or hypoechoic lesions and can demonstrate ringing artifacts (comet tail appearance). On CT, they appear as small cystic lesions of round, oval, or irregular shape without contrast enhancement, although thin rim enhancement may sometimes be present, thus mimicking hypovascular liver metastases [40]. When enhancement is present, it is usually very thin (≤2 mm) and observed only on equilibrium-phase images, related to the fibrous component of the lesions [45]. On MRI, biliary hamartomas appear low signal intensity on T1-weighted imaging and high signal intensity on T2-weighted imaging (Fig.). They are best observed on maximum intensity projections MRCP sequences as high signal intensity foci without connection to or associated abnormalities of the intrahepatic ducts. Occasionally, bile duct hamartomas can

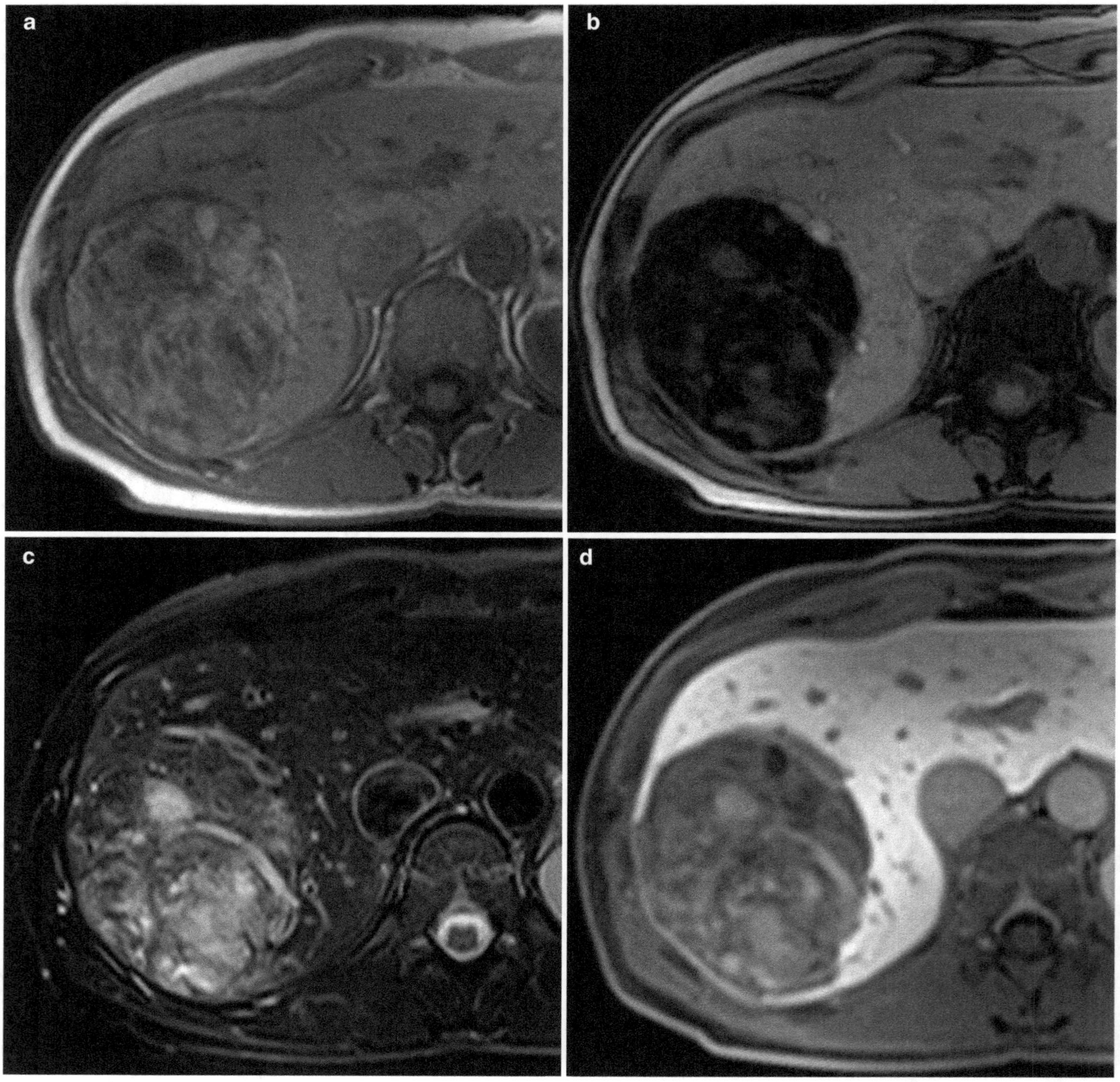

Fig. Adenoma (HNF1A subtype). (**a**) T1-weighted in-phase GRE image demonstrates a very large mass in a young woman. The mass is inhomogeneous and shows bright spots. (**b**) There is typical signal intensity drop on the opposed-phase image indicative of intratumoral fat. (**c**) The T2-weighted TSE shows moderate hyperintensity. (**d**) On the gadoxetic acid-enhanced images in the hepatobiliary phase, there is little to no enhancement

be very large, up to 20 cm, and be symptomatic from internal hemorrhage or pressure on adjacent structures [46]. Differential diagnoses of biliary hamartomas include peribiliary cysts (predominantly perihilar distribution in patients with liver parenchymal disease), polycystic disease, and Caroli's disease (cysts communicate with bile ducts and are associated with bile duct abnormalities). They can also mimic liver abscesses in the appropriate clinical setting.

Hepatic Abscess and Echinococcus

The appearances of hepatic abscesses on imaging depend on etiology (peribiliary abscesses tend to be small and scattered adjacent to the biliary tree; hematogenous distribution via the hepatic artery or via the portal vein in appendicitis or diverticulitis tends to lead to larger lesions diffusely spread in the liver). US reveals a cystic lesion with internal

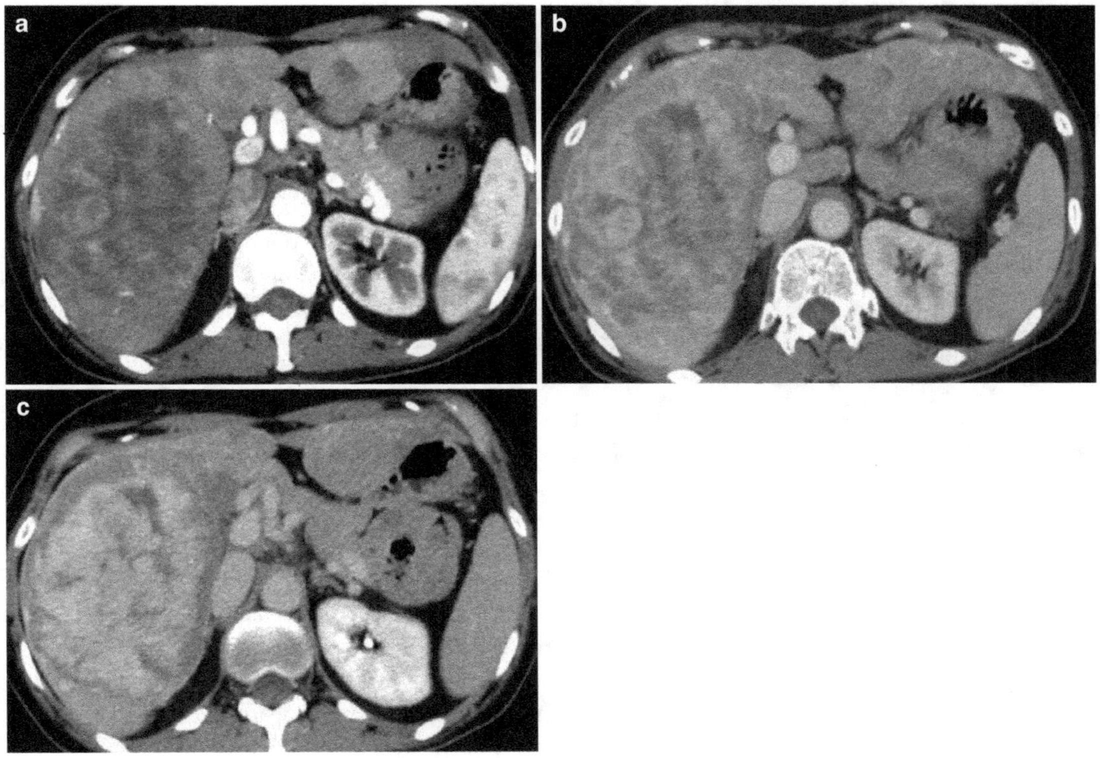

Fig. Adenoma: inflammatory type. (**a–c**) Arterial (**a**) venous (**b**) phase CT shows strong and progressive contrast enhancement of the lesion, which retains enhancement in the delayed phase (**c**), which is typical for peliotic changes in inflammatory adenoma

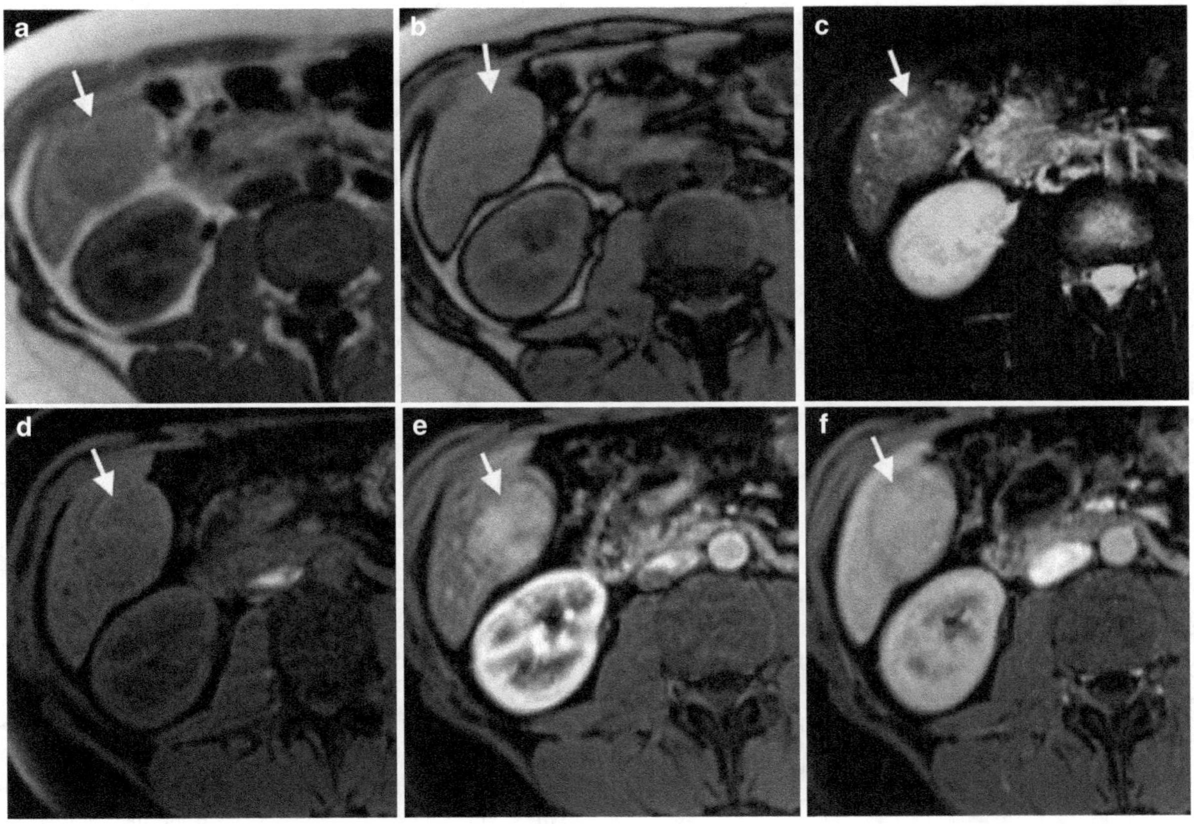

Fig. Adenoma (inflammatory type) in a young female presenting with vague upper quadrant pain. (**a**) In- and (**b**) opposed-phase T1-weighted imaging shows no significant intralesional fat. The nodule is (**c**) mildly hyperintense on T2-weighted imaging. (**d–f**) Pre-contrast, post-contrast arterial phase, and delayed phase images show avid arterial enhancement, which persists. Surgical resection confirmed an inflammatory adenoma

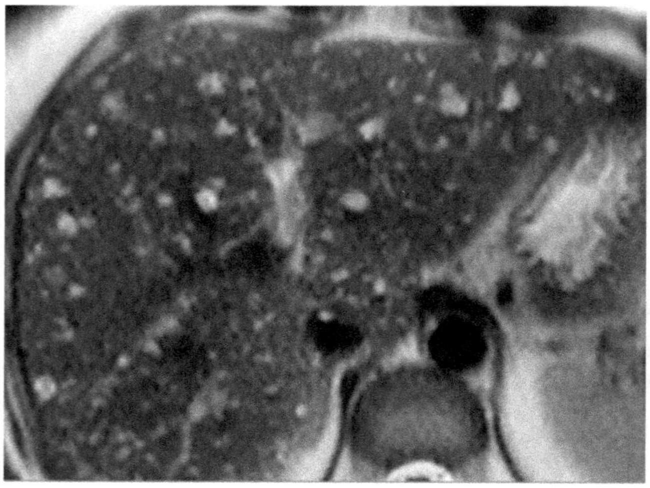

Fig. Biliary hamartomas (von Meyenburg complex). A middle-aged woman was referred to MRI following an ultrasound examination. There are multiple foci of high T2-weighted signal within the liver, suggestive of biliary hamartomas

echoes. On CT, hepatic abscesses are hypodense lesions with capsules that may show enhancement (Fig. 17.11); cluster sign may be noted when multiple abscesses are present [47]. CT appearance of hepatic abscess is nonspecific and can be mimicked by cystic or necrotic metastases. Hence, appropriate clinical and laboratory corroboration is vital toward making the right radiological diagnosis. Though present in only a small minority of cases, central gas is highly specific for abscess. On MR imaging, hepatic abscesses are hypointense relative to liver parenchyma on T1-weighted images and markedly hyperintense on T2-weighted images, often surrounded by a local area of slight T2 hyperintensity representing perilesional edema, which may also show increased enhancement after contrast administration.

Amebic liver abscess is nonspecific. It usually appears as a solitary, hypodense lesion, with an enhancing wall that may be smooth or nodular, and is often associated with an incomplete rim of edema. With MR imaging, lesions are hypointense on T1-weighted images and heterogeneously hyperintense on T2-weighted images [48].

On CT scan, involvement of liver by *Echinococcus granulosus* (hydatid cyst) can manifest as unilocular or multilocular cysts with thin or thick walls and calcifications, usually with daughter cysts seen as smaller cysts, with septations at the margin of or inside the mother cyst (i.e., this appearance is quite different from a "usual" multicystic tumor). On MR imaging, the presence of a hypointense rim on T1- and T2-weighted images and a multiloculated appearance are diagnostic features.

MalignantPrimary Tumors

Hepatocellular Carcinoma

HCC is the most common primary liver cancer, with the highest incidence in Asia and the Mediterranean. In European countries, HCC is found mostly in patients with chronic liver disease (particularly hepatitis B or C, liver cirrhosis, or hemochromatosis). At histopathology, HCC is characterized by abnormal hepatocytes arranged in trabecular and sinusoidal patterns. Lesions may be solitary, multifocal, or diffusely infiltrating.

There is wide varying appearances of HCC on imaging. An early HCC occurring within at risk population is typically small (<3 cm) and has a homogenous appearance. By contrast, late presentation disease (including tumor in noncirrhotic patients) is characterized by more advanced disease, presenting as a larger heterogeneous lesion. US is frequently used for disease screening and surveillance of cirrhosis patients. The appearance of HCC on US is variable, with iso-, hypo-, or hyperechogenicity (increased echogenicity is often due to intratumoral fat). Smaller lesions are typically homogeneous and larger lesions heterogeneous. A surrounding fibrous capsule is often present and characteristic for HCC, appearing as a hypoechoic rim surrounding the lesion.

On unenhanced CT images, most HCCs are hypo- or isodense (the latter particularly if small). The presence of intratumoral fat can lower CT attenuation and is suggestive of primary hepatocellular tumors in the appropriate clinical settings. Due to their altered and predominant arterial supply, HCCs enhance avidly in the arterial phase of contrast enhancement, becoming iso- or hypodense with the liver parenchyma in the portal venous phase of enhancement. Delayed phase images show most HCC lesions as hypodense compared with surrounding liver. The washout of contrast in these tumors is a diagnostic characteristic of HCC (Fig.). Small HCCs may have a nodule-in-nodule appearance on CT and MR images, especially when the disease develops within a regenerative or dysplastic nodule (Fig.). At MR imaging, such a nodule can exhibit higher signal intensity on T2-weighted images and display hypervascularity on arterial-phase images.

Multiphase imaging after contrast administration on CT helps to optimize the detection and characterization of HCC. Late arterial-phase imaging is the most sensitive for detecting small lesions [6, 49, 50]. A venous phase is always necessary for tumor detection/characterization and

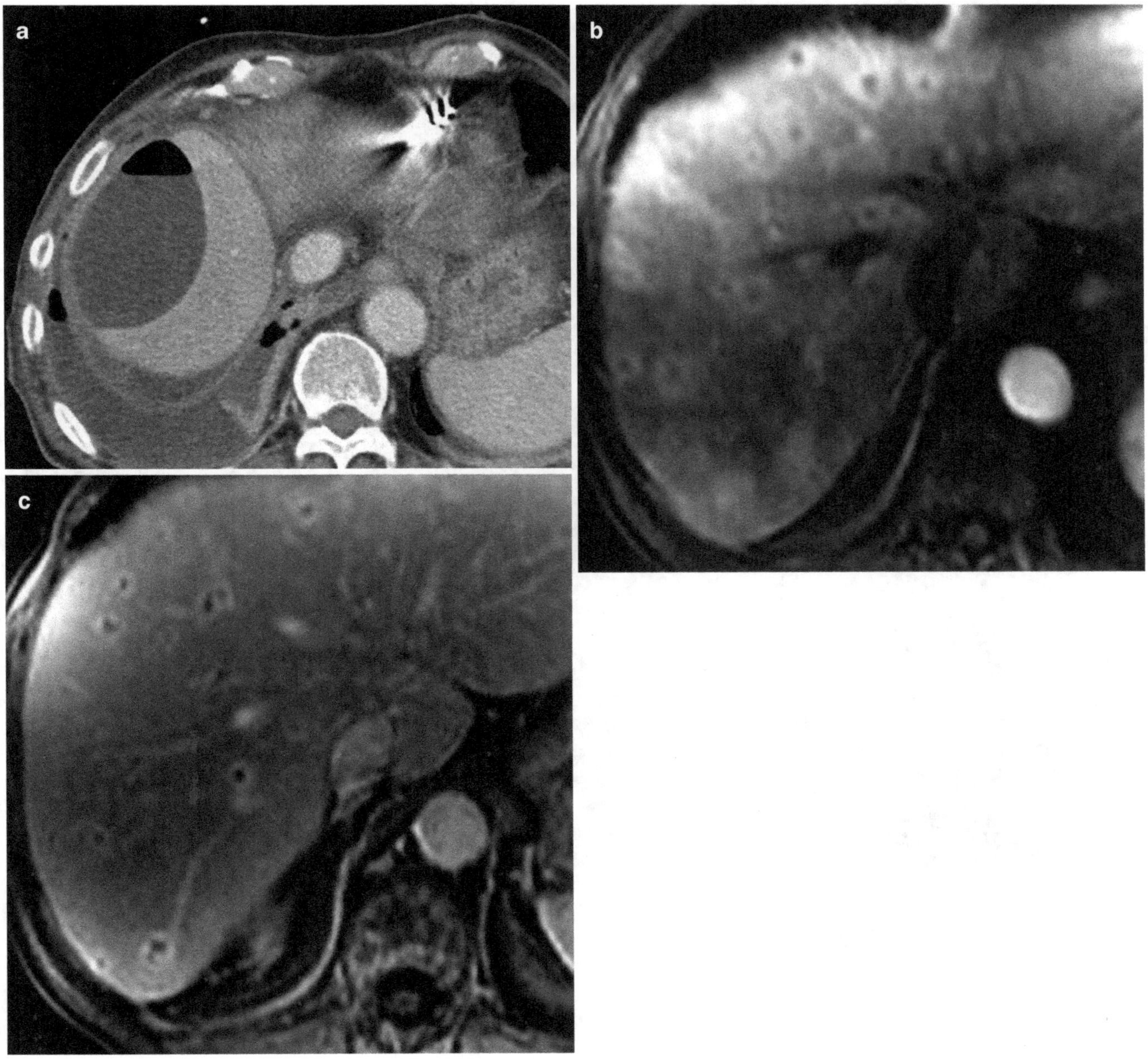

Fig. Abscesses. (**a**) Typical large subcapsular abscess with an air-fluid level and a reactive pleural effusion. (**b**, **c**) Another patient with fever and right upper quadrant pain. T1-weighted contrast-enhanced images in the (**b**) arterial and (**c**) portal venous phase demonstrate multiple ring-enhancing lesions in both lobes of the liver. In the arterial phase, there is also associated increased parenchyma enhancement surrounding many of the lesions. The appearance is consistent with multiple hepatic abscesses

assessment of venous structures (Fig.), as well as other abdominal organs. The delayed phase imaging (e.g., at 2–3 min) can occasionally help to detect a lesion that may be missed [51]. Much more important is that it can help to make a firm diagnosis of HCC by showing typical lesion contrast washout, if it had not been present in the portal venous phase [52]. Unenhanced images are important for identifying hyperdense siderotic nodules and for detecting hypodense intratumoral fat. Unenhanced images are also useful for tumor follow-up after chemoembolization or after tumor ablation. For these reasons, a three- to four-phasic MDCT protocol is utilized at most centers to evaluate HCC.

The reliance on focal hypervascularity in the arterial phase can lead to false-positive diagnosis of HCC [53]. Transient focal enhancement of liver parenchyma during arterial phase, also termed transient hepatic attenuation differences (THAD), can lead to a false diagnosis of HCC. In cirrhotic patients, transient focal enhancement is most often caused by arterial-portal shunting, resulting in inappropri-

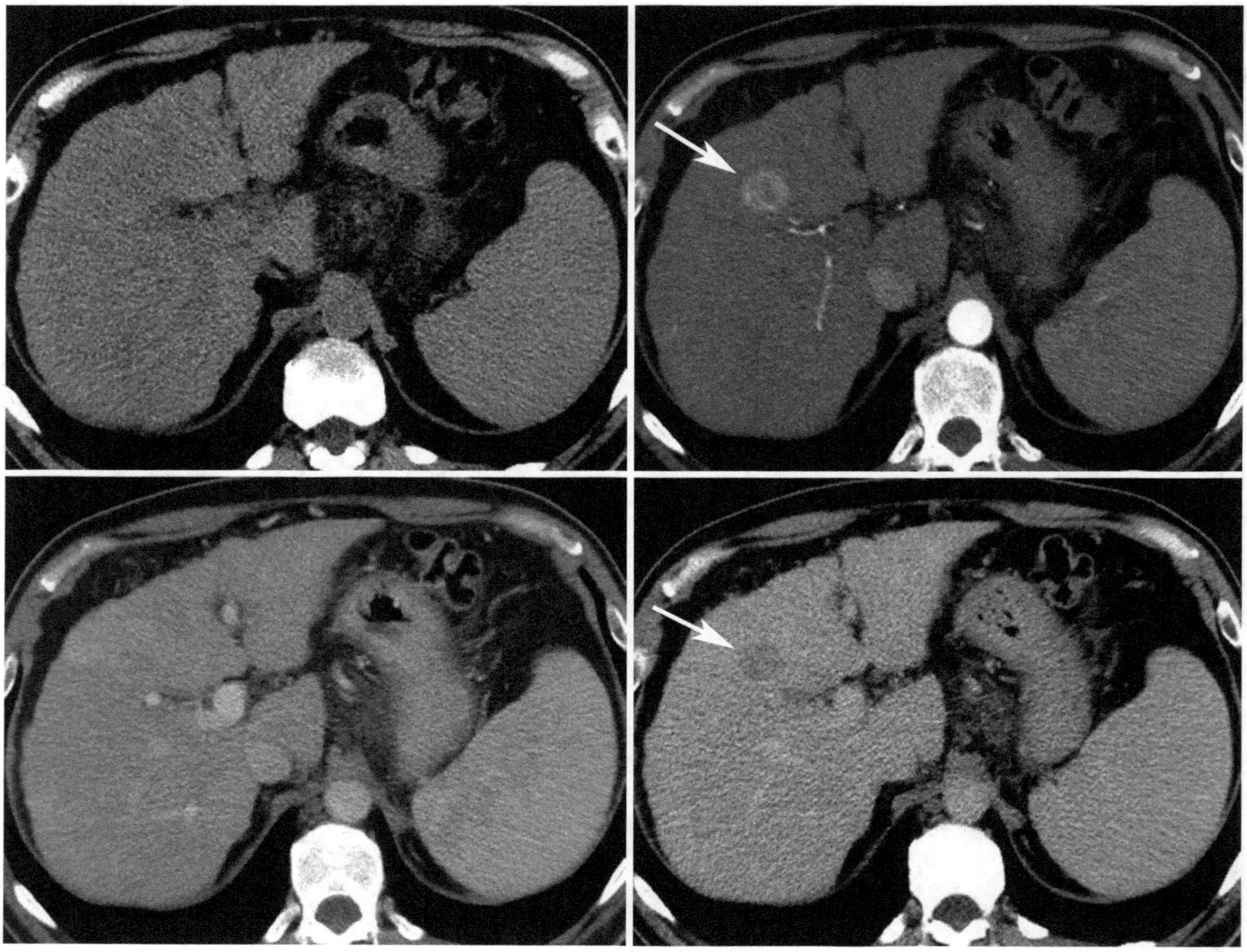

Fig. HCC: quadruple-phasic CT for detection and characteriza-tion. (**a**) Non-contrast CT shows liver cirrhosis and splenomegaly. In segment 4, a lesion is only faintly seen. (**b**) In the late arterial phase, a hypervascular HCC is depicted in segment 4 (arrow). (**c**) In the venous phase, the lesion is not visible. (**d**) The delayed phase scan reveals washout of the lesion, which is now hypoattenuating (arrow). The combination of arterial hypervascularity and washout is a very specific sign of malignancy

ately early focal areas of portal venous distribution enhancement in the liver. THAD are usually peripherally located in the liver, appear wedge shaped, and may be poorly circumscribed. Subcapsular lesions that do not exhibit mass effect or a round nature should be carefully evaluated before suggesting the diagnosis of HCC. THAD are not associated with lesion hypodensity in the portal venous or delayed phases of contrast enhancement.

The combination of hyperdensity on arterial-phase images combined with washout to hypodensity on venous- or delayed phase images, although not sensitive (33%), is highly specific (100%) for the diagnosis of HCC [54] (Fig.). However, a small proportion of HCC can be isovascular or hypovascular compared with the liver, which can be difficult to diagnose. The typical MR imaging features of larger HCC include a fibrous capsule/pseudocapsule, intratumoral septa, daughter nodules, and tumor thrombus (Fig.) [55]. These lesions are often heterogeneous in appearances (mosaic architecture) on both CT and MR [56]. Whereas most large HCC are hyperintense on T2-weighted images, smaller lesions, measuring even 3–4 cm, can appear isointense or hypointense. On T1-weighted images, HCC shows variable signal intensity relative to hepatic parenchyma. A tumor capsule/pseudocapsule may be seen on T1-weighted and, less commonly, as hypointense on Conventional gT2-weighted imaging.adolinium contrast imaging in HCC paral-lels the features described for CT, with characteristic early peak contrast enhancement and delayed phase tumor con-trast washout of the nodular solid components, as well as late T1 enhancement of the capsule/pseudocapsule. Liver- specific MR contrast agents (gadoxetic acid or gadobenate

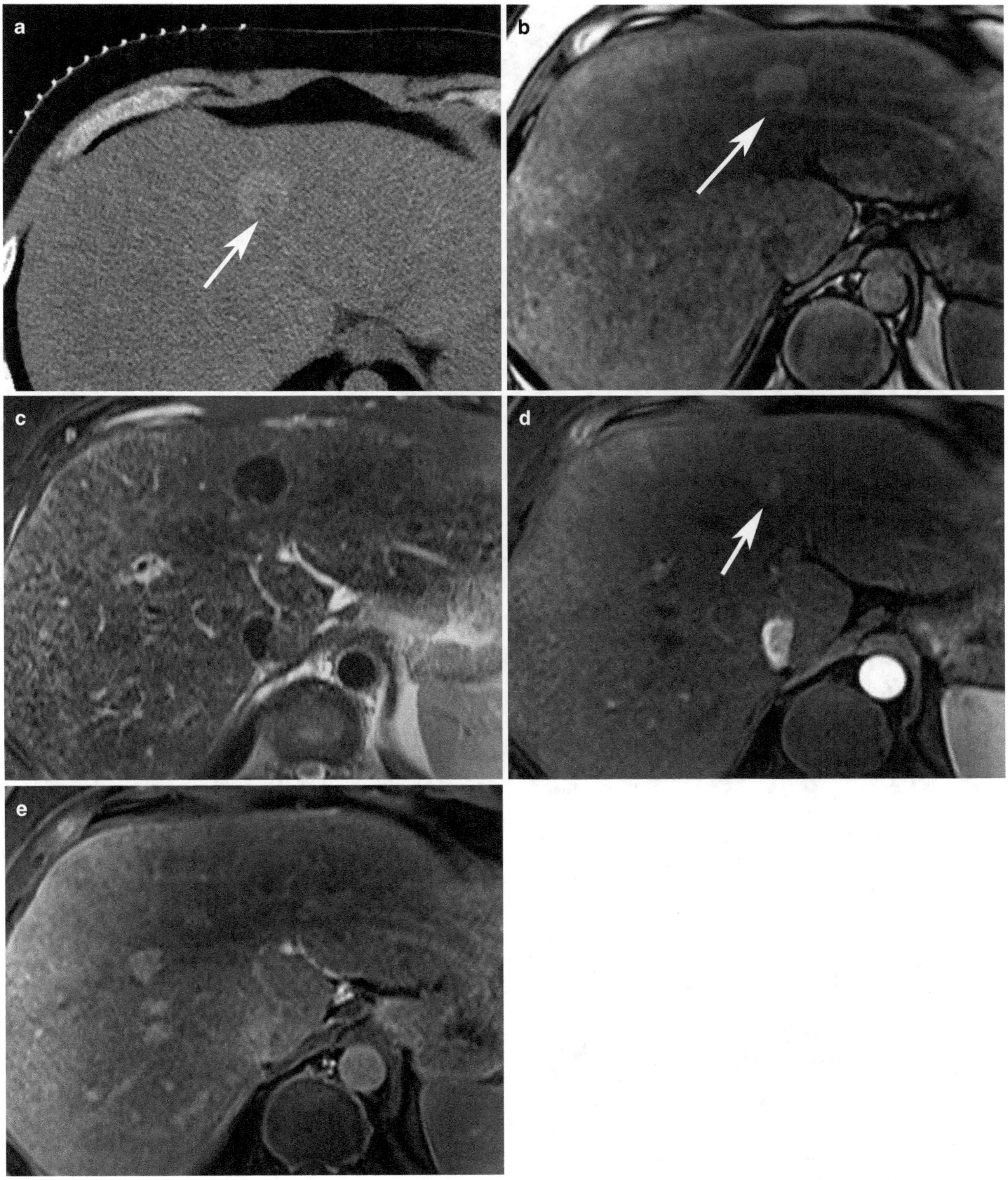

Fig. HCC with nodule-in-nodule appearance. (**a**) Unenhanced CT shows a siderotic (hyperattenuating) large nodule, which contains a low-density (non-siderotic) focus (arrow). (**b**) On T1-weighted GRE opposed-phase image, the marginal nodule shows low signal intensity (arrow). (**c**) The large nodule shows siderosis on T2-weighted TSE images, but the marginal focus displays higher SI. (**d**, **e**) Dynamic gadolinium-enhanced T1-weighted GRE images show (**d**) arterial hypervascularity of the malignant focus (arrow) and (**e**) washout in the equilibrium phase

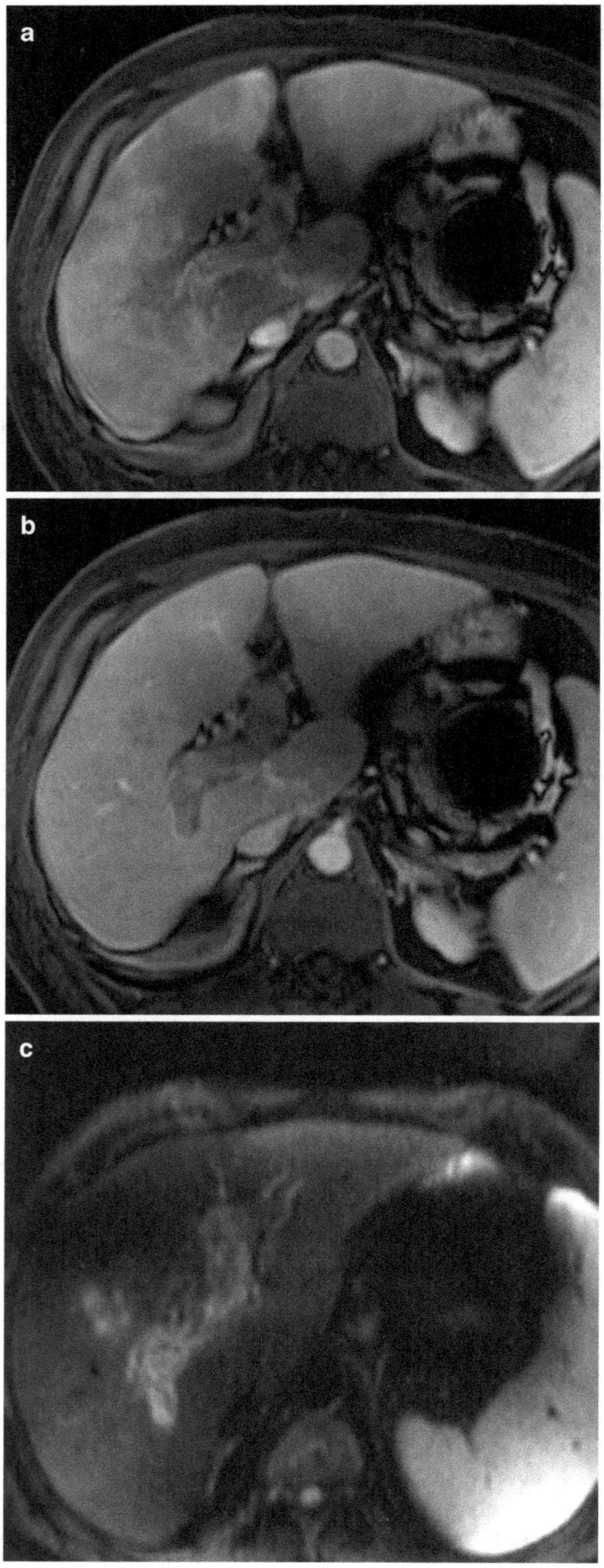

Fig. Diffuse HCC in the right lobe with tumor thrombus in the portal vein. (**a**) Arterial phase and (**b**) venous phase T1-weighted GRE shows inhomogeneous enhancement and expansion of the portal vein. There is inhomogeneous enhancement of the right lobe, but no definite tumor is seen. (**c**) DWI shows a solid mass in the entire intrahepatic portal vein and part of the tumor in the right lobe

dimeglumine) can be administered to provide arterial, portal venous, and equilibrium-phase imaging but has the added advantage of revealing additional characteristics at the delayed hepatobiliary phase of contrast enhancement. HCC typically do not show contrast retention of liver-specific contrast medium in the hepatobiliary phase, which can add confidence toward the detection and characterization of HCC (Fig.) [57]. It has been shown that using gadoxetic acid-enhanced MRI can improve the detection of small or early HCCs, as it is superior for detecting HCC measuring <1–2 cm in size compared with CT [58]. In addition, subcen-timeter lesions detected by gadoxetic acid-enhanced MRI are likely to be or can transform to become HCC within a short interval [59]. Hence, several evolving guidelines for the imaging evaluation of HCC are incorporating the role of liver-specific contrast media for the diagnosis of subcentime-ter HCC. Subcentimeter HCC may be treated by locoregional therapy, thus avoiding the morbidity and mortality associated with radical surgery.

However, it is important to note some potential pitfalls of using liver-specific contrast media for HCC evaluation. Some benign regenerating nodules may appear hypointense at the hepatobiliary phase of contrast enhancement, although the majority appears isointense of the liver [60]. In addition, some well-differentiated or moderately differentiated HCC may appear isointense or hyperintense on delayed images due to higher levels of OATP1B3 and MRP3 receptor expression. For this reason, the use of ancillary imaging features at MRI can improve the confidence of HCC diagnosis. These include mild to high T2 signal intensity and impeded diffusion on high b-value DWI. The use of liver-specific contrast agents may also help toward the identification of isoenhancing or hypoenhancing HCC that do not show typical hypervascularity in the arterial phase of contrast enhancement. With regard to the use of diffusion-weighted MRI for HCC evaluation, higher b-value (e.g., 800 s/mm^2) DWI may help in the identification of disease, particularly if the suspected nodule also demonstrates typical vascularity pattern at contrast-enhanced MRI. Because of background liver cirrhosis, higher-grade/poorly differentiated HCC are more likely to show impeded diffusion and lower ADC values compared with low-grade/well-differentiated HCC.

To summarize, many MR characteristics are often associated with HCC (arterial-phase hyperintensity, T2 hyperintensity, venous- or equilibrium-phase washout, lack of hepatobiliary MR contrast agent uptake on hepatobiliary phase images, and restricted diffusion on high-b-value DWI). However, for each of these findings, there is only ~60–80% sensitivity, and benign lesions show these findings in 16–65% of cases, depending on finding, contrast agent used, and series reported [60, 61]. Based on data from numerous studies, the American Association for the Study of Liver Disease (AASLD) and the European Association for the Study of the Liver (EASL) formed recommendations for the noninvasive

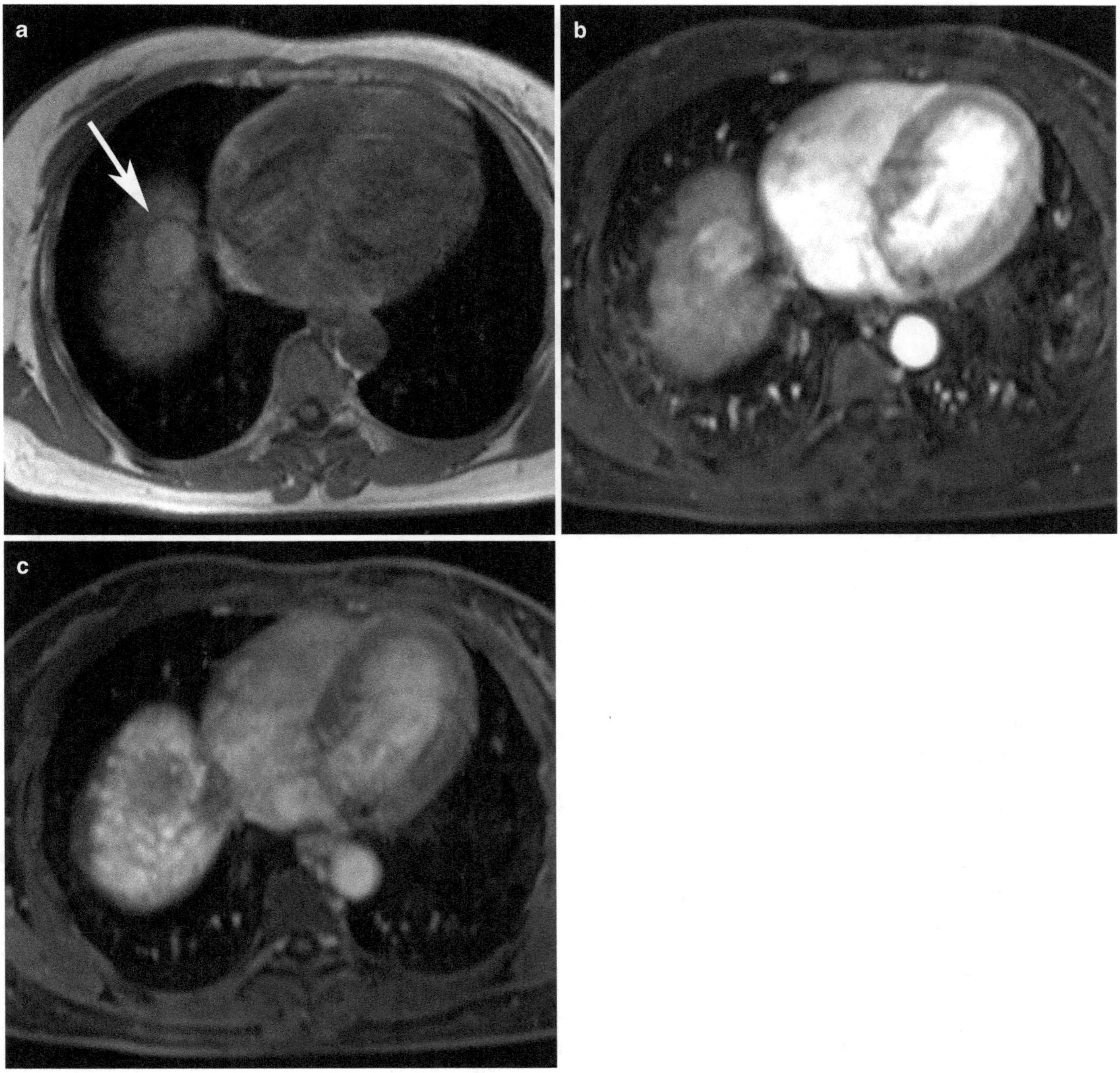

Fig. HCC: MRI with liver-specific contrast agent (gadoxetic acid). (**a**) Axial T1-weighted GRE shows an encapsulated slightly hyperintense mass in the dome of the liver. (**b**) Gadoxetic acid-enhanced image shows strong enhancement in the arterial phase. (**c**) In the hepatobiliary phase after 20 min, the lesion shows hypointensity due to lack of hepatocellular uptake

diagnosis of HCC in patients with chronic liver disease [62]. Lesions more than 1 cm that demonstrate arterial-phase hypervascularity and venous- or delayed phase washout are triaged for treatment with a diagnosis of HCC. If only one of the two findings are present, then the guidelines require obtaining a different modality with contrast imaging to determine whether these findings can be verified. If the lesion remains atypical, then biopsy is recommended. If a suspected lesion is less than 1 cm, the AASLD and EASL guidelines recommend repeating the examination at 3-month intervals, using the same imaging technology used to detect the lesion, to determine whether there is growth or changing in character. In following up patients with chronic liver disease, development of a new nodule with any of the MR signal abnormalities discussed above should be considered worrisome for HCC, even if they do not meet the AASLD [63] criteria for noninvasive diagnosis. These criteria were developed to be specific but are only approximately 70% sensitive [60]. It is essential for radiologists to also document the number and size of all lesions meeting criteria for HCC,

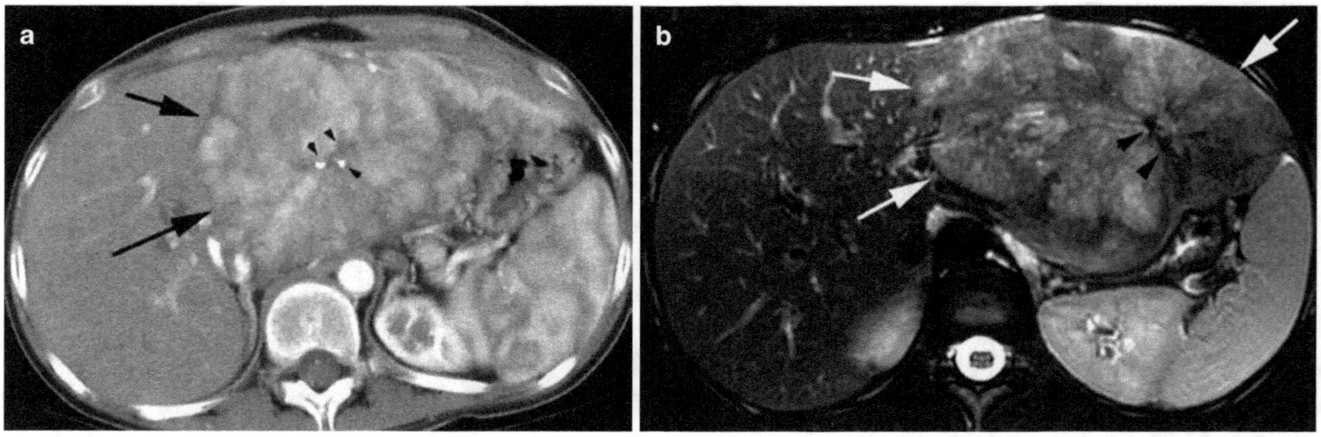

Fig. Fibrolamellar HCC. (**a**) Arterial phase MDCT shows heterogeneously enhancing mass in the left lobe (arrows) with low attenuation central fibrous scar with calcifications (arrowheads). (**b**) T2-weighted MRI shows large left lobe mass (arrows) with heterogeneous appearance and mild to moderately increased signal intensity. Fibrous central scar is of very low signal intensity (arrowheads)

as treatment for these patients varies depending on these factors. It is also important to document whether vascular invasion or distant metastasis is present.

Fibrolamellar HCC

Fibrolamellar HCC (FL-HCC) is a less aggressive tumor with a better prognosis than typical HCC. It consists of malignant hepatocytes separated into cords by fibrous strands. On CT, FL-HCC appears as a large, well-defined vascular mass with lobulated surface and often a central scar and calcifications in up to 70% of cases [64, 65]. On MR imaging, FL-HCC are typically hypointense on T1- and hyperintense on T2-weighted images, with the central scar being hypointense on both sequences (Fig.). This is in contrast to the scar of FNH, which is most often hyperintense on T2-weighted images. The fibrous central zones of both FNH and FL-HCC show delayed retention of CT and extracellular gadolinium MR contrast agents. By comparison with FNH, the contrast enhancement in FL-HCC is usually heterogeneous compared with the often homogeneous contrast enhancement pattern of FNH.

Cholangiocellular Carcinoma

Cholangiocellular carcinoma (CCC) is the second most common primary malignancy of the liver. Intrahepatic CCC originates from the intralobular bile ducts (in contrast to hilar CCC, which arises from a main hepatic duct or from the bifurcation). Intrahepatic CCC often presents late as a large mass [66]. According to the growth characteristics, CCC is classified as mass forming, periductal infiltrating, or intraductal growing, with the mass-forming type being most common in intrahepatic CCC [66]. At CT and MR imaging, lesions tend to be hypodense at unenhanced CT and hypointense on T1-weighted images, with peripheral enhancement at dynamic contrast-enhanced studies [67]. Delayed phase CT/MR imaging (after 5–15 min) may show enhancement homogeneously or in the center of the lesion due to its rich fibrous stroma, which is suggestive of the diagnosis of CCC [68]. Interestingly, the central fibrotic stroma often shows signal suppression on diffusion-weighted MRI and return relatively high ADC value (Fig.). Periductal infiltra-tive CCC causes early segmental dilatation of bile ducts in a stage when the tumor itself may be difficult to discern [67]. In addition, there are morphologic features that can suggest the diagnosis of CCC. Peripheral lesions often demonstrate overlying capsular retraction due to their scirrhous, fibrous matrix (Fig.). Dilated intrahepatic bile ducts proximal to an intrahepatic CCC can also provide clues to the diagno-sis, as biliary obstruction is usual with intrahepatic metasta-ses (with the exception of colorectal cancer [69].

Rare Primary Liver Tumors

Biliary Cystadenoma/Cystadenocarcinomas

These tumors present a similar appearance and morphology as their mucinous counterparts in the pancreas and occur usually in women. Even when benign, these tumors have a propensity for malignant degeneration, and any such tumor should be considered as potentially malignant. They appear as unilocular or multilocular cystic masses, with the typical anechoic and hypoechoic US appearance and near water-like attenuation

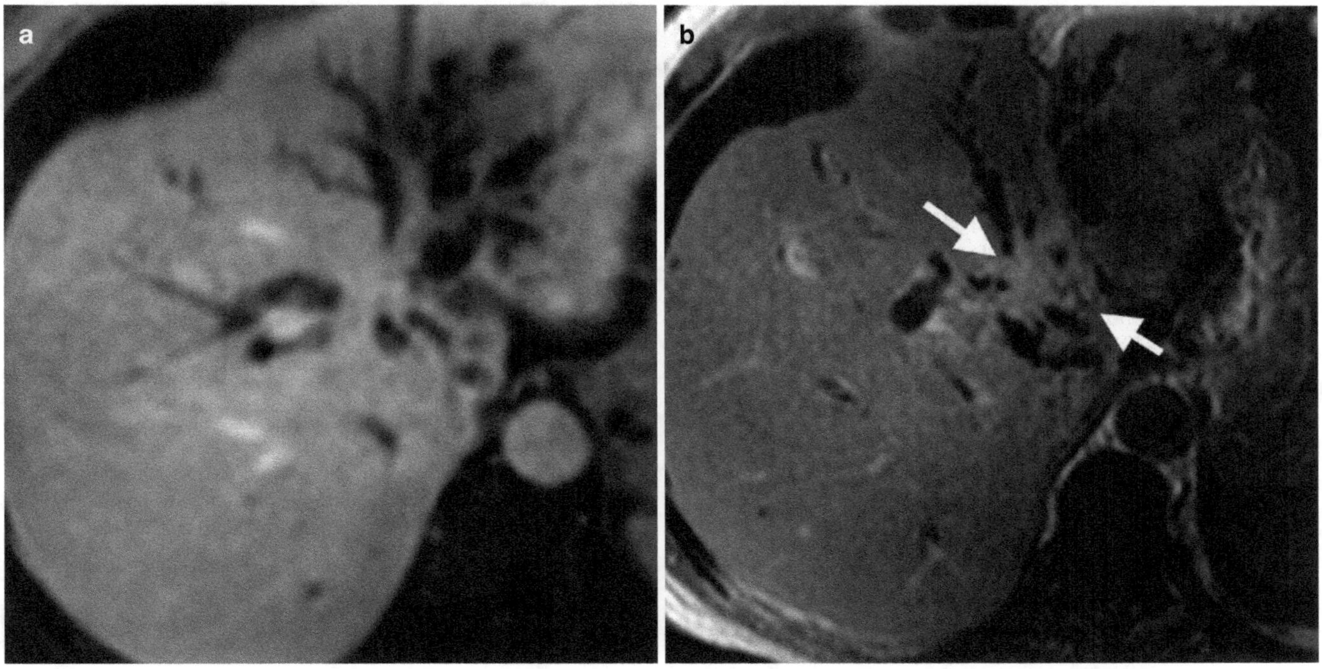

Fig. Hilar cholangiocarcinoma: elderly man with progressive jaundice. (**a**) Contrast-enhanced T1-weighted image in the arterial phase shows dilatation of the intrahepatic ducts, which extend to the hepatic hilum. On the (**b**) 10 mins' delayed image, the tumor demonstrates late enhancement, which allows better delineation of the tumor (arrows) from the surrounding hepatic parenchyma

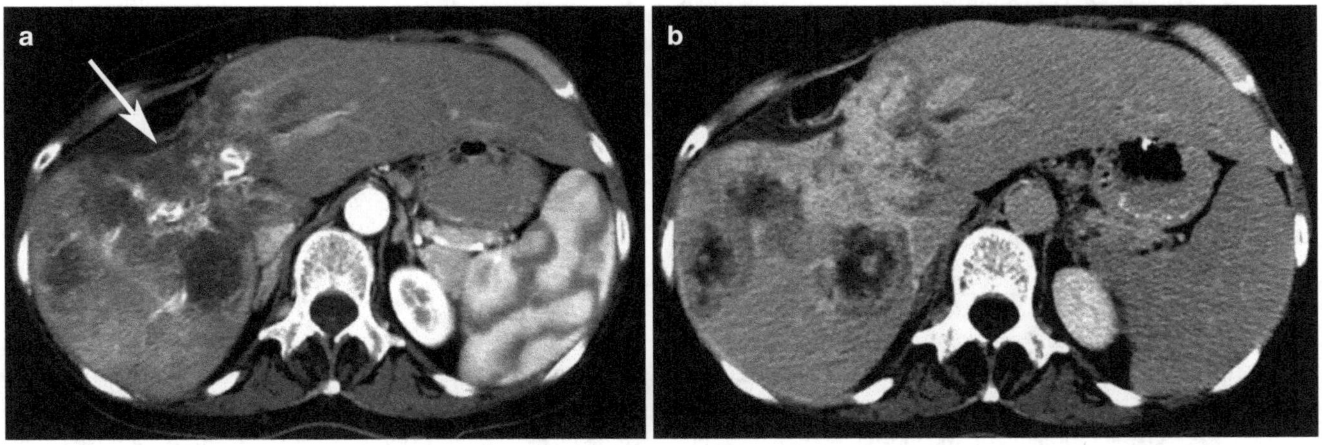

Fig. Peripheral cholangiocarcinoma. (**a**) Contrast-enhanced CT in the arterial phase demonstrates a multicentric hypovascular mass with capsular retraction (arrow). (**b**) Delayed phase demonstrated typical late enhancement due to fibrous matrix

contents on CT, with peripheral soft tissue nodularity and traversing septations. The greater presence of papillary excrescences, soft tissue nodularity or septations, are associated with a higher risk of malignancy [70]. The cystic areas show variable signal intensity at T1-weighted MRI, including being hyperintense to liver related to its proteinaceous content. Coarse calcifications may be observed at US and CT in both cystadenoma and cystadenocarcinoma and is not a sign of benignity.

Hepatic Angiosarcoma

Hepatic angiosarcoma is a rare tumor. There is a strong association with prior exposure to carcinogens such as vinyl chloride and Thorotrast, as well as in patients with hemochromatosis. However, in the majority, the tumor is idiopathic. Pathologically, angiosarcoma presents as large, solitary masses or with multiple tumor nodules of varying size, which contain multiple vascular channels.

The imaging appearance of angiosarcoma is often nonspecific, appearing hypodense on unenhanced CT, hypointense on T1-weighted MR imaging, and mildly hyperintense on T2-weighted imaging (although if prominent sinusoidal vascular spaces are present, these can appear of homogeneous and very high T2-weighted signal intensity). Following iodinated or gadolinium-based contrast administration, most lesions show nonspecific heterogeneous enhancement. Potentially problematic, however, are those tumors with prominent sinusoidal vascular spaces, because they can mimic the appearance of benign hemangioma on CT and MRI. The high MR T2-weighted signal in such lesions further compounds this problem. In most such cases, however, careful evaluation will show that the tumoral enhancement does not follow characteristics of blood pool at all phases or that there are other features, such as multiple lesions, that make the diagnosis of hemangioma unlikely [71, 72].

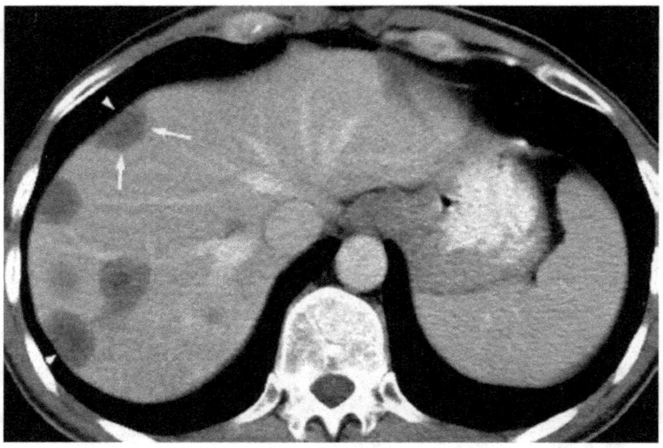

Fig .Epithelioid hemangioendothelioma. Contrast CT (portal venous phase) shows multiple predominantly peripheral-based hypodense lesions. Note that some of the lesions show a laminated appearance (arrows). Early development of capsular retraction is pres-ent with flattening of the capsule overlying some of the lesions (arrowheads)

Epithelioid Hemangioendothelioma

Epithelioid hemangioendothelioma (EHE) is a rare tumor of vascular origin, not to be confused with infantile hemangioendothelioma, which is a very different tumor. These hepatic tumors are characterized by multiple, peripheral-based lesions that progressively become confluent masses. In addition to the unusual peripheral liver distribution, a key characteristic feature is the presence of overlying capsular retraction, due to the presence of fibrosis and scarring [73]. The CT attenuation or MR signal intensity characteristics are nonspecific, although occasional tumoral calcifications m ay b e s een. C ontrast enhancement with CT or MR gadolinium chelates often shows a central zone of decreased enhancement with marked periph-eral enhancement (Fig.). The reverse pattern has also been observed with a central area of increased enhancement and peripheral decreased enhancement. Concentric zones of marked enhancement have also been reported. A visible branch of the portal or hepatic vein terminating at the periph-ery of these lesions t (lollipop sign) has also been described, although this is not pathognomonic of the disease [74]. Lesions often become confluent and may grow large enough to replace nearly the entire liver parenchyma.

Hepatic Metastases

At US, liver metastases can appear hypoechoic, isoechoic, or hyperechoic. On dynamic contrast-enhanced CT, most metastases appear hypovascular and hypodense relative to liver parenchyma on the portal venous phase (Fig.). Hypervascular metastases are most commonly seen in renal cell carcinoma, neuroendocrine tumors, sarcomas, and breast tumor patients (Fig.). These tumors are best seen in the arterial phase and may become isodense and difficult to detect at the later phases of contrast enhancement. At MR, metastases are usually hypointense on T1-weighted and hyperintense on T2-weighted images [75]. Peritumoral edema makes lesions appear larger on T2-weighted images and is highly suggestive of a malignant mass [76]. High signal intensity on T1-weighted sequences is typical for melanoma metastases due to the paramagnetic nature of melanin. Some lesions may have a central area of hyperintensity (target sign) on T2-weighted images, which corresponds to central necrosis. DWI with high b-values (e.g., 600–800) is very helpful for detecting small liver metastases, which may otherwise escape detec-tion (Fig.). On dynamic contrast- enhanced MR imaging, metastases demonstrate enhancement character-istics similar to those described for CT. Metastases may demonstrate a hypointense rim compared with the center of the lesion on delayed images (peripheral washout sign), which is highly specific for malignancy. It has been shown in colorectal cancer that the combination of using DWI, together with liver-specific contrast media, enhanced MRI results in the highest diagnostic accuracy for the detection of liver metastases (Fig.) [77].

Differential Diagnosis of Focal Liver Lesions

The approach to characterizing a focal liver lesion seen on CT begins with determining its density. If the lesion shows near water density, is homogenous in character, and has

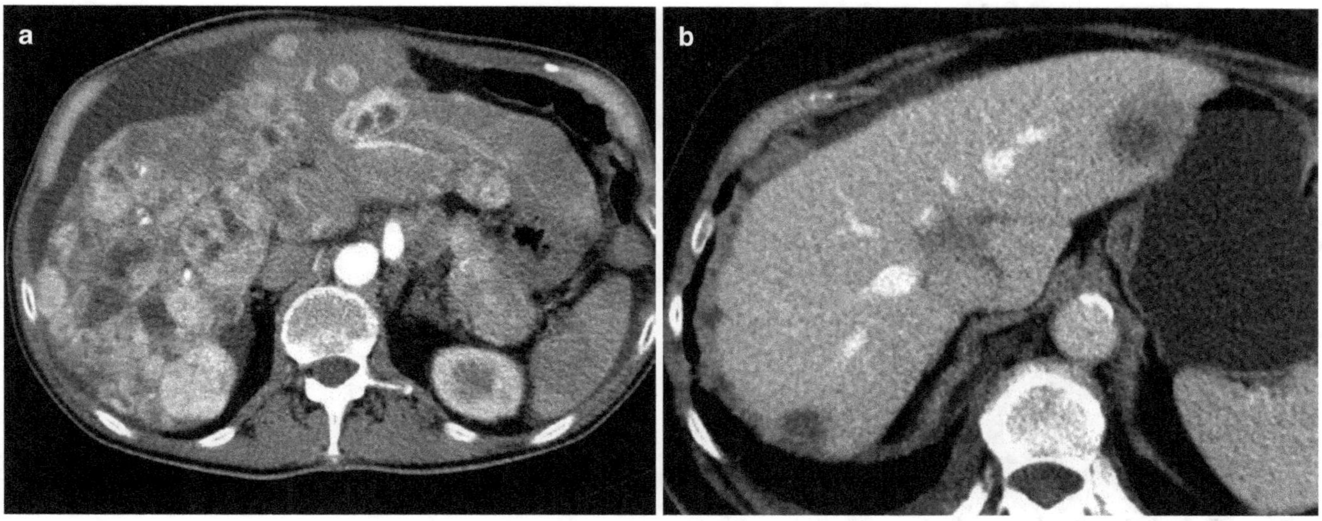

Fig. Metastases. (**a**) Contrast-enhanced MDCT in the arterial phase demonstrates several predominantly hypervascular liver metastases of neuroendocrine cancer of the pancreas. (**b**) Contrast-enhanced MDCT in the venous phase shows typical hypovascular colorectal metastases

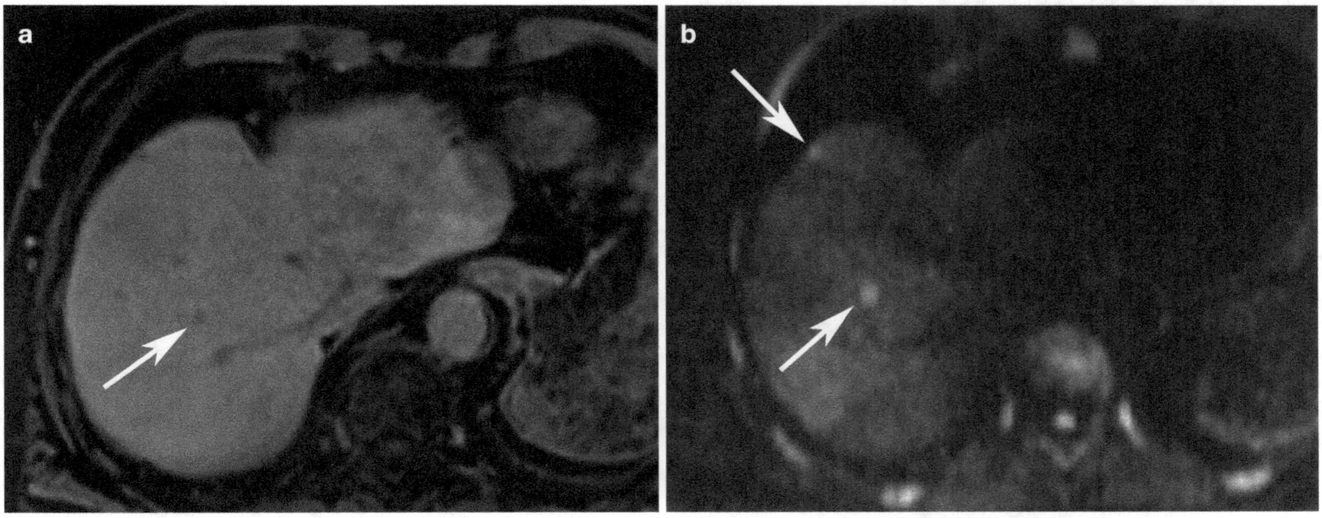

Fig. Value of diffusion-weighted MRI for detection of small metastases. (**a**) Contrast-enhanced MRI shows one small metastasis in the right lobe (arrow). There is a subtle hypointensity in the right lobe in a subcapsular location. (**b**) DWI clearly shows that there is an additional metastasis (arrows)

sharp margins, then a cyst should be considered and can be confirmed with US, equilibrium-phase CT, or even MR imaging (T2 bright and non-enhancing post-gadolinium), which can ensure there are no solid components or mural wall lesions. However, the radiologist should be familiar with the imaging features of other cystic lesions that can mimic simple cysts.

When evaluating solid focal liver lesions, disease characterization is largely reliant on observing the rate and pattern of contrast enhancement. If a lesion shows peripheral and nodular enhancement, with the density of enhancing portions showing the same general levels of blood vessels in the arterial, venous, and delayed phases, a hemangioma can be confidently diagnosed. Arterially hypervascular enhancing

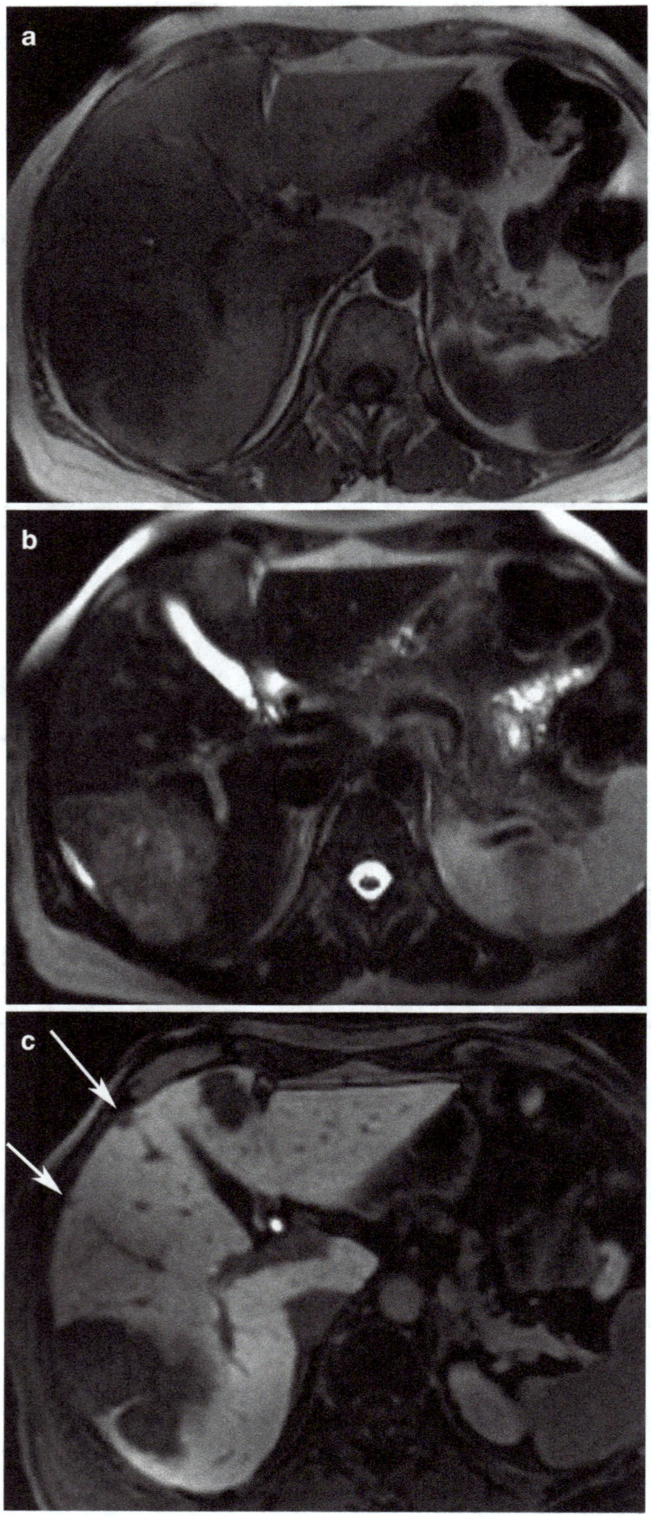

Fig. Colorectal liver metastases at gadoxetic acid-enhanced MRI. (**a**) Unenhanced T1-weighted MRI shows two hypointense lesions in segments 6/7 and 4. (**b**) The T2-weighted TSE image shows the lesions to be moderately hyperintense. (**c**) The gadoxetic-enhanced T1-weighted GRE image in the hepatobiliary phase shows two additional small subcapsular metastases (arrows) not seen on unenhanced MRI or MDCT (not shown)

lesions include FNH, HCA, HCC, and metastases from neuroendocrine tumors, melanoma, renal cell carcinoma, and breast cancer. In general, HCC is considered in a setting of cirrhosis or chronic liver disease. FNH is most likely in young women with a non-cirrhotic liver and if the lesion is homogeneous and near-isodense/near-isointense on unenhanced CT/MR imaging with a central T2-weighted hyperintense scar.

By comparison, thick, irregular, heterogeneous enhancement or the presence of peripheral washout at the delayed phase suggests a malignant mass, such as metastases, CCC, or even HCC. In particular, delayed enhancement is a feature of CC due to is fibrotic stroma.

Liver-specific MR contrast has been shown to improve the characterization of FNH and HCA, increase the detection of suspicious focal lesions in patients with liver cirrhosis, as well as the identification of small focal liver lesions.

DWI is also now routinely performed in liver imaging. Its main clinical benefit is the detection of focal liver lesions, which may be missed on conventional and contrast-enhanced imaging sequences. Quantitative ADC measurements can support the characterization of focal liver lesions, with higher ADC values (e.g., $>1.7 \times 10–3\ mm^2/s$) favoring benign lesions [22]. However, the use of ADC value should be made with the knowledge of the scanner ADC repeatability, as well as in collaboration with all other imaging findings because of the significant overlap of ADC values between benign and malignant lesions.

Take-Home Messages

- Contrast-enhanced liver MDCT for detection and characterization of focal masses should be at least biphasic, with a quadruple-phasic protocol being recommended for HCC detection and characterization in cirrhotic patients.
- MRI protocol should routinely include dynamic contrast-enhanced pulse sequences and DWI.
- Liver-specific MR contrast agents are recommended for evaluation of patients with potentially resectable colorectal liver metastases.
- Liver-specific MR contrast agents are helpful for characterization of FNH and adenoma and may increase the reader confidence in HCC characterization.

References

1. Laghi A. Multidetector CT (64 slices) of the liver: examination techniques. Eur Radiol. 2007;17:675–83.
2. Weg N, Scheer MR, Gabor MP. Liver lesions: improved detection with dual-detector-array CT and routine 2.5-mm thin collimation. Radiology. 1998;209:417–26.
3. Ichikawa T, Nakajima H, Nanbu A, et al. Effect of injection rate of contrast material on CT of hepatocellular carcinoma. AJR Am J Roentgenol. 2006;186:1413–8.
4. Foley WD, Hoffmann RG, Quiroz FA, et al. Hepatic helical CT: contrast material injection protocol. Radiology. 1994;192:367–71.
5. Kim T, Murakami T, Takahashi S, et al. Effects of injection rates of contrast material on arterial phase hepatic CT. AJR Am J Roentgenol. 1998;171:429–32.
6. Schima W, Hammerstingl R, Catalano C, et al. Quadruple-phase MDCT of the liver in patients with suspected hepatocellular carcinoma: effect of contrast material flow rate. AJR Am J Roentgenol. 2006;186:1571–9.
7. Sultana S, Awai K, Nakayama Y, et al. Hypervascular hepatocellular carcinomas: bolus tracking with a 40-detector CT scanner to time arterial phase imaging. Radiology. 2007;243:140–7.
8. Oliver JH, Baron RL. Helical biphasic contrast-enhanced CT of the liver: technique, indications, interpretations and pitfalls. Radiology. 1996;201:1–14.
9. Vardhanabhuti V, Loader R, Roobottom CA. Assessment of image quality on effects of varying tube voltage and automatic tube current modulation with hybrid and pure iterative reconstruction techniques in abdominal/pelvic CT: a phantom study. Investig Radiol. 2013;48:167–74.
10. Singh S, Kalra M, Hsieh J, et al. Abdominal CT: comparison of adaptive statistical iterative and filtered back projection reconstruction techniques. Radiology. 2010;257:373–83.
11. May MS, Wüst W, Brand M, et al. Dose reduction in abdominal computed tomography: intraindividual comparison of image quality of full-dose standard and half-dose iterative reconstructions with dual-source computed tomography. Investig Radiol. 2011;46:465–70.
12. Gonzalez-Guindalini FD, Botelho MP, Töre HG, et al. MDCT of chest, abdomen, and pelvis using attenuation-based automated tube voltage selection in combination with iterative reconstruction: an intrapatient study of radiation dose and image quality. AJR Am J Roentgenol. 2013;201:1075–82.
13. Fuentes-Orrego JM, Hayano K, Kambadakone AR, et al. Dose-modified 256-MDCT of the abdomen using low tube current and hybrid iterative reconstruction. Acad Radiol. 2013;20:1405–12.
14. Altenbernd J, Heusner TA, Ringelstein A, Ladd SC, Forsting M, Antoch G. Dual-energy-CT of hypervascular liver lesions in patients with HCC: investigation of image quality and sensitivity. Eur Radiol. 2011;21:738–43.
15. Luo XF, Xie XQ, Cheng S, et al. Dual-energy CT for patients suspected of having liver iron overload: can virtual iron content imaging accurately quantify liver iron content? Radiology. 2015;277:95–103.
16. Lee MH, Kim YK, Park MJ, Hwang J, Kim SH, Lee WJ, Choi D. Gadoxetic acid-enhanced fat suppressed three-dimensional T1-weighted MRI using a multiecho dixon technique at 3 tesla: emphasis on image quality and hepatocellular carcinoma detection. J Magn Reson Imaging. 2013;38:401–10.
17. Chandarana H, Block KT, Winfeld MJ, et al. Free-breathing contrast-enhanced T1-weighted gradient-echo imaging with radial k-space sampling for paediatric abdominopelvic MRI. Eur Radiol. 2014;24:320–6.
18. Padhani AR, Liu G, Chenevert TL, et al. Diffusion-weighted magnetic resonance imaging as a cancer biomarker: consensus and recommendations. Neoplasia. 2009;11:102–25.
19. Koh DM, Brown G, Riddell AM, et al. Detection of colorectal hepatic metastases using MnDPDP MR imaging and diffusion-weighted imaging (DWI) alone and in combination. Eur Radiol. 2008;18:903–10.
20. Holzapfel K, Reiser-Erkan C, Fingerle AA, et al. Comparison of diffusion-weighted MR imaging and multidetector-row CT in the detection of liver metastases in patients operated for pancreatic cancer. Abdom Imaging. 2011;36:179–84.
21. Vandecaveye V, De Keyzer F, Verslype C, et al. Diffusion-weighted MRI provides additional value to conventional dynamic contrast-enhanced MRI for detection of hepatocellular carcinoma. Eur Radiol. 2009;19:2456–66.
22. Taouli B, Koh DM. Diffusion-weighted MR imaging of the liver. Radiology. 2010;254:47–66.
23. Oudkerk M, Torres CG, Song B, et al. Characterization of liver lesions with mangafodipir trisodium-enhanced MR imaging: multicenter study comparing MR and dual-phase spiral CT. Radiology. 2002;223:517–24.
24. Scharitzer M, Schima W, Schober E, et al. Characterization of hepatocellular tumors: value of mangafodipir-enhanced magnetic resonance imaging. J Comput Assist Tomogr. 2005;29:181–90.
25. Ward J, Robinson PJ, Guthrie JA, et al. Liver metastases in candidates for hepatic resection: comparison of helical CT and gadolinium- and SPIO-enhanced imaging. Radiology. 2005;237:170–80.
26. Hammerstingl R, Huppertz A, Breuer J, et al. Diagnostic efficacy of gadoxetic acid (Primovist)-enhanced MRI and spiral CT for a therapeutic strategy: comparison with intraoperative and histopathologic findings in focal liver lesions. Eur Radiol. 2008;18:457–67.
27. Schima W, Saini S, Echeverri JA, et al. T2-weighted MR imaging for characterization of focal liver lesions: conventional spin-echo vs fast spin-echo. Radiology. 1997;202:389–93.
28. Farraher SW, Jara H, Chang KJ, et al. Differentiation of hepatocellular carcinoma and hepatic metastasis from cysts and hemangiomas with calculated T2 relaxation times and the T1/T2 relaxation times ratio. J Magn Reson Imaging. 2006;24:1333–41.
29. Semelka RC, Brown ED, Ascher SM, et al. Hepatic hemangiomas: a multi-institutional study of appearance on T2-weighted and serial gadolinium-enhanced gradient-echo MR images. Radiology. 1994;192:401–6.
30. Oto A, Kulkarni K, Nishikawa R, Baron RL. Contrast enhancement of hepatic hemangiomas on multiphase MDCT: can we diagnose hepatic hemangiomas by comparing enhancement with blood pool? AJR Am J Roentgenol. 2010;195:381–6.
31. Ba-Ssalamah A, Uffmann M, Saini S, et al. Clinical value of MRI liver-specific contrast agents: a tailored examination for a confident noninvasive diagnosis of focal liver lesions. Eur Radiol. 2009;19:342–57.
32. Vossen JA, Buijs M, Liapi E, et al. Receiver operating characteristic analysis of diffusion-weighted magnetic resonance imaging in differentiating hepatic hemangioma from other hypervascular liver lesions. J Comput Assist Tomogr. 2008;32:750–6.
33. Kehagias D, Moulopoulos L, Antoniou A, et al. Focal nodular hyperplasia: imaging findings. Eur Radiol. 2001;11:202–12.
34. Brancatelli G, Federle MP, Grazioli L, et al. Focal nodular hyperplasia: CT findings with emphasis on multiphasic helical CT in 78 patients. Radiology. 2001;219:61–8.
35. Uggowitzer MM, Kugler C, Mischinger HJ, et al. Echo-enhanced Doppler sonography of focal nodular hyperplasia of the liver. J Ultrasound Med. 1999;18:445–51.
36. McInnes MD, Hibbert RM, Inácio JR, Schieda N. Focal nodular hyperplasia and hepatocellular adenoma: accuracy of gadoxetic

acid-enhanced MR imaging—a systematic review. Radiology. 2015;277:413–23.
37. Purysko AS, Remer EM, Coppa CP, et al. Characteristics and distinguishing features of hepatocellular adenoma and focal nodular hyperplasia on gadoxetate disodium-enhanced MRI. AJR Am J Roentgenol. 2012;198:115–23.
38. Leconte I, Van Beers BE, Lacrosse M, et al. Focal nodular hyperplasia: natural course observed with CT and MRI. J Comput Assist Tomogr. 2000;24:61–6.
39. Mathieu D, Kobeiter H, Maison P, et al. Oral contraceptive use and focal nodular hyperplasia of the liver. Gastroenterology. 2000;118:560–4.
40. Prasad SR, Sahani DV, Mino-Kenudson M, et al. Benign hepatic neoplasms: an update on cross-sectional imaging spectrum. J Comput Assist Tomogr. 2008;32:829–40.
41. Katabathina VS, Menias CO, Shanbhogue AK, et al. Genetics and imaging of hepatocellular adenomas: 2011 update. Radiographics. 2011;31:1529–43.
42. van Aalten SM, Thomeer MG, Terkivatan T, et al. Hepatocellular adenomas: correlation of MR imaging findings with pathologic subtype classification. Radiology. 2011;261:172–81.
43. Bioulac-Sage P, Sempoux C, Balabaud C. Hepatocellular adenoma: classification, variants and clinical relevance. Semin Diagn Pathol. 2017;34:112–25.
44. Nault JC, Paradis V, Cherqui D, Vilgrain V, Zucman-Rossi J. Molecular classification of hepatocellular adenoma in clinical practice. J Hepatol. 2017;67:1074–83.
45. Semelka RC, Hussain SM, Marcos HB, Woosley JT. Biliary hamartomas: solitary and multiple lesions shown on current MR techniques including gadolinium enhancement. J Magn Reson Imaging. 1999;10:196–201.
46. Martin DR, Kalb B, Sarmiento JM, et al. Giant and complicated variants of cystic bile duct hamartomas of the liver: MRI findings and pathological correlations. J Magn Reson Imaging. 2010;31:903–11.
47. Jeffrey RB Jr, Tolentino CS, Chang FC, Federle MP. CT of small pyogenic hepatic abscesses: the cluster sign. AJR Am J Roentgenol. 1988;151:487–9.
48. Barreda R, Ros PR. Diagnostic imaging of liver abscess. Crit Rev Diagn Imaging. 1992;33:29–58.
49. Laghi A, Iannaccone R, Rossi P, et al. Hepatocellular carcinoma: detection with triple-phase multi-detector row helical CT in patients with chronic hepatitis. Radiology. 2003;226:543–9.
50. Ichikawa T, Kitamura T, Nakajima H, et al. Hypervascular hepatocellular carcinoma: can double arterial phase imaging with multidetector CT improve tumor depiction in the cirrhotic liver? AJR Am J Roentgenol. 2002;179:751–8.
51. Monzawa S, Ichikawa T, Nakajima H, et al. Dynamic CT for detecting small hepatocellular carcinoma: usefulness of delayed phase imaging. AJR Am J Roentgenol. 2007;188:147–53.
52. Iannacone R, Laghi A, Catalano C, et al. Hepatocellular carcinoma: role of unenhanced and delayed-phase multi-detector row helical CT in patients with cirrhosis. Radiology. 2005;234:460–7.
53. Baron RL, Brancatelli G. Computed tomographic imaging of hepatocellular carcinoma. Gastroenterology. 2004;127:S133–43.
54. Forner A, Vilana R, Ayuso C, et al. Diagnosis of hepatic nodules 20 mm or smaller in cirrhosis: prospective validation of the noninvasive diagnostic criteria for hepatocellular carcinoma. Hepatology. 2008;47:97–104.
55. Tublin ME, Dodd GD, Baron RL. Benign and malignant portal vein thrombosis: differentiation by CT characteristics. AJR Am J Roentgenol. 1997;168:719–23.
56. Stevens WR, Gulino SP, Batts KP, et al. Mosaic pattern of hepatocellular carcinoma: histologic basis for a characteristic CT appearance. J Comput Assist Tomogr. 1996;20:337–42.
57. Choi JW, Lee JM, Kim SJ, et al. Hepatocellular carcinoma: imaging patterns on gadoxetic acid-enhanced MR images and their value as an imaging biomarker. Radiology. 2013;267:776–86.
58. Chen L, Zhang L, Bao J, et al. Comparison of MRI with liver-specific contrast agents and multidetector row CT for the detection of hepatocellular carcinoma: a meta-analysis of 15 direct comparative studies. Gut. 2013;62:1520–1.
59. Song KD, Kim SH, Lim HK, Jung SH, Sohn I, Kim HS. Subcentimeter hypervascular nodule with typical imaging findings of hepatocellular carcinoma in patients with history of hepatocellular carcinoma: natural course on serial gadoxetic acid-enhanced MRI and diffusion-weighted imaging. Eur Radiol. 2015;25:2789–96.
60. Kim TK, Lee KH, Jang JJ, et al. Analysis of gadobenate dimeglumine-enhanced MR findings for characterizing small (1-2-cm) hepatic nodules in patients at high risk for hepatocellular carcinoma. Radiology. 2011;259:730–8.
61. Lee MH, Kim SH, Park MJ, et al. Gadoxetic acid-enhanced hepatobiliary phase MRI and high-b-value diffusion-weighted imaging to distinguish well-differentiated hepatocellular carcinomas from benign nodules in patients with chronic liver disease. AJR Am J Roentgenol. 2011;197:W868–75.
62. Bruix J, Sherman M. Management of hepatocellular carcinoma: an update. Hepatology. 2011;53:1020–2.
63. McEvoy SH, McCarthy CJ, Lavelle LP, et al. Hepatocellular carcinoma: illustrated guide to systematic radiologic diagnosis and staging according to guidelines of the American Association for the Study of Liver Diseases. Radiographics. 2013;33:1653–68.
64. Ichikawa T, Federle MP, Grazioli L, et al. Fibrolamellar hepatocellular carcinoma: imaging and pathologic findings in 31 recent cases. Radiology. 1999;213:352–61.
65. Ichikawa T, Federle MP, Grazioli L, Marsh W. Fibrolamellar hepatocellular carcinoma: pre- and posttherapy evaluation with CT and MR imaging. Radiology. 2000;217:145–51.
66. Lim JH. Cholangiocarcinoma: morphologic classification according to growth pattern and imaging findings. AJR Am J Roentgenol. 2003;181:819–27.
67. Han JK, Choi BI, Kim AY, et al. Cholangiocarcinoma: pictorial essay of CT and cholangiographic findings. Radiographics. 2002;22:173–87.
68. Lee WJ, Lim HK, Jang KM, et al. Radiologic spectrum of cholangiocarcinoma: emphasis on unusual manifestations and differential diagnoses. Radiographics. 2001;21:S97–S116.
69. Jhaveri KS, Halankar J, Aguirre D, et al. Intrahepatic bile duct dilatation due to liver metastases from colorectal carcinoma. AJR Am J Roentgenol. 2009;193:752–6.
70. Buetow PC, Buck JL, Pantongrag-Brown L, et al. Biliary cystadenoma and cystadenocarcinoma: clinical-imaging pathologic correlations with emphasis on the importance of ovarian stroma. Radiology. 1995;196:805–10.
71. Peterson MS, Baron RL, Rankin SC. Hepatic angiosarcoma: findings on multiphasic contrast-enhanced helical CT do not mimic hepatic hemangioma. AJR Am J Roentgenol. 2000;175:165–70.
72. Koyama T, Fletcher JG, Johnson CD, et al. Primary hepatic angiosarcoma: findings at CT and MR imaging. Radiology. 2002;222:667–73.
73. Miller WJ, Dodd GD 3rd, Federle MP, Baron RL. Epithelioid hemangioendothelioma of the liver: imaging findings with pathologic correlation. AJR Am J Roentgenol. 1992;159:53–7.
74. Alomari AI. The lollipop sign: a new cross-sectional sign of hepatic epithelioid hemangioendothelioma. Eur J Radiol. 2006;59:460–4.

Permissions

All chapters in this book were first published in DTAP, by Springer Nature; hereby published with permission under the Creative Commons Attribution License or equivalent. Every chapter published in this book has been scrutinized by our experts. Their significance has been extensively debated. The topics covered herein carry significant findings which will fuel the growth of the discipline. They may even be implemented as practical applications or may be referred to as a beginning point for another development.

The contributors of this book come from diverse backgrounds, making this book a truly international effort. This book will bring forth new frontiers with its revolutionizing research information and detailed analysis of the nascent developments around the world.

We would like to thank all the contributing authors for lending their expertise to make the book truly unique. They have played a crucial role in the development of this book. Without their invaluable contributions this book wouldn't have been possible. They have made vital efforts to compile up to date information on the varied aspects of this subject to make this book a valuable addition to the collection of many professionals and students.

This book was conceptualized with the vision of imparting up-to-date information and advanced data in this field. To ensure the same, a matchless editorial board was set up. Every individual on the board went through rigorous rounds of assessment to prove their worth. After which they invested a large part of their time researching and compiling the most relevant data for our readers.

The editorial board has been involved in producing this book since its inception. They have spent rigorous hours researching and exploring the diverse topics which have resulted in the successful publishing of this book. They have passed on their knowledge of decades through this book. To expedite this challenging task, the publisher supported the team at every step. A small team of assistant editors was also appointed to further simplify the editing procedure and attain best results for the readers.

Apart from the editorial board, the designing team has also invested a significant amount of their time in understanding the subject and creating the most relevant covers. They scrutinized every image to scout for the most suitable representation of the subject and create an appropriate cover for the book.

The publishing team has been an ardent support to the editorial, designing and production team. Their endless efforts to recruit the best for this project, has resulted in the accomplishment of this book. They are a veteran in the field of academics and their pool of knowledge is as vast as their experience in printing. Their expertise and guidance has proved useful at every step. Their uncompromising quality standards have made this book an exceptional effort. Their encouragement from time to time has been an inspiration for everyone.

The publisher and the editorial board hope that this book will prove to be a valuable piece of knowledge for researchers, students, practitioners and scholars across the globe.

List of Contributors

Refky Nicola
Division of Abdominal Imaging, SUNY-Upstate Medical Center, Syracuse, NY, USA

Christine O. Menias
Department of Radiology, Mayo Clinic in Arizona, Scottsdale, AZ, USA

Jeong Min Lee
Department of Radiology, Seoul National University Hospital, Seoul, Republic of Korea

Daniel T. Boll
Department of Radiology and Nuclear Medicine, University Hospital of Basel, Basel, BS, Switzerland

C. Dan Johnson
Mayo Clinic, Scottsdale, AZ, USA

Perry J. Pickhardt
University of Wisconsin, Madison, WI, USA

Jeanne S. Chow
Department of Radiology, Boston Children's Hospital, Boston, MA, USA

Annemieke S. Littooij
Department of Radiology, University Medical Center Utrecht, Utrecht, The Netherlands

S. O. Schönberg and J. Budjan
Medical Faculty Mannheim, Heidelberg University, Mannheim, Germany

D. Hausmann
Institute of Radiology, Kantonsspital Baden AG, Switzerland

Francesca Maccioni
Department of Radiological Sciences, Oncology and Pathology, Sapienza University of Rome, Rome, Italy

Celine D. Alt
Department of Diagnostic and Interventional Radiology, University Duesseldorf, Medical Faculty, Duesseldorf, Germany

Pablo R. Ros
Department of Radiology, University Hospitals Health System/Case Western Reserve University, Cleveland, OH, USA

Richard M. Gore
North Shore University Health System, Evanston, IL, USA
Pritzker School of Medicine at the University of Chicago, Chicago, IL, USA

Marc S. Levine
Hospital of the University of Pennsylvania, Philadelphia, PA, USA
Perelman School of Medicine at the University of Pennsylvania, Philadelphia, PA, USA

Lejla Aganovic
Department of Radiology, University of California, San Diego, Medical Center, San Diego, CA, USA

Richard H. Cohan
Department of Radiology, University of Michigan Hospital, Ann Arbor, MI, USA

Andrea Rockall
Consultant Radiologist, Department of Radiology, The Royal Marsden NHS Foundation Trust, London, UK
Professor of Radiology, Faculty of Medicine, Imperial College London, UK

Rosemarie Forstner
Faculty of Medicine, Imperial College London, London, UK

Khoschy Schawkat and Caecilia S. Reiner
Institute of Diagnostic and Interventional Radiology, University Hospital Zurich, Zurich, Switzerland

Andrea Laghi
Department of Radiological, Oncological and Pathological Sciences, Sapienza – University of Rome, ICOT Hospital, Latina, Italy

Amy K. Hara
Department of Radiology, Mayo Clinic Arizona, Phoenix, AZ, USA

James A. Brink
Department of Radiology, Massachusetts General Hospital, Boston, MA, USA

Brent J. Wagner
West Reading Radiology Associates, West Reading, PA, USA

Yulia Lakhman
Department of Radiology, Memorial Sloan Kettering Cancer Center, New York, NY, USA

Caroline Reinhold
Department of Radiology, McGill University Health Centre, Montreal, QC, Canada

Emily A. Dunn and Thierry A. G. M. Huisman
Division of Pediatric Radiology, Russell H. Morgan Department of Radiology and Radiological Science, Johns Hopkins University School of Medicine, Charlotte R. Bloomberg Children's Center, Baltimore, MD, USA

Øystein E. Olsen
Radiology Department, Great Ormond Street Hospital for Children NHS Foundation Trust, London, UK

Karen Kinkel
Institut de radiologie, Clinique des Grangettes, Chêne-Bougeries, Geneva, Switzerland

Susan M. Ascher
Department of Radiology, Georgetown University School of Medicine, Washington, DC, USA

Caroline Reinhold
Department of Radiology, McGill University Health Center, Montreal, QC, Canada

Irene A. Burger
Department of Nuclear Medicine, UniversitätsSpital Zürich, Zürich, Switzerland

Regina G. H. Beets-Tan
Department of Radiology, The Netherlands Cancer Institute, Amsterdam, The Netherlands

Andreas G. Wibmer and Hebert Alberto Vargas
Radiology- Memorial Sloan Kettering Cancer Center, New York, NY, USA

Thomas Mang
Department of Biomedical Imaging and Image-guided Therapy, Medical University of Vienna, Vienna, Austria

Philippe Lefere
Department of Radiology, AZ Delta, Roeselare, Belgium

Jay P. Heiken
Mallinckrodt Institute of Radiology, Washington University School of Medicine, St. Louis, MO, USA

Douglas S. Katz and Yves Menu
Hôpital Saint Antoine, Paris, France

Bernd Hamm and Patrick Asbach
Department of Radiology, Charité—Universitätsmedizin Berlin, Berlin, Germany

Wolfgang Schima
Department of Radiology, Göttlicher Heil and Krankenhaus, Barmherzige Schwestern Krankenhaus, Sankt Josef Krankenhaus, Vinzenzgruppe, Vienna, Austria

Dow-Mu Koh
Department of Radiology, Royal Marsden Hospital, Sutton, UK

Index

www.ingramcontent.com/pod-product-compliance
Lightning Source LLC
LaVergne TN
LVHW081036210926
848485LV00004B/1035
* 9 7 8 1 6 3 9 2 7 0 6 9 9 *